Advanced Health Assessment *and* Diagnostic Reasoning

THIRD EDITION

Jacqueline Rhoads, PhD, ACNP-BC, ANP-C, GNP-BE, PMHNP-BE, FAANP
Professor
School of Tropical Medicine
Tulane University
New Orleans, Louisiana

Clinical Professor
School of Nursing
University of North Carolina at Charlotte
Charlotte, North Carolina

Sandra Wiggins Petersen, DNP, APRN, FNP/GNP-BC, PMHNP-BE, FAANP
Professor
Director, Doctor of Nursing Practice Program
College of Nursing & Health Sciences, School of Nursing
The University of Texas at Tyler
Tyler, Texas

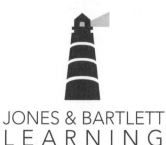

JONES & BARTLETT
LEARNING

World Headquarters
Jones & Bartlett Learning
5 Wall Street
Burlington, MA 01803
978-443-5000
info@jblearning.com
www.jblearning.com

Jones & Bartlett Learning books and products are available through most bookstores and online booksellers. To contact Jones & Bartlett Learning directly, call 800-832-0034, fax 978-443-8000, or visit our website, www.jblearning.com.

Substantial discounts on bulk quantities of Jones & Bartlett Learning publications are available to corporations, professional associations, and other qualified organizations. For details and specific discount information, contact the special sales department at Jones & Bartlett Learning via the above contact information or send an email to specialsales@jblearning.com.

13139-0

Production Credits

VP, Executive Publisher: David D. Cella
Executive Editor: Amanda Martin
Associate Acquisitions Editor: Rebecca Stephenson
Editorial Assistant: Emma Huggard
Production Manager: Carolyn Rogers Pershouse
Production Editor: Vanessa Richards
Associate Production Editor: Juna Abrams
Production Assistant: Brooke Haley
Senior Marketing Manager: Jennifer Scherzay
Product Fulfillment Manager: Wendy Kilborn
Composition: S4Carlisle Publishing Services
Cover Design: Kristin E. Parker
Associate Director of Rights & Media: Joanna Gallant
Rights & Media Specialist: Wes DeShano
Media Development Editor: Troy Liston
Cover & Part Opener Images: © Yevhen Vitte/Shutterstock; © pedrosala/Shutterstock; © everything possible/Shutterstock
Chapter Opener Image: © everything possible/Shutterstock
Printing and Binding: LSC Communications
Cover Printing: LSC Communications

Library of Congress Cataloging-in-Publication Data

Names: Rhoads, Jacqueline, 1948- author. | Petersen, Sandra Wiggins, 1955- author.
Title: Advanced health assessment and diagnostic reasoning / Jacqueline Rhoads, Sandra Wiggins Petersen.
Description: Third edition. | Burlington, Massachusetts : Jones & Bartlett Learning, [2018] | Includes bibliographical references and index.
Identifiers: LCCN 2016031655 | ISBN 9781284105377 (hardcover)
Subjects: | MESH: Nursing Assessment | Diagnostic Techniques and Procedures | Diagnosis, Differential
Classification: LCC RT48 | NLM WY 100.4 | DDC 616.07/5--dc23
LC record available at https://lccn.loc.gov/2016031655

6048

Printed in the United States of America
22 21 20 19 18   10 9 8 7 6 5 4

Contents

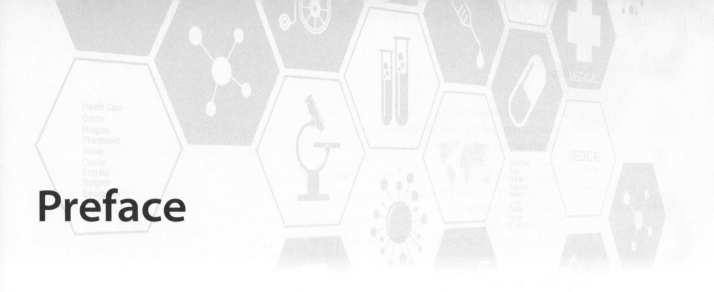

Preface

Daily life activities place physical and emotional demands on people and expose them to a wide variety of diseases and conditions. Consequently, the healthcare provider must be prepared to diagnose and treat a variety of disorders. Health assessment is a complex process, yet many assessment texts address only the physical examination component in any real depth. We developed *Advanced Health Assessment and Diagnostic Reasoning* to include each step of health assessment, demonstrating the links between health history and physical examination and illustrating the diagnostic reasoning process. We wanted to fill in the missing piece in most basic physical examination texts—the thought process one must assume as one assesses an actual case.

Advanced health assessment involves determining existing conditions, assessing capabilities, and screening for disease or other factors predisposing a patient to illness. A thorough health history and physical examination are necessary to correctly diagnose existing conditions and detect risk for other conditions. This text provides the healthcare provider with the essential data needed to formulate a diagnosis and treatment plan.

Organization of the Text

This text provides three introductory chapters that cover general strategies for health—history taking, physical examination, and documentation. The remainder of the text consists of clinical chapters covering assessment of various systemic disorders (e.g., gastrointestinal, cardiovascular, musculoskeletal, etc.). Each clinical chapter includes the following sections:

Anatomy and Physiology Review
Health History
    History of Present Illness
    Past Medical History
    Family History
    Social History
    Review of Systems
Physical Examination
    Equipment Needed
    Components of the Physical Exam
    Inspection
    Palpation
    Percussion
    Auscultation

Key Features

Content in this text is presented in a way that is easy to follow and retain. It is also presented so that all of the pieces of assessment "fit together." Aspects of the health history are given in a two-column format: The first column gives the type of information that the provider should obtain, while the second column provides specific questions or information to note. The second column also takes matters a step further—it gives examples of which conditions the findings may indicate. Aspects of the physical examination are also given in a two-column format: action and rationale. The first (action) column gives the actions clinicians should take (with appropriate steps or strategies), and the second (rationale) column lists normal and abnormal findings and, as applicable, possible indications/ diagnoses associated with those findings. To further demonstrate diagnostic reasoning, every clinical chapter contains a "Differential Diagnosis of Common Disorders" table, which summarizes significant findings in the history and physical exam and gives pertinent diagnostic tests for common disorders.

To demonstrate how various aspects of health assessment are applied, a case study is integrated into the chapter (e.g., the case patient's social history is presented with the general social history content). A case study review concludes the chapter; it recounts the patient's history and provides sample documentation of the history and physical examination. The sample documentation familiarizes students with proper and complete documentation and use of forms. The case study is complete with a final assessment finding, or diagnosis.

Every clinical chapter also includes "Assessment of Special Populations." This section highlights important information on assessing pregnant, neonatal, pediatric, and geriatric patients.

Acknowledgments

We have looked forward to this opportunity to thank the many people who have been instrumental in the development of this text.

We offer a sincere thanks to the contributors and consultants who have worked so hard to make certain that every chapter covered essential content important to every healthcare provider and student. Without their contributions, this text would not have benefited from that special uniqueness that each of them possesses. We are truly fortunate to know them and to have had them play such a critical role in this project.

We wish to thank the peer reviewers who reviewed the chapters, ensuring that the content was valid and essential. Their extensive, constructive criticism enabled us to feel confident that all aspects of advanced assessment are addressed, making the text a scholarly peer-reviewed textbook.

We owe a heartfelt thanks to Rebecca Stephenson, Associate Acquisitions Editor at Jones & Bartlett Learning. Without her encouragement and support, this third edition would not have happened. We would also like to thank Emma Huggard, Editorial Assistant; Juna Abrams, Associate Production Editor; Vanessa Richards, Production Editor; Brooke Haley, Production Assistant; Wes DeShano, Rights & Media Specialist; and Troy Liston, Media Development Editor.

Publisher's Note

Jones & Bartlett Learning would like to thank Melrose-Wakefield Hospital in Melrose, MA for kindly offering their space and equipment for use in this textbook. We would like to acknowledge the nursing staff for their support, expertise, and assistance with the photographs found in this book. We would like to especially thank Donna Harvey for her thoughtful guidance throughout the process and Anthony Alley for reserving the space in Medical 4.

Disclaimer

Care has been taken to confirm the accuracy of the information presented in this text and to describe generally accepted practices. However, the authors, editors, and publisher are not responsible for errors or omissions or for any consequences from application of the information in this book and make no warranty, express or implied, with respect to the content of the publication.

The authors, editors, and publisher have exerted every effort to ensure that the drug selection and dosage information set forth in this text is in accordance with the current recommendations and practice at the time of publication. However, in view of ongoing research, changes in government regulations, and the constant flow of information relating to drug therapy and drug reactions, the reader is urged to check the package insert for each drug for any change in indications and dosage and for added warnings and precautions. This is particularly important when the recommended agent is a new or infrequently employed drug.

Some drugs and medical devices presented in this publication have U.S. Food and Drug Administration (FDA) clearance for limited use in restricted research settings. It is the responsibility of the healthcare provider to ascertain the FDA status of each drug or device planned for use in his or her clinical practice.

Contributors to the First Edition

Gary J. Arnold, MD
Nancy J. Denke, RN, MSN, FNP-C, CCRN
Terry Denny, BSN, MN, CRNA, APRN
Laurie Anne Ferguson, MSN, APRN, FNP, BC
Mary Masterson Germain, EdD, APRN, BC
Willeen Grant-Druley, MS, FNP
Dorothy J. Hamilton, MSN, ACNP-BC, CCRN
Donald Johnson, PhD, CS
Joan E. King, PhD, RNC, ACNP, ANP
Lauren Mustin, BSN, MN, CRNA, APRN
Patricia M. Navin, EdD, APRN, CNS
Marian Newton, PhD, PMHNP-BC
Karen Koozer Olson, PhD, FNP
Cindy Parsons, MS, ARNP, BC
Jacqueline Rhoads, PhD, ACNP-BC, ANP-C, GNP, CCRN
Tina M. Samaha, BSN, CCRN, CRNA-c
Barbara Sinni-McKeehen, MSN, ARNP, DNC
Ardith L. Sudduth, PhD, RN, FNP-C
Chris Trahan, MN, CCRN, CRNA, APRN
Chad A. Trosclair, BSN, CCRN, CRNA-c
Monica Wilkinson, MN, CRNA, APRN

Consultants

Gerontological Consultant
Lynn Chilton, DSN, GNP-C, FNP-C
Professor
University of South Alabama
Mobile, Alabama

Pediatric Consultant
Dawn Lee Garzon, PhD, APRN, BC, CPNP
Clinical Associate Professor
College of Nursing
University of Missouri, St. Louis
St. Louis, Missouri

Cultural Consultant
Jana Lauderdale, PhD, RN
Assistant Dean for Cultural Diversity
Vanderbilt University School of Nursing
Program Coordinator
Fisk-Vanderbilt BSN Program
Nashville, Tennessee

Reviewers

Kathleen Ahern, PhD, FNP-BC
Professor/Program Director
Wagner College
Staten Island, New York

Frank Ambriz, MPAS, PA-C
Department Chair/Clinical Associate Professor
University of Texas Rio Grande Valley
Edinburg, Texas

Renee Andreeff, EdD, PA-C, DFAAPA
Interim Chair/Program Director
D'Youville College
Buffalo, New York

Hannah Bascomb, MSN, RN
Nursing Instructor
Mississippi University for Women
Columbus, Mississippi

Kenneth R. Butler, PhD, MS
Associate Professor
Mississippi College
Clinton, Mississippi

Terry Mahan Buttaro, PhD, AGPCNP-BC, FAANP, DPNAP
Assistant Clinical Professor
University of Massachusetts, Boston
Boston, Massachusetts

Sara Jane "Saje" Davis-Risen, PA-C, MS
Program Director/Assistant Professor
Pacific University
Hillsboro, Oregon

Cheryl Erickson, MA, FNP-BC, CNE
Associate Professor
University of Saint Francis
Fort Wayne, Indiana

Karen L. Fahey, MSN, RN, FNP-BC, DNP (in progress)
Graduate Instructor
Wheeling Jesuit University
Wheeling, West Virginia

Ellen Reilley Farrell, DNP, CRNP, FNP-BC, GNP-BC
Associate Clinical Professor
George Washington University
Washington, DC

Linda Sweigart, MSN, APRN
Instructor
Ball State University
Muncie, Indiana

James Terry Todd, RN, DNP
Instructor
Mississippi University for Women
Columbus, Mississippi

Amber Vermeesch, PhD, MSN, RN, FNP-C
Associate Professor
University of Portland
Portland, Oregon

Christine Verni, EdD, FNP-BC
Assistant Professor
D'Youville College
Buffalo, New York

Donna J. Williams, DNP, RN
Assistant Professor/Nursing Instructor
Mississippi University for Women
Columbus, Mississippi

Part 1

Strategies for Effective Health Assessment

Chapter 1

Interview and History Taking Strategies

"In taking histories follow each line of thought, ask no leading questions. Never suggest. Give the patient's own words in the complaint."

Sir William Osler (1849–1919) (Bean & Bean, 1968)

Functions of the Interview and Health History

Interviewing and taking health histories serve five major functions:

1. Establishing the initial bond between provider and patient (**Figure 1-1**)
2. Laying the foundation for subsequent clinical decision making
3. Providing a legal record of the subjective and objective data (**Box 1-1**) elicited during the clinical interview, which drive clinical judgments
4. Fulfilling a critical component of the documentation required for third-party payer reimbursement for clinical services
5. Serving as an essential element in the peer review process for evaluation of clinical practice, such as application of evidence-based practice and identification of desired patient outcomes

As the primary goal of this text is to help the reader to develop expertise in advanced health assessment, this chapter will focus primarily on functions one and two. Legal and reimbursement requirements mandate meticulous, comprehensive, and complete documentation of all the components of care, including patient teaching and counseling provided at each provider–patient encounter. These include not only the traditional face-to-face encounters, but also other means of care, such as interaction via e-mail and telephone. Meticulous and comprehensive, however, are not necessarily synonymous with lengthy. The skilled clinician strives to record all essential clinical data concisely and to document the clinical decision making that underlies diagnostic and treatment decisions. The objectives are to provide effective communication to all caregivers, to ensure continuity of high-quality care for the patient, to minimize legal vulnerability for the provider, and to maximize reimbursement for clinical services. From a legal perspective, what is not recorded has not been done. Documentation validates performance (see Chapter 3 for further discussion of documentation).

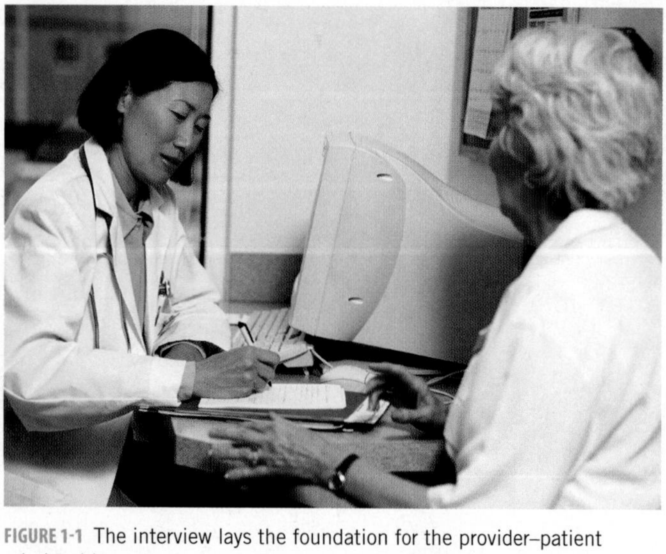

FIGURE 1-1 The interview lays the foundation for the provider–patient relationship.

BOX 1-1 SUBJECTIVE AND OBJECTIVE DATA

Subjective data are the information that the patient or other informant provides during the health history. They are so called because they reflect the patient's perception and recall of his current health need(s) and past health. Perception and recall are subject to many influences that make the information less quantifiable and open to multiple interpretations.

In contrast, *objective data* are measurable and verifiable, such as test results and physical examination findings.

Both types of data are subject to error, and both are critical to the caregiving process. Our perceptions filter all our experiences and significantly influence our behavior. Successful patient outcomes are dependent upon successfully integrating both subjective and objective data to formulate individualized plans of care to which the patient will adhere. The health history contains predominantly subjective data. Data, such as test results or copies of past medical examinations, supplement the information that the patient provides during the interview. The combination of subjective and objective data constitutes the patient's database.

Interviewing

Establishing and Maintaining a Relationship with the Patient

Building a sound provider–patient relationship is essential to effective clinical management of patients with complex health and illness needs. Mutual trust is a critical element in the relationship. Also important is the ethical principle of autonomy, which places ultimate healthcare decision making in the hands of the patient. The ability to exercise self-determination is greatly facilitated by clinicians who actively seek to engage their patients as true partners in the caregiving process. The old adage— knowledge is power—is the key to patient empowerment. Patients must feel involved in their health care. How the clinician conducts the initial health history and subsequent data collection interviews exerts a profound influence on the nature of the provider–patient relationship. The clinician and patient form a dyad. In order to guide the patient's decision-making processes and to facilitate adherence to therapeutic interventions, the clinician and the patient must form an ongoing partnership built on mutual trust and respect for the patient's active role in making healthcare decisions.

Providing Culturally Competent Care

Patient populations are becoming increasingly diverse. *Healthy People 2020,* the fourth report of the United States Department of Health and Human Services on the health of the American people, presents compelling evidence of the relationship between ethnicity, socioeconomic status, and health. This document focuses on two overarching health initiatives.

1. Determinants of health and health disparities: "Biological, social, economic, and environmental factors—and their interrelationships—influence the ability of individuals and communities to make progress on these indicators. Addressing these determinants is key to improving population health, eliminating health disparities, and meeting the overarching goals of *Healthy People 2020.*" (U.S. Department of Health and Human Services, 2014)
2. Health across life stages: "[U]sing a life stages perspective this initiative recognizes that specific risk factors and determinants of health vary across the life span. Health and disease result from the accumulation (over time) of the effects of risk factors and determinants. Intervening at specific points in the life course can help reduce risk factors and promote health. The life stages perspective addresses 1 of the 4 overarching goals of *Healthy People 2020*: 'Promote quality life, healthy development, and health behaviors across all life stages.'" (U.S. Department of Health and Human Services, 2010)

Achieving these goals will necessitate addressing the social determinants of health, making our healthcare delivery system more linguistically and culturally appropriate, and increasing the ability of practitioners to deliver culturally congruent care.

Diverse patient populations present significant challenges to both clinicians and healthcare organizations. As third-party payers and regulatory bodies increasingly look to clinical outcomes data to measure the performance of individual providers and institutions, the impact of culture on standards of care will be profound. New and emerging patient populations represent a kaleidoscopic image of healthcare beliefs, values, and practices—"Equal care cannot be defined as the same care in a culturally diverse society because this care will not be considered equally good or appropriate by all patients" (Salimbene, 1999, p. 24).

In addition to meeting the social contract to provide high-quality health care to all patients, clinicians must develop caregiving skills that are culturally congruent, and which reflect therapeutic interventions that take into account the patient's socioeconomic status. History taking is often the first encounter between patient and provider. Cultural competence requires knowledge of the beliefs, values, and practices of the patient populations being served, as well as willingness on the part of the provider to openly reflect on the impact that his or her own attitudes, beliefs, and behaviors have upon the caregiving process.

Ethnocentrism, the belief in the superiority of one's own beliefs and values, is a major barrier to establishing effective patient–provider relationships. Similarly, ignorance of a cultural group's norms may lead to a negative interpretation of well-meaning caregiver behaviors. These norms include beliefs about personal space, definitions of health, communication, and eye contact, as well as who makes healthcare decisions. Many well-intentioned caregivers breach these norms out of ignorance, thereby adversely affecting the development of patient trust and adherence to treatment interventions. For example, many Western caregivers consider direct eye contact as indicative of a patient's forthrightness and honesty. They may interpret a patient's failure to engage and maintain eye contact as an indication that he may have something to hide. In many cultures, it is considered disrespectful to look directly at an authority figure.

Through the use of cross-cultural theoretical models, the application of relevant research findings, and valuing of our ethnically diverse patients as teachers about their cultures, the caregiver who is committed to providing culturally competent care will come to understand each culture's world view from an *emic*, or native, perspective (Jones, Bond, & Cason, 1998). Many excellent resources have been developed to assist clinicians to become more culturally competent as caregivers. Resources for providing culturally competent care are given at the end of the chapter.

Overcoming Difficulties in Provider–Patient Relationships

Some patient relationships will challenge the provider from their onset, such as initial encounters with patients who are angry or hostile. Even when a strong alliance has been established between the provider and the patient, critical events in the caregiving process and/or the influence of significant others may challenge the stability and effectiveness of the relationship. For example, Platt and Gordon (2004) refer to a phenomenon known as the Two Patient Syndrome in which a family member or significant other serves as the translator for the patient. In such a situation, the answers to the provider's questions may reflect the translator's perceptions of the patient's healthcare needs, status, and goals, rather than those of the patient, especially if the family member or significant other is also the primary caregiver for the patient. Similarly, adverse clinical phenomena such as unexpected fetal loss, chronic pain that is unresponsive to treatment, or the need to inform the patient and family of a terminal diagnosis will test the strength of the most well-established provider–patient relationship.

Recognizing and Reacting to Communication Barriers

In order to successfully navigate challenging situations, recognize the feelings/behaviors being manifested by the patient (e.g., sadness, fear, anxiety, anger, hostility). Recognition requires that the provider be an attentive listener and observer and that he or she take the time to reflect and process what he or she sees and hears. Recognition often begins with a perception of distance or strained communication in a relationship that has previously been characterized by warmth and a free flow of communication. When this occurs, stop the usual routine of the visit and share these perceptions with the patient. Identify the perceived behavior or effect and seek the patient's confirmation as to the accuracy of these observations. If the nature and source of the patient's behavior are still unclear, reassure the patient that you have listened to him or her but remain confused about why he or she feels the way he or she does. Ask the patient to help you to better understand what he or she is experiencing. Do NOT become argumentative and defensive.

Acknowledge and validate the patient's feelings as appropriate through the use of statements that convey understanding and concern, such as "I can see where that would be very frightening. Do you feel any better now?" Demonstrate empathy (**Figure 1-2**). Coulehan and Block (1997) define empathy as "a type of understanding. It is not an emotional state of feeling sympathetic or sorry for someone. . .being empathic means listening to the total communication—words, feelings, and gestures—and letting the patient know that you are really hearing what she is saying" (p. 6). For most if not all challenges to provider–patient relationships, there is no quick fix, and attempts to implement one are usually perceived by the patient as being dismissive of her or his feelings, thereby disrupting the relationship even more. Support and understanding are essential to building and maintaining a relationship.

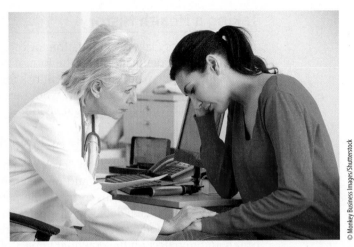

FIGURE 1-2 A healthcare provider displays empathy as a patient discusses an upsetting matter.

Touch may help convey understanding. If it is culturally appropriate and the situation warrants such an action, as in the loss of a loved one or when delivering an unfavorable prognosis, touch can be very therapeutic.

Demonstrate hope. This is particularly important in situations involving poor prognoses. Although the eventual outcome may not be altered, the patient needs to know that the provider will not withdraw because cure is not an option, will remain a consistent source of support, and will help the patient to identify and achieve the life goals that are important in his or her remaining lifespan.

Working with Resistant Patients

Patients who are resistant to therapeutic recommendations represent another challenge to provider–patient relationships. Such resistance often represents a failure of the provider to fully engage the patient as a partner in decisions about his or her health care. Cultural norms and patient ambivalence may also be major factors, as in patients who smoke. Smokers who have not experienced the negative health consequences of smoking often do not perceive themselves to be at risk, and their sociocultural environment may support continuation of this negative health behavior. The provider should continually assess the readiness of the patient to adopt or change a behavior or intervention and be ready to capitalize on any opportunity that may increase the patient's level of readiness. For example, a female smoker previously resistant to smoking cessation interventions may become very responsive if an abnormal Pap smear causes her to be sent for colposcopic examination and she learns about the relationship between smoking and cervical cancer. The grandmother who smokes and cares for her grandchild while his parents work may be resistant to quitting for her own health, but may do so to protect the health of her grandson (e.g., prevention of recurrent ear infections).

Institutional Factors Affecting Patient–Provider Relationships

Most practitioners are employed by healthcare institutions. Many institutional factors affect patient–provider relationships. Cost containment has led to an ever-increasing emphasis on productivity. Increasing patient volume often decreases the time allotted for initial and follow-up patient visits. If the time allocated for the patient sessions is inadequate to obtain all of the necessary historical data, the patient can be asked to complete a linguistically appropriate (appropriate to the patient's primary language) health history form before being seen by the provider.

Prioritization of data collection is essential and is determined by the patient's expressed reason for seeking care (chief complaint), as well as the presenting signs and symptoms. For example, although diet, exercise, and social history influence treatment decisions, past medical history and a focused review of systems take precedence in the acute phase of illness.

Taking a Health History

The health history lays the foundation for care. It guides the relative emphasis placed on each system in the physical examination and the formulation of differential diagnoses and treatment decisions. A weak foundation places the patient at risk for misdiagnosis and inadequate or erroneous treatment; it also identifies the clinician as one who does not practice within acceptable standards of care, making the clinician vulnerable to legal action.

The Health History as a Vehicle for Patient Empowerment

Having the patient participate in developing his or her health history is a powerful tool for building a partnership between patient and provider. A well-designed, culturally and linguistically appropriate health history form helps to move the patient from passive responder to active collaborator in developing the personal database that will drive future decisions about his or her care. It also begins the patient education process. The form requires the patient to complete a review of past and current health and to reflect on the potential impact of healthcare behaviors, beliefs, and values upon his or her health status. Engaging a patient in this reflective process helps to give a sense of ownership over his or her healthcare data and primes receptivity to future patient education.

The ultimate goal of all health care is to maximize the health and well-being of the patient. Whether this involves health maintenance and disease prevention or the actual treatment of a medical or surgical condition, many patients will be asked to make major, sustained changes to their current behaviors in order to acquire or sustain their desired level of health. Adherence to a therapeutic regimen is influenced by multiple factors, including the patient's perception of the severity of the need or condition and the costs–benefits associated with adherence. By actively involving the patient in the development and analysis of a personal health history, the clinician lays the groundwork for active participation in identifying healthcare goals and in designing a culturally congruent plan of care. An ongoing, collaborative process supports patient autonomy, enhances adherence, and increases the likelihood of achieving desired clinical outcomes. Strategies for performing an effective interview and health history are outlined in **Box 1-2**.

BOX 1-2   INTERVIEWING AND HISTORY TAKING POINTERS

The interview and health history lay the foundation for effective patient care. Remember the following tips when conducting the interview and health history:

- Demonstrate professional appearance and behavior. Unkempt, overly casual or inappropriate dress, and/or unprofessional behavior do not inspire confidence.
- Provide for privacy. Health histories contain highly confidential information and should be obtained in settings that maximize the patient's privacy. Adolescents and patients who have engaged in behaviors that may be viewed as socially unacceptable may be particularly reluctant to share information. Try to conduct a portion of the adolescent's health history without the presence of a parent or guardian, especially when exploring sensitive areas such as sexuality, drug and/or alcohol use, etc.
- Provide a quiet and nondistracting environment wherever possible. Distractions include provider behaviors such as answering the telephone and pagers. Unless it is essential to your professional role, turn off cell phones and electronic pagers and do not interrupt the flow of the patient's history by answering the telephone.
- Address the patient by the appropriate title (Mr., Mrs., Ms.).
- Always introduce yourself to a new patient and identify your role. For example: "I'm Ms. Rogers, a nurse practitioner. . ."
- Request the patient's permission to conduct the health history.
- Try to obtain historical data with the patient fully clothed. Clothing is important to a sense of personal integrity and identity. Initial appearance may also give the examiner valuable cultural and diagnostic clues.
- Position yourself at the same level as the patient to avoid establishing the provider as being dominant in the relationship (**Figure 1-3**). Similarly, respect cultural norms about personal space and eye contact.

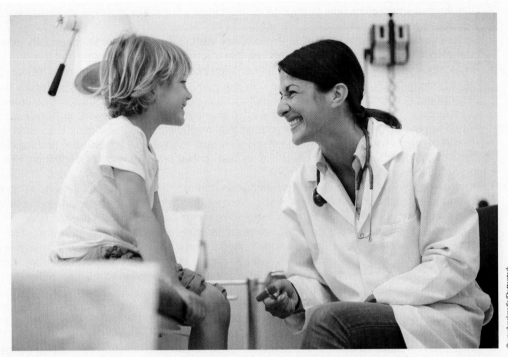

FIGURE 1-3 The healthcare provider positions herself at eye level with the patient, maintaining eye contact.

- Recognize potential biases that may adversely affect your ability to elicit an accurate and complete health history (e.g., ageism or gender bias).
- Observe the patient for any sensory deficits such as hearing or visual loss and adjust your interviewing techniques and positioning accordingly. When interviewing patients with hearing loss, position yourself so that the patient can see your face and speak more loudly and more slowly.
- Prioritize information needs to maximize conservation of the patient's physical and emotional resources. Patients in pain or acute stress require special consideration.
- Know and respect the cultural norms and values of individual patients and adjust interviewing techniques accordingly. Do not impose cultural norms on the interviewee.
- If language barriers necessitate using a translator, address the questions to the patient, not the translator, and allow adequate time for the translation and response.
- Ask the patient if it is acceptable if you take *brief* notes during the interview. Explain that the health history contains critical information that will influence decisions about care and that it is important not to miss any vital piece of information; however; be judicious in note taking. Do not become so focused on recording the data that you cease to relate to the patient.
- Assure the patient that all of the information that is provided will be kept confidential and used as a basis for care decisions. If the information provided by the patient will be used for other purposes, such as to obtain third-party reimbursement, the patient or parent/guardian must asked to sign a release authorizing approval for these additional uses of privileged healthcare data.
- Use open-ended questions, whenever possible, to elicit information during the history taking interview. Do NOT suggest symptoms or descriptors to the patient and/or informant, especially in the initial portion of obtaining the history of present illness (HPI). Ask the patient to describe the illness in his or her own words. How and what he or she focuses on gives valuable insight into the patient's perception of the relative importance of the symptoms the patient is experiencing. If additional data are needed after the patient has responded to open-ended questions, ask specific questions to obtain more detail. Avoid asking questions that suggest a particular response or that can be answered with a simple yes or no. The following is an example of *inappropriate* questioning: Would you describe your pain as sharp and stabbing or dull and achy?
- Help patients to become partners in the caregiving process. Ask about their healthcare goals and expectations about their care.

- Give the patient adequate time to respond; do not create a hurried atmosphere, especially when eliciting sensitive information.
- Do not use technical terms or medical jargon. Every health history presents an opportunity for patient education. Give your explanations in language that the patient can comprehend and use.
- Be an attentive, nonjudgmental listener and an alert observer throughout the health history. Do not interrupt prematurely, and control an urge to fill every pause or silence with another question. Give the patient time to reflect on her or his answers to your questions before intervening with a prompt or a direct question. When a prompt is necessary, often a simple statement of support, such as "Please continue," will encourage a patient to reveal additional information that facilitates clinical decision making.
- Observe nonverbal behaviors throughout the interview, such as significant affective and postural changes. These often occur in areas of the health history that contain sensitive information that requires more in-depth exploration.
- Acknowledge the value of the patient's information through the use of supportive statements during and at the end of the clinical interview. A statement such as "Mr. Jones, you have provided a very clear picture of your symptoms. This will help us to make much wiser choices about what tests to order," speaks to partnership and communicates how much the clinician values and relies on the quality of the information provided by the patient. If mechanisms have been set up at your institution to safeguard the electronic transmission of information, you may also want to invite the patient to e-mail you any additional information pertinent to his or her care that he or she may have forgotten to mention during the health history. Follow-up telephone communication is also an option, provided similar safeguards are in place.
- Validate your perceptions when the patient has completed telling you a piece of information or expressed a particular healthcare preference. Verbally summarize your understanding of the data and ask the patient if that is an accurate portrayal of the information that she or he has provided.
- If the interview yields contradictory information, revisit earlier areas of inquiry to check for consistency of response and/or ask the patient to clarify your perceptions.
- Beware of prematurely cutting off a line of diagnostic inquiry. Although a patient's presenting symptoms may strongly suggest a particular diagnosis, failure to adequately explore alternative explanations may cause the clinician to falsely reject an important differential diagnosis.

Types of Health Histories

Health histories are of two types: comprehensive and focused.

Comprehensive Health History

A comprehensive health history should be performed on all nonemergent, new patients who will be receiving ongoing primary care from a particular provider or group of clinicians. Comprehensive health histories contain all of the following elements:

- **Patient identifiers.** These include name, gender, age, ethnicity, occupation, source of referral, and date and time of the clinical encounter.
- **Reliability.** It is particularly critical to assess the reliability of the individual providing the historical data. In most instances, it will be the actual patient. However, in some clinical situations (e.g., patients with severe trauma, the very elderly, children), a person other than the patient will provide all or most of the data. It is imperative that the clinician identifies the source(s) of the data and records her or his judgment about the reliability of the information provided. For example, a clinician might record the following statement: Reliability—patient has difficulty describing the severity and progression of his symptoms and uses contradictory terms to describe the character of the chest pain.

  In some situations, assessment of the reliability of the information is complicated by language barriers. When a translator is required, the clinician should address questions to the patient and/or caregiver, not the translator, and should allow adequate time for the translator to reformulate the questions for the patient.

  Additional factors may influence the reliability of the information presented, including such patient/informant emotions as fear and shame. The clinician should try to create a supportive, nonjudgmental interviewing environment, which will encourage full disclosure of health and social information by the patient.

- **Chief complaint (CC).** This term reflects a medical or problem-oriented focus to care. Many patients seek care for health maintenance/disease prevention reasons, for example well child visits. A more encompassing term is *reason for seeking care.*
- **History of present illness (HPI).**
- **Past medical history (PMI).**
- **Family history (FH).**
- **Social history (SH).**
- **Review of systems (ROS).**

Focused Health History

A focused health history is performed in emergency situations and/or when the patient is already under the ongoing care of the clinician and presents with a specific problem-oriented complaint. Focused histories include:

- **Identifying data.**
- **Chief complaint.**
- **History of present illness.**
- **Data from the patient's past medical history, family history, and social history that are pertinent to the chief complaint.**
- **Problem-oriented review of systems.** For example, a known adult patient complaining of substernal or epigastric pain would be asked questions related to the cardiovascular, respiratory, musculoskeletal, and gastrointestinal systems. Focusing attention on these systems would help the clinician to formulate and prioritize differential diagnoses based on the most likely origin of the patient's symptoms.

Components of the Comprehensive Health History

Chief Complaint

Use the patient's own words to describe the reason for her visit. Ask the patient to tell you why she has sought care: *"Mrs. Brown, what brings you to the office today?"* Record the patient's response using her actual words; do NOT rephrase the stated reason using medical terminology. For example:

Correct: I've had a runny nose and sore throat for 3 days.
Incorrect: Patient states that she has experienced coryza and pharyngitis × 3 days.

History of Present Illness

These data represent an amplification of the patient's reason for seeking care. The thoroughness and quality of the data in the history of present illness are the driving forces in determining which systems the clinician will focus on in the review of systems and subsequent physical examination. This judgment requires that the clinician think critically in analyzing the data and apply evidence-based research findings.

The goal in obtaining the history of present illness is to get a comprehensive description of the characteristics and progression of symptoms for which the patient seeks care. For several decades, clinicians have used the mnemonic device **PQRST** to help ensure that all the necessary data are gathered regarding the patient's presenting symptoms:

P:	*precipitating* factors (What provokes the symptom?)
Q:	*quality* (Describe the character and location of symptoms.)
R:	*radiation* (Does the symptom radiate to other areas of the body?)
S:	*severity* (Ask the patient to quantify the symptom[s] on a scale of 0–10, with 0 being absence of the symptom and 10 being the most intense.)
T:	*timing* (Inquire about the onset, duration, frequency, etc.)

Although PQRST is useful in accurately describing symptoms, it does not capture many of the elements of health and illness as experienced by the patient. The following mnemonic device integrates ethnocultural considerations into the data gathering process and facilitates the provision of culturally congruent care. It also serves as a reminder to clinicians that patient outcomes determine whether an acceptable standard of care has been met. Successful outcomes are inextricably linked to care that is culturally and linguistically competent. The mnemonic device is **CLIENT OUTCOMES**.

C:	*character* of the symptoms, including intensity/severity
L:	*location*, including radiation (if present)
I:	*impact* of the symptoms/illness on patient's activities of daily living (ADL) and quality of life
E:	*expectation* (client's) of the caregiving process
N:	*neglect* or abuse, including any signs that physical and emotional neglect or abuse plays a role in the patient's condition
T:	*timing,* including onset, duration, and frequency of symptoms
O:	*other* symptoms that occur in association with the major presenting symptom
U:	*understanding/beliefs* (client's) about the possible causation of the illness/condition
T:	*treatment* (medications and other therapies that the patient has used to try to alleviate the symptoms/condition)
C:	*complementary* alternative medicine (CAM), including a description of the patient's use of these agents or practices
O:	*options* for care that are important to the patient (e.g., advance directives)
M:	*modulating* factors, meaning factors that precipitate, aggravate, or alleviate the patient's symptoms/condition
E:	*exposure* to infectious agents, toxic materials, etc.
S:	*spirituality,* including spiritual beliefs, values, and needs of the patient

Past Medical History

This section of the health history collects information about all of the patient's past health and illnesses, with particular emphasis on disease processes, surgical procedures, and hospitalizations. The term is somewhat of a misnomer; although a patient may report having been diagnosed with essential hypertension 4 years ago, the condition will continue to be an active disease process requiring ongoing evaluation and treatment in the present. Thus "past" in many cases refers to the point in time at which a condition was initially diagnosed, not that it no longer affects the patient.

The information gained from this portion of the history often gives the provider important clues about the etiology or contributing factors to the patient's current healthcare need(s). Key elements of the past medical history include:

Patient's definition of health and perception of current health status	Ask the patient to fully describe her or his health.
Childhood illnesses	Record the date, treatment, and any long-term adverse sequelae, especially any that affect the patient's functional abilities (e.g., postpolio syndrome) or current health status (e.g., past history of untreated streptococcal infection, which may contribute to mitral valve disease of the heart). *Illnesses to note include measles/rubella, mumps, pertussis, chickenpox, poliomyelitis, diphtheria, rheumatic fever, scarlet fever, and smallpox.*

Major adult illnesses/ conditions	Record date of diagnosis, treatment, and whether the condition was successfully treated or requires ongoing care. Assess impact on patient's functional ability and quality of life. *Illnesses/conditions to note include tuberculosis; coronary artery disease, especially myocardial infarction; hypertension; dyslipidemia; diabetes mellitus (specify type); cancer; autoimmune disorders, such as lupus erythematosus; osteo- or rheumatoid arthritis; gout; substance abuse; seropositivity for HIV (HIV+); AIDS; hepatitis (specify type); obesity; and sexually transmitted diseases.*
Allergies	Note any allergies to food, beverages (e.g., sulfites in some wines), drugs (see medications below), and environment. Record type and rapidity of symptomatic response to exposure, with particular attention to any respiratory symptoms. Assess the patient's knowledge of potential allergens and identify steps taken to limit exposure. Record treatment, including prescription and over-the-counter (OTC) medications and desensitization therapy. If patient has a history of severe allergic reactions, does she or he carry medical alert data on her or his person at all times? Has the patient been prescribed an emergency treatment product such as an anaphylaxis kit or Epi-Pen, a prefilled, self-injectable epinephrine syringe?
Medications	Elicit and record the name, dosage, and frequency of administration of all current, and, to the extent possible, recent past prescription and nonprescription medications. Many patients do not consider vitamins, laxatives, dietary aids and supplements, herbal products, and common drugs, such as aspirin, acetaminophen, and antacids, as being nonprescription medications and will not report their usage unless specifically questioned about them. Fully describe any drug allergies and adverse reactions experienced by the patient while taking any medication. Do NOT accept the statement "I'm allergic to. . ." at face value. Ask the patient to describe what signs (e.g., hive-like rash) or symptoms (e.g., nausea) were experienced and who determined that he is actually "allergic" to the particular drug. It should be noted that not all adverse drug effects are detectable by the patient. For example, HMG Co-A reductase inhibitors, commonly referred to as statins, are used to treat dyslipidemia and may cause elevated levels of liver enzymes in susceptible patients. Ask if the patient has ever been told to discontinue a medication because of abnormal blood chemistries. Also, inquire and fully document any CAM, including foods and beverages, such as herbal teas that the patient consumes as a treatment. This information will help the provider to develop a culturally appropriate plan of care with the patient and will preclude prescribing medications that could produce adverse interactions or have altered efficacy.
Injuries	Record the nature of the injury; date; cause (e.g., motor vehicle accident); treatment; outcome, including any long-term sequelae, especially if they affect the patient's functional ability or activities of daily living (ADL).
Hospitalizations	Record the reason for the hospitalization, dates, and complications, if any. Obtain the name and address of the facility to obtain the patient's medical records, if necessary.

Transfusions	Elicit and record the date, type, number of units administered, and the nature and severity of any reaction.
Immunizations	Elicit and record date of last immunization by type, such as diphtheria, pertussis, tetanus, polio, pneumococcal vaccine, influenza, smallpox, cholera, typhoid, anthrax, bacilli Calmette-Guérin (BCG). Also, record the date of the patient's last purified protein derivative (PPD) tuberculin skin test, as well as any other skin testing, such as allergy testing.
	Important: If the type of immunization requires serial administration of the vaccine, as with immunization against hepatitis B, record the date of each administration to determine if the interval between doses adheres to the recommendations of nationally accepted clinical guidelines. Also, note any unusual reactions to previous vaccinations. Some localized redness and tenderness at an injection site is considered normal, as are minor flu-like symptoms lasting 2 to 3 days. *People that have been successfully vaccinated with BCG will have positive PPD tuberculin tests; do NOT administer a PPD test to patients who have received BCG.*
Screening exams	Record the date of the following exams, as appropriate to the patient: Pap smear, mammogram, prostate-specific antigen (PSA), digital rectal exam, cholesterol, lipid profile, blood glucose, eye exam, glaucoma testing, hearing test, PPD (if not recorded under immunizations), chest x-ray (CXR), if patient has been immunized with BCG vaccine, and dental prophylaxis.
Psychiatric/mental health	Elicit and record any conditions requiring psychological or psychiatric intervention. Briefly describe treatment interventions. If hospitalization was required, note and cross-reference it to the PMH section on hospitalizations.

When recording the past medical history, it is helpful to end this portion of the health history with a brief statement summarizing those elements of the history that continue to exert a significant influence on the patient's health, functional ability, and/or sense of well-being.

Family History

Many disease processes follow demonstrable hereditary patterns. Knowledge of the current health status or cause of death of the patient's relatives facilitates risk analysis and promotes early intervention to prevent or delay the onset of many diseases. For instance, a patient with a first-degree (mother, father, sibling) blood relative who has experienced premature onset (women younger than 65 years of age and men younger than 55 years of age) of cardiovascular disease (CVD) is at higher risk for the development of CVD than a patient with no such familial history. The family history should extend back for two generations if the patient can provide the data and should note any intermarriage between close relatives. The family history includes:

Major illnesses and health status of relatives	Ask the patient to describe the age, health status, and presence or absence of each of the conditions listed below for each blood relative. If a relative is in good health and has none of the conditions listed below, he can be characterized as being "alive and well" (A&W).
	Conditions to be noted include cancer (specify type); hypertension; stroke; myocardial infarction; coronary artery disease (CAD)/coronary heart

	disease (CHD); neurological conditions, such as epilepsy, Huntington's chorea, and Alzheimer's disease; diabetes mellitus (specify type); tuberculosis; kidney disease; asthma and/or other allergic disorders; arthritis (specify type); anemia (specify type); thyroid disease; and mental illness.
Genetic defects	Inquire about disorders that are genetically transmitted such as cystic fibrosis, Tay-Sachs disease, beta thalassemia, hemophilia, Huntington's disease, and polycystic kidney disease.
Deaths	Note the cause, age at time of death, and relationship of the person to the patient.
Ethnicity	Note the patient's ethnicity, as certain diseases predominate in selected ethnic groups.

In addition to recording the family history in narrative form, most clinicians find it useful to construct a pictorial representation (genogram), which facilitates rapid transmission of data from one caregiver to another (see Chapter 3 for further discussion of the genogram, along with a sample).

Social History

This portion of the health history seeks to create a living picture of the patient as a person. In many instances, the patient's beliefs and practices may not be consistent with those of the provider. Remember, the goals of obtaining the health history are to acquire information to support accurate clinical decision making and to establish a partnership/relationship with the patient that will allow for the development of a culturally appropriate plan of care that maximizes adherence. Avoid being judgmental. A condescending or disapproving manner will close communication and deny the provider current and future access to essential information. Key elements in the social history include:

Personal data	Note place of birth, birth order, description of childhood family (noting family status: intact, separated/divorced, single parent, happy, abusive, and so on), brief description of childhood and young adulthood, level of education, marital status, and description of current family unit.
Occupation	Describe current or former work; work status (full-time, part-time, retired); job training; level of responsibility, if pertinent to the management of the patient's care (such as a hypertensive patient in high-stress position); occupational exposure to health hazards, such as excessive noise, pollution, toxic chemicals or vapors, infectious agents; and availability and use of protective clothing and equipment. As the patient responds to questions about work, try to assess the importance of his or her work to self-image.
Housing	Note type (e.g., private home, walk-up apartment); if the patient owns or rents the residence; type and adequacy of heat, cooling, humidification, refrigeration, cooking facilities; any potential hazards, such as asbestos or lead-based paint (which is found in some homes built before the 1970s); safety of the surrounding neighborhood and, if an apartment, the building itself; telephone access; pets; and single level or multiple levels in home (including information about stairs, number of flights, elevator, and other details). Additional information may be sought based on the particular needs of the patient. For example, if a patient presents with asthmatic symptoms, inquire about the type of floor covering in the home—carpeting may harbor dust mites, mold, and other allergens that can trigger asthmatic symptoms.

Safety	Assess and record data about the patient's actual or potential exposure to environmental hazards as well as her or his safety practices. Environmental considerations include the patient's perception about the safety of her or his neighborhood, work environment, and transportation. It also includes asking about safety needs that are patient specific. For example:

- Does the home have smoke alarms, window guards for child protection in elevated apartments, or a carbon monoxide alarm in a home using fuel oil for heating?
- If the patient has functional limitations, are assistive devices such as bathtub bars in place?

Note safety practices. Practices include such behaviors as use of seat belts and not drinking and driving.

Socioeconomic status	Note the adequacy of personal and/or family income to meet basic requirements for housing, food, and clothing. Does income allow for discretionary expenditures for recreation/travel? Does the patient/family have health coverage? (If so, note type: private, Medicare, Medicaid, and so on.) What is the extent of coverage? Does it include reimbursement for health promotional interventions and dental care? If it includes a prescription plan, is coverage limited to generic drugs or to medications chosen from a preapproved formulary? Other information, such as which diagnostic and treatment procedures (if any) require preapproval, can be determined when a specific expensive test or procedure is being considered.
Diet	Time limitations usually preclude eliciting a comprehensive diet history during the initial health history. Unless management of the patient requires immediate dietary intervention, the patient can be asked to keep a record of food and beverage intake for a typical week, not during vacation or over a holiday. Less extensive diet histories often grossly misrepresent the patient's usual dietary practices and do not facilitate effective clinical management. Ask the patient to record the date, time, type, and amount of food and beverage consumed. Important additional information to be recorded includes:

- Cultural or religious practices that influence dietary practices
- Specific quantities (e.g., Did the patient have a 6-ounce cup of coffee or a 16-ounce mug?)
- How food was prepared (Was it broiled, fried, baked, or prepared some other way? Was it prepared at home or purchased commercially?)
- Use of salt in the preparation or addition as a seasoning
- Use of oil (Was oil used in preparing the food? If yes, specify type. Some oils are very high in saturated fat and trans fatty acids.)
- Type of beverages consumed (Note whether they are caffeinated, alcoholic, or artificially sweetened.)

If at all possible, ask the patient to return the completed diet history to your practice site before the next visit so that you may review it. If the appropriate patient privacy and confidentiality of health information safeguards are in place at your institution, you may be able to receive this information in electronic form.

One more caveat: Dietary practices are influenced by many factors. Some are obvious, as with socioeconomic status. Others are more subtle, as is often the case with many elderly patients living alone. They may have the means to purchase and prepare an adequate diet, but because of loneliness may not do so. Eating is a social experience for most people, and elderly patients living alone, in particular, are at risk for nutritional deficiencies.

Exercise	Note type, intensity, duration, and frequency. Which factors influence the patient's participation or nonparticipation in regular, aerobic exercise (e.g., work, homemaking, childcare responsibilities, access to safe recreational areas, or physical limitations, such as obesity, arthritis, or angina)?
Sleep	Note the usual number of hours per 24-hour period. Does the patient engage in rotating shift work, which can alter sleep–wake patterns? Does she or he experience difficulty falling or staying asleep? Does she or he consume anything before retiring that may interfere with sleep, such as caffeinated beverages, chocolate, or diuretics? Is there any evidence of sleep apnea, such as snoring, excessive daytime sleepiness, or feeling fatigued upon awakening? Is the patient awakened from sleep by pain or by the need to void?
Sexual history	Traditionally, the sexual history has focused almost exclusively on assessing the patient's feelings about and satisfaction with his or her sexual performance. For example, it includes the number and type of partners, frequency of intercourse and other sexual practices, type and use of contraception, ability to achieve and sustain an erection, ability to achieve orgasm, and overall satisfaction. These are important questions and allow for identification of treatable conditions, such as erectile dysfunction. It is also useful to conceptualize sexuality as encompassing a broad range of expressions of intimacy and caring, such as holding, cuddling, and touching.
Drug and alcohol use	For all of the substances addressed in this section, the social conditions of use often play a major role in determining amount and pattern of consumption. Knowledge of the conditions under which and with whom a patient may engage in substance abuse can help the provider to develop more effective interventions. Many patients who engage in substance abuse will abuse more than one substance. Smoking is addressed in this portion of the history because of the addictive properties of cigarettes. If a patient smokes, determine how much, how long, and under which conditions he or she smokes (e.g., all the time, only at work, in social situations). Ask who would be exposed to the patient's secondhand smoke. Smoking cessation interventions, however brief, should be carried out at every patient encounter.
	Inquire about past and current usage of any illicit drugs, such as amphetamines, Ecstasy, cocaine, marijuana, heroin, and steroids. Determine the amount, type, method of administration, and perceived impact on health. If drug administration is by injection, are needles shared? Inquire about alcohol intake, noting type, amount, and frequency. Does the patient drink alone? Some subpopulations may be particularly vulnerable to dependence on alcohol. Alcoholism in the elderly is a growing concern of many healthcare providers and is thought to be related to feelings of loneliness, loss, and decreasing physical and mental ability. If providers suspect alcohol abuse, they can use instruments such as the CAGE questionnaire to further assess the patient's use of alcohol.
Social support	How does the patient perceive her or his level of social support? Who/what are the patient's primary sources of support? To what extent does she or he want these individuals or entities to be involved in her or his care?
Stress and anger management	Ask the patient to identify sources of stress in his or her life and to describe strategies used to cope with stress. Inquire about the patient's anger management strategies.

Recreation/ travel	Which interests or hobbies does the patient have? Does the patient participate regularly in recreational, occupational/professional, or church groups? Note any major travel within the recent past, especially if travel involved potential exposure to untreated water, raw sewage, rodent excrement, contagious disease, and/or parasites.
Cultural beliefs and practices	How do cultural beliefs and practices influence the patient's healthcare behaviors? For example, is the patient comfortable performing breast or testicular self-examination? Discuss patterns of communication about healthcare information within the family unit. Who makes healthcare decisions? If pertinent, what are the beliefs about death and dying? Does the patient utilize folk medicine and culturally based healing practices? If so, how might these be integrated into the plan of care? Will the clinician have to negotiate modification of some of these practices to achieve treatment goals?
Spirituality	What role do spiritual beliefs and practices play in the patient's life? Are they a key source of support for the patient? How can they become a component of the patient's plan of care?
Military service	Note the branch and dates of service, occupational specialty, geographic location of assignment(s), and any potential exposure to hazardous materials or conditions.

Review of Systems

The last component of the health history is the review of systems (ROS), during which the clinician questions the patient about whether or not she or he has experienced symptoms that may indicate possible pathology in one or more body systems. The nature and depth of the questioning are determined by the reason for which the patient is seeking care (chief complaint), as well as the severity of the condition if she or he presents with an acute problem.

Types of Reviews of Systems

In a nonemergent primary care setting, the review of systems follows one of two forms: comprehensive or focused.

Comprehensive ROS. This type of ROS is conducted when a patient presents for general health maintenance/disease prevention care. The provider asks general questions that are designed to identify if the patient is experiencing symptoms that may suggest an actual or potential problem in one or more body systems. Questioning covers *ALL* body systems.

Subsequent chapters in this text provide in-depth information about conducting a focused ROS. Therefore, only the elements of a comprehensive ROS will be presented below.

Before examining the key questions to be asked for each of the body systems, there are important concepts to note: **significant or pertinent positives** and **significant or pertinent negatives.** Disease states usually produce a cluster of symptoms; however, some are considered to be more indicative of a particular condition than others. For example, chest pain is strongly associated with cardiac disease, although it may also occur with gastrointestinal and musculoskeletal disorders.

The questions commonly included in a comprehensive ROS are those to which a **positive** response suggests the existence of pathology in a given system. Thus, when a patient responds that he or she has experienced the symptom about which he or she is being questioned, that is considered to be a significant **positive** response. When such a response is given during the comprehensive ROS, the clinician will then ask additional questions to better describe the characteristics of the symptom and to determine the presence or absence and description of any associated symptoms. For example, if a patient acknowledges that she or he has experienced chest pain, the clinician will probe further to obtain a full description of the pain (PQRST). The provider would ask questions about the presence or absence of radiation of the pain to the left arm, jaw, or area between the shoulder blades and about precipitating and alleviating factors (e.g., if the pain was brought on by exertion or emotional excitement/distress, if it subsided with rest).

The provider would ask the patient about the coexistence of associated symptoms, such as nausea or sweating (diaphoresis). If the patient acknowledged experiencing additional symptoms of nausea and diaphoresis during episodes of chest pain, these would be considered to be other significant **positives** in that they tend to confirm that the pain is of cardiac origin. In contrast, negative responses to questioning about these associated symptoms would be considered to be significant **negatives** because the absence of these symptoms decreases the likelihood that the patient's chest pain is cardiac in nature. Eliciting and recording significant positives and negatives are essential to developing sound differential diagnoses and to assessing the potential severity of the patient's symptoms.

Focused ROS. This type of ROS is conducted when a patient presents with a specific chief complaint. Questioning would be directed toward the systems most likely to be involved in producing the patient's symptoms. The patient would not be questioned about symptoms in the remaining body systems. For example, if a patient presented with a sore throat and a sensation of pain and pressure below both eyes, the clinician would ask problem-specific questions about the head and neck, including the eyes, nose, mouth and throat, sinuses, lymph glands, and respiratory system.

Components of a Comprehensive Review of Systems

General/ Constitutional	Ask about weight loss or gain, changes in appetite, general state of health, sense of well-being, strength, energy level, ability to conduct usual activities, and exercise tolerance, night sweats, and fever.
Skin	Ask about skin changes, including rashes, itching, pigmentation, moisture or dryness, texture; changes in color, size, or shape of moles; changes in hair (growth or loss), and changes of the nails (e.g., clubbing, spooning, or ridges).
Eyes	Inquire about injury; double vision; visual acuity (near and far); sudden loss of vision; tearing (unilateral or bilateral); blind spots; pain; blurring of vision; ability to see at night, especially if the patient operates an automobile; photophobia; haloes around lights and headache (suggestive of narrow angle glaucoma); discharge; seeing spots (may indicate "floaters").
Ears	Question about pain, discharge, injury (including barotrauma associated with air travel, diving); hearing acuity; tinnitus; vertigo; balance (inner ear function); frequency and severity of ear infections (include treatment); care of ears, including wax (cerumen) removal if performed.
Nose	Ask about nosebleeds (including frequency), colds, obstruction, discharge (including color and quantity), changes in sense of smell, polyps, sneezing, and postnasal drainage.
Mouth/Throat	Inquire about dental difficulties, lesions, gingival hyperplasia and bleeding, use of dentures, adequacy of saliva flow, hoarseness, difficulty articulating words (dysarthria), frequency and severity of sore throats (including treatment), and changes in the appearance of the tongue or sense of taste. Ask about neck stiffness, pain, tenderness, masses in thyroid or other areas, and lymphadenopathy (pain or swelling of the lymph nodes).
Cardiovascular	Question about chest pain, substernal distress, palpitations, syncope, dyspnea on exertion, orthopnea, paroxysmal nocturnal dyspnea, edema, cyanosis, hypertension, heart murmurs, varicosities, phlebitis, and claudication, hemoptysis, and coldness of extremities (note severity and conditions under which this occurs).

Respiratory	Ask about pain (including location, quality, and relation to respiration), shortness of breath (SOB), dyspnea, wheezing, stridor, cough (noting time of day and, if productive, amount in tablespoons or cups per day and color of sputum), hemoptysis, respiratory infections, tuberculosis (or exposure to tuberculosis), and fever or night sweats. Note date of last chest x-ray (CXR), if applicable.
Gastrointestinal	Inquire about appetite, dysphagia, indigestion, food idiosyncrasy, abdominal pain, heartburn, eructation, nausea, vomiting, hematemesis, jaundice, polyps, constipation, diarrhea, abnormal stools (e.g., clay-colored, tarry, bloody, greasy, foul smelling), flatulence, hemorrhoids, and recent changes in bowel habits.
Genitourinary	Ask about urgency, frequency, dysuria, colic-like pain in flank area, suprapubic pain, facial puffiness, nocturia, hematuria, polyuria, oliguria, unusual (or change in) color of urine, stones, infections, nephritis, hernias, hesitancy, change in size and force of stream, dribbling, acute retention or incontinence (note type, e.g., stress, overflow), changes in libido, potency, genital sores, discharge, and sexually transmitted diseases.
	Ask male patients about the age of onset of secondary sexual characteristics, achieving and maintaining an erection, ejaculation, fertility, testicular pain or masses, and frequency and technique for performance of testicular self-exam. Ask female patients about age of onset of menses; length and regularity of menstrual cycles; date of last Pap smear; date of last menstrual cycle; dysmenorrhea, menorrhagia, or metrorrhagia; vaginal discharge, vulvar itching; postmenopausal bleeding; dyspareunia; hormone replacement or contraceptive therapy (describe fully and note any possible contraindications to same, such as a history of thrombophlebitis); type and frequency of sexual activity; number of sexual partners; infertility; number and results of pregnancies (gravida, para); complications of pregnancy, delivery, or the postpartum period (e.g., postpartum depression); and type of delivery (e.g., normal, spontaneous vaginal delivery, use of forceps, cesarean section).
Breast	Inquire about breast masses/lumps, lesions, tenderness, swelling, nipple discharge, dimpling/retraction of any area of the breast, and frequency and technique of breast self-examination (BSE).
	Note: Males may also develop breast cancer. They should be questioned about any discharge, masses, etc.
Musculoskeletal	Question about the experience of pain, swelling, redness, or heat of muscles or joints; bony deformity; limitation of motion; muscular weakness; atrophy; and cramps.
Neurologic	Ask about headaches, lightheadedness, convulsions, paralyses, incoordination, sensory changes (such as paresthesia, anesthesia, and hyperesthesia), changes in mentation, fainting, syncopal episodes, loss of consciousness, difficulties with memory or speech, sensory or motor disturbances, or disturbances in muscular coordination (ataxia, tremor).
Mental/Psychiatric	Ask about predominant mood; emotional problems; anxiety; depression (including suicidal ideation if appropriate); difficulty concentrating; if previous historical data suggest, assess for domestic, partner, and/or elder abuse; previous psychiatric care; unusual perceptions; and hallucinations.

Lymphatic	Inquire about local or general lymph node enlargement or tenderness or suppuration.
Hematologic	Question about anemia, abnormal bleeding or clotting tendencies, previous transfusions and reactions, and Rh incompatibility.
Endocrine	Inquire about polydipsia, polyuria, polyphagia, unexplained changes in weight; changes in skin texture or hair texture and distribution; energy level; appetite; changes in mentation; thyroid enlargement or tenderness; changes in size of head or hands; asthenia; hormone therapy; growth; secondary sexual development; and intolerance to heat or cold.

Completion of the review of systems concludes the health history. Before moving on to the physical examination, however, it is desirable to ask the patient if there are any health concerns or issues that were either not identified or not covered adequately during the history taking process. Even if the patient declines to add anything, asking conveys a respect and valuing of the patient's role in decision making about her or his health and helps to reinforce the partnership between provider and patient.

Summary

The health history is the foundation upon which all other components of the patient's care are built. The manner and skill with which the clinician elicits the information has a major influence on the development of the provider–patient relationship and the quality of the data that will drive diagnostic and treatment decisions. The decisions and the patient's responses to treatment will be evaluated in terms of measurable outcomes, cost–benefit analysis, and patient satisfaction. Outcomes and patient satisfaction are intimately connected. The expert clinician is culturally competent and conducts all facets of care with an understanding and respect for the cultural dimensions of care. Such care creates a win–win situation: The patient achieves better clinical outcomes and is highly satisfied with his or her care, and the clinician meets institutional and third-party payer expectations that care will achieve evidence-based clinical outcomes in a cost-effective manner. Remember **C-L-I-E-N-T O-U-T-C-O-M-E-S** as you progress from novice to expert in your history taking knowledge and skill.

Bibliography

Bean, R. B., & Bean, W. B. (Eds.). (1968). *Sir William Osler: Aphorisms from his bedside teachings and writings.* Springfield, IL: Charles C. Thomas. Retrieved from http://www.vh.org/adult/provider/history/osler/intro.html.

Coulehan, J. L., & Block, M. R. (1997). *The medical interview: Mastering skills for clinical practice* (3rd ed.). Philadelphia, PA: F. A. Davis.

Jones, M. E., Bond, M. L., & Cason, C. L. (1998). Where does culture fit in outcomes management? *Journal of Nursing Care Quality, 13*(1), 41–51.

Platt, F. W., & Gordon, G. H. (2004). *Field guide to the difficult patient interview* (2nd ed.). Philadelphia, PA: Lippincott Williams & Wilkins.

Salimbene, S. (1999). Cultural competence: A priority for performance. *Online Journal of Nursing Care Quality, 13*(3), 23–36.

U.S. Department of Health and Human Services (2010). *Healthy People 2020 (Conference Edition, in two volumes).* Washington, DC: Author.

U.S. Department of Health and Human Services, Public Health Service (2014). *Fact sheet—addressing racial and ethnic disparities in health* (AHRQ Publication No. 00-P041). Rockville, MD: Author.

Additional Resources

The National Center for Cultural Competence

http://nccc.georgetown.edu

The National Center for Cultural Competence (NCCC) at Georgetown University's Center for Child and Human Development has developed instruments for both individual and institutional assessment of cultural and linguistic competency.

Culture Clues

http://depts.washington.edu/pfes/CultureClues.htm

"Culture Clues," produced by the University of Washington Medical Center's Patient and Family Education Committee, are of value to a busy clinician. These invaluable clinical tools are designed to allow a caregiver to quickly (in 3 to 5 minutes) acquire a baseline understanding of the defining characteristics, values, and beliefs of a particular cultural group, such as Korean, Latino, Albanian, Vietnamese, and Hard of Hearing. Additional culture clues are under development.

Chapter 2

Physical Examination Strategies

Function of the Physical Examination

The physical examination requires you to use your senses to assess the patient. You collect objective data regarding various aspects of the patient's health through sight, hearing, touch, and smell. Though strategies are discussed separately, it is important to realize that the history complements and validates the physical examination. The history and physical examination are the foundation of the treatment plan. The history obtained provides clues and guides you through the physical examination process. As the examination begins, some components of the examination process may prompt you to return to the history. Discreetly incorporating some history during the examination process facilitates the exposure of the principal, or sometimes underlying, diagnosis.

General Considerations

Interacting with the Patient

When conducting a physical examination, remember that encounters with the human body may be discomforting, embarrassing, and sometimes distressing for the patient. Your comfort level should never become so great that you forget about this often-invasive experience for each individual patient. Respect the integrity of the patient while maintaining a professional, courteous approach (as discussed in Chapter 1).

Gaining the trust and confidence of your patient is essential for obtaining an accurate history and physical examination. As you are examining the patient, the patient is simultaneously examining you (see **Figure 2-1**). The patient will note any hesitation or tone changes in your voice, how long you spend assessing certain body systems, and your facial expressions.

Determining the Scope of Examination

Physical examinations are of two types: comprehensive and focused. As with comprehensive health histories, a comprehensive (or head-to-toe) physical examination should be performed on all nonemergent, new patients who will be receiving ongoing primary care from a particular provider or group of clinicians. Components of a comprehensive physical examination are discussed later in the chapter.

A focused physical examination is performed in emergency situations and/or when the patient is already under the ongoing care of the clinician and presents with a specific problem-oriented complaint. Chapters 4 through 16 discuss focused assessments for various systemic disorders.

Assessment Techniques

Inspection

Inspection involves collecting data through sight and smell. Upon first contact with the patient, you observe mannerisms, gait, stature, and various other physical qualities. Inspection provides significant

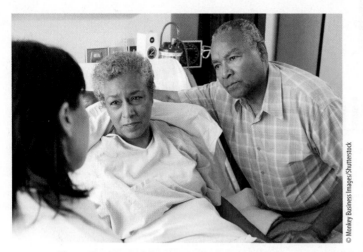

FIGURE 2-1 The patient notes the tone and demeanor of the examiner.

insight into underlying diseases/disorders. Knowing what to look for and what it means helps focus inspection. The systemic disorder chapters that follow give inspection points and relate them to possible diagnoses.

Palpation

Palpation involves using touch to collect data. Palpation is used to determine such characteristics as temperature, texture, tenderness or pain, and sensation. It is also used to establish information about internal characteristics, such as enlargement of the spleen. Depending on the amount of pressure applied, palpation can be characterized as light, moderate, or deep. Various aspects of your hands are used to assess different things.

Percussion

Percussion uses tapping to assess underlying structures. Percussion over a structure causes vibrations, which can be felt and heard. Percussion is used to establish such qualities as location, size, density, and reflex. Percussion may be direct or indirect. With direct percussion, use your finger or hand to strike/tap the surface of the patient's body directly. For indirect percussion, place your hand over the surface of the patient's body and with the other hand, strike the first hand (**Figure 2-2**). Percussion sounds maybe described as tympanic, hyper-resonant, resonant, dull, or flat.

Auscultation

Auscultation entails listening to body sounds and is particularly important for assessing the lungs, heart, and abdomen. Most auscultation requires a stethoscope, so it is critical that the provider invest in a high-quality stethoscope that has excellent sound quality and is comfortable to use. Before you buy one, consider the following:

Eartips. It is important to use an eartip size that best fits your ears. When the eartips are in your ears, they should fit snugly, not loosely, so that the sound/or acoustic performance is clear and loud. All eartips are available in small and large sizes. Poorly fitting ear tips can result in a poor seal, which can lead to missing critical sounds.

The seal. Stethoscopes rely on an airtight seal to transmit body sounds from the patient to the practitioner's ears. Loose parts in the chestpiece and loose or cracked tubing can prevent an airtight seal.

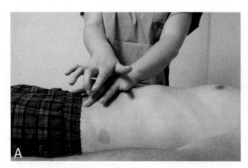
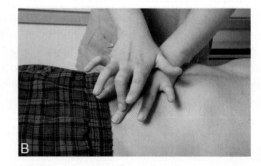

FIGURE 2-2 Indirect percussion.

The bell. When using a double-sided stethoscope, you can use either the bell or the diaphragm. Sound quality and volume depend on a quality bell.

Tubing. The tubing should retain its shape and flexibility even after being folded tightly into a pocket. Ideally, it should be made of material that does not contain materials that would irritate a patient's or provider's skin, especially those with allergies. Make sure the tubing is double lumen so sound is magnified.

Head-to-Toe Examination

Preparing for the Examination

Gather necessary equipment (**Figure 2-3**). **Box 2-1** provides a list of equipment needed for a comprehensive examination. Before beginning the examination, instruct the patient to empty the bladder and remove as much clothing as possible and put on a gown. Remember to respect modesty (close doors, use drapes, and leave the room while patient is dressing/undressing). Allow a third party in the room if that helps the patient feel more comfortable. Upon entering the room, wash your hands (and apply gloves, as appropriate). Make sure to tell the patient what you will be doing before you begin the examination.

Sequencing

Integration of the head-to-toe assessment requires rehearsal and repeated examinations to develop comfort and confidence. It takes time for the procedure to flow naturally. Learn to adapt to a situation and establish a routine that feels comfortable and natural to you. Develop a systematic pattern that is efficient and comfortable for the patient and that will prompt you not to omit parts of the examination.

Of course, there is no one correct way to put an examination together. The goal is to create a sequence that will flow very smoothly, accommodate the patient, and make it easier for the patient in that she or he will not have to make numerous position changes. Any approach may need to be adjusted to patient-specific conditions or disabilities.

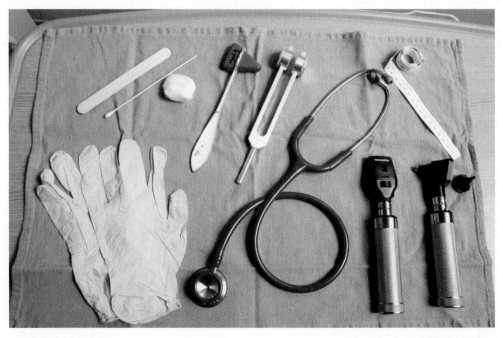

FIGURE 2-3 Basic equipment.

BOX 2-1   COMPREHENSIVE LIST OF EQUIPMENT FOR PHYSICAL EXAMINATION

BASIC EQUIPMENT
- Cotton balls
- Cotton-tipped applicators/sticks
- Drapes
- Flashlight with transilluminator, or penlight
- Gauze squares
- Gloves
- Craves or Pederson speculum
- Lubricant
- Marking pen
- Measuring tape
- Nasal speculum
- Odorous substances
- Ophthalmoscope
- Otoscope with pneumatic bulb
- Penlight
- Percussion hammer
- Sharp and dull testing instruments
- Sphygmomanometer
- Stethoscope with diaphragm and bell
- Taste-testing substances
- Thermometer
- Tongue blades
- Tuning forks
- Visual acuity screening charts

SUPPLIES FOR GATHERING SPECIMENS
- Culture media
- Glass slides
- KOH (potassium hydroxide)
- Occult blood testing materials
- Pap smear spatula and/or brush, fixative, and container
- Saline
- Sterile cotton-tipped applicators

The following is an example of a suggested approach, based on patient positioning.

General Survey

The examination begins as the patient enters the room.
- Assess appearance including age, sex, skin color, facial expressions, dress, eye contact, mood, mental alertness, and orientation.
- Note physical structure including posture, stature, size, contour, and nutritional state.
- Evaluate mobility including gait and movement when sitting and rising.
- Note speech pattern.
- Note hearing deficits or aids.

Measurements

- Measure weight.
- Measure height.
- Assess vital signs: blood pressure, pulse, respirations, and temperature.

Components of the Physical Examination

Patient Seated and Facing Examiner

Head and Face

- Inspect skin characteristics.
- Inspect and palpate scalp and hair for texture, distribution, quantity, masses, parasites, or lesions.
- Inspect face for appearance, expression, symmetry of structure and features, and movements.
- Ask the patient to raise his eyebrows, frown, smile, and open eyes against resistance. Note strength and symmetry of facial muscles (CNs V and VII).
- Evaluate sensation awareness of the forehead, cheeks, and jaw on each side of the face (CN V).
- With the patient's teeth clenched, palpate the masseter and temporal muscles.

Eyes

- Inspect the corneal light reflex for symmetry (Hirschberg's test).
- Perform the cover–uncover test.
- Assess extraocular muscles for movement through the six cardinal fields of gaze.
- Assess position and alignment of the eyes.
- Inspect eyelids and eyelashes.
- Inspect lacrimal apparatus and conjunctiva.
- Inspect the sclera for color and clarity.
- Inspect pupils (pupils equal, round, reactive to light—PERRL).
- Perform fundoscopic assessment:
  - Observe the red reflex.
  - Inspect the optic disc.
  - Inspect for retinal background hemorrhages, exudates, and lesions.

Ears

- Observe for position, size, shape, and symmetry of pinnae.
- Carefully palpate each ear separately; apply pressure to the tragus.
- Inspect the ear canal and tympanic membrane using an otoscope.
- Test hearing acuity (Weber, Rinne, and whisper tests).

Nose

- Inspect the external nose for overall shape, symmetry, and edema.
- Inspect the skin around the nose for lesions, color, and irregularities.
- Palpate the bridge and soft tissues of the nose.
- Inspect the sinus areas for edema; palpate and percuss sinuses.
- Inspect the nasal cavity.
  - Assess the nasal cavity for patency and the nasal septum for continuity.
  - Assess the turbinates for color, texture, and discharge.
  - Inspect the color of the mucous membranes.
- Test sense of smell (CN I).

Mouth and Oropharynx

- Observe movement of the mouth and lips and note any asymmetry.
- Inspect the lips for symmetry, color, edema, and lesions.
- Note odor of the patient's breath.
- Inspect the buccal mucosa and gums for color, ulcerations, lesions, or trauma.
- Observe position, color, and number of teeth.
- Inspect tongue for color and texture.
- Assess the tongue for atrophy and movement (CN XII).
- Inspect the hard and soft palates for color and appearance.
- Ask the patient to say "ah," and stroke the palatal arch with a tongue blade to observe for the presence of the gag reflex (CNs IX and X).
- Note the presence and size of tonsils and any exudate.
- Assess taste (CNs VII and IX).

Neck
- Palpate the lymph nodes in the neck area.
- Palpate carotid pulses one at a time.
- Determine the position of the trachea.
- Palpate thyroid.
- Auscultate carotid arteries and thyroid for bruits.

Upper Extremities
- Inspect the contour of the clavicles, scapulae, and shoulders.
- Palpate the sternoclavicular and acromioclavicular joints, acromion process, clavicles, and greater trochanter of the humerus.
- Test range of motion (ROM) of the shoulder and elbow.
- Assess biceps, brachioradialis, and triceps reflexes.
- Assess radial and brachial pulses.
- Inspect the hand; palpate for tenderness.
- Test ROM of the hand and wrist.

Patient Seated and Facing Away from Examiner with Back Exposed
Posterior Chest and Back
- Inspect skin for lesions.
- Note thoracic configuration.
- Palpate the spine.
- Percuss the kidneys.
- Assess the lungs:
  - Evaluate thoracic expansion.
  - Palpate for tactile fremitus.
  - Percuss the chest.
  - Determine diaphragmatic excursion.
  - Auscultate the posterior thoracic cage; note breath sounds.

Patient Seated and Facing Examiner with Chest Exposed
Anterior Chest
- Determine the shape and symmetry of the thorax.
- Assess the lungs:
  - Establish the respiratory rate and pattern.
  - Palpate for crackles and rubs.
  - Evaluate thoracic expansion.
  - Auscultate for breath sounds.
- Assess the heart:
  - Visualize the apical pulse.
  - Auscultate for heart sounds.
- Assess the breasts. Inspect the breasts with the patient assuming the following positions: arms extended over the head, pushing hands on hips, hands pushed together in front of chest, and leaning forward.
  - Inspect the breasts for size and symmetry.
  - Inspect the skin for texture and color.
  - Inspect the venous system.
  - Inspect for lesions or masses.

Patient Reclining 45 Degrees
Assist the patient to a reclining position at a 45-degree angle. Stand to the side of the patient that allows the greatest comfort.
- Inspect jugular venous pulsations.
- Measure jugular venous pressure.

Patient Supine with Chest Exposed

Assist patient into a supine position. If the patient cannot tolerate lying flat, have him or her maintain head elevation at 30-degree angle if possible. Uncover the chest while keeping the abdomen and lower extremities draped.

Female Breasts

Place a towel or pillow under the patient's back and ask her to raise her arms above her head.
- Inspect and palpate breast.
- Palpate the nipple.

Heart
- Palpate the precordium.
- Palpate the apical pulse.
- Percuss the borders of the heart.
- Auscultate heart sounds.

Patient Supine with Abdomen Exposed

Cover the chest with the patient's gown and expose the abdomen.

Abdomen
- Inspect the abdomen for peristalsis, asymmetry, and abdominal distention.
- Assess skin of abdomen, observing color, scars, rashes, or lesions.
- Auscultate all four quadrants for bowel sounds.
- Auscultate for vascular sounds, bruits, venous hums, and friction rubs.
- Percuss all quadrants for dullness.
- Percuss for tympany and hyperresonance.
- Percuss the liver.
- Percuss the spleen.
- Using light, moderate, and deep palpation, palpate all quadrants.
- Perform fluid wave test.
- Palpate for rebound tenderness.
- Palpate for inspiratory arrest (Murphy's sign).
- Palpate for McBurney's sign.
- Palpate for abdominal aortic aneurysm.
- Palpate right costal margin for liver border.
- Palpate the liver.
- Palpate the kidneys.
- Palpate the spleen.

Male Genitalia
- Inspect and note the distribution of the pubic hair.
- Inspect and palpate the penis for any lesions, sores, rash, or masses.
- Inspect and palpate the urinary meatus.
- Inspect the scrotum for lesions, rashes, color changes, or edema.
- Palpate the testes.
- Assess for inguinal hernias.

Patient Supine with Legs Exposed

Arrange gown and drape so that they are covering the abdomen and pubis.

Hips
- Palpate the bony areas anteriorly.
- Test ROM.

Lower Extremities
- Inspect the knees for swelling, deformity, muscle tone, and alignment of patellae.
- Palpate the knees and test ROM.
- Inspect the ankles and feet for edema, ecchymosis of deformity.
- Palpate and test ROM of the ankles and feet.

Patient Seated Facing Examiner
Neurologic System
- Test rapid alternating movements (RAM).
- Observe for leg dystaxia using the heel-to-shin test.
- Assess exteroceptive sensation.
  - Assess the patient's ability to sense superficial pain.
  - Test temperature sensation.
- Assess proprioceptive sensation.
  - Test motion and position sense.
  - Test vibratory sense.
- Assess cortical sensation.
  - Test stereognosis.
  - Assess graphesthesia.
  - Test two-point discrimination.
  - Assess extinction.
- Test plantar and Achilles reflexes.

Patient Standing
Neurologic
- Observe patient standing, walking regularly, walking on heels, walking on tiptoes, and walking toe to heel.
- Instruct the patient to walk forward a few steps with eyes closed.
- Perform Romberg's test.
- Test for pronator drift.

Spine
- Assess posture.
- Palpate the spinal column.
- Palpate the paravertebral muscles.
- Observe ROM. Have the patient flex as if she or he were trying to touch her or his toes, extend, and move side to side.

Female Patient in Lithotomy Position
Remember to drape appropriately.
- Assess the mons pubis for general hygiene, pubic hair distribution, and condition of underlying skin.
- Inspect the vulva for lesions, edema, color, or discharge.
- Inspect the clitoris, urethral orifice, and vaginal introitus.
- Palpate the Bartholin's glands for masses, tenderness, or edema.
- Using a speculum, inspect the internal genitalia:
  - Inspect the cervix; note color and texture.
  - Inspect the cervical os.
- Perform bimanual examination:
  - Palpate the vagina.
  - Palpate the cervix.
  - Palpate the uterus, including the fundus.
  - Palpate the ovaries.
- Perform rectovaginal examination.

Physical Examination of Special Populations

Considerations for the Pregnant Patient

The examination sequence for the pregnant woman is the same as for the adult but requires a more inclusive assessment of the abdomen and pelvis. Remember, it is more difficult for a pregnant woman to assume the supine position. The preferred method is the side-lying position. Use the supine position only when necessary. Have the pregnant woman empty her bladder prior to examination. Abdominal assessment may be particularly uncomfortable for a pregnant woman because of associated urinary urgency and frequency.

Considerations for the Neonatal Patient

Newborns require special considerations in regard to physical assessment. Assessment techniques may vary related to age, wakefulness, and/or illness. With neonates, it is important to look carefully before touching. Inspecting without disturbing the baby is the key. Visual assessment provides many clues in determining the diagnosis (**Box 2-2**). Assessment sequence for newborns should be head/fontanels, extremities, abdomen, and the rest of the body. Always save invasive procedures, such as otoscopic examination, for last.

Considerations for the Pediatric Patient

Remember to consider developmental stages while performing assessment. Know that children are unpredictable, so you may need to alter the sequence of the assessment to suit the moment. For example, a sleeping baby enables a good assessment of the heart, lungs, and abdomen, while a crying infant allows visualization of the oropharynx. If necessary, allow the parent to be the "examination table" for the comfort of the infant and parent. (**Figure 2-4**).

To win cooperation of children, establish comfort prior to examination. Take a few minutes to establish a relaxed environment. Give a 1-year-old an object to hold in his hands. With a toddler, use a gentle pat, pleasing words, or interactive play. Allow children to touch the equipment used during the examination. For example, allow the child to use the stethoscope to listen to his parent's heart (**Figure 2-5**).

Considerations for the Geriatric Patient

The assessment sequence for older adults is the same as for the younger adult; however, there are several special considerations when examining the elderly. The elderly may have difficulty assuming certain positions (e.g., lithotomy position, knee-chest position, or lying supine) or may have decreased sensory capabilities. Assist the geriatric patient with position changes as needed to conserve energy or ensure safety. In addition, reaction time maybe longer. Remember to maintain patience and assist in any way possible. You may have to assist the patient to the table, speak a little slower, or repeat yourself. The key with the elderly is to remain patient to ensure accuracy of the physical examination.

With the elderly population, it is necessary to obtain a functional assessment to determine the ability of the patient to perform day-to-day tasks (**Box 2-3**). The use of a functional assessment can determine:

- Ability of the elderly to deal with the daily demands of life
- How to shape your management plan
- Level of instruction you can provide
- Ability of the patient to comply with the management plan

BOX 2-2   VISUAL ASSESSMENT OF THE NEWBORN

Inspection of the newborn should include these key characteristics:
- Awareness, alertness, responsiveness, and playfulness
- Posture
- Flaccidity, tension, and spasticity
- Gross deformities
- Spontaneity in behavior
- Obvious and subtle interactions between parent(s) and child
- Feeding, sucking, and swallowing

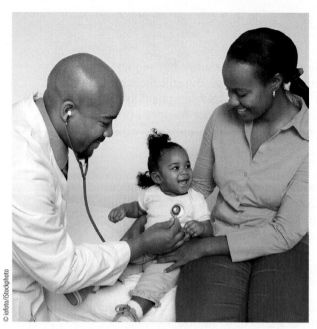

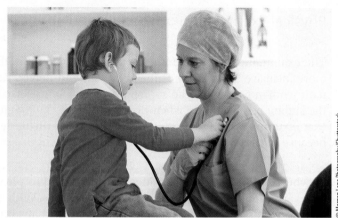

FIGURE 2-5 Allaying a child's fears by letting him use a stethoscope

FIGURE 2-4 Allowing the mother to hold the infant during examination.

BOX 2-3   FUNCTIONAL ASSESSMENT OF THE ELDERLY

Evaluate the following:

- Ability to perform basic activities of daily living (ADL), such as bathing, dressing, toileting, and feeding
- Ability to perform instrumental ADL, such as housekeeping, money management, grocery shopping, and meal preparation
- Mobility (use of cane, walker, wheelchair)
- Communication, including speech, ability to dial a phone, hearing acuity
- Safety (does the patient need assistance to get in and out of home, shower, car, etc.)
- Medication status, including regimen, acquisition, compliance, and ability to access health care
- Mental status and mood impairment

Bibliography

DeGowin, R. L., & Brown, D. D. (2014). *DeGowin's diagnostic examination* (8th ed.). New York, NY: McGraw-Hill.

Kuczmarski, M. F., Kuczmarski, R. J., & Najjar, M. (2001). Descriptive anthropometric reference data for older Americans. *Journal of the American Dietetic Association, 100,* 59–66.

Lipman, T. H., Hench, K., Logan J. D., DiFazio, D. A., Hale, P. M., & Singer-Granick, C. (2000). Assessment of growth by primary healthcare providers. *Journal of Pediatric Health Care, 14*(4), 166–171.

Purnell, L. D., & Paulanka, B. J. (2003). *Transcultural health care: A culturally competent approach* (2nd ed.). Philadelphia, PA: F. A. Davis.

Chapter 3

Documentation Strategies

Functions of Documentation

Documentation is a critical step in the health assessment process. The healthcare provider can perform an excellent examination; however, the documentation that follows determines the worth of the examination. The documentation of the patient–provider encounter not only provides the background necessary for follow-up with the patient but it also serves as a legal account of the patient–provider interaction and subsequent interactions. If the documentation just indicates that the healthcare provider found "no problems," it is unclear to the next provider what areas were truly assessed and what questions were asked. For example, if a history of the respiratory system is taken but the documentation merely states "no problems," it is unclear to the next healthcare provider, or to a person performing a legal review of the chart, if the patient has been successfully queried about tuberculosis, chronic obstructive pulmonary disease, asthma, or sleep apnea. It also fails to provide sufficient data to justify the cost of any specific tests or treatments that require third-party reimbursement. From a more practical perspective, giving a more detailed list of the items or questions reviewed with the patient also provides documentation for the provider himself, and it facilitates management of the patient in future encounters (**Figure 3-1**). Once a provider has documented specifics about the past medical history, he does not need to repeat the same questions in future encounters. Instead, the provider is able to focus on any changes in the history since the last appointment. This facilitates continuity of care and helps the patient to feel that her past history is well known and her current needs are being met.

General Considerations

As a healthcare provider begins to document the history and physical examination, it is important to keep some simple strategies in mind. If a preprinted (check-off) form is being used, it is appropriate to fill out the form while interviewing or examining the patient. Be sure to record vital signs as you take them and do not rely on your memory. Also remember the basic rule: If the examiner forgets to assess anything in the history or physical, he or she can come back to it later in the process, but the examiner must only record data that he or she has truly obtained. If the provider is using an open format, or a nonprinted form, it is helpful to take detailed notes while assessing the patient and then combine and transfer the notes into formal written format as soon as possible (**Figure 3-2**). Again, if any assessment parameters

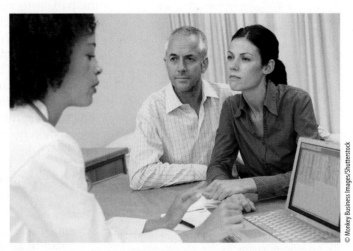

FIGURE 3-1 The healthcare provider listens to a patient's history of present illness, documenting pertinent data.

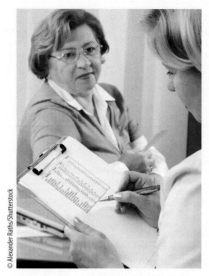

FIGURE 3-2 The healthcare provider takes brief notes during the interview.

have been omitted in either the history or the physical, it is appropriate to indicate "not assessed"; be sure not to fabricate any findings or data. Instead, make a note in the plan of care of additional areas that need to be covered during the next appointment. For example, if one forgets to assess the thyroid and the patient's chief complaint includes fatigue, then it would be appropriate to make a notation in the plan that the thyroid should be assessed and a thyroid-stimulating hormone (TSH) level drawn at the next encounter.

Although accuracy is foremost in each provider's mind when performing a history and physical examination, speed of documentation is also important. One strategy that ensures both accuracy and speed is the use of drawings. Frequently, healthcare providers use a stick figure to document pulses and deep tendon reflexes **(Figure 3-3)** and use an anatomical drawing of the body or a body part to document the size and location of skin lesions, rashes, or wounds. In many institutions both the stick figures and anatomical drawings of the body are already on the preprinted forms, whereas in other institutions, the provider must draw each item. The goal is to provide the best "picture" of the patient's condition, either in written format or with a drawing, in order to serve as a comparison for future assessments.

In the documentation process, it is important to only use standard abbreviations. Institutions will have different policies about the use of abbreviations. One institution may severely restrict the use of abbreviations, especially if it has found that the abbreviations have led to medication or treatment errors. Therefore, each provider should check with her specific institution to determine which abbreviations are acceptable. As a reference, both commonly used abbreviations and symbols can be found in many medical dictionaries. Although abbreviations facilitate the speed of recording the history and physical examination, remember that the data and information need to be recorded in such a manner that others reading the write-up can clearly understand the information presented.

Although many methods of documentation are available, such as direct computer written reports, each new method provides potentially new concerns. As of April 2003, federal guidelines, called the Health Insurance Portability and Accountability Act (HIPAA), have been implemented to restrict the sharing of patient information, either direct or indirectly. Although data can easily be recorded directly into an institution's computer database, this process places an added responsibility upon the provider that computer screens are not left unattended, where patient data can be seen or reviewed by unauthorized individuals. The new guidelines also regulate with whom a provider can share patient information. In addition, HIPAA regulations require the patient to provide consent for his medication information to be disclosed to other individuals. The challenge for the provider is to write an appropriate record of the history and physical examination, using the latest technology available without violating the patient's right to confidentiality. The use of e-mail and faxes to share patient information poses an additional problem. Most institutions advise that a disclaimer be inserted at the bottom of any patient-related communication that indicates that the following information is confidential. For example, if information needs to be shared electronically, the following disclaimer may be used:

HIPAA Notice: The information transmitted within this email or in any attached documents is intended solely for the individual or entity to which it is addressed. That information may contain confidential and/or privileged material. If you believe you have received this email in error, please immediately contact the sender and delete the material from your system.

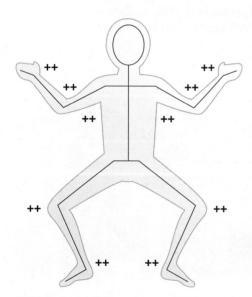

FIGURE 3-3 A stick figure can be used to document deep tendon reflexes. 0, no response; 1+, sluggish; 2+, expected response; 3+, slightly hyperactive; 4+, hyperactive.

SOAP Approach

The most common approach for documenting a history and physical is the SOAP format. The SOAP format stands for Subjective data, Objective data, Assessment, and Plan. In documenting the history and physical examination, you should remember that the **Subjective** section includes any information or facts that the patient presents or that the chart provides. Standard sections within the Subjective section include chief complaint, history of present illness, past medical history, medications, allergies, last menstrual period for women, family history, social history, nutritional assessment, and the review of systems. The **Objective** section consists of data and information obtained by the examiner with his or her eyes, ears, and hands. If obtained at the time of the examination or immediately afterwards, laboratory findings and diagnostic test results are also recorded in the Objective section. Previous test results belong in either the history of present illness or in the review of systems. **Assessment** refers to the final assessment; it pulls together the findings presented in the subjective and objective sections to form a diagnosis. The **Plan** outlines the treatment plan related to the chief complaint, current comorbidities, and/or additional problems that have become evident during the examination. (For further explanation of subjective and objective data, see Box 1-1 in Chapter 1.)

Two broad subclassifications of the SOAP format are a comprehensive health history and physical examination and a focused, or episodic, health history and physical examination. Both a comprehensive and focused history and physical use the same format, but the extent of the information obtained varies. (See Chapter 1 for a detailed description of the components of each type of history.) The reason for the patient's visit and the extent of the illness dictate which approach is used. If a patient is presenting to the healthcare provider for a specific problem, such as a sore throat, then a focused history and physical is completed. If a patient presents for an annual physical examination or is a new patient, then the provider should use a comprehensive format, which explores all the systems. Part of the role of the healthcare provider is to determine which SOAP format is to be used, what questions are pertinent to explore, and how the data can be integrated into an appropriate list of diagnoses, differential diagnoses, and problems. This organization of data presents the stepping stone for the next phase, the development of the treatment plan or plan of care.

Documentation Tips

Each component of the health history contains information that is important for making diagnosis and treatment decisions (for more information, see Chapter 1). Just as the right questions must be asked, the right data must be documented. This section provides tips for ensuring proper documentation. There are a number of different formats that can be used for documentation, including a preprinted form that requires checking off the correct box and an open format in which no preprinted information appears. Both systems have advantages and disadvantages. The preprinted formats are easy and quick to use. They help to ensure that all the desired areas are assessed, and they eliminate the struggle over wording. However, the preprinted forms frequently limit the amount of extra information that can be added, so in some cases when positive findings are obtained, it is difficult to individualize the form to accurately document the data. On the other hand, the open format is similar to a blank page, where no headings or prompts are included. With the open format, the provider can include as much information as she or he wishes; however, a provider may fail to include all the necessary data because prompts or choices were not provided. In addition, the open format is more time consuming because each provider must individually write each finding in the history and physical examination, and word selection may become an issue.

Whether you are using a "check-off" format or an open format, it is important that each system is covered completely and the data accurately reflect both what the patient stated and the provider's physical findings. Note that frequently the patient will provide additional information scattered throughout the examination process. It is important for the documentation process that the subjective information, the information the patient tells you, is properly recorded in the subjective component of the write-up, and that any physical findings that the provider finds are documented in the objective component. It is also important to accurately listen to the information the patient is providing, and then document the information in the most accurate medical terminology possible. Usually only the chief complaint is provided as a direct patient quote. For example the patient may state that she or he had a "heart attack," but the provider's documentation should indicate the patient had a myocardial infarction. Also with respect to the physical examination, it is important to realize that the examination itself is performed region by region, or area of the body by area of the body, but the data are documented according to systems. For example, when examining the neck, assess the thyroid and the carotid arteries. However, documentation of the thyroid occurs under the system heading "endocrine," and carotid artery findings are documented under "cardiac" or "cardiovascular."

Subjective Data

Patient Identifiers and Chief Complaint

The provider should first document patient identifiers, including the patient's name, date of birth, and the date and time of examination. This is followed by the "chief complaint" (CC). The chief complaint must be expressed in the patient's own words and is written in quotation marks. For example, if a patient presents to a clinic with a chief complaint of abdominal pain and expresses it as "my stomach is killing me," then the phrase "my stomach is killing me" is documented in the chief complaint. Documenting the patient's chief complaint in his or her own words serves to highlight the patient's reason for presenting to the healthcare facility.

History of Present Illness

Along with the chief complaint, the history of present illness is documented. The history of present illness (HPI) is a concise description of the patient's recent history. The opening sentence should contain key pertinent data that both the provider and any other healthcare professional should know, including age, gender, and significant comorbidities. For example, if the patient presents with a chief complaint of a "lump in her breast" and is 10 weeks' pregnant, the opening sentence of the history of present illness should state "a 26-year-old female who is 10 weeks pregnant presents with a recent history of a lump in the upper outer quadrant of her left breast." This information alerts the provider and all other healthcare workers that the patient is pregnant, a key factor that must be considered when developing the patient's treatment plan. If in fact this patient has breast cancer, then the typical treatment guidelines for breast cancer will need to be altered. The patient will not be a candidate for any treatment or medication that would be harmful to the fetus. Failure to document this information would have significant legal implications.

Once the opening sentence is developed, the clinician then documents the patient's presenting signs and symptoms. For each sign or symptom, the clinician should fully explore each topic by asking pertinent questions using the mnemonic PQRST or CLIENT OUTCOMES, as discussed in Chapter 1. These are important factors that guide this patient's plan of care and help to identify future teaching needs.

If a patient describes more than one sign or symptom, each one should be explored. For example, if the patient states that she has a severe headache as well as nausea and vomiting, each component needs to be described or explored in depth. The clinician never wants to make the assumption that the signs and symptoms are related. The headache may be a long-term problem that the patient always has, but the nausea and vomiting may be a new onset.

For situations in which the patient has an extensive recent history, such as a trauma patient admitted into the hospital, the key pertinent data are summarized in the history of present illness, so all healthcare providers who are involved in the patient's care understand what has happened to the patient, and what treatment modalities have already been implemented. In addition, all recent diagnostic tests, along with the outcome of any intervention taken during this recent hospitalization should be summarized. For example, if a patient is intubated in the emergency room, the practitioner should record whether the initial intubation effort was successful, what size tube was inserted, where the ET tube markings are in relationship to the patient's lips, and what was suctioned from the lungs. If it was a traumatic intubation, this should be documented in an effort to alert other healthcare workers that the patient may have bloody oral secretions as well as hemoptysis. It also alerts others that the patient may develop laryngeal edema upon extubation.

The history of present illness should include any pertinent recent test results and test dates. For example, if a patient presents with chest pain but indicates that he had a negative stress test 2 weeks ago, these data should be incorporated into the history of present illness, as they have a direct bearing on the patient's chief complaint. However, if the same patient presents for evaluation of hematuria, then a recent stress test result should be incorporated into the past medical history. Test results should be summarized, providing other healthcare workers, physicians, nurses, and other practitioners with an overview of results and indications. The history of present illness should not be a repetition of the formal diagnostic reports. Dates also help other healthcare workers understand previous occurrences, but it is important to summarize the information in the history of present illness and not just list the dates in a bulleted format. Thus, the history of present illness should be a concisely written paragraph (or paragraphs) that describes the patient's signs and symptoms and the course of events up until the present encounter. A guiding rule of thumb is to consider the record to cost "a dollar a word"; hence it is important to be concise, but also to be accurate and document all pertinent data. The key for the novice provider is to determine what is pertinent information and what is superficial information.

Past Medical History

Once the history of present illness is concisely documented, describe the patient's past medical history (PMI). The past medical history should include significant information about previous or current illnesses, hospitalizations, surgeries, injuries, immunizations, medications, and allergies (for a complete list, see Chapter 1). Also, document information about transfusions and any transfusion reactions, immunizations, and results of any screening examinations. When recording this information, it is important that dates, or approximate dates, are included in order to provide an accurate perspective of the patient's past history. For females, last menstrual period (LMP) should be documented. Although the history of present illness is written in paragraph form, the past medical history is typically presented as bulleted information with appropriate dates included. If a preprinted form is being used, it is important to add the appropriate dates and outcomes in addition to the finding itself. For example, if the patient has a history of hypertension (HTN), and the preprinted form has a selection for HTN, not only should HTN be checked, but it should indicate either the year it was diagnosed, or the number of years the patient has had the condition, and if the hypertension is well controlled. If the patient does not have allergies or if she or he is not taking any medications, it is important that the word "none" is listed beside the heading. This eliminates a question as to whether the clinician forgot to ask about allergies or medications.

Family History

Following the past medical history, the family history (FH) is documented. The family history should include pertinent negatives, as well as positive findings. Broad categories that are usually explored in this section include a family history of cancer, diabetes, cerebrovascular accidents, myocardial infarctions, and genetic defects. Within each of these categories it is appropriate to further explore positive findings. For example if a patient has a family history of cancer, the clinician should document the type of cancer and which family member. For cardiovascular diseases it is also appropriate to document the family member's age at the time of the event. For example, it makes a difference in terms of cardiovascular risk factors if a patient's father had a myocardial infarction at the age of 54 and died from it or whether the father had a myocardial infarction at the age of 84.

In some cases, a genogram may be included. The genogram provides a rapid way to condense the data and indicates whether immediate relatives are alive or have died, and what type of comorbidities each individual has or had. Symbols are used to represent family members when developing the genogram. An open circle refers to female relatives, an open square represents male relatives;

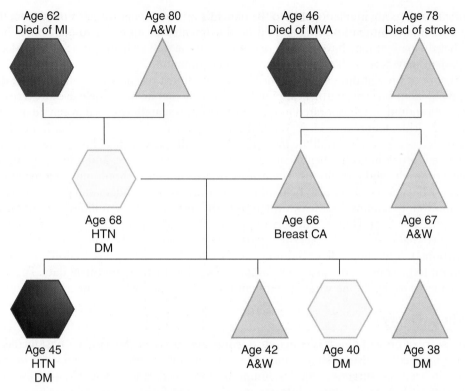

FIGURE 3-4 Genogram. This patient is a 45-year-old man who has hypertension (HTN) and diabetes mellitus (DM). He has three siblings: two sisters and a brother. One sister and his brother have DM. The patient's parents are alive. His father has HTN and DM and is 68 years old. His mother is 66 years old and has had breast cancer (CA). His aunt is age 67 and alive and well (A&W). Maternal grandparents are both dead. His grandfather died in a motor vehicle accident (MVA) at age 46, and his maternal grandmother died of a stroke at age 78. Paternal grandparents were divorced. His paternal grandfather died of a myocardial infarction (MI) at the age of 62, and his paternal grandmother is A&W.

if either the circle or square is colored in, it indicates that the individual is deceased. Lines are used to indicate both marriages and children, and a broken line indicates a divorce. In developing a genogram, it is important to indicate the patient's position within the genogram with an arrow. **Figure 3-4** depicts a genogram.

Social History

Following family history, the provider should document the patient's social history (SH), including the nutritional history. Social history should include the patient's marital status, highest level of education, and use of alcohol, tobacco, and recreational drugs (see Chapter 1 for a more inclusive list). Other items can be included such as sleep habits, exercise habits, and religious preference. In obtaining this information it is important to be concise and summarize the pertinent points in order to individualize the patient's plan of care. Hence, although a patient may exercise daily and do a number of different types of sports or exercises, a brief summary of the patient's exercise pattern is all that is needed. For example unless the patient is presenting for a sports-related injury, it is sufficient to state, "Patient exercises for 45 minutes three times per week." On the other hand, if the patient's history indicates that he has a limited income, poor housing, and no running water, these details belong in the written social history because they may have a direct impact on the patient's plan of care. Nutritional history can be documented as a summary statement, and does not need to include a 24-hour recall unless nutritional status is a pertinent problem for the patient. For example, if a patient is homeless and has an open wound that has been healing poorly, then a more complete documentation of that patient's dietary intake may be appropriate in order to document her or his need for further assistance or social services.

Review of Systems

The next broad category under the subjective findings is the review of systems (ROS). Within each system, the clinician should document the data that were sought, including pertinent negatives. The term "no significant findings" or "negative" should be avoided. Such forms of documentation fail to provide any specific information as to what was asked or not asked. Also fully describe any positive findings. For example if the patient's chief complaint is a "cold," but the review of systems reveals he or she has a history of asthma, the clinician should determine how many years the patient has had asthma, what seems to trigger the asthma, how the attacks present themselves, what makes it better, what makes it worse, and when the last attack was. Subsequent chapters discuss the specific questions related to each system that need to be explored in further detail. Chapter 1 lists the broad categories. Which systems are explored is determined by the patient's chief complaint, list of comorbidities, and whether the examination is a comprehensive history and physical or a focused history and physical. For a comprehensive examination, all the systems should be appropriately explored in the review of systems, and for the focused examination only those systems pertinent to the history of present illness and past medical history are explored.

Determining which systems are explored in the review of systems is an important clinical decision that guides the remainder of the physical examination and the documentation process. The review of systems represents the end of the subjective component of the SOAP.

Objective Data

Physical Examination

The objective component begins with the physical examination; the review of systems and physical examination should match each other (i.e., if all systems are evaluated in the review of systems, then all systems should be evaluated in the physical examination). If a focused examination is being done, and if only the general, respiratory, and cardiac systems are explored in the review of systems, then the physical examination should focus on these same three components. Conversely, if the physical examination included general, respiratory, cardiovascular, and gastrointestinal, then these same four systems should have been explored in the review of systems. Concise accurate documentation of all findings is imperative in the physical examination. Correct terminology, accurate descriptions, appropriate legends, and completeness are vital components within the physical examination. Legally, the standard rule is: If it is not documented, it either was not assessed or not done. Hence, omissions can be critical. If the clinician fails to document that all lobes of the lung are clear to auscultation, then one cannot assume that all lobes were assessed. Also, if in the documentation of the cardiac assessment, the provider does not comment about rate, rhythm, or pulse deficit, then one cannot derive that these aspects were evaluated or assessed.

Diagnostic Tests

The last component of the objective section is diagnostic tests (laboratory findings). In some institutions, the laboratory findings are integrated into the appropriate system. For example arterial blood gases and the most current chest x-ray may be documented in the respiratory section. In other institutions, laboratory findings, such as a basic or complete metabolic panel, are listed separately. Again abbreviations and symbols may be used, if approved by the institution or facility.

Assessment

Once the subjective and objective data are completed, the clinician then organizes the findings into an appropriate section called assessment, or final assessment findings. The final assessment findings

BOX 3-1   SAMPLE PROBLEM LIST FOR A PATIENT IN HEART FAILURE

Atrial fibrillation
Hypokalemia
Potential hyperkalemia (secondary to the use of a potassium-sparing diuretic)
Fluid overload
Shortness of breath
Skin breakdown
Anxiety (secondary to shortness of breath)
Potential for deep venous thrombosis (secondary to inactivity)
Potential for respiratory failure
Potential for cardiogenic shock

can be divided into three categories: (1) all new diagnoses, as well as any preexisting diagnoses; (2) differential diagnoses, or those diagnoses that require further testing in order to confirm them; and (3) a problem list. When this approach is used, the final assessment findings include any additional findings that may or may not be directly related to the history of present illness. For example, if the patient has a history of smoking, cigarette abuse should be listed. If the patient is a type 2 diabetic, then type 2 diabetes should be listed, in addition to any diagnoses related to the patient's chief complaint. Many times, however, the diagnosis is not firmly established; in this case possible diagnoses are listed as "differential diagnoses." Some individuals may label these as "rule outs." For example, consider a 54-year-old man who presents with a 2-hour history of chest pain that is epigastric in nature, does not radiate, and is relieved by antacids. These symptoms may lead the novice practitioner to think about gastro-esophageal reflux disease (GERD), but another more significant differential is acute coronary syndrome, which needs to be "ruled out" before the diagnosis of GERD can be focused upon.

A third component of the assessment section is called the problem list. Not all patients will have a problem list, but for many hospitalized patients, the problem list includes other issues that are not true diagnoses, but issues that need to be addressed as the result of either the diagnosis or the plan of care. For example, if a patient is hospitalized for heart failure and her basic metabolic panel indicates that she is hypokalemic, then the diagnosis is "heart failure," and hypokalemia would appear in the problem list. Typically, items in the problem list are conditions that can be treated and, it is hoped, resolved. For example, with heart failure, the heart failure will be treated, but not cured. However, with appropriate potassium replacement, the hypokalemia can be eliminated as a problem. It may need to be continually reassessed; hence developing a problem list helps to guide further treatment and care. It documents in a readily retrievable format other issues that need to be potentially re-evaluated. **Box 3-1** provides a sample problem list.

Plan

The last component of the findings is the plan. There are five components of the plan. These are non-pharmacological interventions, pharmacological interventions, educational needs for both the patient and his family, follow-up, and referrals. Which components are included in the plan are determined by both the data obtained in the subjective and objective components of the write-up as well as the diagnosis and differentials. Not every patient will have a non-pharmacological section to the treatment plan. This component is frequently reserved for hospitalized patients, and it represents the "orders" for the staff nurses to follow. Also depending upon the patient's diagnosis, medications may not be ordered. Under "education," it is critical to document any instructions that have been given to the patient and/or family. This includes any instructions in terms of when to seek additional medical attention. One common legal problem that frequently surfaces is the patient or family's comment "we were not told." In order to avoid these situations, the clinician should document (1) what was taught or explained, (2) to whom it was told, (3) if the patient or family stated that he/she or they understood the information presented, (4) and what was the format. For example, were they given written instructions as well as verbal instructions?

Summary

Documentation of the patient's health history and physical examination is vital in order to guide the care and treatment of the patient, to provide ongoing feedback to other healthcare providers, and to provide a sound basis for legal review. The provider must complete documentation that is accurate, concise, and confidential. It is an important aspect of assessment that should not be overlooked. **Figure 3-5** demonstrates documentation of a sample case. This format is used to demonstrate cases throughout the rest of the text.

Name JS		Date 1/19/13	Time 0845
		DOB 1/16/48	Sex M

HISTORY
CC "I have chest pain."
HPI 57-year-old Caucasian male in acute distress presents with a 2-hour history of chest pain. Mr. S woke up and felt a new "heaviness" in his chest. He took two Tums, which did not relieve the pain. Pain has gotten worse and is radiating down his left arm. He rates the pain an 8 (out of 10). He states he feels nauseated and slightly short of breath.
Medications Vasodec: 10 mg qd for HTN. Last dose 1/18/13. ASA: 81 mg qd for "blood thinner." Last dose 1/18/13.
Allergies NKA
PMI Illnesses No history of angina or MI. History of hypertension for 5 years. History of GERD, self-treats with Tums.
Hospitalizations/Surgeries No history of hospitalizations or surgeries.
FH Father died of MI at age 52. No history of cancer or diabetes mellitus.
SH Mr. S is married (for 25 years) and has two grown children living in the area. Mr. S is self-employed as a consultant and has insurance. He exercises 1–2 times per month. Mr. S tried to follow a low-fat diet. He smokes 2 packs per day (for 25 years).

ROS	
General No history of recent weight change or dietary changes.	Cardiovascular History of HTN. Chest pain, radiating to left arm (see HPI).
Skin Denies history of scars, eczema, psoriasis, or cancer.	Respiratory Smokes 2 ppd (≈ 25 years); slight SOB.
Eyes Nearsighted and wears glasses. No history of glaucoma.	Gastrointestinal Nausea started with chest pain. History of GERD, well controlled with PPI.
Ears Denies hearing problems.	Genitourinary/Gynecological Difficulty starting stream for past year. Has noctura » 2 nightly. 6 months ago, diagnosed with benign prostate hypertrophy.
Nose/Mouth/Throat Denies oral problems; wears dentures, upper and lower.	Musculoskeletal Denies history of fractures, arthritis, or trauma.

FIGURE 3-5 Sample documentation.

(continues)

Breast	Neurological
Denies problems.	Denies history of seizures, strokes, or syncope. No history of Parkinson's, tremors, paralysis, headaches, falls, or vertigo. Denies depression, memory impairment, dementia, or speech impairment.

PHYSICAL EXAMINATION

Weight 195 lb	Temp 98.0	BP 92/78
Height 6'	Pulse 118	Resp 24 and labored

Skin
Cool and pale; turgor, brisk recoil.

HEENT
Eyes: No erythema of the sclera; pink conjunctiva, no discharge; EOMs intact w/o lid lag or nystagmus; fundoscopic exam revealed no AV nicking or cotton wool patches. Ears: Tympanic membrane pearly gray with no discharge. Mouth: Buccal mucosa pink, without lesions.

Cardiovascular
S1 and S2 heard with no splitting or murmurs. S3 audible predominantly at apex. PMI 5th ICS midclavicular line. No JVD noted. Carotids equal bilaterally with no bruits. No bruits over aorta, renal, iliac, or femoral arteries. Capillary refill brisk. Pretibial edema +1 bilaterally.

Respiratory
Respirations labored. Clear to auscultation in all lobes.

Gastrointestinal
Bowel sounds active in all quadrants. Abdomen soft and without tenderness. No hepatomegaly or splenomegaly noted.

Genitourinary
Not examined.

Musculoskeletal
Muscle strength 5/5 in upper and lower extremities bilaterally. Full ROM in all joints. No atrophy noted. No crepitus over joints noted. Gait deferred.

Neurological
Awake, alert, and orient $\approx$ 3. Moderately anxious. PERRLA. Speech clear. CN II–XII intact. All DTRs bilaterally 2+.

Other

Lab Tests
Tropin I, CK-MB, basic metabolic panel, PT, PTT drawn but not back from lab.

Special Tests
12 lead ECG indicates ST segment elevation in leads II, III, and AVF. No Q wave present; good progression of R wave leads V_1–V_3. Chest x-ray clear.

Final Assessment Findings
1. Acute coronary syndrome
2. HTN
3. Cigarette abuse

FIGURE 3-5 Sample documentation (*continued*).

Bibliography

DeGowin, R. & Brown, D. (2014). *DeGowin's diagnostic examination*. New York, NY: McGraw-Hill.
Venes, D. & Thomas, C. (2013). *Taber's cyclopedic medical dictionary* (19th ed.). Philadelphia, PA: F. A. Davis.

Additional Resource

HIPAA Regulations

http://www.hhs.gov/ocr/privacy/hipaa/understanding/
This website gives national standards about maintaining patient privacy.

Part 2

Advanced Assessment of Systemic Disorders

Chapter 4

Mental Health Disorders

All clinicians will assess, diagnose, and treat psychiatric conditions, either as a primary or a concurrent diagnosis. Furthermore, psychiatric problems such as anxiety disorders, depression, and substance abuse may be "masked" or hidden by a presenting complaint of pain, insomnia, or gastrointestinal symptoms. It is essential, therefore, that practitioners develop the skills and insight to detect and identify both covert and overt psychiatric disorders.

Anatomy and Physiology Review of the Brain

Mental health assessment involves an assessment of the organic functioning of the brain. The human brain consists of the cerebrum, cerebellum, and brain stem (see **Figure 4-1**). Mental health assessment focuses primarily on assessment of cerebral function. The cerebrum is divided in two hemispheres, which are further subdivided into lobes (see Chapter 16). The outer layer of cerebrum is called the cerebral cortex. The cerebral cortex houses higher mental functions and is responsible for general movement, visceral functions, perception, behavior, and integration of these functions. Commissural fibers interconnect the counterpart areas in each cerebral hemisphere, unifying and coordinating higher sensory and motor function.

Lobes of the Brain

The lobes of the cerebrum are responsible for perceptual and motor functioning. The frontal lobe contains the motor cortex, associated with voluntary skeletal movement and speech formation (Broca's area). The areas related to emotions, affect, drive, and awareness of self also originate here.

The parietal lobe is primarily responsible for processing sensory data (visual, tactile, gustatory, olfactory, and auditory). It also governs the functions of comprehension of written language and proprioception (awareness of body parts and position).

The temporal lobe is responsible for perception and interpretation of sounds and determination of their source. It also houses the Wernicke speech area, which controls the comprehension of written and spoken language. In addition, the temporal lobe is involved in integrating sensations such as smell, taste, and balance; the integration of behavior, emotion, and personality occurs here as well.

The occipital lobe is primarily responsible for processing vision and provides interpretation of visual input.

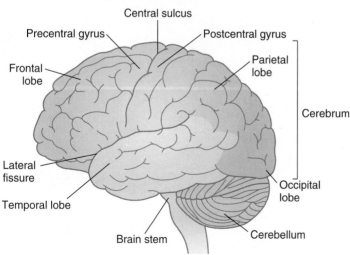

FIGURE 4-1 The brain.

Limbic System

The limbic system, or "emotional brain," mediates certain patterns of behavior that determine survival, such as fear, aggression, and mating. Short-term memory and the ability to retain and recall information are also governed by the limbic system. The affective response is modulated by connections between the limbic system and frontal lobe. Important limbic structures include the hippocampus (memory), amygdala (confusion, fear, anger), cingulate gyrus (attentive behavior and sexual activity), septal area, medial forebrain bundle (pleasure), and hypothalamus, which contains connections to the autonomic nervous system, limbic system, and endocrine system. An emotion (feeling and affect) depends upon the functioning and coordination among the limbic system, cortex, and hypothalamus.

The cranial nerves are peripheral nerves that arise from the brain and are responsible for sensory and motor functions of the head and upper body. A person's ability to perceive and interpret sensation (sound, taste, vision) is an important component of mental health. Evaluation of the functioning of the cranial nerves is an integral component of a neurological examination, but a brief assessment should be incorporated into the mental status examination. The cranial nerves are responsible for the five senses and are expected to be intact in a well-person examination. Deviation from normative functioning can be indicative of trauma or lesion in the cerebral hemisphere or local injury to the nerve.

A brief cursory examination of the cranial nerves will include observation of the person's facial muscle tone and strength. Drooping of the mouth or eyes, changes in facial tone or muscle strength, or loss of any of the senses indicates a deviation from normal and warrants a more comprehensive neurological examination (see Chapter 16).

Health History

Certain basic principles guide the clinician in obtaining the most accurate mental status assessment. A quiet, private, and unhurried environment will reduce barriers and facilitate conversation about more personal psychosocial issues. Appropriate eye contact, attentive body language (**Figure 4-2**), a pleasant and natural vocal quality, impeccable listening skills, and continual evaluation of whether verbal reports match or reveal discrepancies are essential. Using an unhurried pace, exhibiting well-developed listening skills, and attempting to clarify for the patient what he has stated communicate caring, empathy, and compassion.

The environment, setting, and the mind frame of both patient and clinician must be factored into assessment of mental status. Warmth, genuineness, confidence, appropriate use of humor, and an empathic link felt by patient from the clinician can enhance the assessment. On the other hand, barriers include interrupting, belittling, moralizing, failing to provide privacy, and lacking consideration. Environmental temperature, fear, anxiety, hunger, pain, or a rushed schedule can also negatively affect the mental status data. For example, performing the assessment at the time of admission, discharge, or following negative news may cause mental status examination results that do not typically represent the patient. Interview technique and communication is especially important when assessing mental health. See Chapter 1 for a review of strategies for effective interviewing and communication.

In addition, it is important for the practitioner to reassure the patient who presents psychosocial (psychiatric mental health) information that she considers symptoms to be understandable and within a normal range. For example, the clinician may say, *"Some people have experienced sexual side effects from this medicine, but never mentioned it. Please let me know if this medicine causes such a problem so we can explore other medication options and ways to cope."* An additional strategy is to make transitional statements connecting information from the medical part of the interview to a current psychosocial topic. For example, if the

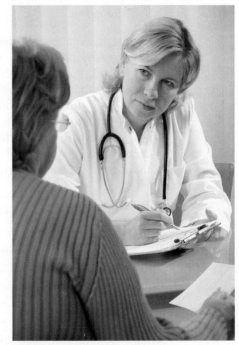

FIGURE 4-2 The healthcare provider displays attentive and empathetic body language.

patient speaks of how difficult it is to "go on" and cope with certain types of illness, the practitioner can follow up with questions about levels of depression and thoughts of suicide. If a patient speaks of "needing alcohol to get to sleep," follow-up questions about amount and history of alcohol use can follow. Even if the patient denies presence of mental health issues, "seeds have been planted" regarding the clinician's interest and willingness to listen and intervene in such issues. The patient may feel relieved that the practitioner is interested in a holistic approach regarding both medical and mental health issues.

The Diagnostic and Statistical Manual of Mental Disorders, Fifth Edition (*DSM-5*; 2015) is the authoritative book that provides a common and definitive language for mental health practitioners to evaluate, treat, and monitor psychiatric problems. It includes guidelines for assessing selected mental health conditions, some questions to use if abnormal mental status is suspected, and specific criteria used for further evaluation.

Chief Complaint and History of Present Illness

"I'm overtired and can't sleep or eat."

> JD is a 31-year-old female biology graduate student. She reports, "I'm overtired and can't sleep or eat." Ms. D has lost 15 pounds over the past month and wakes up unusually early each morning. She no longer is interested in her hobby of tennis because she feels tired most of the time. Ms. D is a "good" student, but she has not been attending classes on a regular basis for the past month and feels guilty about this. She denies suicidal ideas, because it is against her religion, but feels depressed for most of each day and says that nothing is fun.
>
> This feeling has been present for 5 to 6 weeks. She states, "I would like to feel better enough to resume playing tennis and attending classes. I just have to get myself going. Maybe a vitamin would help." She provides little detail to questions and talks in mumbled tones. She denies hearing voices and blames no one but herself for this condition.

Common chief complaints (CCs) related to mental health disorders include such symptoms as sleep disturbances, mood/emotional alterations, weight loss or gain, cognitive difficulties, personality changes, and delusions or hallucinations. Sleep disturbances and personality changes are discussed in detail below.

Fatigue, Insomnia, and Other Sleep Disturbances

Sleep patterns provide clues to interpret mental status, and they often signal that mental health problems are present. Problems with falling asleep, staying asleep, and waking up frequently or early in the sleep cycle should be identified. Frequently, the depressed person may wake up early feeling depressed whereas the anxious person may have difficulty falling asleep. When persons with schizophrenia or mania have problems with sleep, this may indicate that their illness is worsening. The person with post-traumatic stress disorder may not experience deep levels of sleep and thus feel chronically fatigued. Lack of sleep may affect all components of the mental status examination; thus, it is important to ask about quantity, patterns, and quality of sleep when discussing the history of present illness (HPI).

Onset	Was the onset sudden or gradual?
Quality	Do you have trouble falling asleep? Do you have trouble staying asleep? Are you always tired? Are you tired even when you get a full night's sleep?
	Knowing the nature of the insomnia or fatigue helps narrow diagnosis. Depression may present with trouble falling asleep and always feeling fatigued.
	Patients with generalized anxiety disorder may be easily fatigued and may have difficulty falling asleep or staying asleep. Patients with bipolar disorder may feel as if they do not need to sleep.

Duration	How long have you been experiencing this symptom?
	Dysthymia is a depressive disorder lasting 2 years or longer.
Associated symptoms	Ask about associated symptoms, including difficulty concentrating, loss of pleasure or interest in hobbies, loss of appetite, guilt, suicidal ideation, excessive worrying or uncontrolled anxiety, elevated mood, or hyperactivity.
	*Patients with depression may present with difficulty concentrating, disinterest in hobbies, guilt, suicidal ideation, and anorexia (**Box 4-1**). Suicidal ideation should be assessed (**Box 4-2**). Generalized anxiety disorder may present with difficulty concentrating and excessive worrying (see **Box 4-3** for other defining characteristics).*
	*Patients with bipolar disorder often experience elevated mood, grandiose ideas, and hyperactivity (see **Box 4-4** for more information on bipolar disorder).*
Medications	Are you taking any medication?
	Some medications may cause sleep disturbances.

BOX 4-1   DIAGNOSING DEPRESSION

The neurovegetative signs of depression, which correlate with the *DSM-IV-TR* diagnostic criteria, can be assessed by the mnemonic "SIGECAPS" scheme devised by Dr. Carey Gross at Massachusetts General Hospital. Four symptoms plus either depressed mood or anhedonia (absence of pleasure) for at least 2 weeks must be present to diagnose major depression. Dysthymia is a depression lasting 2 years or longer, which can be assessed by simply questioning the patient as to how long it has been since he has *not* felt depressed. People with dysthymia have two SIGECAPS symptoms plus depressed mood for 2 years. The SIGECAPS acronym represents:

Sleep: *"How well do you sleep?"*
Interest: *"How is your interest in hobbies?"*
Guilt: *"Do you feel very guilty about anything?"*
Energy: *"Do you feel like you have enough energy to do things you like and need?"*
Concentration: *"You said you were a student, so how is your concentration to study?"*
Appetite: *"How is your appetite and weight—have you had any big changes?"*
Psychomotor activity: *"I noticed you were pacing and wringing your hands out in the waiting room. How are you feeling?"*
Suicide: *"Have you had any thoughts about harming or killing yourself?"*

BOX 4-2   ASSESSING SUICIDE RISK

To assess for suicide risk, the clinician asks depressed patients if they ever feel they would be better off dead. Patients will usually answer, "no," but if they say, "yes," then questions should follow regarding their ideation, intent (seriousness), plan, and whether they possess the means to attempt suicide. Risk factors in addition to seriousness and having a means to commit suicide include:

- History of suicide attempts and depression
- Family history of suicide
- Acute overuse of alcohol or other central nervous system depressants
- Severe hopelessness and/or helplessness (Ask, "What do you see as a cause for hope?")
- Attraction to death
- Losses or separation
- Serious medical condition (perceived or real)
- Age, such as teens and males age 80 and older
- Giving away special possessions

Despite myths to the contrary, persons feel relieved by the clinician asking about suicide.

BOX 4-3   COMMON SIGNS OF GENERALIZED ANXIETY DISORDERS

- Excessive anxiety and worry about a number of topics on most days for at least 6 months
- Difficulty controlling worry
- Anxiety and worry associated with three or more of following on most days for at least 6 months:
  - Restless, feeling tense and "keyed up"
  - Being easily fatigued
  - Difficulty concentrating or mind going blank
  - Irritability
  - Muscle tension
  - Sleep disturbance: difficulty falling asleep, staying asleep, restless sleep

---

BOX 4-4   DIAGNOSING BIPOLAR DISORDER

Bipolar disorder affects 1% to 2% of the population, and it is often overlooked, especially when the patient presents in the depressed mood phase. A prescription for an antidepressant drug alone without a mood stabilizer drug in such a person can precipitate a manic episode. A key screening question is to ask whether the patient experiences times of feeling so happy or full of energy that friends of the patient report that the patient talks too fast or displays hyperactivity. A positive response to this query can be followed with assessment by the mnemonic "DIGFAST" scheme, which represents the *DSM-IV-TR* signs of mania. A manic episode includes at least 1 week of irritable or elevated mood plus three of the following seven "DIGFAST" symptoms for at least 1 week:

Distractibility: inability to concentrate on specific tasks and work projects

Indiscretion: overinvolvement in pleasurable activities: *"How would you describe your money spending these days?"*

Grandiosity: unfounded self-claims of superiority and authority

Flight of ideas: *"It appears your thoughts come faster than you can get them out."*

Activity increase: continually and simultaneously adding new projects and interests

Sleep deficit: *"It sounds as if you feel you do not need to sleep."*

Talkativeness: nonstop speech that is fast and abnormally animated and loud

---

Personality Change

Family or significant others accompanying a patient may report a personality or behavioral change. A careful history of the nature of the change, onset, and associated symptoms helps determine the underlying cause.

Onset	Was the onset sudden or gradual?
	Delirium has an acute onset, whereas dementia has a slow, gradual onset.
Quality	Describe the change in personality.
	Patients with dementia may exhibit extreme personality changes. For example, the meticulous dresser will care little about her attire and often dress in wrinkled and mismatched outfits. Patients with dementia may present with emotional outbursts. With delirium, emotions may fluctuate, ranging from severe anxiety, depression, and euphoria to apathy.
	Patients with schizophrenia may exhibit flat or inappropriate emotion and paranoia.
	Patients with bipolar disorder may exhibit elevated mood and delusions of grandeur.
Associated symptoms	Ask about associated symptoms including cognitive difficulty, such as disorganized thoughts or speech and impaired memory; change in the level of consciousness; insomnia or sleep deficit; hyperactivity; delusions; hallucinations; or paranoia.

Symptoms of delirium include distractibility; difficulty focusing and attending to tasks; speech that is rambling, irrelevant, pressured, and incoherent; and thought process that is disorganized as it shifts from topic to topic.

Dementia often presents with cognitive difficulties, including impaired short-term and long-term memory, aphasia, agnosia, and sleep disturbances.

Schizophrenia often presents with hallucinations, delusions, and disturbed thought processes.

Patients with bipolar disorder may have difficulty concentrating, sleep deficits, flight of ideas, and hyperactivity.

Precipitating factors	Ask about recent illnesses or trauma. What medication is the patient taking? *Delirium is usually associated with some type of neurological insult such as a medication reaction, abuse of illicit substances, or an injury to the brain.* *Dementia can be either a primary disorder or secondary problem that results from an illness, such as HIV, or from cerebral trauma.*

Past Medical History

> JD denies having a history of eating disorders, sexual or physical abuse, or depression. Ms. D denies recent trauma, illness, hospitalization, or surgery. She takes only aspirin for the occasional headache or muscle ache.

Past health conditions or surgeries	Ask about past or ongoing health conditions. *Some conditions, such as HIV or AIDS, may contribute to mental health disorders.* Question about a history of mental health disorders, such as depression, generalized anxiety disorder, schizophrenia, bipolar disorder, dissociative disorder, anorexia, and bulimia. Ask about past surgeries.
Trauma	Ask about past trauma, such as head trauma, CNS insult, birth trauma, spinal cord injury, and peripheral nerve damage. If the patient has a history of trauma, how and when did it happen? Was she or he treated? If so, how? *Head trauma may result in neurological damage.*
Abuse	Ask about a history of sexual, emotional, or physical abuse (**Box 4-5**). *Abuse has been linked to many mental health disorders.*
Medications	Does the patient take any medications? *Variables affecting mental status include medications such as anticholinergics, corticosteroids, heart and blood pressure drugs (propranolol), central nervous system depressants (benzodiazepines, alcohol), illicit drugs, herbals, over-the-counter medications, nicotine and/or caffeine, and unknown home remedies.*

Family History

Many mental health disorders are related to genetics; the healthcare provider should ask the patient about a family history (FH) of mental health disorders. Patients with a mental health disorder often have family members who have experienced the same or similar disorders.

> Ms. D's mother died of cancer about 6 months ago, but she believes she is over the death because of her return to school following the death. Her father has no known medical or psychiatric problems. She is the oldest of three sisters; both her sisters are alive and well. Her paternal grandmother was treated for "change of life depression," and her maternal grandfather was a secret ("behind the barn") drinker.

BOX 4-5   ASSESSING FOR VIOLENCE

The healthcare provider should assess patients for signs of abuse and neglect perpetrated by one person in a relationship attempting to control or hurt the other. Such patterns are found across socioeconomic, ethnic, gender, and age groups and consist of domestic violence, sexual abuse, or coercion against elderly adults, teens, children, or intimate partners. Abuse also includes neglect, consisting of physical deprivation of care or emotional failure to provide verbal and behavioral expressions of love. Caring, empathetic questions by practitioners may open the door for later disclosure by the patient. Sensitivity to the patient's answers to questions about abuse is essential, and talking face to face is more effective than written patient questionnaires. The clear message must be communicated that the patient is not alone, is not to blame, does not deserve violent treatment, and that help is available. Following are some potential questions (modified from Campbell and Humphreys, 1993) to identify and evaluate domestic abuse:

- Since our last visit, during the past year, or during your pregnancy: Have you been hit, slapped, kicked, or otherwise physically hurt by someone? If yes, by whom? The number of times? The description?
- Have you ever been emotionally or physically abused by someone close to you?
- Within the past year has anyone made you do something sexual that you did not want to do? (If yes, who?)
- Are you afraid of your partner or anyone else?

In addition to physical signs of abuse, the advanced practice clinician should be sensitive to emotional or verbal clues to abuse, such as the following:

- Wearing out-of-season clothing
- Family who will not allow patient to speak with practitioner alone
- Victim sits in a position that suggests fear or discomfort
- Sleep disturbances
- Attempt to avoid a particular person
- Fear of being alone or going home
- Recent weight change
- Passive or overly pleasing behaviors
- Post-traumatic stress behaviors, such as hyperarousal (startle reflex), nightmares, and numbness to emotions
- Other signs of anxiety or depression, drug abuse, or eating disorders from the *DSM-IV-TR*

The following elements of the SAFE acronym (Ashur, 1999) will also guide the assessment of domestic abuse and risk of danger.

S: Stress in relationship, is it **s**afe with your partner?

A: What happens when your partner is **a**ngry? Are you **a**fraid at times? Have you been **a**bused?

F: What **f**inancial resources do you need? Is a **f**irearm present at home? What do **f**riends and **f**amily know of your situation?

E: Emergency situation now? What **e**mergency plan for escape do you have if necessary?

Domestic abuse is one of the most common causes of complications during pregnancy. One in four pregnant women is physically abused, and the rate is higher when the female is a teenager. Be sensitive and alert to this domestic abuse, and ask questions regardless of the setting or the reason for the healthcare visit.

Age of living relatives	Include relationship and health of parents, siblings, and children.
Deaths	Ask about relationship of deceased to patient and cause of death; specifically explore disorders that may have mental health implications.
Chronic diseases; neurological or mental health disorders	Ask about chronic diseases and mental health disorders. Is there a history of mental health disorders in the family? If so, what is the relationship of the family member with the mental health disorder? What disorder did he have?
	Specifically, explore the patient's family history of depression, dementia, panic disorder, obsessive–compulsive disorder, and schizophrenia, as these tend to run in families.

Social History

Ms. D is a graduate student. She is single and lives alone. She states that lately she has had trouble "making it to class" and keeping up with her studying. Ms. D used to enjoy playing tennis, but no longer has the energy to do so. She denies nicotine use, drinking more alcohol than two glasses of wine per weekend, and illicit drug use. She had enjoyed friendships with other graduate students in class, but has been keeping to herself lately. Ms. D used to attend church regularly, but has been missing Mass frequently.

In addition to the below categories, culture, religion and spirituality, and sexuality are also assessed as part of the social history (SH), during the mental health assessment, because these areas affect or are affected by mental status. Asking the patient about these topics after initial data are collected may facilitate relationship building and make the patient feel secure to discuss them. Also, clues such as inability to perform activities of daily living (ADL) provide insight into the severity of the patient's diagnosis.

Family	Ask to describe current family unit.
Occupation	What does the patient do for a living? Has the patient had any recent trouble functioning at work?
	A change in ability to focus and complete work may indicate impaired cognitive status or altered level of consciousness.
	Ask about physical and emotional stress.
Hobbies	Ask about use of leisure time. Does the patient no longer want to do activities that once were enjoyable?
	Depression often causes the patient to no longer enjoy hobbies.
	Patients with anorexia may exercise excessively.
Activities of daily living (ADL)	Ask about diminished ability to carry on ADL, such as proper hygiene and eating.
	Dementia may interfere with ADL; patient's hygiene, nutrition, and safety often suffer. Patients with depression may exhibit poor hygiene.
	For patients with schizophrenia, delusions, hallucinations, and paranoia may affect their ability to carry on ADL.
Use of tobacco	Ask about tobacco use including types, amounts, duration of use, amount, and exposure to secondary smoke.
Use of alcohol	Does the patient drink alcohol? If so, what type and how much does she or he drink? Refer to the CAGE questionnaire (see Appendix A).
	Alcohol abuse is often linked to mental health disorders, such as depression.
Use of recreational drugs	Is the patient using recreational drugs? If so, which drugs and how much?
	Certain mental health disorders can be linked to drug use.
Sexual practices	Ask the patient about his sexual history.

Review of Systems

Many mental health disorders have manifestations in various body systems. A comprehensive review of systems (ROS; see Chapter 1) should be performed whenever possible; however, due to time and other types of constraints, the provider may be able to perform only a focused review of systems. During a focused review of systems, the provider focuses questioning on the systems in which mental health problems are most likely to have manifestations. Below is a summary of common manifestations of mental health problems.

System	Symptom or Sign	Possible Associated Diseases/Disorders
General	Sleep disturbances	Depression, generalized anxiety disorder, bipolar disorder
	Weight loss	Anorexia nervosa, bulimia, depression, dementia, drug abuse
	Weight gain	Depression, schizophrenia
	Dizziness	Panic disorder
Skin	Cracked, dry skin; fine, downy hair on extremities, trunk, and face	Anorexia nervosa
	Abrasions on the hands (from inducing vomiting)	Bulimia
	Dry, cracked hands (from repeated handwashing)	Obsessive–compulsive disorder
Eye	Visual disturbances/difficulty	Dementia
Mouth	Tooth erosion	Bulimia
Respiratory	Hyperventilation	Generalized anxiety disorder, panic disorder
Cardiovascular	Tachycardia, palpitations	Generalized anxiety disorder, panic disorder
	Bradycardia	Anorexia nervosa
Gastrointestinal	Vomiting (self-induced)	Bulimia
	Loss of appetite	Depression, dementia
	Nausea	Generalized anxiety disorder
Genitourinary	Loss of sexual interest	Depression, anorexia nervosa
	Amenorrhea	Anorexia nervosa
Musculoskeletal	Growth arrest	Anorexia nervosa
	Muscle tension	Generalized anxiety disorder
	Weakness	Bulimia
Neurological	Speech difficulties, impaired memory, seizures	Dementia
	Disorganized speech	Schizophrenia
	Decreased level of consciousness	Delirium

Mental Status Examination

Equipment Needed

- Paper and a pencil
- Common objects, such as watch, paper clip, and coin

Comprehensive Mental Status Examination

The mental status examination (MSE) includes assessment of appearance and behavior, cognitive abilities, emotional response, and speech and language. The assessment results may be obtained through direct questions and observations, and less obviously during other parts of obtaining the patient's history information. The mental status review includes several parts that reflect the ability of the person to interact with the environment. These components have also been called ego functions. The clinician should provide clear examples with any terms used to describe the patient to avoid the patient feeling "labeled" and "stereotyped," and to ensure that accurate and truthful responses are obtained.

The assessment of cognitive function is an integral part of the MSE. Impairment in cognitive processes can be indicative of neurological disorders, organicity, developmental delays, or signs of mental illness. A large portion of the assessment of the patient's cognitive abilities can be accomplished through the history-taking interview.

Action	Rationale
1. Assess appearance and behavior. The information collected should be documented so clearly that someone who has not met the patient could easily identify him or her in a crowded room.	

Action	Rationale
a. Observe the patient for hygiene and clothing.	**a.** The patient should display good hygiene and appropriate clothing. Patients with depression, dementia, and schizophrenia may display poor or lapsed hygiene. Patients with bipolar disorder may present with bizarre or inappropriate dress. Patients with dementia may also present with inappropriate dress.
b. Note body size and stature of the patient.	**b.** Patients with anorexia are often underweight. Anorexia may also cause growth arrest. Patients with bulimia may be slightly overweight, average weight, or slightly underweight. Dementia and depression may also cause weight loss.
c. Inspect hair and skin tone.	**c.** Skin tone should be even and consistent with ethnicity. Anxiety or panic disorder may present with flushing. Patients with anorexia may have a fine, downy hair on their extremities, trunk, and face.
d. Note the patient's overall cooperativeness, hostility, or withdrawal behaviors.	**d.** These all provide clues to mental health. Depression may cause a patient to be withdrawn. Schizophrenia, delirium, and dementia may cause a patient to be uncooperative or hostile.
2. Evaluate sensorium (level of consciousness), which determines the patient's ability to participate in the interview.	**2.** Levels of consciousness can be thought of in terms of orientation and responsiveness. Responsiveness reflects the activity of the subcortical reticular activation system, involving awareness of internal and external stimuli. Levels of consciousness can vary from alert (the normal finding) to coma (see **Table 4-1**).
3. Assess mood and affect.	**3.** These subjective parameters are frequently considered at the same time, but they differ in some respects. Mood is *what* feeling is conveyed, and affect is *how* the mood is conveyed.

TABLE 4-1	Levels of Consciousness
Level	**Description**
Alert	Awake and spontaneous
Confused	Decreased attention span and memory; answers questions inappropriately
Lethargy	Drowsy; falls asleep easily; when aroused, answers appropriately
Delirium	Confused with disordered perceptions, decreased attention span, inappropriate reactions to stimuli
Stupor	Slow responses; can be aroused for short periods of time to visual, verbal, or painful stimuli
Coma	Not awake or alert, decerebrate posturing to painful stimuli

Action	Rationale
a. Ask about the patient's spirits to help define the mood of the patient. It may also help to ask the patient's significant others about the prevailing mood.	**a.** Mood consists of a sustained feeling expressed by the patient, which includes impressions such as sad, euphoric, depressed, and angry. For example, a patient with bipolar disorder may feel euphoric during mania.
b. Note affect, the observable prevailing emotional tone or expression of mood in voice, facial expression, and demeanor.	**b.** Affect may be described with terms such as flat, inappropriate (laughing about a sad event), and labile (rapid shift from one extreme to another, like euphoric to irritable). Patients with depression may display a flat affect. Schizophrenia may present with inappropriate affect. Dementia may present with labile affect.
4. Evaluate speech patterns. Assess the quantity, content, and speed. Note unusual words or characteristic patterns the person uses, such as ending every response with "that's just the way it is."	**4.** Patterns may be described as rambling, pressured, slow, fast, loud, garbled, and well articulated. Mutism occurs when the patient does not speak, but appears to follow the discussion. Blocking occurs when a patient abruptly stops talking for no obvious cause. Some patients may make up a word that has special meaning to them, but which is not known to anyone else, called a neologism. In schizophrenia, the patient may speak a lot, but convey little information; speech maybe disorganized. Patients with delirium may have slurred speech. With progressive dementia, patients may present with aphasia and confabulation.
5. Assess motor behavior. Note pacing, hyperactivity, retarded movement (little movement or underactivity), rigidity (little spontaneous movement), hand wringing, picking at clothes, abnormal startle reflex, tics, and tremors.	**5.** Dementia may present with rigidity. Depression may present with psychomotor retardation or agitation. Patients with anxiety may be restless and wring their hands, pace, and fidget.
6. Evaluate judgment and insight.	
a. Judgment and insight are closely related terms; judgment involves the ability to make decisions appropriate to a particular situation after comparing and evaluating the alternatives. When assessing judgment, evaluate the ability of the patient to meet family and social obligations, how realistic the patient's plans for the future are, and patient's ability to solve hypothetical problems.	**a.** Abnormal findings for judgment include impulsive, indecisive, and lacking in reality testing (i.e., ability to distinguish and validate what is from what is not based in reality). Patients with dementia may demonstrate deteriorated and impulsive judgment. During a manic episode, a patient with bipolar disorder may also demonstrate impulsive judgment. Patients with depression and anxiety disorders may be indecisive.

Action	Rationale
b. Assess insight. Insight, in contrast, involves the ability to connect problems with personal behaviors, learn from mistakes, and understand consequences of behaviors and illness.	**b.** Patients with little insight often fail, for example, to comply with proper instructions to take their medications. It may be difficult for them to understand that taking medication, such as psychotropic drugs, can prevent psychotic symptoms from re-emerging.
7. Evaluate thought patterns. This area assesses "how" the patient thinks relative to logic and coherence, and the content, or "what," the patient thinks about. Note how the patient's thoughts/responses relate to your conversation.	**7.** Thought may be described with terms such as negative, delusional (fixed false beliefs), persecution, grandiosity, ideas of reference, and somatic. Other thought descriptors include racing, paranoid (suspicious), loose associations, flight of ideas, circumstantial (delay in reaching point because of unnecessary detail), perseverance (persistent repetition of words or ideas), thought broadcasting, and obsessions. Patients with bipolar disorder may experience grandiose and racing thought patterns. Schizophrenia often presents with delusional and paranoid thoughts. Patients with obsessive–compulsive disorder may experience persevering and obsessing thought patterns.
8. Assess perception. Perception relates to information taken in through the five senses: auditory, visual, tactile, olfactory, and taste.	**8.** Perception may be external or internal. For example, hallucinations in which there is no known object in the environment are internal, and illusions consisting of a misidentification of objects in reality are external. Abnormal perceptions include auditory or visual hallucinations; depersonalization, consisting of feelings of unreality with extreme anxiety; derealization, in which the person experiences a loss of ego boundaries of where self ends and the world begins; a distorted sense of the world, as may occur in schizophrenia; and a distorted body image, as may occur in schizophrenia and eating disorders.
9. Assess memory (the ability to register or record and store information).	
a. Assess recent (short-term) memory by asking the patient to identify common facts and relationships, such as his or her name, address, marital status, number and names of children, occupation, and what he or she ate for breakfast.	**a.** Patients with delirium or dementia may have impaired short-term memory. Amnesic disorders cause impairment in new learning or immediate recall ability.

Action	Rationale
b. Evaluate remote (long-term) memory by inquiring about birthdays, schools attended, jobs held, or past historical events that are common knowledge.	**b.** Remote memory is most often impaired in late-stage dementia.
c. Assess orientation to time, place, and person. • What is today's date? • What is the season of the year? • What is the name of this place or building? • Who is the president of the United States? • Who is the governor of this state?	**c.** Orientation may be reversibly altered by drugs, electrolyte imbalance, infection, and hypoxia or irreversibly altered related to cognitive decline, such as Alzheimer's dementia. Disorientation to "place" can occur with psychiatric and organic brain syndromes, whereas disorientation to "person" can follow head trauma, seizures, and amnesia. Problems with orientation to time are indicative of anxiety and depressive disorders as well as organic mental syndromes. Problems in orientation to person may indicate cerebral trauma and organic or psychotic disorders.
d. Test short-term recall and attention. Have the patient say a five-letter word, such as world, and then spell it backwards. Have him or her name three unrelated objects, such as pencil, orange, and truck; then have the patient repeat them immediately and again about 5 minutes later.	**d.** Normally people are able to perform these without difficulty. One of the first signs of impaired consciousness is a decreased attention span. These aspects of memory maybe altered in depression, anxiety, cognitive disorders, and confusion states.
e. Ask the patient to perform some simple math tasks, such as the following: • Serial 7s: subtract 7s from 100 until reaching 79. • Adding a short series of numbers, such as $17 + 24 + 31$. • Completing a few multiplication tasks, such as 2×3, 4×3, 5×7.	**e.** Patients of average intelligence and healthy mental status should easily perform these simple calculations. However, difficulties with calculations occur with severe depression and diffuse brain disease. Impairments in recent memory that are detectable by these questions are seen in persons with delirium or dementia.
10. Assess general intelligence. This is measured by performance on intelligence quotient (IQ) tests.	
11. Measure adaptive functioning by having the patient perform simple calculations or verbal reasoning tasks. Test abstract reasoning. Abstract reasoning is the process of drawing conclusions or inferences from pieces of information, and it is evaluated by having the patient explain metaphors or complete analogies or sentences.	**11.** Persons of average intelligence and healthy mental status should be able to perform these tasks easily. Problems with performance may be indicative of cerebral lesions (left or dominant hemisphere), brain damage, organic syndromes, or low-level intellectual functioning.

Action	Rationale
12. Assess writing and fine motor ability. Have the patient write her or his name and a few words or simple phrases. Ask the patient to draw a clock with complete numbers and hands, and set the time at 10 minutes before 2. Ask the patient to copy shapes on a piece of paper (**Figure 4-3**).	**12.** The ability to coordinate and complete fine motor tasks is indicative of an intact central nervous system. For example, sloppy or incorrect clock construction, including incorrect spacing of hour numbers and incorrect hand placement, suggests dementia or parietal lobe damage. When a patient omits or adds letters and shapes, or misuses words, this can indicate aphasia. Problems with geometric and common figures or uncoordinated writing point to cerebellar lesions or peripheral neuropathy. Patients with mental retardation will probably exhibit impaired performance on all these tasks.

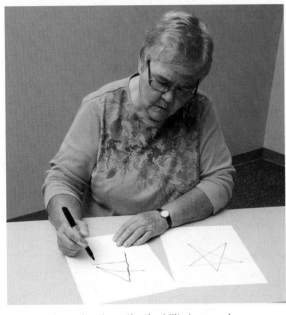

FIGURE 4-3 Assessing the patient's ability to copy shapes.

Table 4-2 discusses common mental health disorders in relation to the mental status examination.

Mini-Mental Status Examination

The Folstein Mini-Mental Status Examination (see Additional Resources at the end of the chapter) is a relatively common and brief screening tool used to quantitatively assess cognitive functioning or document cognitive changes. It consists of 11 questions that can be completed in 5 to 10 minutes. The test score depends upon summing the numbers derived from each correct response. Each item

TABLE 4-2	Common Mental Health Disorders and Associated Findings					
Diagnosis	Affect/Emotion	Thought	Perception/View	Judgment	Motor Behavior	Speech
Depression	Sad	Negative, slow	Low self-esteem	Indecisive	Slow, retarded	Soft
Mania	Elated, angry outbursts	Racing	Grandiose	Impulsive	Hyperactive	Pressured
Schizophrenia	Flat, inappropriate	Delusions, paranoia	Auditory hallucinations	Indecisive	Rigid, withdrawn	Disorganized
Anxiety	Anxious, fearful	Obsessive, hard to concentrate	Worry, fear	Indecisive	Pacing, tense	Fast
Delirium and dementia (short-term memory)	Labile	Confabulation, delusions	Visual or tactile hallucinations	Impulsive, difficult because of cognitive loss	Wandering, pacing	Varies

TABLE 4-3 Differential Diagnosis of Fatigue			
Differential Diagnosis	Significant Findings in the Patient's History	Significant Findings in the Patient's Mental Status Examination	Diagnostic Tests
Depression	Fatigue, insomnia, loss of appetite, anhedonia, suicidal ideation, symptoms occurring for at least 2 weeks	Flat affect, difficulty concentrating, indecisiveness, psychomotor retardation or agitation	CBC, CMP, TFTs (to rule out other systemic causes)
			HAMD, Beck Depression Inventory
Dysthymic disorder	Fatigue or chronic fatigue, anhedonia, loss of appetite, perceived inability to cope with responsibilities, suicidal ideation	Flat affect, difficulty concentrating, indecisiveness	CBC, CMP, TFTs (to rule out other systemic causes)
			HAMD, Beck Depression Inventory
Generalized anxiety disorder	Fatigue, insomnia, excessive anxiety or worry, nausea	Restlessness (hand wringing, pacing), difficulty concentrating, indecisiveness, fast speech	CBC, CMP, TFTs (to rule out other systemic causes)
			HAMA

Abbreviations: CBC, complete blood count; CMP, comprehensive metabolic panel; HAMA, Hamilton Anxiety Scale; HAMD, Hamilton Depression Scale; TFTs, thyroid function tests.

has a specific number of points. This is a clinician-administered instrument of questions or tasks that test the client's cognitive functioning, such as orientation to time, place, and person; recall; short-term memory; and arithmetic skills. The cutoff point to indicate cognitive impairment is generally 23–25. There is evidence that older and poorly educated patients may give false-positive scores when they do not have mental or neurological disease and that it may miss mild impairment. Test scores of 20 and less are common in patients with dementia, schizophrenia, or delirium, but scores in the 24-to-30-point range are common in patients with affective disorders.

Diagnostic Reasoning

Based on findings in the health history and mental status examination, the clinician should formulate his assessment and plan. For example, a patient may report symptoms that suggest many possible diagnoses; however, findings in the past medical history (PMI) and during the mental status examination narrow the possible diagnoses down to one or two. Sleep problems exemplify common chief complaints, which must be assessed further to determine the diagnostic formulation. **Table 4-3** illustrates differential diagnosis of common mental health disorders associated with sleep disturbances.

Mental Health Assessment of Special Populations

Considerations for the Pregnant Patient

- Be sensitive to pregnant patients regarding signs and symptoms of depression and anxiety.
- As a part of routine care, healthcare providers should assess mental health postpartum. During the postpartum period, a major depressive episode can occur within 4 weeks after delivery and last for months thereafter. A history of depression increases potential for and length of postpartum depression. The SIGECAPS criteria of depression symptoms (discussed in Box 4-1) will identify if postpartum depression is present and differentiate it from the "baby blues," which peak from 3 to 5 days after delivery and which may last up to 10 days. The "baby blues" appear as anxiety, fatigue, tearfulness, irritability, and mild depression. The Edinburgh Postnatal Depression Scale (EPDS) assists primary healthcare professionals to detect postnatal depression, which affects up to 10% of mothers, many of whom are untreated. The EPDS is a self-rated, 10-question scale with a 0–3 scoring range, where 3 indicates the most severe depressive response to each question. A total number of points from 12 to 15 indicates mild depression; a total greater than 16 indicates severe depression. During the postpartum period, the father should also be assessed for signs of

depression, anxiety, or irritability and assisted, as needs dictate. Undetected depression can have longstanding effects on the family.

- Postpartum psychosis, in contrast, occurs several days following delivery and may last for days to several weeks. Mothers' delusions and hallucinations focus on hurting themselves and their babies. Other symptoms of this disorder include anger, paranoia, fear of being alone, hostility, overactivity, and severe depression. Postpartum psychosis requires immediate medical attention.

Considerations for the Pediatric Patient

- When performing mental status assessment, focus the data collection to be developmentally appropriate. Adults and older adolescents are capable of participating in an interview with open-ended questions, but young children may be anxious or not have the language capabilities to answer many questions in a useful manner. To ease the anxiety of a young child, clinicians should maintain eye contact, place themselves at the child's body level, and maintain a therapeutic distance. It may be helpful to have an adult family member present throughout the assessment process to calm the child and to observe family interactions.
- Young children are often not adept at identifying and verbalizing their feelings. Using a feelings chart or poster can help children pinpoint their feelings. Also, allowing children to draw, color, or use figures to describe family interactions or roles is a technique that can improve assessment results (**Figure 4-4**).

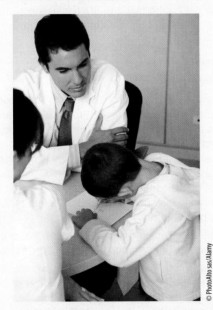

FIGURE 4-4 Having a pediatric patient draw a picture of his family to illustrate familial roles and interactions.

Considerations for the Geriatric Patient

- Age-related changes affect all physiologic systems, including central nervous system neurotransmitters, vision, mobility, and hearing. Reduced hearing, for example, can be a barrier to obtaining accurate mental status information.
- Use of multiple medications for multiple disease states complicates assessment of mental status. Use of alcohol, nicotine, caffeine, herbals, and over-the-counter medications may also adversely affect mental status examination results.
- Older patients may lack knowledge of what the clinician is asking and feel embarrassed to ask questions about their nonunderstanding. The clinician may normalize problems by queries, such as stating, *"Sometimes people have questions about_____. I wonder if you do."*

- Approaching the elderly with an attitude of respect and dignity, and not assuming all elderly persons have the same needs, is a positive approach to performing the MSE.
- Geriatric patients may have a diagnosed psychiatric condition that can be assessed by the Geriatric Depression Scale, Hamilton Rating Scale for Depression, Beck Depression Inventory, Brief Psychiatric Rating Scale, CAGE, MMSE, or Quality of Life Scale.
- Direct questions about mood, suspicions, and fears can be incorporated during the assessment. The initial examination may also point to the need for referral to a social worker, clergy, or other mental health professionals.
- Always ask if any change in mental function, such as cognition, thinking, and memory, was sudden or gradual, and then assess if the patient may also be depressed.
- Personality does not normally change with aging, but existing personality traits may become more pronounced during aging. Paranoia exemplifies this trend, and the clinician must evaluate whether paranoia exists or there is a reason based in reality that someone is trying to inflict injury to the patient.
- Alzheimer's disease accounts for 35% to 50% of dementia cases, and it is present in 5% of persons 65 to 85 years old and 20% of persons older than 85 years.

Case Study Review

Throughout this chapter, you have been introduced to JD. This section of the chapter pulls together her history and demonstrates the documentation of her history and mental status examination.

Chief Complaint

"I'm overtired and can't sleep or eat."

Information Gathered During the Interview

JD is a 31-year-old female biology graduate student. She reports, "I'm overtired and can't sleep or eat." Ms. D has lost 15 pounds over the past month and wakes up unusually early each morning. She no longer is interested in her hobby of tennis because she feels tired most of the time. Ms. D is a "good" student, but she has not been attending classes on a regular basis for the past month and feels guilty about this. She denies suicidal ideas, because it is against her religion, but feels depressed for most of each day and says that nothing is fun. This feeling has been present for 5 to 6 weeks. She states, "I would like to feel better enough to resume playing tennis and attending classes. I just have to get myself going. Maybe a vitamin would help." She provides little detail to questions and talks in mumbled tones. She denies hearing voices and blames no one but herself for this condition.

JD denies having a history of eating disorders, sexual or physical abuse, or depression. Ms. D denies recent trauma, illness, hospitalization, or surgery. She takes only aspirin for the occasional headache or muscle ache.

Ms. D's mother died of cancer about 6 months ago, but she believes she is over the death because of her return to school following the death. Her father has no known medical or psychiatric problems. She is the oldest of three sisters; her sisters are alive and well. Her paternal grandmother was treated for "change of life depression," and her maternal grandfather was a secret ("behind the barn") drinker.

Ms. D is a graduate student. She is single and lives alone. She states that lately she has had trouble "making it to class" and keeping up with her studying. Ms. D used to enjoy playing tennis, but no longer has the energy to do so. She denies nicotine use, drinking more alcohol than two glasses of wine per weekend, and illicit drug use. She had enjoyed friendships with other graduate students in class, but has been keeping to herself lately. Ms. D used to attend church regularly, but has been missing Mass frequently.

Clues	Important Points
Fatigue and insomnia	Many mental health disorders are associated with sleep disturbances.
Says that nothing is fun and feels guilty	Anhedonia and guilt are symptoms of depression.
Loss of appetite and weight loss	These are associated with depression.
Denies hearing voices	Suggests she is not schizophrenic.

| Name JD | Date 6/17/15 | Time 1015 |
| | DOB 4/4/84 | Sex F |

HISTORY

CC

"I'm overtired and can't sleep or eat."

HPI

Over the past 5-6 weeks, a history of depression, guilt, fatigue, insomnia (wakes up early), loss of appetite, and weight loss (15 lb in past month). Having trouble making it to class (graduate student). No longer enjoys hobby. Denies hearing voices. Mother died 6 months ago (may not have taken time to grieve).

Medications

ASA for occasional ache

Allergies

NKDA

PMI

Illnesses

Denies history of trauma, eating disorders, abuse, or depression.

Hospitalizations/Surgeries

None

FH

Mother died of breast cancer (age 60). Father has no known mental health or medical problems. Paternal grandmother treated for depression during menopause. Maternal grandfather abused alcohol. Two sisters, alive and well.

SH

Graduate student, not attending class regularly. Used to be a good student. Keeping to herself. No longer attending church regularly. Denies nicotine and drug use. Drinks 1–2 glasses of wine on the weekend.

ROS

General	Cardiovascular
Fatigue, weight loss.	Denies palpitations or other problems.
Skin	**Respiratory**
Denies rash.	Denies hyperventilation and other problems.
Eyes	**Gastrointestinal**
Denies problems.	Poor appetite.
Ears	**Genitourinary/Gynecological**
Denies problems.	Denies problems.
Nose/Mouth/Throat	**Musculoskeletal**
Denies problems.	Feels some muscle weakness.
Breast	**Neurological**
Denies lumps.	Denies headache.

PHYSICAL EXAMINATION

| Weight 110 lb | Temp 98.4 | BP 110/70 |
| Height 5'6" | Pulse 74 | Resp 20 |

General Appearance

Cooperative, thin, tired-looking Caucasian female

Skin

Warm, dry

HEENT

PERRL; hearing grossly intact

Cardiovascular

Apical pulse palpated; regular rate and rhythm. S1 and S2 auscultated. No murmurs, rubs, or bruits.

Respiratory	
Respirations even and unlabored	
Gastrointestinal	
Not examined	
Genitourinary	
Not examined	
Musculoskeletal	
No involuntary movements noted	
Neurological	
A J O X 3	
Other	
Flat affect, provides little detail in answers, indecisive, has difficulty concentrating.	
Lab Tests	
CBC: within normal range	T3 total: 100 ng/dL
TSH: 2.1 uIV/L	T4 total: 7.1 ug/dL
Special Tests	
Hamilton's Depression Rating Scale: met requirements for depression.	
Final Assessment Findings	
Depression	

Bibliography

American Psychiatric Association. (2015). *Diagnostic and statistical manual of mental disorders* (5th ed.). Washington, DC: American Psychiatric Press.

Ashur, M. L. (1999). Advisor Forum: SAFE questions about domestic violence. *The Clinical Advisor,* July–August, 52.

Bear, M. F., Connors, B. W., & Paradiso, M. A. (2015). *Neuroscience: Exploring the brain* (4th ed.). Philadelphia, PA: Lippincott Williams & Wilkins.

Black, M. C., Basile, K. C., Breiding, M. J., Smith, S. G., Walters, M. L., Merrick, M. T., . . . Stevens, M. R. (2011). *The National Intimate Partner and Sexual Violence Survey (NISVS): 2010 summary report.* Atlanta, GA: National Center for Injury Prevention and Control, Centers for Disease Control and Prevention. Retrieved from http://www.cdc.gov/violenceprevention /pdf/nisvs_report2010-a.pdf.

Breiding, M. J., Smith, S. G., Basile, K. C., Walters, M. L., Chen, J., & Merrick, M. T. (2014). Prevalence and characteristics of sexual violence, stalking, and intimate partner violence victimization— National Intimate Partner and Sexual Violence Survey, United States, 2011. *Morbidity and Mortality Weekly Report. Surveillance Summary 6*(Suppl 8), 1–18.

Campbell, J. C., & Humphreys, J. (1993). *Nursing care of survivors of family violence.* Saint Louis, MO: Mosby.

Cox, J. L., Holden, J. M., & Sagovsky, R. (1987, June). Detection of postnatal depression. Development of the 10-item Edinburgh Postnatal Depression Scale. *British Journal of Psychiatry, 150,* 782–786.

Erikson, E. H. (1963). *Eight stages of man in childhood and society.* New York, NY: W. W. Norton.

Ewing, J. A. (1984). Detecting alcoholism: The CAGE questionnaire. *Journal of the American Medical Association, 252*(14), 1905–1907.

Folstein, M. F., Folstein, S. E., & McHugh, P. R. (1975). Mini-mental state examination: A practical method of grading cognitive state of patients for the clinician. *Journal of Psychiatric Research, 12,* 189.

Markin, P. A., & Schneidman, M. E. (2014). Evaluation of psychiatric illness. In J. T. Dipiro, R. L. Talbert, G. C. Yee, et al. (Eds.), *Pharmacotherapy: A pathophysiological approach* (8th ed., pp. 1137–1148). New York, NY: McGraw-Hill.

Maslow, A. H. (1968). *Toward a psychology of being.* New York, NY: D. Van Nostrand.

Matzke, H. A., & Foltz, F. M. (1979). *Synopsis of neuroanatomy.* New York, NY: Oxford University Press.

Piaget, J. (1963). *The child's conception of the world.* New York, NY: Littlefield, Adams.

Sajatovic, M. S., & Ramirez, L. F. (2004). *Rating scales in mental health* (2nd ed.). Hudson, OH: Lexi-Comp.

Wise, M. G., & Gray, K. F. (2014). Delirium, dementia and amnestic disorders. In R. E. Hales, S. C. Yudofsky, & J. A. Talbott (Eds.), *The American Psychiatric Press textbook of psychiatry* (4th ed.). Washington, DC: American Psychiatric Press.

Additional Resources

Mini-Mental Status Examination

Holstein, M. F., Holstein, S. E., & McHugh, P. R. (1975). Mini-mental state: A practical method for grading the cognitive state of patients for the clinician. *Journal of Psychiatric Research*, *12*(3), 189–198. http://dx.doi.org/10.1016/0022-3956(75)90026-6

National Institute of Mental Health

http://www.nimh.nih.gov

This government site provides resources and studies related to a variety of mental health disorders and issues.

Chapter 5

Integumentary Disorders

Anatomy and Physiology Review of the Integumentary System

The skin, long recognized as the largest organ, is responsible for providing the first line of defense to the entire body. While many body systems interact closely, the skin is a highly dynamic structure that achieves many specific functions within its individual structures. These functions include:

- Preventing fluid loss
- Providing a barrier to invading organisms
- Relaying sensations of touch, temperature, and pain
- Regulating body temperature and blood pressure
- Synthesizing vitamin D
- Excreting sweat, urea, and lactic acid

Skin

The skin structure is comprised of the epidermis, the dermis, and the subcutaneous tissue (see **Figure 5-1**). The functional layers are clearly stratified; however, they may vary in depth depending upon location in the body.

The **epidermis** is the outermost, avascular layer of the skin. It contains four to five layers: stratum corneum, stratum lucidum (mostly found in skin on the hands and feet), stratum granulosum, stratum spinosum, and stratum germinativum. Keratinocytes, found in the basal layer (stratum germinativum), produce and synthesize waterproof protein keratin cells, which protect the skin. The early germinal keratinocytes multiply and migrate upward in an unorganized fashion through the epidermal layers until they lose their nucleus and form the tough layer of dead keratinocytes of the stratum corneum. The average epidermis differentiates upward from the basal layer to the stratum corneum every 30 days. After 14 days, the topmost level sheds and is replaced with the next level. In addition to keratinocytes, the epidermis contains melanocytes, pigment-producing cells that give skin its color.

Sometimes referred to as the "true" skin, the **dermis** is composed of two layers: a thin upper layer, the papillary dermis, and a thicker lower layer, the reticular dermis. The reticular dermis lies between the papillary dermis and the subcutaneous tissue. As a connective tissue layer, the dermis provides strength and stability. The fibrous matrix of collagen and elastin is set in a disorganized fashion so that movement and resistance can occur. The dermis is composed of cells, nerves, and blood vessels. Most hair follicles originate in this level.

The **subcutaneous layer** of skin, which binds the dermis to underlying body tissue, is composed of fat and connective tissues. Some sweat glands and deep hair follicles extend into this layer of skin. Adipose deposition provides a cushioning base for the subcutaneous layer.

Skin Appendages

In addition to the layered skin, the skin appendages—the nails, hair, eccrine glands, and apocrine glands—make up the full complement of the integument.

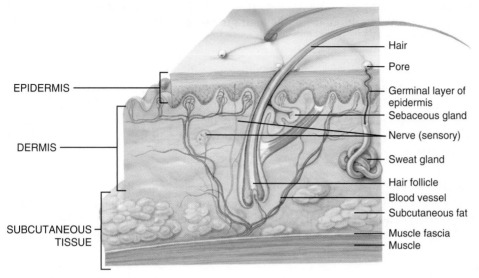

FIGURE 5-1 Structure of the skin.

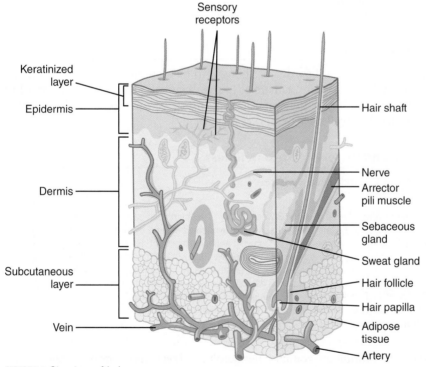

FIGURE 5-2 Structure of hair.

Hair

The structure of hair consists of the follicle, shaft, sebaceous gland, and arrector pili muscle (**Figure 5-2**). Blood vessels in the hair papilla in the bulb nourish and maintain the follicle. As with the skin, melanocytes, found in the bulb, provide the color.

The hair shaft is a shaft of dead protein. It originates in the living cells of the matrix, which then multiply and arise from the hair follicle. The hair growth cycle continuously evolves through three stages: the anagen (growth) stage, the catagen (transitional follicular regression) stage, and telogen (resting) stage. Recognizing the hair biology and growth phases of hair aids in the understanding of the hair loss disorders.

Nails

Nails, found on the fingers and toes, are keratinized plates. The anatomy of the normal nail unit includes the hard keratin nail plate, the nail bed, the proximal nail fold, and nail matrix. Nails serve to protect the fingers and toes. They grow out of the nail groove. The nail matrix, the germinal region of the nail plate, forms the floor of the nail groove. The nail bed attaches the nail plate to the underlying epidermis.

Eccrine Glands

Eccrine sweat glands originate in the dermis. Under control of the hypothalamus, they regulate body temperature through water secretion and evaporation. They are distributed and open directly to the surface of the skin in all areas but the lip margins, nail beds, inner surface of the prepuce, and the glans penis.

Apocrine Glands

Apocrine glands are located deep in the dermal layer in the areas of the axilla, nipple, areola, eyelids, external ears, and in the anogenital regions. Apocrine secretions are clear and odorless and are released under cholinergic and hormonal control. When mixed with bacteria on the surface, the secretions produce body odor.

Health History

While much of assessing skin disorders is thought to be identification by recognition, good history taking, as in any other assessment, is crucial to the diagnosis. The immediate skin history cues the examiner to the contributing or precipitating features of a skin problem. Careful history alerts the potential for localized as well as general disease.

Chief Complaint and History of Present Illness

"I've got spots, and I'm itchy everywhere."

LK is a 42-year-old man who presents with a 3-week history of erythematous papules and plaques of the lower anterior, medial, and lateral legs that have developed slowly and persisted. The condition worsened while using an over-the-counter neomycin antibiotic ointment. He has since discontinued use of the ointment and his legs have slightly improved. Mr. K has experienced recurrent similar episodes. He complains of moderate lower leg pruritus. Slight tenderness and straw-colored, odorless drainage has developed over the past 5 days. The patient describes other scattered pruritic areas of the arms and back as severe. He denies chemical exposure at work or in or outside of his home. He has not traveled or been exposed to persons with similar problems. He denies changes in the appearance of hair or nails.

Growths, rashes, and pruritus are common dermatologic chief complaints (CC). Specific information and questions about lesions/rashes and pruritus (regarding the history of present illness [HPI]) are given here.

Lesions/Rashes

Any growth should be evaluated for potential malignancy. Any complaint of a "spot," especially in a new patient, requires a thorough history and risk factor evaluation. Histologic evaluation (biopsy) may be performed whenever there is clinical suspicion of skin malignancy or neoplasm of undetermined origin. Rashes are particularly puzzling and should be systematically evaluated. History of morphologic presentation/changes, as well as major constitutional symptoms of fever, chill, lethargy, and toxic appearance, are important.

Onset	Was the onset sudden or gradual?
Duration	How long has the lesion or rash been present?
Quantity and location	Does the patient have a single lesion or multiple lesions?
	Where is/are the lesion(s) located?
	Rash or lesions confined to the genital area suggest a sexually transmitted disease.
	Herpes zoster is commonly confined to the thoracic, trigeminal, and lumbosacral areas.
	Impetigo is most often found on the face.
	Rosacea is usually confined to the middle third of the face.
Quality	Describe the size, shape, elevation, and color of the lesion. Ask about exudate, crusting, and pain.
Changes in quality since onset	Has the size, shape, elevation, location, or color changed since the onset?
	Varicella (chickenpox) begins as red macules and quickly progresses to papules and vesicles to crusts. Varicella, rubella (German measles), and rubeola (measles) usually begin on the face and spread to the trunk and extremities.
Associated symptoms	Ask about associated symptoms including fever, pruritus, malaise, headache, chills, and anorexia.
	Fever, malaise, and anorexia are often seen in varicella. Patients with mumps often experience headache, anorexia, and fever.
	In addition to the rash, patients with rubeola often present with fever, cough, and fatigue.
Precipitating factors	Has the patient experienced a previous malignancy?
	Has the patient experienced any recent injuries or trauma to the skin?
	Has the patient traveled recently or been exposed to chemicals?
	Exposure to chemicals may result in irritant contact dermatitis.
	Has the patient recently spent time outdoors or been exposed to poison oak or ivy?
	Is the patient taking any medications?
	An adverse reaction to a drug often manifests as a rash.
	Has the patient eaten any new foods recently?
Alleviating and aggravating factors	What alleviates and aggravates the symptoms? Has the patient taken any medications? Has the patient applied any topical creams or gels? Have any other measures, such as applying heat or cold, alleviated the symptoms?

Pruritus

Pruritus (itching) is actually a form of pain. Many localized and generalized conditions present with the symptom of itch. In addition, pruritus is associated with many environmental factors, which should be evaluated as potential contributing features. Occasionally systemic illness may be associated with pruritus; therefore, a careful history must precede the physical examination.

Onset	Was the onset sudden or gradual?
Quality and location	Describe the intensity of the pruritus.
	Where is the patient experiencing pruritus?
Pattern and duration	Is the pruritus worse at night or during particular seasons?
	Pruritus associated with scabies is often worse at night.
Associated symptoms/ conditions	Ask about associated symptoms/conditions including rash or lesions, asthma, and allergies.
	Patients with atopic dermatitis often have a history of asthma or chronic allergies.
	Pruritus often occurs at the site of a rash or lesion.
Precipitating factors	Ask about the presence of insect bites or exposure to insects.
	Many insect bites are very pruritic.
	Is the patient taking any medications, specifically aspirin, hormones, opiates, phenothiazine, B_{12}, quinidine, CNS stimulants, beta blockers, or warfarin?
	Has the patient traveled recently?
Alleviating and aggravating factors	What alleviates the symptom (e.g., cold compresses, topical or oral medications)?
	What aggravates the pruritus (e.g., low humidity, certain fabrics, stress, cleansers)?
Bathing habits	How frequently does the patient bathe? What products does he use?

Past Medical History

Mr. K has a 14-year history of generalized pruritus, often severe. He reports chronic, relapsing, localized, intensely pruritic lesions of the lower leg. He denies systemic diseases. Allergy patch testing was performed and, according to the patient, yielded no valuable results. The patient has tried multiple oral antihistamines; he currently takes none. The patient denies a history of childhood eczema, skin cancers, or precancers. He states that he had varicella as a child. Mr. K reports he is mildly tolerant to sunlight. He denies previous surgeries or blood transfusions.

Past medical history (PMI) of the patient with a skin disease/disorder should be as comprehensive as that for any other medical complaint. Careful history reveals recurrences or flare patterns linked to triggers and modifying factors.

Past health conditions or surgeries	Ask about health conditions, including diabetes, thyroid or other endocrine dysfunction, HIV, atopic conditions (allergic asthma, hay fever, and eczema), and thromboembolism.
	These conditions may provide a clue to skin diagnoses or may modify treatment of the skin. Related systemic complexes such as the immune response of allergy, asthma, and tissue inflammatory reaction are connected to atopic dermatitis (eczema), psoriasis, and viral infections.
	Has the patient had any surgeries?
	Previous medical treatments, surgery, and trauma interrupt the natural defense of the skin barrier, providing hospitable ground for infection and inflammation.

Skin, hair, or nail conditions	Does the patient have or has the patient had any skin, hair, or nail disorders? Ask about treatment. Does the patient have a history of skin cancer or precancers? *A past history of skin cancer or precancerous dermatoses increases the patient's risk for skin cancer.* **Box 5-1** *provides additional risk factors for skin cancer.*
Tolerance to sunlight	Ask the patient about her or his tolerance to sunlight and history of sunburns. *The Fitzpatrick sun sensitivity skin typing scale* **(Table 5-1)** *is used as a tool for classifying skin type to provide uniform assessment of potential risk.* *One blistering sunburn causes a two-fold risk of developing melanoma.*
Allergy testing	Has the patient been tested for allergies?

BOX 5-1 SKIN CANCER RISK FACTORS

Men over age 50	Personal history of skin cancer
Blue or green eyes	Continuous exposure to sun at work or play
Blonde or red hair	Light skin that burns, freckles, or easily gets red
Family history of skin cancer	Certain types and larger number of moles

---

Table 5-1 Fitzpatrick Skin Type Classification

Type	Sun Reaction*
I	Always burns easily; never tans
II	Usually burns; tans minimally
III	Burns moderately; tans gradually
IV	Burns minimally; tans readily
V	Rarely burns; tans profusely
VI	Never burns; darkly pigmented

*Note: Reaction is based on 30 minutes of exposure to summer sun.

Family History

> Mr. K has a negative family history of arthritis, eczema, psoriasis, heart disease, diabetes, and skin cancer. He is an only child; both parents are alive and well. His mother is sensitive to cosmetics and sunscreens and has a childhood history of itch and rashes. His parents and he all have fair skin and blue eyes.

Inherited color of eyes, hair, and skin tone reveal signs of the skin's natural protection or lack of it. Many skin disorders are familial or genetic, so it is important to explore the family history (FH) of such disorders.

Age of living relatives	Include relationship and health of parents, siblings, and children.
Deaths	Includes relationship of the deceased to the patient and cause of death (specifically disorders that affect the skin).
Chronic diseases; skin disorders	Ask about chronic diseases in the family; include the relationship of the patient to the family member with the disease. Focus on inherited skin disorders or disorders that have skin manifestations.

Inherited skin disorders are divided into several broad classifications. The disorders of keratinization are attributed to X-linked ichthyosis or excessive scaling of the skin. Neurocutaneous disorders are isolated to chromosome 17 and are characteristically recognized in early life by café-au-lait patches. **Mechanobullous** *disorders, specifically epidermolysis bullosa, are caused by defects of keratin proteins and collagen genes that are responsible for structural integrity of the cells.*

Immune-mediated diseases such as atopic dermatitis, psoriasis, and seborrheic dermatitis are not inherited disorders specifically, but follow familial patterns. Decreased cell-mediated immunity may allow the skin to exhibit inflammation as a result of physical or emotional stressors.

Family history relative to skin immune response includes asthma, hay fever, environmental allergens, and persistent rashes.

Genetic defects	Is there a history of congenital birth defects?

Social History

Mr. K does not smoke or drink. He is employed as a social worker. He lives in a single-family home with his wife and two children. Currently, 10 puppies, 1 dog, and 1 cat reside in the patient's home. He denies outdoor vocations or avocations. Mr. K reports that he wears an SPF of 15 when outdoors for prolonged periods. He had remote exposure to Agent Orange in Vietnam.

Cumulative exposure to ultraviolet radiation is the strongest predictor for lifetime risk for developing a skin cancer. Statistically, greater than half of all patients over age 60 will develop some form of cutaneous malignancy. Therefore, known risk factors should be evaluated (see Box 5-1). Aspects of a patient's social history (SH) provide pertinent information for determining his or her risk for skin cancer. For example, those who live in tropical climates and did not practice photoprotection have a greater incidence of skin cancers than their counterparts that reside in northern climates.

Family	Ask to describe current family unit.
Occupation	Ask about the patient's occupation.
	Outdoor occupations with prolonged sun exposure, such as farmer and landscaper, greatly increase the risk for skin cancer.
	As few as three summers of outdoor employment are considered a risk, as is any repeated intense exposure that is more damaging than multiple chronic exposures.
	Certain occupations have exposure to chemicals.
Hobbies	Ask about hobbies and activities.
	Outdoor hobbies, such as golfing and sailing, involve increased sun exposure.
Use of tobacco	Ask about tobacco use including types, amounts, duration of use, and exposure to secondary smoke.
	Habits suppressive to the immune system, such as smoking, inhibit ability to repair cell damage after an intense ultraviolet exposure.
Use of alcohol	Does the patient drink alcohol? If so, what type and how much does she drink?
	Excessive consumption of alcohol increases the risk for skin cancer.

| Use of recreational drugs | Does the patient use recreational drugs? If so, what type and how much? |
| | *Drug use may cause skin-related problems. Amphetamine use can result in dry, itchy skin.* |

Review of Systems

Many skin diseases/disorders have manifestations in systems other than the integumentary system. A comprehensive review of systems (ROS; see Chapter 1) should be performed whenever possible; however, due to time and other types of constraints, the provider may only be able to perform a focused review of systems. During a focused review of systems, the provider focuses questioning on the systems in which skin problems are most likely to have manifestations. Below is a summary of common manifestations of skin problems.

System	Symptom or Sign	Possible Associated Diseases/Disorders
General	Fever, malaise	Herpes zoster, varicella, erythema nodosum, roseola, rubéola
HEENT	Red eyes	Rosacea
	Conjunctivitis	Rubeola
	Upper respiratory infection symptoms	Erythema nodosum
Respiratory	Asthma, allergies	Atopic dermatitis
	Cough	Rubeola
Cardiovascular	Varicosities, pedal edema	Stasis dermatitis
Gastrointestinal	Anorexia, abdominal pain	Roseola
Musculoskeletal	Arthritis, joint stiffness	Psoriasis, erythema infectiosum

Physical Examination

Equipment Needed

- Gloves
- Ruler
- Magnifying glass
- Good lighting source

Components of the Physical Examination

Inspection

It is important to be specific and descriptive about all skin findings. Recognition of primary and secondary skin lesions is the basis of the skin evaluation. Assessment begins with the identification of the basic skin lesion (primary) including description of size, shape, configuration, color, texture, elevation, depression, and pedunculation. Secondary lesions may be superimposed on the primary lesion, obscuring its identification, or may exist in the absence of a primary lesion. A systematic approach describing localized and generalized skin findings by morphology, arrangement, and distribution of specific skin findings increases the likelihood of arriving at an accurate diagnosis.

Visual examination should take place in a well-lit room allowing an appreciation of distribution and regional characteristics of lesions. Distinguishing features of primary lesions, examined with hand magnification when needed, are often sufficient to establish a diagnosis.

Diascopy, or the use of compression usually accomplished with a microscope slide, interrupts arteriole distention and can be helpful in identifying lesions of vascular origin. In areas of widespread discoloration caused by superficial engorged capillaries, application of diascopy forces blood out of surface vessels so that other colors in the skin are less visually obscured.

Action	Rationale
1. Begin with a general inspection of the overall skin. Observe general color.	1. Overall skin color should be consistent throughout and usually reflects the patient's genetic background. Patients with dark skin tones may have lighter skin tone on their palms and soles of their feet. Abnormal findings include regions of color change, such as pallor, cyanosis, erythema, or jaundice.

2. Inspect the skin for lesions (**Figure 5-3**).

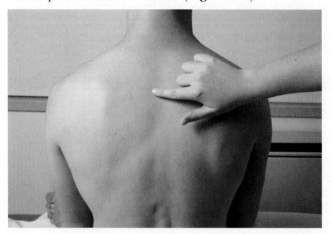

FIGURE 5-3 Inspecting for lesions.

a. Identify the morphology of the lesion, including elevation, shape, and size. Use a magnifying glass, as necessary. A ruler helps the examiner determine size.

a. Gross morphology, or the structure and form of a skin lesion, is the core of dermatologic diagnosis. Assessment begins with primary lesions. Secondary skin lesions are not pathologic, but are the result of manipulation or infection, or simply the natural evolution of the primary process. Occasionally, a pathologic lesion exists that cannot be described as primary or secondary. These special lesions are unique and readily identified. See **Tables 5-2**, **5-3**, and **5-4** for descriptions and examples of primary, secondary, and special lesions

b. Inspect the lesions for color and arrangement.

b. Critical thinking about skin lesion evaluation begins with the identification of size and elevation; the differential diagnosis quickly narrows with the consideration of color and arrangement. Multiple lesions in particular arrangements can be extremely helpful in providing specific pathognomonic signs of a particular disease. For example, the Christmas tree arrangement of pityriasis rosea or the dermatomal arrangement of herpes zoster is among the many important arrangement patterns.

    Table 5-5 describes arrangement patterns with common examples.

Table 5-2   Primary Lesions

Type	Description	Examples	Illustration
Macule	< 1 cm in diameter, flat, non-palpable, circumscribed, discolored	Brown: freckle, junctional nevus, lentigo, melasma Blue: Mongolian spot, ochronosis Red: drug eruption, viral exanthema, secondary syphilis Hypopigmented: vitiligo, idiopathic guttate hypomelanosis	
Patch	> 1 cm in diameter, flat, non-palpable, irregular shape, discolored	Brown: larger freckle, junctional nevus, lentigo, melasma Blue: Mongolian spot, ochronosis Red: drug-eruption viral exanthema, secondary syphilis Hypopigmented: vitiligo, idiopathic guttate hypomelanosis	
Papule	< 1 cm in diameter, raised, palpable, firm	Flesh, white, or yellow: flat wart, milium, sebaceous hyperplasia, skin tag Blue or violaceous: venous lake, lichen planus, melanoma Brown: seborrheic keratosis, melanoma, dermatofibroma, nevi Red: acne, cherry angioma, early folliculitis, psoriasis, urticaria, eczema	
Nodule	> 1 cm in diameter, raised, solid	Wart, xanthoma, prurigo nodularis, neurofibromatosis	
Plaque	> 1 cm in diameter, raised, superficial, flat-topped, rough	Psoriasis, discoid lupus, tinea corporis, eczema, seborrheic dermatitis	
Tumor	Large nodule	Metastatic carcinoma, sporotrichosis	
Vesicle	< 1 cm in diameter, superficially raised, filled with serous fluid	Herpes simplex, herpes zoster, erythema multiforme, impetigo	

(continues)

Table 5-2 Primary Lesions (*continued*)

Type	Description	Examples	Illustration
Bulla	> 1 cm vesicle	Pemphigus, herpes gestationis, fixed drug eruption	
Pustule	Raised, superficial, filled with cloudy, purulent fluid	Acne, candidiasis, rosacea, impetigo, folliculitis	
Wheal	Raised, irregular area of edema, solid, transient, variable size	Hives, cholinergic urticaria, angioedema, dermatographism	
Cyst	Raised, circumscribed, encapsulated with a wall and lumen, filled with liquid or semisolid	Digital mucus, epidermal inclusion, pilar	

Table 5-3 Secondary Skin Lesions

Type	Description	Examples
Scale	Irregular formation of exfoliated, keratinized cells, irregular shape and size	Psoriasis, tinea versicolor, pityriasis rosea, seborrheic dermatitis
Crust	Dried serum, blood, or exudate, slightly elevated	Impetigo, tinea capitis, acute eczematous inflammation
Lichenification	Thickened epidermis with accentuated skin lines caused by rubbing	Lichen simplex chronicus
Scar	Thin or thick fibrous tissue, following dermal injury	Burns, acne, keloid, herpes zoster, hidradenitis
Fissure	Linear break in skin through epidermis and dermis	Hand dermatitis, intertrigo
Excoriation	Hollowed-out area of all or portion of epidermis with depressed appearance	Eczema, insect bite, acne excorié
Erosion	Localized loss of epidermis, heals without scarring	Herpes simplex, perléche
Ulcer	Loss of epidermis and dermis, variations in size	Decubitus or stasis ulcer, factitial ulcer, pyoderma gangrenosum
Atrophy	Depression resulting from loss of epidermis and/or dermis	Morphea, striae, aging, dermatomyositis, topical and intralesional steroids

Table 5-4   Special Skin Lesions

Type	Description	Examples
Burrow	A narrow, elevated channel produced by a parasite	Scabies
Telangiectasia	Superficial dilated blood vessel	Rosacea, side effect of topical steroid
Petechiae	< 1.0 cm circumscribed deposit of blood	Gonococcemia, meningococcemia
Purpura	> 1.0 cm circumscribed deposit of blood	Senile traumatic purpura

Table 5-5   Arrangement Patterns

Arrangement Pattern	Description	Examples
Nummular	Coin-shaped	Nummular eczema
Annular	Circular or ring shape	Tinea corporis
Linear	Line formation	Coupe de sabre
Arciform	Arch-shaped	Drug reaction
Grouped	Occurring closely together	Herpes zoster
Gyrate	Convoluted, serpiginous shape	Creeping eruption

Action	Rationale
c. Inspect for regional involvement and distribution.	**c.** Most skin diseases exhibit a preference for area of involvement. The structure, function, and physical nature of the skin in specific body regions are more favorable for some diseases. For example, opposing skin folds favor hidradenitis and candidiasis. Photo-exposed areas of the head and neck are frequent sites of skin malignancy, such as basal cell carcinoma (**Figure 5-4**) and squamous cell carcinoma (**Figure 5-5**). Areas of heavy follicular distribution, such as the chest and back, are subsequently prone to folliculitis and cystic structures.

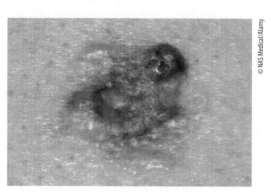

FIGURE 5-4 Basal cell carcinoma.

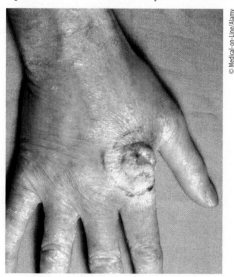

FIGURE 5-5 Squamous cell carcinoma.

Action	**Rationale**
	Similarly, the term *distribution* is used in describing skin findings. Terms of distribution commonly used in describing skin disease include generalized, localized, discrete, or confluent.
	While not always as helpful as a regional approach, certain distribution patterns such as the localized areas of involvement in allergic contact dermatitis are crucial characteristics of the diagnosis.
	Terms used to describe distribution patterns include flexor, extensor, and dermatomal.
3. Inspect the hair.	
a. Observe color, texture, and distribution.	**a.** If you find localized alopecia, assess for a scarring versus a nonscarring appearance. Scarring (cicatricial) alopecia is caused by diseases that destroy and scar the hair follicles. Smooth, shiny, scarred areas on the scalp with no obvious follicle visible suggest deep inflammatory conditions where the follicles are destroyed, such as discoid lupus erythematosus and lichen planus.
	Nonscarring alopecia found in singular or multiple patches may represent hair breakage as seen in traction alopecia and trichotillomania. Both result from manipulation, unlike the breakage of hair seen in tinea capitis that is caused by a fungal infection. Chronic conditions, such as diffuse androgenic alopecia (**Figure 5-6**), can develop insidiously during the second or third decade of life.
	With telogen effluvium, a generalized hair loss usually related to an internal stressor, evident hair loss begins 3 months after a stressful encounter.
	Alopecia areata (**Figure 5-7**), an autoimmune cell-mediated problem, may affect any hair-bearing surface and usually occurs as 1- to 5-cm round or oval patches of hair loss.
	Unexplained patchy hair loss, especially at the occiput, should always be evaluated as a secondary finding of syphilis.
b. Inspect the scalp for lesions or infestations.	**b.** Head lice (pediculosis capitis) lay white eggs on the hair shaft and cause severe pruritus.

Action

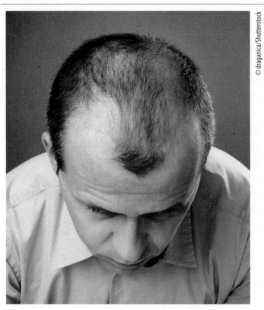

© draganica/Shutterstock

FIGURE 5-6 Androgenic alopecia.

c. Note any excessive hair.

4. Inspect the nails.

a. Observe the consistency/texture. Note any separation of the plate from the nail bed.

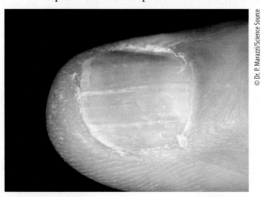

© Dr. P. Marazzi/Science Source

FIGURE 5-8 Longitudinal ridging, a normal finding associated with aging.

Rationale

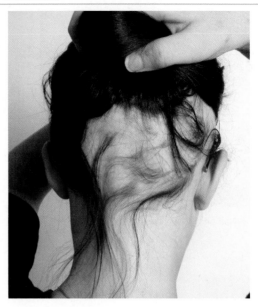

FIGURE 5-7 Alopecia areata.

c. Hirsutism is excessive hair in females that occurs in regions where males commonly have hair, such as the beard area, upper back, shoulders, sternum, axillae, and pubis. Causes include endocrinologic disorders and androgen-related disorders (and therefore are related to the ovary). Polycystic ovary disease is the most common cause of hyperandrogenism and mild hirsutism. Serious disease should be considered in the presence of rapid progression of hirsutism, balding, and deepening of voice. If an extensive evaluation proves negative, hirsutism may be classified as idiopathic.

a. Nail surface should be smooth and consistent. The nail plate should be adhered to the nail bed.

Longitudinal ridging (**Figure 5-8**) and loss of the lunula are age related and do not signal disease. Habitual picking may also cause distortion of the nail plate but does not interrupt the adherence of the nail.

Psoriasis usually presents with nail pitting (**Figure 5-9**), subungual thickening, and distortion.

Nails affected with lichen planus exhibit longitudinal grooves.

Action

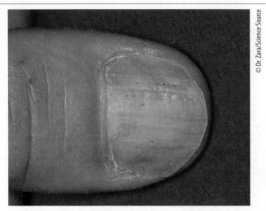

© Dr. Zara/Science Source

FIGURE 5-9 Nail pitting of psoriasis.

b. Inspect nails for color.

Rationale

Fungal nail infections are described according to the pattern of the infection entry point; these include distal subungual onychomycosis (most common), white superficial onychomycosis, proximal subungual onychomycosis, and candidal onychomycosis. Thickening, opacification, nail crumbling, and distortion (dystrophy) are common exam findings of fungal infections. Diagnosis is made by performing KOH (potassium hydroxide) preparation, culturing of scrapings from under the nail plate, or nail biopsy for PAS (periodic acid-Schiff).

Herpetic whitlow, a viral infection caused by transference of the herpes simplex virus (HSV) and frequently acquired by healthcare workers, can be exquisitely edematous and painful.

Separation of the nail plate from the nail bed can occur after trauma or may be related to psoriasis or *Pseudomonas* infection.

b. The nails should be translucent, not opaque.

Pigmented longitudinal bands are a common finding among blacks, but should be carefully evaluated for a differential diagnosis of acral melanoma.

Candidal infection of the nail may be yellow-green in color but maintain the integrity of the nail plate. *Pseudomonas* infections, by contrast, most commonly present with a green-black discoloration and onycholysis of the nail plate.

Palpation

While much of the skin examination can be accomplished through visualization, valuable information maybe gained by palpating and manipulating the skin. The palpated epidermal and/or dermal features of a lesion can be demonstrated with relative ease, assisting in formulation of a diagnosis. Consistency, turgor, temperature, mobility, and tenderness are among the valuable findings of palpation. **Remember to wear gloves when palpating lesions and open skin.**

Action

1. Assess the temperature, level of moisture, and texture of the patient's skin.

Rationale

1. Skin should be cool or warm to the touch. The temperature of the examination room may affect the temperature.

Skin should not be overly moist or dry. Overly moist skin may indicate temperature regulation problems. Dry skin may represent hyperthyroidism.

Action	Rationale

Skin should feel smooth. Very rough skin could suggest a keratinization disorder. Extremely cracked or fissured skin may be chemically injured or xerotic. Very smooth or slightly depressed skin with absence of superficial features is usually a scar.

2. Test skin turgor (**Figure 5-10**). Gently pinch the patient's skin between your thumb and finger and then release it.

    2. The skin should spring back into place.

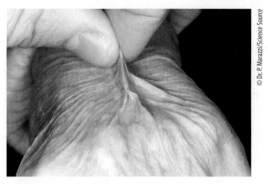

© Dr. P. Marazzi/Science Source

FIGURE 5-10 Testing skin turgor.

3. Palpate lesions. Depending on the type of primary or secondary lesion identified during inspection, use the following technique.

    a. Squeeze or apply lateral pressure to localize the level of a lesion. The dermis is fibrous and can be picked up and moved over the subcutaneous nodules of deeper lesions of muscles or bone.

    a. Squeezing can sometimes force fluid or semisolid matter out of the skin, which can help with diagnosis (i.e., squeezing an edematous extremity).

    b. Scrape the skin surface to provide information about superficial lesions.

    b. Dermatophyte and psoriasis plaques are of epidermal location and shed scale very easily when scraped with a #15 blade. Plaques of granuloma annulare that often mimic a dermatophyte do not shed scale when scratched. Thick crusts overlying ulcers can mask the depth of dermal involvement. Removal of surface crusts improves assessment.

    c. Apply linear pressure or rub the skin surface with a blunt, narrow object to release the inflammatory mediators in cutaneous mast cell disorders exhibiting characteristic dermatographism or an urticarial wheal.

    c. Lateral pressure applied to perilesional normal skin of active pemphigus blisters causes shearing away of the epidermis (Nikolsky's sign).

    d. Use paring to aid in the differential diagnosis of corns and warts.

    d. Paring the surface of a corn reveals a smooth, often shiny keratin kernel. A pared wart will exhibit small dark vessels.

Action	Rationale
4. Perform a hair pull test. Grasp about 60 hairs between the thumb and finger. Apply slow, constant traction.	**4.** Tractions against the scalp should not yield more than six hairs. If it does, inspect the bulbs for stage.
5. Palpate nails.	
a. Assess texture, temperature, and tenderness.	**a.** Nails should be smooth and firmly adhered to the nail bed. Palpation should not elicit tenderness. Bacterial infections of acute and chronic paronychia are easily distinguished by the warmth, tenderness, swelling, and erythema that are present.
b. Paring the nail bed may be helpful.	**b.** Paring the surface keratin of a nail enables the assessment of a nail bed, or confirms the presence of blood in a suspected subungual hematoma.

The distinguishing feature of a skin disease/condition is usually readily identifiable. If the primary lesion is accurately identified, most disorders can be recognized by hallmark features. **Tables 5-6 through 5-14** describe the hallmark features of many common skin disorders.

Table 5-6 Papulosquamous Diseases			
Diagnosis	Location of Lesions	Physical Examination Findings	Photograph
Seborrhea and dandruff	Head and trunk at sites of sebaceous gland, rich skin	Erythematous plaques with dry or oily scales	© Dr. P. Marazzi/Science Source
Psoriasis	Knees, elbows, buttocks	Chronic, well-demarcated, erythematous plaques with silver scale	© Christine Langer-Pueschel/Shutterstock

Table 5-6 Papulosquamous Diseases (*continued*)

Diagnosis	Location of Lesions	Physical Examination Findings	Photograph
Pityriasis rosea	Following natural skin lines of trunk	Single 3- to 4-cm oval plaque at onset that is followed by numerous smaller (< 1 cm) plaques with collarette scale	Courtesy of CDC
Rosacea	Face	Papules; pustules; no comedones	© Hercules Robinson/Alamy
Lichen planus	Extremities	Pruritic, polyangular, planar, purple papules; lacy surface	Courtesy of Susan Linsley/CDC

Table 5-7 Vesiculobullous Diseases

Diagnosis	Location of Lesions	Physical Examination Findings
Impetigo	Face, neck, extremities	Thin, erythematous bullous vesicles or pustules that heal with honey-colored crust
Herpes simplex (initial and recurrent)	Orolabial, genital	Expanding erosions with pain; an active vesicular border and scalloped periphery
Herpes zoster	Dermatomal distribution of thoracic, cranial, trigeminal, lumbar, and sacral nerves	Sequential pain; crops of erythematous papules and plaques followed by erosive blisters
Dyshidrosis	Symmetrically, palms, lateral fingers and toes, soles	Sudden eruption of highly pruritic vesicles that are deep-seated with clear fluid, followed by ring of scale and peeling
Erythema multiforme, minor	Extensor surfaces of extremities, oral mucosa	Successive crops of target lesions with well-defined borders and three zones of color
Erythema multiforme, major	Widespread trunk and mucosal involvement	Raised, flat, erythematous macules and papules; two-color zones with a poorly defined border; extensive eruption, epidermal detachment and systemic symptoms

Table 5-8   Dermatitis

Diagnosis	Location of Lesions	Physical Examination Findings	Photograph
Allergic contact dermatitis	Exposure site; often hands, forearms, face, and tops of feet	Vesicles, edema, redness and extreme pruritus	© Cavallini James/age fotostock
Atopic dermatitis	Flexural in children; extensor in adults	Abrupt onset; erythematous, oozing, vesicular acute rash with severe pruritus, redness, and scale	© iStockphoto/Thinkstock
Nummular dermatitis	Extremities and trunk	Sharply demarcated, scaling, annular plaques with eczematous inflammation	© Custom Medical Stock Photo/Alamy
Stasis dermatitis	Leg with varicosities and dilated veins and edema	Eczematous dermatitis with fissuring, chronic venous congestion, hyperpigmentation	© Medical-on-Line/Alamy
Diaper area dermatitis	Infant buttock/genitalia, convex surfaces contacting diaper	Red base with satellite pustules; fringe of moist scale	© Medical-on-Line/Alamy

Table 5-8   Dermatitis (*continued*)

Diagnosis	Location of Lesions	Physical Examination Findings	Photograph
Seborrheic dermatitis	Scalp, brow, paranasal, postauricular, and flexural areas	Greasy, adherent scale on coalescing macules, papules, and patches	© Hercules Robinson/Alamy

Table 5-9   Nodules

Diagnosis	Location of Lesions	Physical Examination Findings
Erythema nodosum	Extensor aspect of extremities	Often bilateral, poorly defined, red, nodule-like swelling over shins
Dermatofibroma	Legs	Solitary, dome-shaped, fixed, pink to brown; lateral pressure causes dimpling
Granuloma annulare	Lateral or dorsal surfaces of hands/feet	Asymptomatic, flesh-colored or red papules that progress to annular ring without scale
Cysts	Back, neck	Circumscribed lesion with wall and lumen that is filled with fluid or solid

Table 5-10   Inflammatory Disorders

Diagnosis	Location of Lesions	Physical Examination Findings
Acne	Face, neck, back, chest	Comedones and inflammatory papules, pustules, and nodules
Boil (furuncle)	Hair-bearing body part: head, neck, axilla, buttock	Red, hard, tender, then fluctuant
Hidradenitis	Axilla, inguinal, and perianal	Inflammatory subcutaneous nodules, perforate, drain, and form sinus with healing
Pyogenic granuloma	Head, lips, neck, hands	Friable vascular papule arising at site of previous trauma

Table 5-11   Hyperplasia

Diagnosis	Location of Lesions	Physical Examination Findings
Verruca	Hands, elbows, knees, feet	Epidermal proliferations, single, multiple, or confluent
Molluscum	Trunk, extremities, face	White, firm, flesh-colored, dome-shaped papule with central umbilication
Corn	Feet	Occurring over a bony prominence
Epidermal cyst	Head, neck, trunk	Dermal nodule with small overlying punctum
Xanthelasma	Eyelid skin	Yellow plaques
Skin tag	Neck and skin fold areas	Fleshy, compressible papules

Table 5-12   Benign Neoplasia

Diagnosis	Location of Lesions	Physical Examination Findings
Seborrheic keratosis	Anywhere	Variable color, waxy surface, stuck-on appearance
Mole	Anywhere; sun-exposed areas	Clusters of nevus cells arranged at various levels in the skin
Lipoma	Anywhere	Solitary, soft, well-defined tumor
Dermatofibroma	Legs	Solitary, dome-shaped, fixed, pink to brown lesions; lateral pressure causes dimpling
Keloid	Anterior chest, shoulders, neck	Large, raised scar that extends into adjacent normal skin
Hemangioma	Head and neck	Rapid growth, stabilization, and involution of red to purple vascular neoplasm
Neurofibroma	Follow course of peripheral nerves	Dermal and subcutaneous tumors increase with age

Table 5-13   Premalignant Disease

Diagnosis	Location of Lesions	Physical Examination Findings
Actinic keratosis	Head, neck, dorsal hands	Poorly defined hyperemia with adherent scale
Keratoacanthoma	Dorsal hands	Solitary, dull, red nodule with central keratotic plug
Dysplastic nevus	Anywhere; trunk and upper extremities	Multiple, atypical nevi with increased incidence of melanoma

Table 5-14   Malignant Disease

Diagnosis	Location of Lesions	Physical Examination Findings
Basal cell carcinoma	Face, scalp, ears, neck, sun-exposed areas of trunk, extremities	Pearly white, dome-shaped papule with ulcerative crusted, bleeding center
Squamous cell carcinoma	Head, neck, hands, sun-exposed areas of skin	Red, poorly defined base with raised, necrotic, crusted center
Melanoma	Back, chest, legs	Color and appearance vary considerably; pigmented and nonpigmented lesions
Paget's disease	Breast, extramammary	Red, sharply demarcated, irregularly outlined plaque or papule
Cutaneous T-cell lymphoma	Trunk, hip, buttocks, upper thigh, inner arms or legs	Red, scaly, eczematous or psoriasis-like eruption
Kaposi's sarcoma	Feet and lower legs	Raised, oval, poorly demarcated, rust or purplered patch, plaque, or nodule
Metastasis to the skin	Head, neck, chest, abdomen	Discrete, firm, painless nodule

Diagnostic Reasoning

Based on findings in the health history and physical examination, the clinician should formulate his or her assessment and plan. For example, a patient may report symptoms that suggest many possible diagnoses; however, findings in the past medical history and during the physical examination narrow the possible diagnoses down to one or two. Rash is a common chief complaint. **Table 15-15** illustrates differential diagnosis of common disorders associated with rash.

Diagnostic tests may help examiners with diagnosis. **Box 5-2** describes common laboratory and other tests used to diagnose disorders of the skin.

Table 5-15 Differential Diagnosis of Pruritic Rash

Differential Diagnosis	Significant Findings in the Patient's History	Significant Findings in the Patient's Physical Examination	Diagnostic Tests
Allergic or contact dermatitis	New onset, no known injury	Pruritic, papulovesicular rash confined to affected area of contact	Patch testing
Atopic dermatitis	History of childhood eczema, allergic rhinitis, family history of allergic rhinitis and eczema	Pruritic rash; erythematous, confluent papules and plaques affecting extensor areas; scarring	Biopsy, serum total IgE, KOH scraping
Arthropod bites	History of hypersensitivity reactions, outdoor exposure	Isolated, erythematous, pruritic papules and vesicles	None

Note: All scaling rashes should be scraped for potassium hydroxide (KOH) preparation to rule out fungus.

BOX 5-2 COMMON LABORATORY AND DIAGNOSTIC STUDIES USED TO DIAGNOSE SKIN DISORDERS

In the event that physical examination narrows the differential diagnosis but does not provide the final diagnosis, other diagnostic aids provide valuable information. In-office diagnostic testing includes skin surface microscopy, Wood's light exam, dermoscopy, cytologic smears, swab or tissue cultures, patch testing, and skin biopsy for histologic examination.

WOOD'S LIGHT EXAM

Description

Wood's light, or long ultraviolet (UV) light, is used mainly in the examination of epidermal pigmentary disorder and cutaneous infections. Applying long UV light to the skin in a dark room causes epidermal pigment to appear accentuated while dermal pigmentary disorders with normal epidermal findings are obscured. Depigmentation will similarly be exaggerated against normal skin, appearing chalky white.

Findings During the Wood's Light Exam

Fungal Diseases
- *Microsporum audouinii:* Bright blue-green
- *M. canis:* Bright blue-green
- *M. distortum:* Bright blue-green
- *Tinea tonsurans:* Nonfluorescent
- *T. versicolor:* Dull golden yellow

Bacterial Diseases
- Erythrasma: Brilliant coral, red-pink, orange
- *Pseudomonas aeruginosa:* Yellowish green

Pigmentary Disorders
- Epidermal: Accentuates pigment deposition
- Dermal: Unchanged pigment visibility
- Depigmentation: No pigment visible, white

SURFACE MICROSCOPY

Pigmented lesions may be better evaluated with in vivo skin surface microscopy. Surface microscopy or epiluminescence is an oil emersion technique; the epidermis is rendered translucent providing an enhanced exam with the aid of an illuminated 10× magnifier to evaluate the epidermal-dermal junction and melanocytic activity. Pigmented lesions should be evaluated utilizing the ABCDE mnemonic: examining for **A**symmetry, **B**order irregularity, **C**olor variegation, **D**iameter > 6 mm, and **E**levation or **E**nlargement. Following evaluation by the ABCDE mnemonic, histologic substrates are then examined for pattern analysis of the pigmented network. This process is complex and requires clinical experience and proficiency.

SCRAPING

For nonspecific fungal identification, scrapings taken from the skin or nails require scraping skin from the active border, using a #15 scalpel blade, placing onto a microscope slide, a cover slip, and applying 20% potassium hydroxide (KOH). Direct examination with the condenser on low light will aid in the identification of hyphae and spores.

Scraping for herpes virus infection via a Tzanck smear requires placing the scrapings of the base of a vesicle onto a slide and application of Giemsa or Wright's stain. Identification of multinucleated giant cells confirms the diagnosis. Because false negatives can occur, comparison with viral culture is suggested.

(continues)

**BOX 5-2   COMMON LABORATORY AND DIAGNOSTIC STUDIES USED TO DIAGNOSE
SKIN DISORDERS** *(continued)*

Scraping for mites at characteristic flexural sites of serpiginous burrows requires placing the scraping with mineral oil onto a glass slide to produce the female parasite, eggs, or mite fecal pellets (scybala).

CULTURES
Wounds or draining tissue can be cultured to identify the various potential microbial offenders. Correct organism identification is mandatory for complete treatment of an infected area. Bacterial, viral, and fungal cultures are collected and grown in appropriate media for the identification of specific organisms. Dermatophyte test medium (DTM) is a culture medium that will grow dermatophytes over 7 to 21 days.

PATCH TESTING
To diagnose allergic contact (not irritant) dermatitis, the patch test is the best way to expose the patient to the most common allergens in a prepared format. Patches containing the 20 most common allergens are applied, and then removed after 2 days. A papulovesicular eruption at the site of allergen exposure will prove positive reaction.

BIOPSY
Commonly, skin biopsy is required to accurately identify the pathology of a skin finding. The superficial or shave skin biopsy is indicated when pathologic diagnosis can be made from a small sample of tissue. Generally, perform shave biopsies for pedunculated, papular, or exophytic lesions. For evaluating inflammatory skin conditions potentially involving disease at depths from the epidermis down to the subcutaneous fat, perform a punch biopsy. This technique produces a cylinder of tissue varying in size from 2 mm to 10 mm, depending on the equipment used. Punch biopsies examine the depth of involvement and allow for special tissue staining. Excisional biopsy provides a deeper specimen when it is desirable to remove the entire lesion. This biopsy technique results in a larger defect and requires suturing for closure.

Skin Assessment of Special Populations

Considerations for the Pregnant Patient

- Note that the common dermatoses of pregnancy—pruritic urticarial papules of pregnancy (PUPP), intrahepatic cholestasis of pregnancy (ICP), and prurigo gravidarum— all include the common symptom of pruritus.
- Distinguish between herpes gestationis (HG) and PUPP. Herpes gestationis, more appropriately termed pemphigoid gestationis, is a pruritic condition of pregnancy that occurs with much less frequency (1:50:000) than PUPP. It should be distinguished from PUPP, as treatment commonly includes the use of oral corticosteroids. **Table 5-16** compares the clinical course and presentations of HG and PUPP.
- Recognize two other common pruritic conditions of pregnancy: prurigo gravidarum and ICP. Prurigo gravidarum (recurrent cholestasis of pregnancy) occurs late in pregnancy without any visible primary skin lesion. Signs of jaundice may develop, in addition to the generalized excoriations resulting from pruritus. An associated incidence of low birth weight and prematurity may occur. Recurrence may be seen in subsequent pregnancies. Symptoms resolve soon after delivery. ICP develops generally after 30 weeks and recurs in greater than 50% of subsequent pregnancies. The patient with ICP has a greater chance of developing cholelithiasis.

Table 5-16 Comparison of Herpes Gestationis (HG) and Pruritic Urticarial Papules of Pregnancy (PUPP)		
Feature	HG	PUPP
Etiology	Autoimmune	Urticaria, reaction pattern
Incidence of occurrence	1:50,000	1:160–300; greater in primigrávidas
Symptom	Intense pruritus	Pruritus
Morphology	Tense vesicles and bullae	Coalescing papules
Regional involvement	Trunk, buttock, extremities	Abdominal, rarely umbilical
Onset	Anytime, usually 2nd trimester	Last trimester, commonly
Clinical course	Exacerbations and remissions	Fixed eruption, clear postpartum
Histopathology	Dermal eosinophils	Perivascular infiltrate
Postpartum prognosis	Recurs in subsequent pregnancy	Does not recur in subsequent pregnancy
Infant mortality	Some prematurity, small for age	No fetal effect

Considerations for the Neonatal Patient
- Recognize possible congenital patches of color and their significance.
- Note nevus flammeus (stork bite at back of the neck).
- Recognize Mongolian spots. These appear as areas of deep pigmentation in the sacral and gluteal regions of neonates with dark skin.

Considerations for the Pediatric Patient
General
- Note the following:
  - Pediatric patients present with an array of acute infections and infestations, as well as chronic dermatosis. The care of infections (bacterial, viral, and dermatophyte) is an important aspect of pediatric care.
  - Due to underdeveloped hygiene habits and multiple frequent contacts, the pediatric population harbors a plethora of organisms, which are readily identifiable and treatable.
- When taking the history remember the following:
  - Many families diagnose and treat children with readily available over-the-counter treatments prior to medical evaluation. When you are assessing the child with a skin condition, it is imperative that prior treatments be clearly identified.
  - Ask about all close personal contacts.

Common Skin Conditions/Diseases
- Bacterial infections: A superficial skin infection, impetigo (bullous and nonbullous), results from infection of primarily *Staphylococcus aureus,* and to a lesser extent, streptococci. Rarely, the organisms invade skin more deeply and cause erysipelas, cellulitis, and lymphangitis. In a superficial bacterial infection, the clinical course begins with an area of broken skin on the face or body, followed by localized vesiculobullous enlargement and rupture and ooze of serum from inflamed central bullae followed by the formation of a honey-colored crust. A mildly erythematous border may occasionally develop. Postinflammatory hyperpigmentation or hypopigmentation may follow the healed lesions. Careful history should be elicited regarding the duration of occurrence; for example, an increased incidence of nephritic involvement has been noted where streptococcus was responsible for a skin infection that has lasted longer than 1 week.
- Viral infections: Cutaneous viral infections are another frequent finding of the pediatric skin exam. Verruca vulgaris (common warts), verruca plantaris (plantar warts), and verruca plana (flat warts) are common visible manifestations of human papillomavirus, which can be seen in children and adolescents as firm hyperkeratotic papules and plaques of the epidermis. Molluscum contagiosum, a cutaneous viral infection caused by the poxvirus, also exhibits firm, raised, benign growths on the skin surface. **Table 5-17** distinguishes these common types of cutaneous viral illnesses and their clinical presentation. The varicella virus, commonly identified as chickenpox, is transmitted by the respiratory system. Varicella exhibits multiple teardrop-shaped vesicles on an erythematous base that develop 10 to 14 days after exposure.
- Superficial fungal infections: Superficial fungal infections exist in the uppermost, keratinized layer of skin. In childhood, superficial fungal infections frequently arise on the scalp, trunk, extremities, and feet. Generally, the fungi, belonging to several genera, create varying degrees of inflammatory response and exhibit a typically active scaly border. **Table 5-18** describes common superficial fungal infections of childhood with their usual presentations and causative organisms.
- Infestations: The pediatric population may exhibit the cutaneous manifestations of infestation. Mites *(Sarcoptes scabiei)* burrow in body folds, skin creases, and feet to produce

Table 5-17   Viral Skin Infections

Diagnosis	Virus Type	Location of Lesions	Physical Examination Findings	Arrangement	Hallmark Features
Molluscum	Poxvirus	Face, trunk, extremities	Dome-shaped, umbilicated papules, 1–5 mm	Single or grouped	Waxy appearance
Verruca vulgaris (common)	Human papillomavirus (HPV) 1, 2, 4, 7	Hands, extremities	Hyperkeratotic papules, may enlarge to plaques	Single or grouped	Black dots of thrombosed capillaries
Verruca plantaris (plantar)	HPV 1, 4, 63	Plantar surface of foot	Hyperkeratotic papules or plaques	Numerous small warts may fuse to mosaic surface	Lateral pressure causes pain
Verruca plana (flat)	HPV 1, 4, 63	Face, hands, legs	Flat-topped papules, 1–3 mm	Linear or grouped due to trauma of scratch/shave	Multiple, slightly elevated

a significant degree of pruritus. Another burrowing infestation, cutaneous larvae migrans (CLM), commonly known as creeping eruption, usually presents as burrows in the foot. Blood-sucking lice that inhabit the body *(Pediculus humanus)*, head *(Pediculus capitis)*, and genital regions *(Pediculus pubis)* puncture the skin and create irritation and pruritus with their saliva. Tick infestations, while a somewhat less common mite and more geographically predictable, can transmit the spirochete *Borrelia burgdorferi*, causing significant morbidity and potential mortality, and therefore should remain in the differential diagnosis of any insect bite or infestation. **Table 5-19** gives clinical features of infestations.

- Chronic relapsing conditions
  - *Atopic dermatitis:* Although the onset of atopic dermatitis (AD) occurs in the newborn period, it is regarded as a very common chronic disease (affecting approximately 10% of the pediatric population) and remains an underdiagnosed and often poorly managed disease. Often, the clinician is able to obtain an accurate history, identify typical skin findings, and secure the diagnosis of atopic dermatitis with very little challenge. In other cases, however, the dynamic process of acute, subacute, and chronic atopic dermatitis confuses the examination with multiple morphologies and the variations of age.
  - *Acne:* Acne is another multifactoral, challenging chronic disease of childhood and adolescence. Although not exclusive to adolescence, acne affects 85% of those aged between 12 and 24 years. Contributory factors include a hereditary predisposition, androgenic hormones, and inflammatory factors. **Table 5-20** presents acne subtypes. Two broad categories of acne exist: noninflammatory and inflammatory. Noninflammatory acne consists of the formation of open and closed comedones, frequently referred to as blackheads and whiteheads, respectively. Inflammatory lesions are characterized by morphologic description; acne lesions vary in size (papules less than 5-mm diameter, nodules greater than 5 mm) and may have purulent contents (pustules). Severity is graded as mild, moderate, or severe, as determined by the number of lesions present and the amount of inflammation. Assessment of the psychosocial impact of acne patients follows the physical assessment of the acne lesions. It is important to stress the goals of acne treatment, which are to control new acne and minimize scarring.
  - Similar-appearing lesions that are commonly mistaken for acne include perioral dermatitis, rosacea, hidradenitis suppurativa, and true keratinous cysts. Perioral dermatitis is an intolerance reaction; it often presents in young women as papules and pustules on the chin and nasolabial fold. Rosacea is of vascular origin. Patients with rosacea often have flushing, papules, pustules, telangiectasia, and tissue swelling. No comedones are present with rosacea. Hidradenitis, an epithelialization disorder, presents with communicating sinus tracts under inflammatory cysts.

Table 5-18   Superficial Fungal Infections

Diagnosis	Location of Lesions	Hallmark Features	Causative Organism	Clinical Subtypes
Tinea pedís	Soles, toe webs	Scale, inflammation, maceration	*Trichophyton rubrum* or *T. mentagrophytes*	Interdigital, moccasin, vesiculobullous
Tinea capitis	Hair shaft	Fine scale, kerion	*T. tonsurans* *T. schoenleinii*	Endothrix, ectothrix, favus
Tinea corporis	Non-hairy extremities, trunk	Arciform with advancing border	*T. rubrum* *T. mentagrophytes* *Microsporum canis*	Cranulomatous, verrucous, tinea incognito
Tinea versicolor (pityriasis versicolor)	Trunk, neck, arms, shoulders	Finely scaling, hypopigmented and hyperpigmented flat plaques	*Pityrosporum orbiculare*	
Cutaneous candidiasis	Diapered region	Bright erythema with satellite papules	*Candida albicans*	

Table 5-19   Infestations

Diagnosis	Method of Transmission	Incubation	Life Cycle	Symptoms	Clinical Highlight
Pediculosis	Shared clothing or bedding	30 days	25 days	Irritation, pruritus	It most commonly affects Caucasian children with straight hair.
Pubic louse	With or without person-to-person contact	Eggs are viable for 10 days	25 days, can live off host for 36 hours	Irritation, pruritus	There is a 95% chance of acquiring from an infected partner after one sexual exposure.
Ticks	From trees, grass, bushes, and animals; attach to human skin	Engorged after 7–14 days	Female feeds, engorges, and drops off after 1 to 2 weeks	Site marked by a round, crusted ulcer; bites often unrecognized	Rickettsial, viral, and spirochetal transmission is possible.
Scabies	Personal contact, clothing, linen, furniture	Usually 3–4 weeks; up to 8 weeks	Female can survive off human for 96 hours	Severe nighttime pruritus	It is highly communicable. There is cross antigenicity with house dust mites.

Table 5-20   Acne Subtypes

Acne Subtype	Inflammatory Features/Contributing Factors
Acne mechanica	Mechanical pressure over skin (i.e., chin straps, hats)
Steroid acne	Oral corticosteroids
Drug-induced acne	Anabolic steroids, antiepileptics, isoniazid
Acne neonatorum	Large sebaceous glands stimulated by maternal androgen
Acne excorié	Self-manipulation/excoriation
Acne cosmetica	Layers of cosmetics, aggressive cleansing with scrubs encourages inflammatory papules, masques

Considerations for the Geriatric Patient
General
- Note that an impaired epidermis, often seen in geriatric patients, is more susceptible to outside irritants.
- Remember visible skin signs of age can be attributed to intrinsic and extrinsic aging. Features of intrinsic and extrinsic aging may overlap but can usually be distinguished by inspection and palpation.
  - Inspect for signs of intrinsic aging. Intrinsic aging, or the changes due to normal maturity, include most noticeably a decreased number of sweat glands and hair follicles, decreased pigment of hair (thinning, graying hair), decreased dermal collagen and decreased number of dermal elastic fibers (fine wrinkling), thinning and ridging of nails, and loss or increase in subcutaneous fat deposition.
  - Inspect for signs of extrinsic aging (i.e., resulting from external insults), most significantly sunlight, but can occur secondary to ultraviolet light exposures in tanning booths and secondary to therapeutic ultraviolet light treatment. Environmental

pollution and smoking negatively impact cellular immunity and function also. In the epidermis, early changes of sun exposure take the form of freckling and solar lentigines. These changes demonstrate the effects of increased melanin production in an increased number of melanocytes. Epidermal thickening can be seen as early as the third decade of life (leathered appearance). Deeper papillary dermal effects of long-term sun exposure include wrinkled skin, telangiectasia, senile purpura, lentigo senilis, senile comedones, and skin cancers. Ultraviolet light exposure degrades dermal collagen, weakening the skin, resulting in atrophy and production of abnormal elastotic fibers. The examiner often finds that loss of dermal collagen surrounding blood vessels combined with minor trauma produces the common solar purpura. Sharply demarcated purpuric areas are commonly found on the arms. Telangiectasia, commonly seen on the facial skin and venous lakes of the lips, are isolated vascular formations found on sun-exposed areas where incidental sun exposure eventually affects perivascular collagen.

- Inflammatory skin conditions common to geriatric patients (including xerosis, dermatophytosis, stasis dermatitis, seborrheic dermatitis, and rosacea) can occur at any time in the life cycle but occur with increased frequency in this population.

Common Skin Conditions/Diseases

- Xerosis: Impaired keratinocyte formation, which results in abnormal epidermal cell turnover, is responsible for xerosis, the most common cause of itch in the elderly.
- Stasis dermatitis: Dry, itchy skin of the lower extremities warrants special evaluation for advancing vascular changes. Superficial varicose veins with the underlying vascular impediments of edema and pressure manifest as an eruption of the lower leg seen in stasis dermatitis. The inflamed, sometimes ulcerated skin of acute stasis dermatitis maybe accompanied by the chronic changes of stasis dermatitis including hyperpigmentation, lichenification, and scars of healed ulcers.
- Rosacea: While not limited to the geriatric population, rosacea is an underdiagnosed and misdiagnosed inflammatory condition, which is chronic and progressive. The hallmark of rosacea in the geriatric population is in the bulky tissue (phymatous) and dilated telangiectatic vessels commonly seen after years of persistent redness and flushing. Another common variant of rosacea in the elderly is ocular rosacea, often overlooked in the ocular examination.
- Skin tumors: Geriatric patients often seek evaluation because they have been "growing things," and should remain under a high index of suspicion for cutaneous malignancies as a result of cumulative ultraviolet exposure. Many skin tumors, however, are not malignancies. **Table 5-21** describes common geriatric benign tumors, with hallmark features that aid in their identification.

Table 5-21 Geriatric Benign Skin Tumors			
Benign Epidermal Growth	Location of Tumors	Hallmark Features	Differential Diagnosis
Seborrheic keratosis	Face, trunk	Stuck-on appearance, varying color and degrees of dryness, waxy with pebbly or verrucous surface	Pigmented basal cell and squamous cell carcinomas, malignant melanoma, lentigo, wart, actinic keratosis
Cherry angioma (senile angioma)	Trunk	Smooth, firm, deep red, few or hundreds, increasing with age	Petechiae
Acrochordon (skin tag)	Neck, axillae, groin, eyelids	Soft compressible, pedunculated, or projectile	Seborrheic keratosis, dermal nevi, warts
Venous lake	Vermilion border of lip, ear	Compression collapses lesion	Blue nevus, malignant melanoma, tattoo
Sebaceous hyperplasia	Face—glabella	1- to 2-mm soft, dome-shaped, pale yellow with central umbilication	Basal cell carcinoma, HSV, molluscum
Chondrodermatitis nodularis chronica helicis	Lateral surface of the helix, antihelix	Single, firm, 2- to 6-mm painful, red to white nodule	Actinic keratosis, keratoacanthoma

Case Study Review

Throughout this chapter, you have been introduced to Mr. K. This section of the chapter pulls together his history and demonstrates the documentation of his history and physical examination.

Chief Complaint (Present Illness)

"I've got spots and I'm itching everywhere."

Information Gathered During the Interview

Mr. K is a 42-year-old man who presents with a 3-week history of erythematous papules and plaques of the lower anterior, medial, and lateral legs, which have developed slowly and persist. The condition worsened while using an over-the-counter neomycin antibiotic ointment. He has since discontinued use of the ointment and his legs have slightly improved. Mr. K has experienced recurrent similar episodes. He complains of moderate lower leg pruritus. Slight tenderness and straw-colored, odorless drainage gas developed over the past 5 days. The patient describes other scattered pruritic areas of arms and back as severe. He denies chemical exposure at work or in or outside his home. He has not traveled or been exposed to persons with a similar problem.

Mr. K has a 14-year history of generalized pruritus, often severe. He reports chronic, relapsing, localized, intensely pruritic lesions of the lower leg. He denies systemic diseases or change in appearance of hair or nails. Allergy patch testing was performed and, according to the patient, yielded no valuable results. The patient has tried multiple oral antihistamines; he currently takes none. The patient denies a history of childhood eczema, skin cancers, or precancers. He states that he had varicella as a child. Mr. K. reports he is mildly tolerant to sunlight. He denies previous surgeries or blood transfusions.

Mr. K has a family history of allergy, eczema, heart disease, and diabetes but no skin cancer. He is an only child; both parents are alive and well. His mother is sensitive to cosmetics and sunscreens and suffered from eczematous rashes in childhood. All family members have fair skin and blue eyes.

Mr. K does not smoke or drink. He is employed as a social worker. He lives in a single-family home with his wife and two children. Currently, 10 puppies, 1 dog, and 1 cat reside in the patient's home. He denies outdoor vocations or avocations. He had remote exposure to Agent Orange in Vietnam.

Clues	Important Points
Atrophic patches with loss of surface characteristics	Scar formation is the visible and tactile result of healed repeated injury.
Hyperpigmentation	Indicative of postinflammatory pigmentary alteration.
Erythematous, raised, poorly defined papules	Inflammatory reaction induces localized edema and erythema without margination.
Erosions	Initial scratching excoriates epidermis with central superficial tissue loss. Repeated trauma such as scratching or rubbing results in tissue thickening or *lichenification.* Often occurs at sites of easy access such as arms, legs, and upper back.
Dry, cracked skin of lower extremities	Dry skin, commonly found where sebaceous activity is minimal, is the frequent cause of pruritus. Interrupted/excoriated skin is easily attacked by allergens and infectious organisms.
Scattered, isolated pustules surrounded by erythematous halo	Pustules indicate bacterial process with inflammation at site of friction.

Name LK		Date 2-1-16	Time 1000
		DOB 7-12-74	Sex M
HISTORY			
CC			
"I've got spots and I'm itching everywhere."			
HPI			
3-week history of pruritic erythematosus papules, plaques of lower legs; now tender with straw-colored drainage; worsened with neomycin topical antibiotic			

Medications
None. Previously ordered nasal steroids and oral antihistamines; self-discontinued

Allergies
Peanuts, sulfa drugs, seasonal environmental allergies

PMI
14-year history of dry, sensitive skin with generalized pruritus, with chronic, relapsing, localized intensely pruritic areas of the lower leg in the last year.

Illnesses
Childhood varicella; patient experiences recurring pruritic areas.

Hospitalizations/Surgeries
None

FH
Unknown family history of asthma. Mother has been sensitive to cosmetics and sunscreens and had eczematous rashes in childhood. FH includes allergy, eczema, heart disease, and diabetes. Denies FH of skin cancer.

SH
Lives with wife, 2 children, 1 dog, 10 puppies, 1 cat. Works as social worker. Denies outdoor hobbies.

ROS	
General	Cardiovascular
Denies recent constitutional changes.	Unremarkable.
Skin	Respiratory
Relapsing episodes of inflamed, pruritic papules, plaques of lower extremities.	No asthma. Positive for environmental allergies.
Eyes	Gastrointestinal
No deficits, no correction.	Denies nausea and vomiting.
Ears	Genitourinary/Gynecological
No deficits.	Denies presence of rash or recent changes.
Nose/Mouth/Throat	Musculoskeletal
Dentition intact.	Osteoarthritis of knees.
Breast	Neurological
Negative.	Denies changes in mental status.

PHYSICAL EXAMINATION				
Weight 158 lb		Temp 98		BP 132/70
Height 5'9"		Pulse 82		Resp 20

General Appearance
Alert, well-developed, normal habitus. In no acute distress

Skin
Multiple moderately erythematosus, isolated and confluent papules and plaques, loosely arranged, with central erosions on xerotic skin of lower extremities. No warmth; minimal drainage; some crust and slight tenderness at singular area. Multiple lichenified, hyper-pigmented and atrophic patches scattered over lower extremities.

HEENT
Normocephalic. Increased ocular lacrimation. Slight, clear nasal drainage

Cardiovascular
RRR, normotensive

Respiratory
No wheeze or cough

Gastrointestinal
Deferred

Genitourinary
Deferred

Musculoskeletal
Stable gait
Neurological
Grossly intact
Other
Lab Tests
KOH of scaly plaque
Special Tests
Consider culture and/or tissue biopsy if not responsive to treatment.
Final Assessment Findings
1. *Atopic dermatitis with impetiginization*
2. *Possible allergy or sensitivity to topical neomycin*

Bibliography

American Academy of Family Physicians (AAFP). (1999). AAFP core educational guidelines: Conditions of the skin. *American Family Physician, 60*(4), 1258–1264.

Arndt, K. A. (1997). *Primary care dermatology.* Philadelphia, PA: W. B. Saunders.

Boguniewicz, M. (2002, September). Introduction to immunology (the A's, B's, and T's). *Adapt: Evolving strategies for the management of atopic dermatitis,* 1–24.

Burkhart, C. G. (2001, July/August). Case 4: Oh boy! *Clinical Advisor,* 76–86.

Callen, J. P., Greer. E., Paller, A. S., Swinyer, L. J. (2000). *Color atlas of dermatology* (2nd ed.). Philadelphia, PA: W. B. Saunders.

Grin, C. M. (2001). Can you identify these disorders in black skin. *Consultant, 41*(4), 550–562.

Habif, T. (2015). *Clinical dermatology: A color guide to diagnosis and therapy* (6th ed.). Edinburgh, UK: Saunders/Elsevier.

Porth, C. M. (2013). *Pathophysiology: Concepts of altered health states* (9th ed.). Philadelphia, PA: Lippincott Williams & Wilkins.

Additional Resource

The Skin Cancer Foundation

http://www.skincancer.org
This site provides extensive information about detection, prevention, and treatment of skin cancer.

Chapter 6

Eye Disorders

Anatomy and Physiology Review of the Eye

The eyes are responsible for transmitting visual stimuli to the brain for interpretation via the optic nerve (cranial nerve II). Four of the twelve cranial nerves (CN) directly mediate ocular function. Pupillary constriction, opening the eye, and most ocular movements are controlled by CN III. Rotation of the eyeballs in their orbits to allow focused image is controlled by CN III, IV, and VI. The bony orbit protects the eyes. The anterior aspect of the eye is exposed, while the remainder is protected within the skull.

External Eye

The external eye is comprised of the eyebrows, eyelids, eyelashes, conjunctiva, and lacrimal apparatus (see **Figure 6-1**). These structures, along with the extraocular muscles, protect and support the eye.

Eyelids protect the eye and maintain moisture. The upper eyelid normally covers a portion of the iris but does not overlap the pupil. The opening between the eyelids is called the palpebral fissure. Eyelashes normally curl outward from the lid margins. Firm strips of connective tissue called tarsal plates lie within the eyelids. Each plate contains rows of meibomian glands. The meibomian glands secrete an oily lubricating substance at the lid margins that prevents excessive evaporation of tears and provides a seal when the lids are closed. The oculomotor nerve innervates the levator palpebrae muscle, which raises the upper eyelid. The levator muscle originates superior and posterior to the eye and inserts into the upper eyelid margin. Sympathetic nerves control Müller's muscles. Contracted during wakeful periods, they relax with fatigue or sleep, allowing the eyelids to close.

The conjunctiva is a transparent or clear membrane that covers the anterior portion of the eyeball. The palpebral portion of the conjunctiva lines the eyelids while the bulbar portion lies over the sclera. The two conjunctiva portions meet the cornea at the limbus. Glands in a healthy conjunctiva produce a tear film, which is essential to maintaining a healthy corneal surface.

The lacrimal glands lie in the bony orbit temporally and lateral to the eye. Meibomian, conjunctival, and lacrimal glands produce tear fluid that protects the conjunctiva and cornea from drying, prevents microbial growth, and promotes a smooth surface to the cornea. Tear fluid drains medially through two tiny holes called the lacrimal puncta and pass into the lacrimal sac and into the nose through the nasolacrimal duct. The puncta are found just superior to the lower lid margin medially. The medial fold in the conjunctiva is the plica semilunaris. The lacrimal caruncle is an elevated mass that resembles both skin and conjunctiva. Tear fluid from the nasolacrimal duct passes through the medial wall of the maxillary sinus and empties into the nose (which is why when people cry, they need to blow their nose). An imbalance between tear production and tear drainage via the nasolacrimal ducts causes "dry eye" or keratitis sicca.

Internal Eye

Intraocular structures include the sclera, cornea, iris, pupil, anterior chamber, lens, ciliary body, choroid, and retina (**Figure 6-2**). The eyeball is a spherical structure that focuses on the neurosensory fibers within the retina. There are three tunics of the eye: the fibrous, consisting of the sclera

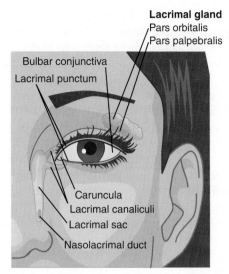

Lacrimal gland
Pars orbitalis
Pars palpebralis
Bulbar conjunctiva
Lacrimal punctum
Caruncula
Lacrimal canaliculi
Lacrimal sac
Nasolacrimal duct

FIGURE 6-1 Extraocular structures.

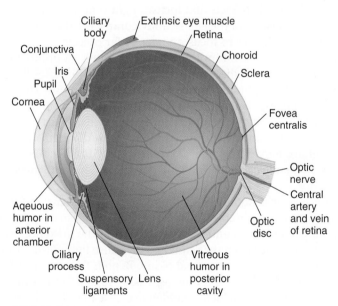

Ciliary body
Extrinsic eye muscle
Retina
Conjunctiva
Iris
Pupil
Cornea
Choroid
Sclera
Fovea centralis
Optic nerve
Central artery and vein of retina
Aqeuous humor in anterior chamber
Ciliary process
Suspensory ligaments
Lens
Optic disc
Vitreous humor in posterior cavity

FIGURE 6-2 Intraocular structures.

and cornea; the vascular, consisting of choroids and ciliary body; and the sensory, consisting of the retina.

The sclera, sometimes referred to as the "white" portion of the eye, forms the outer layer of the globe of the eye. It merges with the cornea on the anterior portion of the eye at the limbus. The sclera and the episclera are composed of connective tissue that provides a protective coat for the eye. In addition, the rigid structure of the sclera is necessary to maintain vision during eye movements. Inserted into the sclera are three pairs of muscles (the superior rectus, the lateral rectus, and the medial rectus). In addition, the oblique muscles (superior oblique and inferior oblique), together with the rectus muscles, rotate the eyeball in the orbit and allow images to be focused at all times on the fovea.

The cornea is a smooth, moist tissue that covers the area over the pupil and iris. It is continuous with the conjunctiva. The cornea is transparent and richly innervated with sensory nerves via the trigeminal nerve (CN V). The constant wash of tears protects its surface from drying. The cornea allows light transmission through the lens to the retina and separates fluid from the anterior chamber from the external environment.

The anterior chamber lies posterior to the cornea. It is bordered anteriorly by the cornea, laterally by the sclera and the ciliary body, and posteriorly by the iris and the portion of the lens that is within the papillary opening. The anterior chamber is filled with aqueous humor. Aqueous humor, a fluid that is continuously produced by the ciliary body, circulates from the posterior through the pupil into the anterior chamber and drains out through the canal of Schlemm. The relationship between the rate of production of aqueous humor and the resistance to the aqueous outflow at the anterior chamber angle determines the intraocular pressure (normally 15 mm Hg ± 3 mm Hg).

The iris is the circular disc containing pigment that gives the eye its distinctive color. Iris color is due to variable amounts of eumelanin (brown/black melanins) and pheomelanin (red/yellow melanins) produced by melanocytes. Brown-eyed people have more eumelanin and blue- and green-eyed people have more pheomelanin.

The pupil is a black-appearing aperture that allows light to enter the eye. It dilates and constricts, controlling the amount of light entry. The pupil also constricts in response to accommodation, which is the change in focus from a distant to a near object.

The lens lies behind the iris. It refracts and focuses light onto the retina. The muscles of the iris control pupillary size, while muscles of the ciliary body control the thickness of the lens. Changes in the thickness of the lens allow the eye to focus on near or far objects.

The fundus, or the posterior portion of the eye seen through an ophthalmoscope, includes the retina, choroids, fovea, macula, optic disc, and retinal vessels. It translates light images into a series of impulses or visual stimuli to the brain. **Figure 6-3** depicts the fundus. The optic nerve and retinal vessels are found on the optic disc. Lateral and inferior to the disc is a small depression in the retinal surface that marks the point of central vision. The darkened circular area surrounding this depression is the fovea (centralis). The macula surrounds the fovea; it distinguishes fine detail and colors.

The inner retina contains nerve fibers, which synapse in the brain along with vascular structures. The vascular structures are manifest primarily in the nerve fiber layer and are seen clinically as opacifications in the inner retina.

The vitreous humor is a clear liquid that is found between the lens and the retina, forming the vitreous body. In a newborn, the vitreous has an egg-white consistency and is firmly attached to the retina. With age, the vitreous thins and may separate from the posterior eye, usually a harmless condition. As the vitreous detaches from the retina, it may cause light flashes or floaters. Floaters are caused by tiny bits of vitreous tugging on retinal tissue. Benign floaters must be distinguished from retinal tears or detachment, particularly if following a head injury. Flashes may have a neurological origin, as experienced in a migraine headache. Sudden decrease in vision, associated with flashes and floaters or a veil or curtain that obstructs part or all of the vision, and a sudden increase in floaters are symptoms indicating a more serious etiology.

Vision

Light reflected from an object must pass through the normally transparent structures for perception of a clear image. Light enters the eye and is refracted by the cornea through the pupil to the lens. The ciliary body controls the thickness of the lens, adjusting to accommodate so that a clear, focused image (light) is refracted onto the retina. Rods and cones in the retina translate the light into electrical impulses. The optic nerve carries these images to the occipital cortex of the brain, where the image is interpreted.

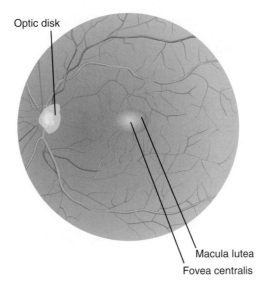

Optic disk

Macula lutea
Fovea centralis

FIGURE 6-3 Fundus.

To focus on near objects, the eye increases the curvature of the lens, constricts the pupil, and converges to allow for accommodation. Divergent light rays must be bent to form a clear image on the retina. Contraction of the ciliary muscles causes the elastic lens to bulge and change curvature for focus.

Pupillary constriction is accomplished as a result of contraction of the circular fibers of the iris. Pupillary constriction directs the light focus, resulting in a clearer image of near vision. The pupils constrict to see near objects and to protect ocular structures in the presence of bright light.

Convergence, the movement of the eyes inward, brings images together. Single binocular vision requires that light rays from an object fall on the same corresponding points on each retina so that a person sees one object instead of two. Extraocular muscles maintain the balance required to hold the two images parallel.

Visual Pathways

Images are reflected in reverse from right to left and upside down; thus an object in the upper nasal field of vision is formed on the lower temporal quadrant of the retina. The fovea centralis is the point of greatest visual acuity; it focuses everything that is closely and critically viewed. Light stimulates nerve impulses, which are conducted through the retina, optic nerve, and optic tract on each side, and then through a curving tract called the optic radiation, ending in the visual cortex, a part of the occipital lobe of the brain. **Figure 6-4** depicts visual pathways.

Visual Fields

The field of vision is the area that can be visualized when the eye is not moving. Visual fields are described as circles from the patient's point of view. The center of the circle represents the focus of gaze with a 90-degree circumference from that point of gaze. Each visual field is divided into quadrants for descriptive purposes. The fields extend farthest on the temporal sides. Visual fields are normally limited by the eyebrows above, the zygomatic bone below, and the nose medially. The lack of retinal receptors at the optic disc produces an oval blind spot in the normal field of each eye, at 15 degrees temporally to the line of gaze. When a person is using both eyes, the visual fields overlap, creating binocular vision. Peripheral vision (or lateral vision) is monocular.

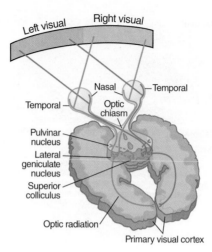

FIGURE 6-4 Visual pathways.

Health History

Essential to successful diagnosis and treatment is a careful history of present illness (HPI), past medical history (PMI), social and family history, and review of systems; this includes pertinent positives and pertinent negatives appropriate to the system.

Chief Complaint and History of Present Illness

"My eye hurts; I may have gotten something in it."

> LP is a 44-year-old woman who presents with a 1-day history of right eye pain, photophobia, and loss of vision. She relates that yesterday she was working in her garden when she began to experience tearing and discomfort. Ms. P attempted to wash her eye with an eyewash solution at home. She has no relief with over-the-counter eyedrops for redness. She wears extended-wear soft contact lenses.

Before the healthcare provider begins any assessment process, it is important to determine the main reason for the clinic/hospital visit. This allows the healthcare provider to focus her or his assessment activities, which would include a careful review of the chief complaint (CC) and symptom analysis. Common chief complaints related to the eye include pain, foreign body sensation, red eye, and vision loss/change. Patients often present with various combinations of these symptoms. Different combinations suggest different underlying disorders. For example, red eye without pain or visual impairment may suggest conjunctivitis or blepharitis, whereas red eye with pain and vision impairment may suggest glaucoma, scleritis, or keratitis. Pain and foreign body sensation are discussed in detail below.

Eye Pain
Eye pain is a common ocular symptom. The examiner must distinguish between pain with acute loss of vision and pain with tearing caused by a foreign body.

Onset	Is onset sudden or gradual?
	How did pain start? What was patient doing just prior to onset of symptom?
Quality	Is this eye pain or irritation?

Location and radiation	Is the pain in the right eye, left eye, or both eyes? Does the pain extend beyond the eye?
	Herpetic lesions on the cornea may start with a painful dermatitis surrounding the eye.
Severity	Ask the patient to rate the pain on a scale of 1 to 10.
	Severe eye pain may indicate corneal ulcer, uveitis, acute angle-closure glaucoma, and endophthalmitis.
Timing	When did the pain start?
Precipitating factors	Has the patient experienced any trauma?
	Has the eye been exposed to foreign bodies or extreme light, such as a welder's arc?
	Has the patient applied anything to his or her eye?
	Various products may irritate the eye. Neosporin is sensitizing to the eye and should be avoided.
Associated symptoms	Is there blurring of the entire visual field or part of it?
	Is there diplopia (double vision) or photophobia?
	Does the patient complain of halos?
	Glaucoma often presents with eye pain, photophobia, and visualization of halos.
Alleviating factors	What relieves the pain?

Foreign Body Sensation

Foreign body sensation, or the feeling that something is in the eye, is a common ocular complaint. It can result from "dry eyes," conjunctival abrasion/irritation to conjunctiva, or corneal foreign bodies.

Onset	Ask about the onset. Was it sudden or gradual?
	When did discomfort start?
	Patients presenting 24 hours after onset of pain may indicate that a formerly pinpoint metal foreign body is now a "rust ring."
Location and radiation	Is foreign body sensation in one or both eyes?
	Is the foreign body felt in a specific location in the eye?
	A specific location of the foreign body is highly suggestive of an actual foreign body.
	A slight delay in using anesthetic medication can assist with direct visualization.
Severity	Ask the patient to rate the discomfort.
Associated symptoms	Ask about associated symptoms, including pain, redness, and vision loss or changes.
Precipitating factors	Ask about activities with exposure to foreign bodies, such as sanding or welding.
Alleviating factors	What relieves the symptoms?

Past Medical History

> Ms. P wears extended-wear soft contact lenses for refraction. She sees an ophthalmologist annually for screening. She has no history of past eye surgeries, trauma, or problems, including glaucoma. Ms. P does not have a history of diabetes, hypertension, or heart disease. She has never received a blood transfusion.

The healthcare provider should ask detailed questions focusing on all past medical illnesses and traumatic events, including elective surgeries. This information will provide critical information that will aid in the formulation of a detailed and comprehensive plan of care.

Past health conditions or surgeries	Ask about health conditions, including hypertension, diabetes, hyperthyroidism, and seasonal or perennial allergies. *Diabetes as well as heart and thyroid disease may be evidenced by visualization of the retinal structures. They may also directly affect vision.* Ask about eye surgeries, including information regarding the condition, date, and outcome. *Previous surgery could suggest an underlying pathology or disease state (e.g., lens implant for keratoconus).*
Traumas or injuries to the eyes	Inquire about history of incident, structures damaged, efforts to correct damage, and degree of success of those efforts. *For instance, corneal trauma may have resulted in permanent loss of vision in affected eye.*
Use of glasses or contact lenses	Does the patient wear eyeglasses or contact lenses? *The patient's response provides information regarding baseline visual acuity, refraction, and infection risk associated with soft contact lenses or extended-wear lenses.* *For example, soft contact lens wearers are at higher risk for* Pseudomonas *infection.*
Last ocular examination	Ask about the date and findings of the last ocular examination.

Family History

> Ms. P's family history is positive for hypertension and negative for coronary artery disease, asthma, diabetes, and cancer. Her parents and siblings are alive and well. There is no history of genetic defects. Ms. P has no children.

Many pathological conditions "run in families"; diseases that might be rare have more significance in the history if there is a genetic link. A family history (FH) of open-angle glaucoma is associated with a five- to sixfold increase in the risk of glaucoma development.

Age of living relatives	Include relationship and health of parents, brothers, sisters, and children.
Deaths	Include relationship of deceased to patient and cause of death (specifically illnesses that affect the eye).
Chronic diseases	Ask about chronic diseases in the family; include relationship of the patient to the family member with the disease and how long that family member has had the disease. Focus on eye diseases that maybe familial or genetic, such as glaucoma and albinism.
Genetic defects	Is there any history of genetic disorders or congenital birth defects?

Social History

In taking the social history (SH), determine your patient's ability to interact with others in healthy ways. Therefore, in addition to inquiring about hobbies and social interactions, examine patient's use of alcohol and ask directly about the use of tobacco and illegal drugs because they can affect the physical examination and visual findings.

> Ms. P denies tobacco or drug use. She reports alcohol use of one to two glasses of wine on weekends. Ms. P is single and works as a kindergarten teacher. She enjoys working in her garden.

Family	Ask to describe current family unit.
Occupation	Ask about occupation.
	Some occupations put patients at higher risk for eye trauma and foreign bodies. For example, welders may have ultraviolet keratoconjunctivitis, a painful condition from exposure to ultraviolet light, especially if eye protection is ill fitting or not worn.
	Determine the patient's need for specific visual acuity and color discrimination.
Hobbies	Ask about hobbies and activities, including welding, grinding, and sanding.
	Fine dust or metallic particles can become imbedded in the cornea.
	Inquire about other possibilities of noxious or traumatic exposure.
Use of tobacco	Ask about tobacco use, including types, amounts, duration of use, and exposure to secondary smoke. Also, inquire about efforts to quit smoking, including factors influencing success or failure.
	Assessment of the fundus can reveal the vascular changes that occur with long-term tobacco use.
Use of alcohol	Does the patient drink alcohol? How much?
	What type (i.e., wine, beer, liquor)?
	See Appendix A: CAGE Assessment.
	Alcohol use increases the risk of injury.
Use of recreational drugs	Does the patient use recreational drugs? If so, inquire as to how much, what type (e.g., ecstasy, PCP, cocaine, heroin), and patterns of use.
	Drugs have systemic effects that may be observed during the eye exam. *Cocaine and amphetamines may cause mydriasis (pupil dilation). Heroin may cause miosis (pupil constriction). Heroin, alcohol, benzodiazepines, cocaine, and amphetamines may cause slow, delayed, sluggish, or absent pupil response.*

Review of Systems

Many eye diseases/disorders have manifestations in systems or parts other than the eyes. A comprehensive review of systems (ROS; see Chapter 1) should be performed whenever possible; however, due to time and other types of constraints, the provider may only be able to perform a focused ROS. During a focused ROS, the provider focuses questioning on the systems in which eye problems are most likely to have manifestations. Below is a summary of common manifestations of eye problems.

System	Symptom or Sign	Possible Associated Diseases/Disorders
Endocrine	Diabetes (polyuria, polydipsia, obesity, frequent infections)	Diabetic retinopathy, vascular disease
Cardiac	Increased blood pressure	Ocular hemorrhage
Neurologic	Headache	Papilledema (increased intracranial pressure) Glaucoma (increased intraocular pressure)
	Nystagmus (congenital)	Hydrocephalus, diencephalic tumors, medication toxicity, Arnold–Chiari malformation, brain tumors or anomalies
	Nystagmus (acquired)	Blindness, multiple sclerosis, peripheral vestibular disease, cerebellar or brain stem disease, drug use

Physical Examination

Equipment Needed

- Snellen eye chart or E chart
- Handheld near-vision screener (Rosenbaum or Jaeger)
- Cover card (opaque)
- Penlight
- Ophthalmoscope
- Color vision plates—Ishihara or Hardy-Rand-Ritter (optional—for specific screening, e.g., Department of Transportation physicals)
- Allen figures

Components of Physical Examination

Physical examination of the eye involves testing visual acuity, visual fields, and extraocular movements; inspection; palpation (to a lesser extent); and ophthalmoscopic examination.

Testing Visual Acuity, Visual Fields, Extraocular Movements, and Color Discrimination

Visual acuity is the "vital sign" in ophthalmology. **Box 6-1** describes the technique for testing acuity. Examination of the eyes also involves testing visual fields, which is described in **Box 6-2**.

BOX 6-1   TESTING VISUAL ACUITY

TESTING CENTRAL VISION

Test acuity of central vision with a Snellen eye chart, which tests the optic nerve. Patients who wear glasses (other than for just reading) should use them for testing.

Technique
- Position the patient 20 feet from the chart.
- Ask the patient to cover one eye with a card and read the smallest line possible.
- Determine the smallest line of print from which the patient can identify more than half the letters or symbols.
- Record the visual acuity designated at the right of each line.

Expressing and Documenting Visual Acuity

Acuity is expressed as two numbers (e.g., 20/40). The first number describes the patient's distance from the chart (20 feet), and the second describes the distance at which the normal eye can read the line of letters or symbols. Vision 20/200 means that at 20 feet the patient can read print that a person with normal vision could read at 200 feet. A larger second number corresponds to a worse vision. As the second number increases, the vision becomes worse. Legal blindness is usually defined as 20/200 or less. Note: Inability to test or decreased visual acuity requires immediate referral to an ophthalmologist.

The following are examples of documented findings, along with explanations.

"20/40 corrected" refers to a patient's acuity (20/40) while wearing a corrective device, such as contact lens or glasses.

"20/40 −2" refers to acuity with the number of errors. In this case, the patient misread two letters, which is documented as −2. The minus number reflects the number of errors the patient missed per line of visual acuity. Usually, if a patient misses more than 2 per line, the next larger line up is used.

OTHER TESTING

Testing near vision with a special handheld card helps identify presbyopia. With age (past the age of 40), eyes lose their ability to accommodate (presbyopia). The patient may need to move the card farther away to focus it more clearly. The special handheld card may be useful at the bedside for vision screening. If charts for visual acuity screening are not available, substitute available print (e.g., newspaper).

BOX 6-2   TESTING VISUAL FIELDS

Screening tests the patient's visual fields. To perform this test, face the patient, gazing eye to eye. Imagine a sphere or bowl encircles the patient's head; place your outstretched hands lateral to the patient's ears about 2 feet apart. Ask the patient to touch your fingers as they come into his or her line of vision. Slowly move your fingers along the imaginary sphere or bowl and toward the patient's line of gaze until the patient identifies them. Repeat this pattern in the upper and lower temporal quadrants. Most common defects occur in the temporal visual fields. If the patient sees the fingers on each side simultaneously, his or her fields of vision are normal.

If you find a defect in the visual fields, test further. Instruct the patient to cover one eye, leaving the eye with the suspected defect uncovered. Face the patient and mirror the patient, covering the opposite eye and looking directly into the patient's uncovered eye. Slowly move your fingers from the defective area to the patient's better field of vision, noting where the patient first responds. Repeat at different levels, thus mapping the area of visual field loss. Often a temporal defect in the visual field of one eye indicates a nasal defect *associated with* the other eye. Repeat the test on the opposite eye to check for a nasal defect.

Color vision is generally assessed to screen for any defects that might impair safety and performance. In addition, loss of color vision is specific for central retinal or optic nerve dysfunction. Discrimination of color is a major safety consideration for certain occupations (e.g., a taxi driver needs to be able to correctly identify traffic signals). Several screening measures are available, including identifying numbers of different colors on Ishihara plates.

Inspection and Palpation

Action	Rationale
1. Inspect extraocular muscle function.	
a. Inspect the corneal light reflex for symmetry (Hirschberg test). Ask patient to stare straight ahead with both eyes open. In a lighted room, stand at a distance of 12 to 15 inches (30 to 38 centimeters) from the patient and shine a penlight toward the bridge of her nose.	a. Light reflections should appear symmetrically in both pupils. When an imbalance is found in the corneal light reflex, perform the cover-uncover test to confirm (see step b). If the Hirschberg test or the cover-uncover test is abnormal, it may indicate a condition called *amblyopia* or, most commonly, *strabismus*.
b. To perform the cover-uncover test, ask the patient to stare straight ahead on a particular object. (A small toy is often helpful when assessing children.) Cover one of the patient's eyes with an opaque card. Assess the uncovered eye's position, noting any deviation from a steady, fixed gaze. Then remove the card and assess the now uncovered eye for movement or deviation. It should not move. Repeat the test on the other eye.	b. If covered eye moves to focus after removing its cover, it is the weaker eye. This requires further investigation by an ophthalmologist.

Action

c. Assess extraocular muscles for movement through the six cardinal fields of gaze. **Box 6-3** describes the technique.

Rationale

c. Normally there is parallel, conjugate movement of both eyes. Mild nystagmus (an involuntary movement of the eyeball in a horizontal, vertical, rotary, or mixed direction) at the extreme lateral gaze is normal but should not persist beyond a few beats.

Eye movement that is not parallel or conjugate indicates an extraocular muscle weakness or dysfunction of CN III, IV, or VI.

BOX 6-3   TESTING EXTRAOCULAR MOVEMENTS

To test extraocular movements in the six cardinal directions of gaze, ask the patient to follow your finger (without turning the head) as you move it *slowly* from up to down and midline, forming an invisible "H" with your movements. Look for loss of conjugate movements. Assess for convergence. Identify any nystagmus and the direction of gaze in which it occurs. Describe the nystagmus in the plane that the movements occur (e.g., horizontal, vertical, rotary, or mixed).

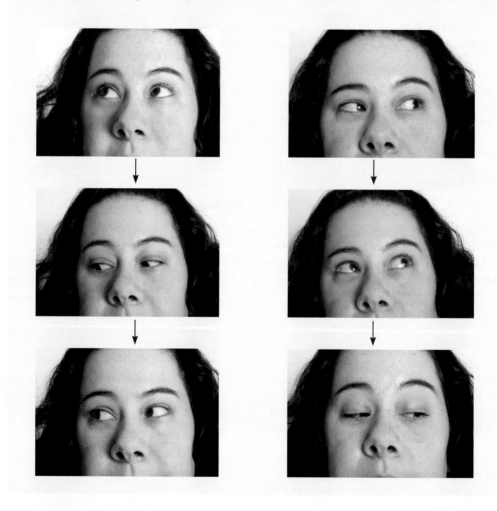

Action

2. Assess position and alignment of the eyes.

3. Inspect the eyebrows for quality, hair distribution, and symmetry. Note the underlying skin.

4. Inspect eyelids and eyelashes.
   a. Assess symmetry, position, and closure.

   b. Inspect eyelids for color, swelling, lesions, nodules, styes, and discharge.

Rationale

2. Inward or outward deviation of the eyes or abnormal protrusion (proptosis) may indicate Graves' disease.

3. Flakiness, hair loss, scaling, and unequal alignment are abnormal findings.
   Loss of the lateral portion of the eyebrow may be seen in hypothyroidism.

a. Eyelashes should be symmetrical and curve slightly outward. Palpebral fissures should be equal, and the upper lid margins should cover part of the iris but not the pupil. Lid closure should be completed without difficulty. Ptosis (eyelids appear droopy) may be seen with third nerve palsy and myasthenia gravis. **Figure 6-5** demonstrates ptosis.

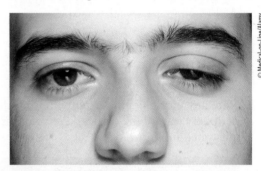

FIGURE 6-5 Congenital ptosis of the left upper eyelid.

b. Lid margins should be pink without edema, exudates, lesions, nodules, or redness.
   Xanthelasma are creamy yellow plaque on the eyelids (**Figure 6-6**). These may indicate abnormal lipid deposits.

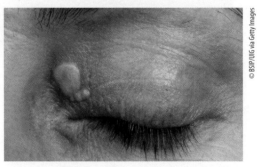

FIGURE 6-6 Xanthelasma.

A stye, or external hordeolum, is an abscess in the eyelash follicle (**Figure 6-7**). Styes are painful.

A chalazion is an inflammatory granuloma of a meibomian gland.

Crusting of the eyelids, thickening of the eyelids, and plugging of the meibomian glands suggest blepharitis (**Figure 6-8**).

Action	Rationale
© Heiko Barth/Shutterstock FIGURE 6-7 Stye.	© Western Ophthalmic Hospital/Science Source FIGURE 6-8 Infectious blepharitis.
c. Inspect the margins of the eyelid for entropion (infolding) and ectropion (rolling outward).	c. Entropion and ectropion may cause burning and irritation.
d. Assess blinking.	d. Blinking normally occurs bilaterally and involuntarily at about 15 to 20 blinks per minute.
5. Inspect lacrimal apparatus and conjunctiva.	
a. Assess for swelling of the lacrimal sac.	a. Swelling may be present with lacrimal duct obstruction.
b. Note any pterygium (tissue growth from the periphery toward the cornea). Pterygium is illustrated in **Figure 6-9**.	b. Commonly, pterygia develop in response to chronic irritation of the cornea, such as wind.
© BSIP SA/Alamy FIGURE 6-9 Early pterygium.	
c. Note any lesions, nodules, or foreign bodies.	c. All foreign bodies (except for those removed easily by irrigation), lesions, and nodules should be referred to an ophthalmologist.
d. Assess color of conjunctiva. Inspect for erythema, exudate, and hemorrhages.	d. Conjunctiva should be pink, not red or pale. Redness may indicate infection or irritation; paleness may indicate severe anemia. Viral conjunctivitis often presents with lid swelling and conjunctival redness; bacterial conjunctivitis (**Figure 6-10**) presents with conjunctival injection, lid swelling, and discharge. Bright red blood with defined borders indicates a subconjunctival hemorrhage.

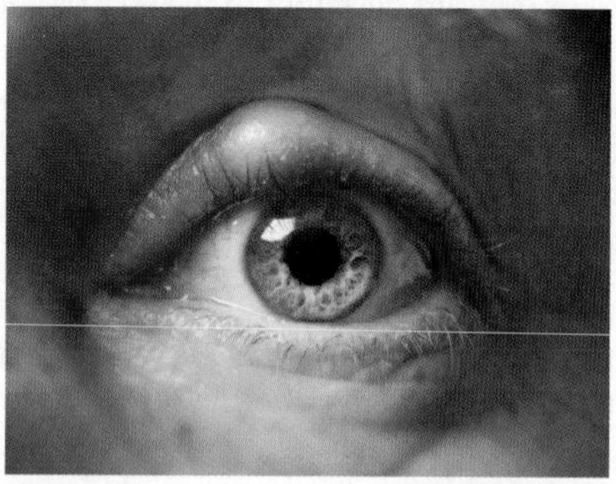

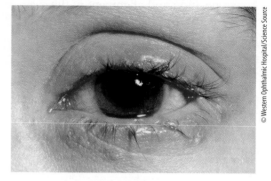

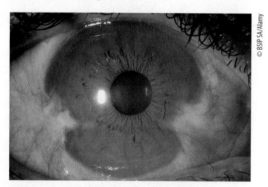

Action

Rationale

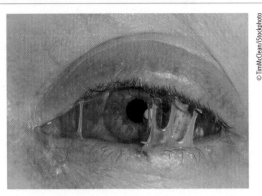

FIGURE 6-10 Acute bacterial conjunctivitis.

e. Pull down and evert the lower lid and ask the patient to look up. Assess the palpebral conjunctiva.

f. Inspect blood vessels on the sclera and conjunctiva.

g. Press on the lower lid close to the medial canthus. Assess for any fluid secreted out of the puncta into the eye.

6. Inspect the sclera for color and clarity.

7. Inspect the cornea for transparency and surface characteristics. *Using oblique lighting*, slowly move the light reflection over the corneal surface. Observe for a transparent, smooth surface that is clear and shiny.

   The ophthalmoscope at +20 diopter may be used to magnify any lesions if a slit lamp is not readily available. (See **Box 6-4** for slit lamp use.)

8. Use fluorescein to stain the eye and irrigate to highlight any lesions or some foreign bodies. All eye complaints without globe penetration should be evaluated with fluorescein. Fluorescein paper strips, not liquid, should be used to avoid contamination. Cobalt blue light in darkened room highlights lesions.

e. The palpebral conjunctiva should be opaque, pink, and vascular.

f. Blood vessels should not be congested. Congestion indicates irritation.

g. Secretion of mucopurulent fluid from the puncta suggests an obstructed lacrimal duct.

6. Sclera should be white and moist. Yellow sclera may indicate jaundice due to hepatic or biliary disease.

7. Note any opacities or irregularities in the corneal surface.

   A white opaque ring around the limbus is called *arcus senilis* (**Figure 6-11**). Whereas arcus senilis may be found commonly in the elderly, investigate for hyperlipidemia if found in a patient under 40.

   Metal foreign bodies may leave a rust ring (**Figure 6-12**).

8. Yellow-orange stain fluoresces with corneal lesions. Painful herpetic lesions of the cornea will absorb fluorescein to facilitate visualization (**Figure 6-13**).

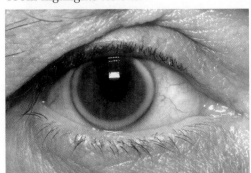

FIGURE 6-11 Arcus senilis.

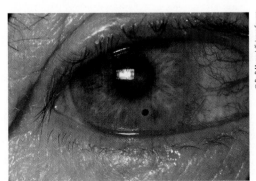

FIGURE 6-12 Corneal rust ring.

BOX 6-4   USING A SLIT LAMP FOR EXAMINATION

The anterior portion of the eye is best examined with a slit lamp biomicroscope. Ask the patient to place his or her chin on the chin rest and forehead against the forehead rest. Once the patient is in position, the slit lamp magnifies the anterior and posterior segments of the eye for more in-depth assessment by moving the binocular lens and a light source at 45 degrees to the patient/examiner axis. The beam can delineate separate layers of the cornea and intraocular content.

Action

Rationale

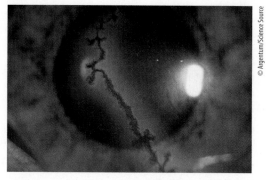

FIGURE 6-13 Fluorescein staining reveals herpetic lesions.

9. Evaluate the depth of the anterior chamber by shining a light from the side and assessing for the presence of a crescent shadow.

9. A shadow is not normally seen. A flat iris and adequate chamber depth allow light to pass without creating a shadow. (See further discussion below, in lid.)

10. Assess for hyphema (blood in the anterior chamber).

10. Hyphema (**Figure 6-14**) is usually the result of trauma or surgery.

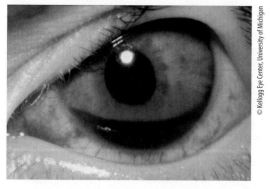

FIGURE 6-14 Hyphema.

11. Inspect pupils.

a. Assess for size and shape.

a. Pupils should be round and equal in size. Abnormal pupil size or reaction may indicate drug use, change in intracranial pressure, congenital anomalies, or prior surgery.

Action	Rationale
b. Test reaction to light. The constricting response of the pupils to a bright, direct light is a papillary reflex. Shine a penlight onto the pupil; it should constrict briskly with a consensual reaction of the other pupil. Check each eye for direct and consensual reaction.	**b.** Failure of pupils to constrict briskly indicates dysfunction of cranial nerve III. Direct reaction refers to the constriction of the pupil receiving the light. The constriction of the pupil that is not receiving increased light is the consensual reaction. As a general rule, a pupil reacting poorly to direct light is an abnormal reaction. Poor papillary reaction occurs with a variety of conditions, including increased intracranial pressure to local instillation of mydriatics. It should always be explored and referred if necessary. Pupils should be equal, round, and reactive to light (PERRL). Because the examiner cannot directly assess accommodation, only convergence (the pupillary constriction and focus medially as object is brought near), only the abbreviation PERRL is accurate.
c. Assess convergence by asking the patient to focus on a distant object and then shift her or his gaze to a near object.	**c.** Pupils normally dilate when focusing on a distant object. When patient shifts gaze to a near object the pupils constrict and converge. Poor convergence maybe seen in hyperthyroidism.

d. Inspect each iris.	**d.** Iris marking should be clearly visible.
	
	  In acute narrow-angle glaucoma, increased intraocular pressure diminishes the normal spatial relationship between the iris and cornea. This occurs when drainage of aqueous humor is blocked. The patient will present with a complaint of a painful eye that appears "steamy" to the observer and is usually unilateral. Shining a penlight on the iris laterally creates a crescent shadow, indicating increased intraocular pressure as seen in acute narrow-angle glaucoma.
	
	  (The more common type of glaucoma is open-angle glaucoma, which is often without symptoms but may cause some decreased vision. Diagnosis is made by measuring intraocular pressure.)

Special Tests

Action	Rationale
12. Assess corneal reflex in selected patients only (usually unconscious patients). Lightly touch cornea with wisp of cotton. **Figure 6-15** demonstrates technique.	**12.** The lids of both eyes will normally close when either eye is touched. Failure of both eyes to close indicates increased intracranial pressure, which impairs the sensory branch (CN V) and motor branch (CN VII).

Action

Rationale

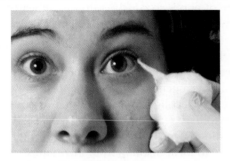

FIGURE 6-15 Testing corneal reflex.

13. **If patient complains of eye pain or foreign body sensation, evert the upper lid.** Gently grasp upper eyelashes and pull downward. Place a cotton-tipped applicator midway on the upper lid. Using slight pressure, evert lid over the applicator. **Figure 6-16** demonstrates technique. Examine the lid for swelling, tenderness, and foreign bodies.

To thoroughly irrigate the eye, evert both upper and lower eyelids on their respective tarsal plates and use an eyewash or normal saline solution to gently irrigate the entire eye.

To return the lid to normal, gently pull on the lashes and ask patient to look up and blink. The lid easily returns to normal.

13. Eversion is necessary to evaluate foreign body sensation.

Eversion of both tarsal plates is necessary to adequately irrigate. Individuals cannot adequately irrigate their own eyes.

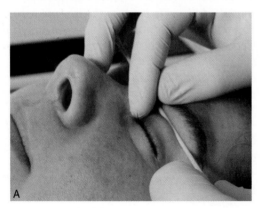
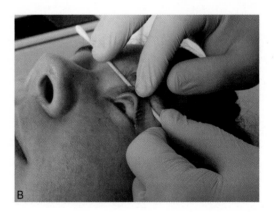

FIGURE 6-16 Everting the upper eyelid.

Fundoscopic Assessment

Fundoscopy in the primary care setting is generally performed on nondilated pupils, which limits the adequacy of the examination. Mydriatic drops are rarely used in the primary care setting. Contraindications for the drops include increased ocular pressure (glaucoma) and susceptibility to angle-closure glaucoma. Use caution in infants and young children because of increased susceptibility to systemic effects of the drugs. Techniques for using ophthalmoscopes are described in **Boxes 6-5** and **6-6**.

BOX 6-5   OPHTHALMOSCOPIC EXAMINATION TECHNIQUE

For ophthalmoscopic examination, use the following technique:

1. If the patient is wearing glasses, ask him or her to remove them; contact lenses may be worn during the examination.
2. Darken the room to dilate the patient's pupil.
3. Have the patient focus on a distant object on the wall.
4. Adjust the lens of the ophthalmoscope to focus on a near object, such as a watch, or set the lens to 0 diopter. Place the index finger on the selection wheel to change settings in order to adjust focus.
5. Begin at about 10 inches away from the patient at a 15-degree angle lateral to the patient's line of vision.
6. To examine the patient's right eye, use your right hand to hold the ophthalmoscope and your right eye to look through it. Conversely, use your left hand and eye to examine the patient's left eye.

Tip: Hold your breath during ophthalmoscopic examination of each eye; this minimizes prolonged examination, which is irritating and uncomfortable for patients.

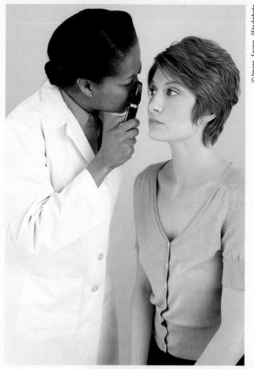

Patient having eyes examined.

BOX 6-6   TECHNIQUE FOR USING A PANOPTIC OPHTHALMOSCOPE

To use a PanOptic Ophthalmoscope, employ the following technique:

1. Explain to your patient that the eyecup will touch the brow. Instruct patient to try not to move her or his head and to focus straight ahead.
2. Although not required, it is recommended that you (the examiner) remove your eyeglasses so that the scope can be brought closer to your eye for a better view.
3. Look through the scope with your thumb on the dynamic focusing wheel and focus on an object in the room that is at least 10 to 15 feet away. Focus the scope on the object so that it is clear and sharp.
4. Next, make sure that the aperture dial is set to the small aperture or "home" position. The setting is marked with a green indicator line on the dial. It is the ideal setting for a typical undilated pupil.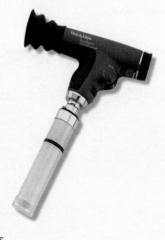
5. Using any standard Welch Allyn 3.5-volt power source, turn the scope on. Adjust the light intensity rheostat to its maximum position.
6. Shine the light at the patient's eye and look for the red retinal reflex. Slowly follow the red reflex toward the patient and into the pupil.
7. The eyecup should be compressed about half its length to maximize the view.
8. At this point, a large view of the entire optic disc and surrounding vessels should be visible. This wide view makes it much easier to see important funduscopic features and to follow the vessels out to the periphery.
9. After examining the right eye, just repeat the procedure for the left eye. Another unique feature of the PanOptic Scope is that it is not necessary to switch your eye. If you are right eye dominant, for example, you can use your right eye to examine both of your patient's eyes.

Content and photograph courtesy of Welch Allyn, Skaneateles Falls, New York.

Action	Rationale
1. Observe the red reflex bilaterally created by light illuminating the retina.	1. An absence of a red reflex may indicate retinal detachment, chorioretinitis, or retinoblastoma. A white retinal reflex is called leukokoria. Visualizing the red reflex is especially important for screening newborns and infants to determine the absence of leukokoria or congenital cataract.
2. Move closer to the eye, adjusting the diopter of the lens to inspect the optic disc for shape and color.	2. The optic disc should be round or oval with distinct clear margins. Its color should be creamy yellow to pink. **Figure 6-17** depicts a normal fundus. Papilledema refers to bilateral optic disc edema characterized by blurring of disc margins, which indicates elevated intracranial pressure.
Note the appearance of the physiological cup.	The physiological cup is the small depression just lateral to the disc's center. The cup is lighter than the disc and its diameter is less than half the diameter of the disc. Cupping may be observed in patients with glaucoma (**Figure 6-18**). The cupping is a result of increased intraocular pressure. Asymmetry of the size of physiological cups bilaterally also suggests glaucoma (**Figure 6-19**).

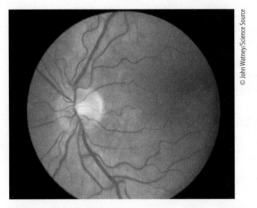

FIGURE 6-17 Normal fundus.

© John Watney/Science Source

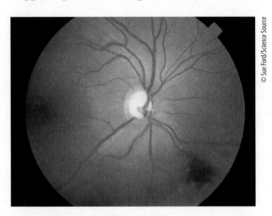

FIGURE 6-18 Glaucomatous cupping.

© Sue Ford/Science Source

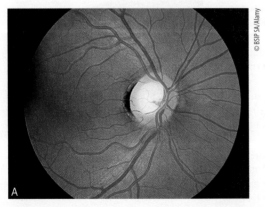

A

© BSIP SA/Alamy

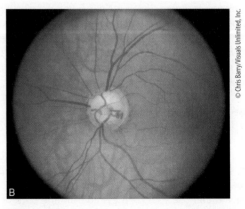

B

© Chris Barry/Visuals Unlimited, Inc.

FIGURE 6-19 Asymmetry of the physiological cups, indicating glaucoma.

Action	Rationale
3. From the optic disc, follow the retinal vessels in four directions from the disc, noting their relative sizes and characteristics at arteriovenous crossings.	3. When compared to veins, arteries are lighter red and may have a narrow band of light in the center. Veins are darker red and about 25% larger than arteries. In hypertensive retinopathy, there may be narrowing of the retinal arteries and changes in arteriovenous crossings.
4. Inspect for retinal background hemorrhages, exudates, and lesions.	4. Hypertensive retinopathy also presents with retinal hemorrhages, hard exudation, and cotton-wool spots (**Figure 6-20**). Microaneurysms, exudate, and edema occur in nonproliferative diabetic retinopathy (**Figure 6-21**). Numerous retinal hemorrhages, venous abnormalities, and neovascularization of the disc suggest proliferative diabetic retinopathy (**Figure 6-22**). Superficial retinal whitening along with a cherry red spot indicates central retinal artery occlusion (**Figure 6-23**).

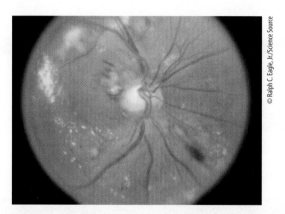

FIGURE 6-20 Grade III hypertensive retinopathy.

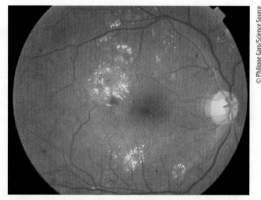

FIGURE 6-21 Nonproliferative diabetic retinopathy.

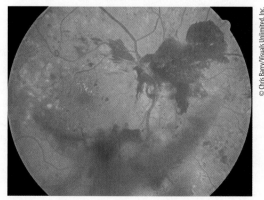

FIGURE 6-22 Proliferative diabetic retinopathy.

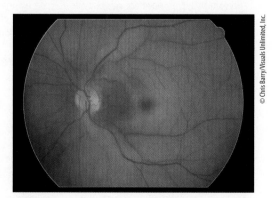

FIGURE 6-23 Central retinal artery occlusion.

Action	Rationale
5. Inspect the macula for color and surface by having the patient focus directly on the light.	5. A small reflex of light seen directly over the macula (foveal light reflex) is an indicator of normal foveal anatomy. It should always be recorded as positive (normal) or negative. If it is diminished, you should record it as + but diminished or small. A negative foveal light reflex may be the result of drusen, retinal pigment epithelium migration, edema, or age-related macular degeneration.

Box 6-7 provides several clinical tips that are helpful in assessment of eye disorders.

Diagnostic Reasoning

Based on findings in the health history and physical examination, the clinician should formulate an assessment and plan. For example, a patient may report symptoms that suggest many possible diagnoses; however, findings in the past medical history and during the physical examination narrow the possible diagnoses down to one or two. Eye pain is a common chief complaint. **Table 6-1** illustrates differential diagnosis of common disorders associated with eye pain.

BOX 6-7   POINTS TO REMEMBER

- Soft contact lens wearers are at higher risk for *Pseudomonas* infection.
- Neosporin is sensitizing to the eye and should be avoided.
- All eye complaints without globe penetration should be evaluated with fluorescein.
- Painful herpetic lesions of the cornea will absorb fluorescein to facilitate visualization.
- Steroid eyedrops should never be used in the primary care setting where ocular pressure cannot be adequately measured.

Table 6-1   Differential Diagnosis of Eye Pain

Differential Diagnosis	Significant Findings in the Patient's History	Significant Findings in the Patient's Physical Examination	Diagnostic Tests
Foreign body	Known foreign body or participation in activity with high possibility of foreign body	Tearing, visualization of foreign body, relief of pain after thorough irrigation with tarsal plates everted	Fluorescein stain, examination with cobalt blue light, ophthalmic or slit lamp examination
Corneal abrasion	Eye pain, especially if following known foreign body or injury	Tearing, photophobia, corneal defect	Fluorescein stain, examination with cobalt blue light, ophthalmic or slit lamp examination
Hyphema	Eye pain and history of trauma	Blood in the anterior chamber	Observation and referral to ophthalmology
Herpetic lesions	Eye pain, herpetic rash on face may be present, no history of trauma	Vesicular rash seen in the distribution of the first division of CN V. (If tip of the nose is involved [Hutchinson's sign], ocular involvement is likely.) Epithelial dendrite stains green with fluorescein dye.	Fluorescein stain, examination with cobalt blue light, ophthalmic or slit lamp examination

Eye Assessment of Special Populations

Considerations for the Pregnant Patient

Remember a pregnant woman's eyes become more sensitive and dry due to a small change in lacrimal duct function; this makes contact lens use more difficult.

Considerations for the Neonatal Patient
General

- Note that during the first 8 weeks of gestation, the fetus's eyes are formed, making them particularly vulnerable to intrauterine drug exposure or maternal infection, both of which can cause eye malformations.
- Note the following physiological variations:
  - Neonates have a visual acuity of 20/200.
  - Peripheral vision is fully developed at birth; however, central vision develops later.

Inspection and Ophthalmoscopic Examination
- Assess red reflex.
- Assess ocular mobility by having the infant follow a brightly colored object or toy.

Considerations for the Pediatric Patient
General

- Recognize changes occurring at various ages:
  - At 2 to 3 months of age, the infant begins to have voluntary control over eye muscles.
  - At about 2 to 3 months of age, the lacrimal ducts begin carrying tears into the nasal meatus.
  - At 8 months, the infant can distinguish colors.
  - At 9 months, the eyes are able to perceive a single image, reflecting the eye muscle's ability to coordinate.
  - Young children's eyes are more spherical, making vision myopic.
  - Adult visual acuity is achieved around the age of 6.
  - Children who have a family history of amblyopia, "lazy-eye," or "crossed eyes"; who are developmentally delayed (e.g., trisomy 21); or who have cerebral palsy are at higher risk of vision problems and should be referred to an ophthalmologist for screening.
- Include the following during the health history:
  - Note any prophylactic gonococcal antibiotic administration.
  - Ask about history of maternal vaginal infection, including the type and treatment.
  - Question regarding a history of mechanical ventilation with high oxygen.
  - Note child's achievement of developmental milestones regarding vision.
  - Inquire about vision screening in school each year. Determine whether the child is able to see chalkboard or classroom instructive devices clearly. Ask if the child has difficulty reading.

Inspection and Ophthalmoscopic Examination
- Assess red reflex.
- Assess ocular mobility by having the child follow a brightly colored object or toy.
- After 6 months of age, perform the cover-uncover test.
- Begin visual acuity screening after age 3.
- Assess binocular vision (stereoacuity).

Considerations for the Geriatric Patient
General

- Note the following physiological changes:
  - Tearing is diminished, resulting in "dry eyes."
  - Decreased corneal sensitivity leads to diminished sensation of infection or injury.

- Color perception becomes altered (difficulty with blue, violet, and green).
- The lens becomes more rigid (around age 45), causing presbyopia.
- Increased density of the lens and degeneration of iris cells, cornea, and lens cause light scattering and sensitivity to glare.

Inspection and Ophthalmoscopic Examination
- Observe changes in the external structure of the eye, including graying of eyebrows and eyelashes, along with loss of tone and decreased elasticity of eyelid muscles.
- Note corneal reflexes may be decreased or absent.
- Test visual acuity in older adults to assess for diminished vision.
- Perform ophthalmoscopy during routine health assessments in older adults.
- Screen for glaucoma.

Case Study REVIEW

Throughout this chapter, you have been introduced to Ms. P. This section of the chapter pulls together her history and demonstrates the documentation of her history and physical examination.

Chief Complaint

"My eye hurts; I may have gotten something in it."

Information Gathered During the Interview

Ms. P is a 44-year-old woman who presents with a 1-day history of right eye pain, photophobia, and loss of vision. She relates that yesterday she was working in her garden when she began to experience tearing and discomfort. She attempted to wash her eye with eyewash solution at home. She has no relief with over-the-counter eyedrops for redness. She wears extended-wear soft contact lenses.

Ms. P wears extended-wear soft contact lenses for refraction. She sees an ophthalmologist annually for screening. She has no history of past eye surgeries, trauma, or problems, including glaucoma. Ms. P does not have a history of diabetes, hypertension, or heart disease.

Ms. P's family history is positive for hypertension and negative for coronary artery disease, asthma, diabetes, and cancer. Her parents and siblings are alive and well. There is no history of genetic defects. Ms. P has no children.

Ms. P denies tobacco or drug use. She reports alcohol use of one to two glasses of wine on weekends. Ms. P is single and works as a kindergarten teacher. She enjoys working in her garden.

Clues	Important Points
One-day history of chief complaint	Acute onset
One eye involved	Not likely a systemic problem
History of working in garden at onset	Increased probability of foreign body and/or corneal abrasion secondary to trauma
No relief with previous treatment or eye irrigation	Individuals cannot adequately irrigate their own eyes
Wears extended-wear contact lenses	Higher risk for pseudomonal infection

Name LP		Date 09-20-15	Time 1340
		DOB 12-14-71	Sex F

HISTORY

CC
"My eye hurts; I may have gotten something in it."

HPI
44-year-old woman with a 1-day history of right eye pain, photophobia, and loss of vision. Yesterday she was working in her garden when she began to experience tearing and discomfort. Attempted to wash her eye with an eyeglass and eyewash solution at home. She has no relief with OTC eyedrops for redness. She wears extended-wear soft contact lenses.

Medications
None.

Allergies
Penicillin, sulfa.

PMI
No significant past medical history. Uses extended-wear soft contact lenses for refraction. Sees ophthalmologist annually for screening. No history of past eye surgeries or trauma. No history of blood transfusions.

Hospitalizations/Surgeries
None.

FH
Positive for HTN and negative for coronary artery disease, asthma, diabetes, and cancer.

SH
Patient denies tobacco or drug use. Reports alcohol use to 1–2 glasses of wine on weekends. Works as a kindergarten teacher.

ROS	
Skin	Respiratory
Burns easily with ultraviolet exposure.	No history of cough or shortness of breath.
Eyes	Gastrointestinal
See chief complaint, no history of other symptoms.	No history of constipation, diarrhea, nausea, or vomiting.
Ears	Genitourinary
No history of otalgia, drainage.	No history of dysuria or polyuria.
Mouth/Throat	Gynecological
No history of symptoms.	Menses regular; no history of dysmenorrhea. LMP, 9/1/15.
Breast	Musculoskeletal
No history of masses, discharge.	No history of arthralgias or myalgias.
Cardiovascular	Neurological
No history of chest pain, weight gain, or edema.	No history of vertigo, difficulty with concentration or memory, or headache.

PHYSICAL EXAMINATION		
Weight 178 lb (BMI 28)	Temp 98.6	BP 100/60
Height 5'7"	Pulse 80	Resp 18

General Appearance
Well-developed Native-American who keeps her right eye covered with her hand, but no other apparent distress

Skin
Warm and dry

HEENT
Head normocephalic; neck supple. TMs neutral, grey, transparent, +/- mobility.
Visual acuity: 20/20 OD, 20/30 OS, 20/20 OU with correction (contact lenses).
Pupils equal, round, reactive to light (PERRL).
Extraocular movements intact (EMOI).
+ 4 injection of conjunctiva.
Anterior chamber normal depth.
Cornea with small defect at 3 o'clock OD.

Cardiovascular
RRR, No S3, S4, murmur.

Respiratory
Normal AP to lateral diameter. Lungs clear to auscultation.

Gastrointestinal
+ bowel sounds; no tenderness; no hepatosplenomegaly.

Genitourinary
No CVA tenderness.

Musculoskeletal	
Full range of motion (FROM); no tenderness; neurovascular intact.	
Neurological	
Awake and alert, oriented × 3. CN II–XII grossly intact. Romberg negative. No ataxia, 5/5 strength. No sensory deficits. DTRs +2 upper/lower extremities.	
Other	
Lab Tests	Special Tests
None	Irrigation of OD with tarsal plates everted.
	+Fluorescein uptake. Ophthalmic/slit lamp.
	→ small corneal defect. No foreign body.
Final Assessment Findings	
Corneal abrasion OD at 3 o'clock.	

Bibliography

Chern, K., & Zegens, M. (2011). *Ophthalmology review manual* (2nd ed.). Philadelphia, PA: Lippincott Williams & Wilkins.

Eagling, E. M., & Roper-Hall, M. J. (1986). *Eye injuries: An illustrated guide*. Philadelphia, PA: J. B. Lippincott.

Tasman, W., & Jaeger, E. (Eds.). (2001). *The Wills Eye Hospital atlas of clinical ophthalmology* (2nd ed.). Philadelphia, PA: Lippincott Williams & Wilkins.

Additional Resources

Ophthalmic Examination Instruments

http://see.eyecarecontacts.com/instruments.html
This website describes and provides photographs of various instruments used in eye assessment.

Family Practice Notebook

http://www.fpnotebook.com
Clinicians can search for information on various disorders and examination techniques.

Diseases and Conditions Simulation

http://www.visionsimulations.com
This site provides simulation of the progression of various eye disorders, helping clinicians to understand them and explain them to patients.

Ask NOAH About: The Eye

http://www.noah-health.org/
This site provides a multitude of links related to eye assessment, including information on various disorders, clinical trials and new treatments, and assessment techniques.

Martindale's "Virtual" Medical Center

http://www.martindalecenter.com/MedicalAudio_2_C.html
The site features tutorials and simulations, helping practitioners refine their skills.

Welch Allyn PanOptic Ophthalmoscope

https://www.welchallyn.com/en/students/ophthalmoscopy-pathologies.html
Common normal and abnormal fundoscopic findings are depicted.

Chapter 7

Ear Disorders

Anatomy and Physiology Review of the Ear

The ears are a pair of complex sensory organs of hearing and balance that lie on either side of the head at approximately eye level. The ears contribute to the appearance of the head and face due to their prominent location on the head. The ears are responsible for:

- Interpreting and identifying sound
- Detecting the direction of sound through identification of the intensity and time lag between hearing the sound in one ear and then the other ear
- Maintaining equilibrium

These functions are described in detail below. The ear is divided into three major parts: the outer or external ear, the middle ear, and the inner ear. **Figure 7-1** illustrates the structures of the ear.

Outer Ear

The external ear consists of the pinna (also called the *auricle*) and the ear canal. The pinna is the visible portion of the outer ear and is composed primarily of elastic cartilage covered with skin and very fine hair. Sebaceous glands are located on the skin surface. The lower part of the pinna (the lobule) is composed of fat and subcutaneous tissue. The posterior, anterior, and superior auricular

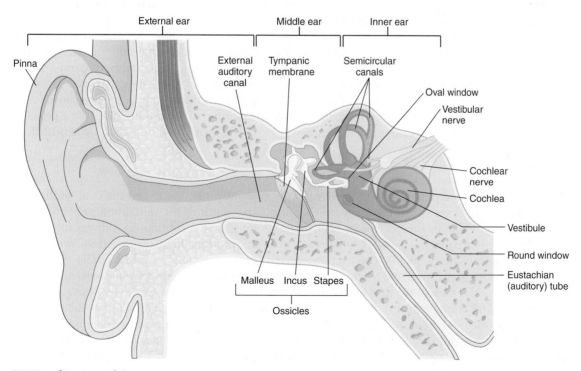

FIGURE 7-1 Structures of the ear.

muscles (which are innervated by a branch of the facial nerve) fasten the cartilaginous ear to the skull. The tragus, a small cartilaginous projection, lies just in front of the opening to the external ear. Also lying near the opening to the external ear canal is the temporomandibular joint (TMJ). Pain in the TMJ may be referred to the ear.

The ear canal is irregular, about 1 inch long, and part of the external ear. It begins at the concha, the deepest part of the pinna, and extends in an inward, forward, and downward direction after age 3; before age 3 the ear canal points upward. The ear canal constricts about midway and again near the tympanic membrane, being narrowest where the cartilage begins its transition to bone. This bending requires the ear canal to be straightened before examining it or the tympanic membrane.

The outer two-thirds of the ear canal are cartilaginous and covered with skin containing sebaceous glands and fine hair follicles. The inner one-third of the ear canal is composed of bone covered with thin, highly sensitive skin containing ceruminous glands. The sticky consistency of cerumen and the fine hairs in the canal provide protection by helping to cleanse the auditory canal of foreign matter. The type of cerumen found in the ear is genetically determined and is one of two major forms: dry cerumen, which is gray and flaky and may form a thin mass in the ear canal, and wet cerumen, which is dark brown and moist. Dry cerumen is found in over 80% of Asians and native North Americans, including Eskimos. Wet cerumen is found in approximately 97% of Caucasians and 99% of African Americans.

Sound waves may be conducted directly though the bones of the skull to stimulate afferent nerve fibers. Most hearing occurs from air conduction through the external, middle, and inner ear. The funnel shape of the external ear begins the hearing process by collecting sound waves and channeling them through the ear canal toward the tympanic membrane, where they are converted into physical vibrations. The pair of ears allows binaural hearing, which is important in the detection of sound direction and for maintaining equilibrium. Determining the direction of sound is accomplished by the brain's capacity to identify the intensity of the sound and the time lag between hearing the sound in one ear and then the other ear.

The tympanic membrane is a thin, translucent, pearly gray oval membrane with blood vessels at the periphery. It is approximately 7–9 mm in diameter and separates the outer ear from the middle ear. **Figure 7-2** illustrates the landmarks of the tympanic membrane. It is composed of an outer skin layer (that is continuous with the skin of the external ear canal), fibrous middle layer, and an inner mucosal layer (that is continuous with the lining of the middle ear). Landmarks that are visible on the surface of the normal tympanic membrane are the annulus, or thickened border that attaches the membrane to the temporal bone; the umbo, seen as the most depressed point on the tympanum where the first ossicle fastens to the tympanic membrane; the pars flaccida, a small triangular area above the short process of the malleus; and the pars tensa, the largest portion of tympanum. The central area of the pars tensa provides the active vibrating surface in response to sound. Because it is a growing structure, punctures to the tympanic membrane will close and ventilation tubes can be extruded.

Middle Ear

The middle ear, or tympanic cavity, lies between the tympanic membrane and the oval window of the cochlea. It functions as a conduit for hearing and as regulator of the ventilation pressure in the middle ear. The tympanic cavity is an air-filled chamber lined with a continuous mucous membrane from the nasopharynx to the mastoid, which nourishes and protects the structures in the middle ear.

All of the walls of the middle ear are bony except for the tympanic membrane. The middle ear consists of three ossicles, oval and round windows, and the superior opening for the eustachian tube, which connects the middle ear to the nasopharynx. The ossicles, known as the malleus (hammer), incus (anvil), and stapes (stirrup), join together to form a movable link that connects the tympanic membrane to the oval window. **Figure 7-3** depicts the auditory ossicles. Muscles, ligaments, and joints hold the ossicles in place. The malleus attaches to the tympanic membrane, and the stapes footplate attaches to the oval window, a membrane that separates the middle ear from the perilymph of the inner ear. The incus connects the malleus and stapes bones.

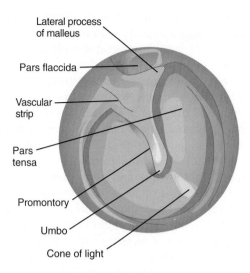

Lateral process
of malleus

Pars flaccida

Vascular
strip

Pars
tensa

Promontory

Umbo

Cone of light

FIGURE 7-2 Right tympanic membrane.

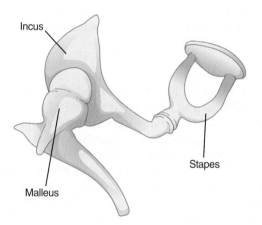

Incus

Stapes

Malleus

FIGURE 7-3 Auditory ossicles.

Sound enters the middle ear through the pars tensa, which vibrates in response. As the sound pressure increases, the vibrations increase in a circular pattern and are transmitted to the malleus, incus, and stapes. This allows airborne acoustic energy to be transmitted to the fluid of the inner ear. Because the surface area of the tympanic membrane is larger than the surface area of the base of the stirrup, sound pressure applied to the stapes in the oval window is magnified. The middle ear bones, acting as mechanical levers, also increase the pressure of the sound at the entrance to the cochlea. Hearing requires the middle ear to be filled with air and the three ossicles to work smoothly as a unit; any alteration will result in a decrease or loss of hearing.

The inner ear (discussed below) contains the tensor tympani muscle, which is attached to the malleus and is innervated by the trigeminal nerve, or fifth cranial nerve. The stapedius muscle, attached at the neck of stapes, is innervated by the facial, or seventh cranial nerve. High-intensity sound causes both muscles to contract. The eustachian tube (channel), approximately 1.5 inches long, connects the middle ear with the nasopharynx. It functions to equalize the pressure in the air-filled middle ear with the air pressure of the environment; this pressure balance allows the tympanic membrane to vibrate freely. The eustachian tube also functions to drain the middle ear and mastoid bone and to protect the middle ear from excessive nasopharyngeal sounds and secretions.

In adults, the eustachian tube consists of two portions: a lateral third (consisting of a bony portion arising from the anterior wall of the tympanic cavity) and a medial fibrocartilaginous two-thirds section that enters the nasopharynx. In infants, the bony portion is relatively longer and wider; the cartilaginous portion lies lower, and the tube is more horizontal compared with that of the adult. At the nasopharyngeal opening, the eustachian tube is lined with respiratory epithelium, including columnar ciliated cells, goblet cells, and mucous glands, which are integrated into the middle ear mucosa in the bony portion of the tube. The bony portion is always open; the cartilaginous portion is closed at rest to prevent sounds of the voice and nasal breathing from passing up the eustachian tube into the inner ear. The eustachian tube opens only on swallowing, yawning, or forceful inflation.

By opening, the eustachian tube allows air into the middle ear to replace air absorbed by the mucous membrane lining or to equalize pressure changes in the middle ear that are a result of altitude changes. The eustachian tube drains normal secretions of the middle ear by a mucociliary transport system and by repeated active tubal opening and closing, which allows the secretions to drain into the nasopharynx. Interference with the opening and closing of the eustachian tube may result in hearing impairment or other ear symptoms.

The mastoid process of the temporal bone lies at the base of the skull, directly behind the pinna, where it is felt as a bony prominence. The mastoid is composed of cuboidal air cells that are surrounded by a bony cortex. Each cell is lined by a mucous membrane of thin epithelial cells that are continuous with the epithelium of the tympanic cavity. The air-filled cells give lightness to the temporal bone and provide a reservoir of air for the middle ear.

Inner Ear

The inner ear contains the structures for balance and hearing through a series of connecting chambers and tubes. The inner ear, housed in the petrous section of the temporal bone, is a fluid-filled labyrinth that contains the cochlea, three semicircular canals, and the vestibule (**Figure 7-4**). The highly compact bone protects these structures from mechanical damage. Each structure consists of a protective bony labyrinth, an inner membranous labyrinth similar in shape to the bony labyrinth, and a space between the two. The inner membranous labyrinth contains endolymph, a fluid similar to intracellular fluid that is high in potassium and low in sodium. The space between the membranous and bony labyrinths contains perilymph, a fluid similar to extracellular fluids that is high in sodium and has an osmolarity similar to plasma.

The organs of hearing and balance branch from the central chamber, the vestibule. The cochlea is located on one side of the vestibule and the semicircular canals on the other. Two additional organs of balance, the utricle and saccule, are located adjacent to the vestibule.

The cochlea, lying in a horizontal plane, is a snail-shaped chamber consisting of 2¾ turns that contains the end organ of hearing known as the organ of Corti. Sound vibrations are transmitted from the stapes to the oval window, resulting in a fluid wave by the perilymph in the labyrinth that then vibrates the round window in a complementary rhythm. This wavelike motion of the fluid is transmitted to the endolymph resulting in movement of the hair cells lining the organ of Corti. The hair cells convert the mechanical energy to electrochemical energy to be transmitted by the acoustic branch of the eighth cranial nerve to the brain stem and brain to be interpreted as sound.

Body balance is the result of a complex relationship between multiple sensorial systems, including the proprioceptive, vestibular, and visual systems. The most significant system for equilibrium and balance is the vestibular system (comprised of the semicircular canals, the saccule, and utricle), which interprets motion and position of the head. When the system is functioning successfully, the brain can interpret the signals from the vestibular system to determine the direction the body is moving or turning or if the body is standing still. The signals from the contralateral ear are connected in the brain stem by the vestibular branch of the eighth cranial nerve.

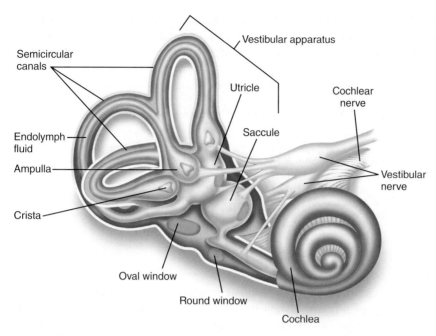

Semicircular canals

Vestibular apparatus

Utricle

Cochlear nerve

Saccule

Endolymph fluid

Ampulla

Vestibular nerve

Crista

Oval window

Round window

Cochlea

FIGURE 7-4 Inner ear.

Rotation of the head is detected by the three semicircular canals in the inner ear that are oriented posteriorly, superiorly, and horizontally. At the base of each semicircular canal is a dilated area containing hair cells that detect the motion of the endolymph-filled canal and send electrical impulses to the vestibular branch of the eighth cranial nerve.

Another function of the semicircular canals is to exert control over the eyes to allow the eyes to remain still in space as the head moves. The muscles of the eyes are aligned with the planes of the three semicircular canals; thus a single canal interacts with a single muscle pair of the eyes. This compensatory reflex is known as the vestibular-ocular reflex (VOR).

The utricle and saccule are sensory organs located in the vestibule. The cilia are located in a gelatinous mass (macula) into which are imbedded small crystals (otoliths). When the head moves, the otolith-gel mass drags on the hair cells. However, when the head is moving at a constant speed such as in a car, the otoliths come to equilibrium and motion is no longer perceived. The utricle, lying horizontally in the inner ear, can detect motion in the horizontal plane. The saccule, oriented vertically, can detect motion in the sagittal plane (that is, up and down, forward and back). The utricle and saccule are also important in maintaining the body vertically with respect to gravity. When the head and body tilt, the vestibular nuclei compensate with postural adjustments.

The anatomical and physiological relationships among the ear, the brain, the visual apparatus, and the upper airway must be understood and examined in order to avert such diverse consequences as poor language development, poor performance in school, social isolation, hearing loss, risk for falls, and missed diagnoses of respiratory and oral infections.

Health History

As in any clinical evaluation, the health history portion of ear assessment is an essential first step in enhancing the accuracy of diagnosis. In addition to careful investigation and documentation of the chief complaints (CCs) and history of present illness (HPI), vital information about ear disease–related impairments can be deduced from a detailed review of systems (ROS) and social history (SH).

Details of the family history (FH) often provide explanations for congenital as well as some acquired causes of hearing loss. A simple analysis of the prevalence of otitis, vertigo, and hearing loss among the U.S. population will evince the importance of an accurate and detailed assessment of the ear.

Chief Complaint and History of Present Illness

"My daughter is pulling at her right ear and cried all night."

> JB is a 12-month-old female child who presents with a 5-day history of "cold" symptoms, including yellow/green nasal discharge, cough, and poor appetite. Last night, she developed a fever of 102 to 103°F, which was taken using the family's tympanic thermometer. She was very irritable and intermittently pulled at her right ear. Mrs. B, the child's mother, gave the child two doses of acetaminophen. Child has had the usual falls and head bumps from learning to stand and trying to walk; mother denies loss of consciousness or evidence of any significant head injury at any time since birth.

Otalgia (Ear Pain)

Ear pain can be primary (originating within ear structures) or secondary (referred to the ear from other regions). Causes of primary otalgia include infections and inflammations of middle and external ear structures and mastoid tissues. Causes of secondary otalgia include TMJ problems; dental and periodontal problems; infections in the sinuses and nasopharyngeal areas; lesions of the tongue; cervical musculoskeletal problems; and neuralgias involving cranial nerves V, VII, IX, and X and cervical nerves I, II, and III.

Onset	Is the pain sudden or gradual?
Quality	Is the pain dull, boring, sharp, burning, or lancinating?
Location	Where is the patient experiencing pain (e.g., pinna, external ear canal, deep inside ear [head], or mastoid area)?
	Pain in the pinna only or pinna and external ear canal suggests external otitis.
	Does the pain radiate/refer to the ear?
	Does the pain occur in the left or right ear, or bilaterally?
Frequency of occurrence; regularity	Is the pain episodic, continuous, or intermittent?
Severity	When appropriate, ask the patient to rank the pain using a pain scale.
Precipitating factors	Is the pain related to certain circumstances, actions, or specific times?
	For example, intensification of otalgia may be associated with the act of chewing or swallowing, possibly indicating dental or TMJ problems, or nasopharyngeal infections. Primary otalgia associated with acute otitis media is also intensified with swallowing. Otalgia intensified or worsened by a head-dependent position (i.e., bending, stooping, or recumbency) usually indicates an infection or inflammation of the middle or external ear.
	Has the patient experienced an associated trauma, such as blunt trauma to head, barotrauma, or direct ear trauma?
Aggravating and alleviating factors	What aggravates the pain (e.g., environmental factors, activity, loud acoustic factors, such as sudden or continuous noises)?
	What alleviates the pain? Ask about both medications and nonpharmacologic measures.

Associated symptoms	Ask about associated symptoms, including dizziness, drainage, itching, hearing loss, tinnitus, fever, seizure, pharyngitis, laryngitis, sinusitis, appetite loss, dental disorders, neck complaints, and fullness in the ear (nonpainful pressure sensations).
	Drainage, itching, and fever are typically associated with acute infections in the ear (acute otitis media, external otitis, or chronic suppurative otitis media). Fever can also be associated with infections in nearby structures (nasopharyngeal or dental) with referred pain to the ear.
	Itching and pain may also indicate fungal infections (otomycosis) or allergic reactions with secondary bacterial infections, usually involving the external ear and/or the ear canal.

Hearing Loss

Hearing loss is third only to arthritis and hypertension as a chronic health problem, with at least 28 million Americans affected. More than 30% of adults over 65 years of age have some type of age-related hearing loss. Hearing loss can be gradual (most common) or sudden. Loss may result from lesions in the brain (cochlear nucleus of the pons or auditory cortex of the temporal lobe) or lesions of the inner, middle, or external ear. Poor transmission of sound waves through the external and/or middle ear causes conductive hearing loss. Diseases of the cochlea and/or poor conduction of sound-generated impulses along the eighth cranial nerve to the brain stem cause sensorineural hearing loss. Mixed hearing loss is a combination of both conductive and sensorineural hearing loss in the same ear.

Onset	Is the onset gradual (over months or years) or sudden?
	Causes of gradual onset include presbycusis, ototoxic drugs, chronic infection, otosclerosis, and brain attack. Examples of causes of sudden onset include acute infections (acute otitis media); nasopharyngeal infections (meningitis); sudden occlusion of external ear canal (edema, foreign body, bleeding); sudden accumulations of middle ear fluid or blood (acute serous otitis, basilar skull fracture); acute perforations of tympanic membrane (acoustic trauma; barotrauma; self-instrumentation with probes); ear and head trauma; acute ototoxic drug toxicity; viral infections of cochlea; brain tumors; neuromas of acoustic nerve; sudden occlusive vascular problems in inner ear or brain; and autoimmune or allergic disorders.
Location	Does the loss occur in the right or left ear or bilaterally?
Frequency of occurrence; regularity	Is the loss episodic, continuous, or intermittent?
Type	Is the loss congenital or acquired?
Patterns	Ask about patterns of the deficit, such as speech (male or female voices), music, high-pitched sounds, low-pitched sounds, telephone, or television.
	Does it occur in certain settings?
	Does it occur at certain times (early morning, late in the day)?
	Does the patient compensate by speaking more loudly or softly than normal?
Severity	Ask the patient to estimate the degree of difficulty (minor, moderate, severe).

Precipitating factors	Is the loss related to certain circumstances, environments, or specific times (e.g., noisy environment, telephone conversations)?
	Has the patient experienced an associated trauma, such as blunt trauma to head, acoustic trauma, barotrauma (injury resulting from sudden change in air pressure), or direct ear trauma?
	Ask about occupational factors (e.g., past or present noise exposure or military noise exposure).
	Ask about hobby or activities with excessive noise exposures.
	Inquire about drug (ototoxic agent) exposure, including current or past, type, amount, duration, dates of exposure, doses (see Past Medical History, Medications).
Aggravating and alleviating factors	What aggravates the loss (e.g., environmental, activity, and acoustic factors [types and volumes of noise sounds])?
	What alleviates the loss, including medications or nonpharmacologic measures?
Associated symptoms	Ask about associated symptoms, including dizziness, drainage, tinnitus, fever, and fullness in the ear.

Tinnitus

Tinnitus originates in the central auditory system and affects approximately 10% of the population. It can be transient or continuous and mild, moderate, or severe. Tinnitus can be subjective (audible only to patient) or objective (sound also audible to examiner as a bruit). Incidence of tinnitus increases with age.

Onset	Is the onset gradual or sudden?
	Examples of causes of gradual onset include advancing age, Ménière's disease, otosclerosis, metabolic conditions (diabetes, hypothyroidism), and TMJ disease.
	Causes of sudden onset include acoustic trauma and barotrauma, acute occlusion of external ear canal, environmental allergies, sudden alteration of blood pressure up or down, head and neck injury, acute therapy with ototoxic drugs, and ear and nasopharyngeal infections.
Location	Does it occur in the right ear, left ear, bilaterally, or is it nonlocalizable?
Frequency of occurrence; regularity	Is it episodic, continuous, intermittent, or progressive over time?
	Inquire as to specifics related to time when tinnitus occurs (daily cycle).
Quality	Is it pure, clicking, blowing, humming, hissing, buzzing, popping, pulsatile, whirring, squeaking, or roaring?
	Buzzing or roaring is typically associated with otosclerosis or Ménière's disease. Pulsatile sounds may be associated with a vascular problem.
Pitch	Is the pitch high, low, or variable?
	Most patients with sensorineural hearing loss experience high-frequency tinnitus, whereas low-frequency tones are more often associated with conductive hearing loss.
Intensity	Is it loud, soft, or variable?
Severity	Is the tinnitus mild (only noticed in quiet environments), moderate (constantly present and noticeable when attempting to sleep and when mentally focusing on tasks), or severe (constantly present and disruptive of sleep and ability to concentrate)?

Precipitating factors	Has the patient experienced an associated trauma, such as blunt trauma to head, barotrauma, or direct ear trauma?
	Question the patient about specifics related to circumstances and place when tinnitus occurs. Ask about drug (ototoxic agent) exposure, including current or past, dates of exposure, type, amount, duration, and doses.
Aggravating and alleviating factors	Ask the patient about aggravating factors (e.g., environmental, activity, acoustic). Ask the patient about alleviating factors, including medications and nonpharmacologic factors.
Associated symptoms	Ask about associated symptoms, including dizziness, drainage, itching, hearing loss, otalgia, fever, seizure, and fullness in the ear.

Otorrhea

Otorrhea may result from acute or chronic infections in the external or middle ear. It may also result from traumatic injury from self-instrumentation to the ear (insertion of rigid probes such as cotton-tipped applicators, paper clips, foreign objects, etc.) or from blunt head trauma. Otorrhea is often associated with tympanic membrane perforation.

Onset	Is the onset gradual or sudden?
Duration	Ask the patient how long the otorrhea has been present (e.g., days, months, or years).
Frequency of occurrence; regularity	Has it been episodic, continuous, or intermittent?
Location	Is it occurring in the right ear, left ear, or bilaterally?
Color; consistency	Is the discharge clear, yellow, green, white, red (bloody), brown, or gray? Is the discharge thin and watery, thick, or mucoid?
	Yellow or green fluid almost always indicates infection in the external or middle ear. Clear fluid with a mucoid consistency is associated with chronic otitis media with a tympanic membrane perforation. Clear watery fluid may indicate cerebral spinal fluid associated with basilar skull fracture with tympanic membrane perforation or possible dermatologic conditions of the external ear such as eczema. White fluid usually indicates fungal infection or possible dermatologic conditions of the external ear canal. Bloody (red) otorrhea is an indication of trauma or chronic infections. Brown or gray fluid may simply be liquefied cerumen.
Odor	Is the discharge odorless or malodorous?
	Foul-smelling otorrhea, especially if purulent, is typical of destruction of the temporal or mastoid bone from anaerobic infection.
Precipitating factors	Has the patient experienced an associated trauma, such as blunt trauma to the head, acoustic trauma, barotrauma, or direct ear trauma?
	Does the patient participate in hobbies or activities associated with barotrauma, especially swimming, deep-sea diving, mountain climbing, or high-altitude flying?
Alleviating factors	Ask about medications or nonpharmacologic measures.
Associated symptoms	Question about associated symptoms, including dizziness, pain, headache, itching, tinnitus, fever, or fullness in the ear.

Vertigo

Dizziness is second only to low back pain as a medical complaint prompting about 40% of all adults to seek medical help. Vertigo is one type of dizziness. It results from disorders of the inner ear or central vestibular pathways. Vertigo is a sense of spinning or turning and may occur while the head and body are not moving or when there is a sudden positional change of the head.

Onset	Is the onset gradual or sudden?
Duration	Ask the patient how long she or he has experienced vertigo (days, weeks, months, years).
Frequency of occurrence; regularity	Has it been episodic, continuous, or intermittent? If episodic, ask the duration of each episode (seconds, minutes, hours, days).
	Brief (seconds or minutes) episodes of vertigo associated with head movement are typically noted with benign paroxysmal positional vertigo (BPPV). Vertigo lasting for hours at a time is usually associated with inner ear disorders such as Ménière's disease, viral labyrinthitis, and perilymph fistula. Longer periods of vertigo (days or continuous) are usually associated with vertebrobasilar insufficiency, other central nervous system conditions, systemic autoimmune disease (rheumatoid disease), and systemic metabolic disease (diabetes, hypothyroidism).
Severity	Ask the patient to rate the severity. Is it mild, moderate, or severe?
Precipitating factors	Has the patient experienced an associated trauma, such as blunt trauma to the head, barotrauma, or direct ear trauma?
	Ask the patient for specific information related to circumstances and place when vertigo occurs.
	Question about the time when vertigo occurs. Is there a pattern?
	Ask the patient about drug (ototoxic agent) exposure (current or past, dates of exposure, type, amount, duration, doses).
Aggravating and alleviating factors	Ask the patient about aggravating factors (e.g., environmental, activity, positional changes).
	Inquire about alleviating factors including medications, nonpharmacologic measures, and positional changes.
	Sudden vertigo associated with nose blowing, straining, coughing, sneezing, or sudden Valsalva maneuver may indicate rupture of the round window and perilymph fistula.

Past Medical History

JB has had multiple upper respiratory infections (URIs), which were treated with antibiotics. She has experienced only one other problem with her ears. The earache occurred 2 months ago; however, she was not treated with antibiotics and recovered without incident. Her immunizations are up to date. JB has never been hospitalized for an illness. She appears to have a close relationship with mother; no evidence of child abuse visible. JB speaks single words, such as mama, dada, ba (for ball), and babbles sounds as though conversing—language development appropriate to age. Her birth was a normal vaginal delivery at 38 weeks after a normal pregnancy, with a weight of 7 lb, 8 oz and no visible birth defects. JB crawls without difficulty and pulls self up to examining table; has had the usual falls and head bumps from learning to stand and trying to walk. She has never lost consciousness or evidenced any significant head trauma.

JB takes a liquid multivitamin daily. Her mother is unaware of any exposure to ototoxic drugs during her pregnancy. There is no history of ototoxic drug use in the child. JB has four deciduous teeth in good condition. She may be allergic to amoxicillin (she developed a "rash" over body after treatment of URI several months ago).

This portion of the interview consists of a combination of open-ended and focused questions covering any/all past medical illnesses and traumatic events, including elective surgery. This information will provide the healthcare provider with critical details of past and present illnesses and conditions that will aid in the formulation of a plan of care.

Past health conditions and/or surgeries	Ask about previous illnesses and diagnoses.
	Illnesses that are associated with ear symptoms or that should be considered in the differential diagnosis include Ménière's disease, diabetes, hypertension, hypothyroidism, migraine syndrome, TMJ conditions, dental conditions, cytomegalovirus infections, seizure disorders, stroke, (orthostatic) hypotension, polycythemia, anemia, arrhythmias, Stokes-Adams attack, syphilis, ear and respiratory infections, acute and chronic sinusitis, metastatic carcinomas, brain tumors, atherosclerosis, vision problems, hyperlipidemias, collagen vascular disorders, psychiatric problems, multiple sclerosis, Parkinson's disease, Lyme disease, systemic lupus erythematosus, sun-induced dermatologic conditions of the external ear, seasickness, eczema (especially involving external ear), and cutaneous fungal diseases.
	Ask about previous surgeries, including diagnoses, dates, names of hospital and surgeons, name of surgical procedure, results of surgery, and complications.
	Especially note any ear surgery, vascular surgery, intracranial neurosurgery, surgery for head trauma, neck surgery (orthopedic or neurosurgical), other types of nose and throat surgery, dental surgery, and TMJ surgery.
	Such surgical procedures, if recent, can result in secondary otalgia and acute onset of tinnitus and hearing loss.
Childhood illnesses	Ask about acute or chronic ear, upper respiratory, or oral/dental infections (especially otitis media, serous otitis, chronic otitis media, mastoiditis, pharyngitis, tonsillitis, meningitis, encephalitis, congenital syphilis) and cytomegalovirus infections.
	Ask about the patient's communicable disease history, including measles, mumps, rubella, tuberculosis.
	Ask about child abuse.
	It frequently involves blows to the side of the head, which may result in ear disorders.
	Inquire about delayed language development, prematurity, hospitalization in neonatal intensive care unit (NICU), and congenital diseases.
	A history of prematurity, early hospitalizations, or the presence of other congenital defects may indicate congenital defects in the ear leading to a diagnosis of hearing impairmerit. A history of delayed or inappropriate language development frequently indicates hearing impairment.
	Note any history of foreign body insertions into ear canal. Did the patient have any behavioral disorders as a child?
	Behavioral problems could result from social isolation associated with hearing loss. Impaired hearing could be the explanation for failure to follow instructions, for inattentiveness, or for lack in progress in school. Undiagnosed chronic otalgia, vertigo, and tinnitus may result in behavior patterns that are mislabeled neurologic or psychiatric illness. Interrupted or delayed social interactions resulting from repeated school absences caused by ear-related illness can be a source of behavior problems.
Hospitalizations	Inquire about previous hospitalizations, noting diagnoses, dates, names of hospital and providers, therapies provided, and results.

Injuries	Has the patient experienced any of the following injuries: head or brain trauma, trauma resulting from an auto accident, acoustic trauma, barotrauma, direct ear trauma (inquiry about habits of self-instrumentation for ear cleaning), injury from examiner manipulation of ear canal, neck injury (whiplash), child abuse, or head injury?
Immunizations	Ask about immunizations, including types, dates, and responses.
	Failure to be adequately immunized against infectious disease could result in central nervous system infections and subsequent inner ear damage. This is especially true of vaccines for haemophilus B; measles, mumps, rubella (MMR); and pneumococcal disease.
Medications	Inquire about use of medications.
	Question about ototoxic drug exposures, especially aminoglycosides, salicylates, loop diuretics, some antineoplastic drugs (nitrogen mustards, bleomycin, cisplatinum, vincristine), heavy metal exposure (mercury, gold, lead, arsenic), and quinine derivatives.
	Drugs related to tinnitus include angiotensin-converting enzyme inhibitors, macrolides, quinolones, sulfa antibiotics, tricyclic antidepressants, antihistamines, beta blockers, calcium channel blockers, some narcotics, and nonsteroidal anti-inflammatory drugs (NSAIDs).
Allergies	In addition to medication allergies, inquire about reactions to contact allergens to the ear (shampoos, nickel, hairsprays, perfumes, cosmetics).
	Inquire about environmental allergies leading to sinusitis, otitis, vertigo, and hearing loss.
Intrauterine exposure	Inquire about any hearing loss and/or exposure to any ototoxic drugs during mother's pregnancy.
	Ask about intrauterine exposure of fetus to infections (especially rubella, cytomegalovirus, and herpes simplex).
	Note any history of birth trauma.

Family History

JB lives with her parents and two siblings (sister age 4 and brother age 7); all are in good health. Father, age 35, is in good health; he has a history of "many ear infections" as a child and had "tubes" in his ears at age 18 months. Mother, age 30, is obese but in otherwise good health. Paternal grandmother, age 60, has diabetes, hypertension, and heart disease. Paternal grandfather died at age 65 in a car accident; he did not have major health problems. Maternal grandmother, age 65, is obese and has hypertension and macular degeneration. Maternal grandfather, age 65, was diagnosed with otosclerosis at age 45; he does not have other health problems. JB's sister is in excellent health. Her brother has been diagnosed with attention-deficit/hyperactivity disorder (ADHD), which is controlled with medication; his general health is excellent.

The family history establishes a pattern of ear diseases/conditions within a family. Many conditions are inherited or genetically determined, and many congenital syndromes are associated with hearing loss or defective anatomical development of ear structures. This assessment should include determination of ear and renal pathology.

Age of living relatives	Include relationship and health of parents, brothers, sisters, and children.
Deaths	Include relationship, age, and cause of death.

Chronic diseases	Ask about chronic diseases in the family; include relationship of the patient to the family member with the disease and how long that family member has had the disease.
Patterns of hearing loss in the family	Inquire about other family members with congenital or acquired deafness. Establish familial relationships of index subject using a genogram.
	Ask about age-related hearing loss within the family. Note gender, age, and related diseases in affected members.
Congenital syndromes/ genetic defects	Inquire about genetic disorders.
	Note family members with possible inherited ear conditions (otosclerosis, Ménière's disease, chronic otitis media, and presbycusis).
	Congenital syndromes associated with ear conditions include Down syndrome, Usher syndrome, Treacher Collins syndrome, fetal alcohol syndrome, Crouzon syndrome, Alport syndrome, hemifacial microsomia, Stickler syndrome, branchio-oto-renal syndrome, Pendred syndrome, CHARGE association, neurofibromatosis type II, Waardenburg syndrome, congenital rubella syndrome, Pierre Robin syndrome, trisomy 13, and cleft lip/cleft palate.

Social History

> JB lives at home with parents in a single-family, middle-class dwelling with modern conveniences. Both parents work outside the home, and the family is covered by health insurance. JB spends most of the day at a day care center. Both parents smoke about a pack of cigarettes per day but report that they smoke outdoors to protect their children; they deny smoking in the car with children. JB continues to sleep with a bottle at night to "help her go to sleep." When child is not ill, she sleeps from 8:00 PM until 6:00 AM without waking. JB feeds herself with fingers. For the past 2 to 3 days, she has not been eating well. For the last 24 hours, she has been drinking poorly (using 2 to 3 diapers/ 24 hours). JB's social interaction with family appears to be appropriate for a 12-month-old child.

This information will aid in an explanation for some symptoms and will form a basis for therapeutic interventions for many ear conditions and illnesses. Exposure to cigarette smoke is a significant risk for recurrent childhood middle ear infection.

Family	Ask to describe current family unit.
Occupation	Inquire about employment in high-noise areas, such as sites with machinery, construction work, employment in factories, airports, concert venues, or in indoor sports arenas. Establish whether the increased noise exposure is prolonged and continuous or episodic and brief.
	Question about the use of ear protection in such employment areas.
Education/ day care	Inquire about highest grade achieved in school and difficulty learning.
	Lack of progress may be related to hearing difficulty. Educational level may be predictive of success in therapeutic regimens for ear-related conditions.
	Inquire about the number of missed days of school (or work) because of ear problems.
	For children, note teacher comments about inattentiveness or misunderstanding of directions. Ask about day care attendance.
	There is an increased incidence of ear and respiratory infections among children attending day care.

Military history	Inquire about exposure to gunfire or other loud noises (motor pool, aircraft engines, and engine rooms—acoustic trauma).

Ask about assignment in jungle areas where fungal diseases are prevalent. |
| Activities of daily living | Has the patient experienced disruptions or alterations to the activities of daily living caused by hearing loss, otalgia, tinnitus, or vertigo?

Inquire, especially, about limitations of telephone use and ability to converse (asking others to repeat themselves), conversational inappropriateness, ambulation and potential for falls, inability to hear doorbells, social isolation, inability to concentrate, poor job performance, and confusion.

These questions help identify the severity of impaired hearing and vertigo.

Obtain information, usually from people other than the patient, about changes in the intensity of patient's voice in conversation (speaking more loudly or more softly than usual).

Family and associates of patients frequently are the first to notice changes in vocal intensity. Patients with conductive hearing loss tend to speak in low-intensity tones whereas patients with nerve deafness tend to speak with increased intensity. |
| Leisure activities | Inquire about relationship between exercise habits and ear symptoms, especially any physical activity that intensifies otalgia or vertigo.

Ask about any limitations to physical exercise caused by ear symptoms, including forced sedentary lifestyle as a result of otalgia, tinnitus, vertigo, or hearing loss.

Does the patient participate in leisure activities that involve exposure to excessive noise levels, such as hunting, target shooting, attending rock concerts, auto/drag racing, woodworking, go-cart/snowmobile riding, etc.?

Inquire about the need to have the TV or radio louder than normal.

Note any tendency to avoid social interaction. |
| Nutritional status | Question about any dietary or eating impairment related to nausea or vomiting, secondary to vertigo.

Inquire about poor appetite, as a related factor to ear problems (especially infections). |
| Sleep patterns | Inquire about patterns of sleep including limitations in duration of sleep caused by tinnitus, otalgia, or vertigo.

Middle ear pain often is worse when people lie down and improves when upright.

Note any difficulty falling asleep, the need for white noise (background noise such as soft music, radio, etc.) in order to fall asleep, required head positions for sleep, awakening from sleep with vertigo or because of otalgia, ability to become fully rested after sleep, and sleep interruptions because of ear symptoms. |
| Use of tobacco | Ask about tobacco use including types, amounts, durations of use, and exposure to secondary smoke.

The irritant effects of smoke on the throat cause edema and obstruction of the eustachian tube with increased pressure and fluid accumulation in the middle ear. This may be a contributing factor in children with frequent acute otitis media. |

Use of alcohol	Question about type, amount, and duration of alcohol consumption; try to establish a relationship between levels of alcohol consumption and ear symptoms.	
Use of recreational drugs	Inquire about types, frequency of use, and effects. Also, inquire about the amount of caffeine consumption. *Drug history (other than medications) may reveal exposure to ototoxic substances or an alternative explanation for symptoms of dizziness or tinnitus.*	

Review of Systems

Ideally, a complete review of systems will provide a thorough and detailed account of a patient's past and present symptoms. When time does not allow for such a discussion, a focused ROS could be substituted with attention focused on signs and symptoms possibly related to the patient's chief complaint. There are many signs and symptoms usually associated with other body systems that are possibly related to ear diseases and conditions. The following table highlights some of the more important points to cover in a focused review of systems.

System	Symptom or Sign	Possible Associated Diseases/Disorders
General/ Constitutional	Weight loss Fatigue	Nausea/vomiting related to vertigo Poor sleeping related to discomfort from otalgia or tinnitus
	Fever	Ear infections
Skin	Itching (in the ears) Rashes (during pregnancy)	Ear fungal infections (otomycosis) Potential for congenital ear abnormalities in the offspring
Eyes	Nystagmus Used to lipread Excessive tearing	Related to vertigo Deafness Possible sinusitis as cause of secondary otalgia
Nose	Nasal stuffiness, discharge	Allergies and head colds associated with many ear conditions
Mouth/Throat	Sore throat, dental/periodontal pain or inflammation	Serous otitis Dental/periodontal infections as cause of secondary otalgia
Cardiovascular	Headache, hypertension, angina, transient ischemic attacks	Central nervous system vascular explanation for tinnitus and/or vertigo
Respiratory	Cough, shortness of breath, bronchitis, pleurisy, excessive sputum production	Respiratory infections associated with ear infections
Gastrointestinal	Anorexia	Vertigo
Genitourinary	Urinary symptoms (dysuria, hematuria, incontinence, flank pain)	Congenital ear abnormalities associated with common congenital urinary system abnormalities
Musculoskeletal	Weakness, muscle atrophy, joint swelling and pain	Rheumatoid disease associated with vertigo
	Temporomandibular (TMJ) joint pain	TMJ arthralgia as a cause of secondary otalgia
Neurologic	Ataxia, focal neurologic deficits (paresthesias, focal paresis/paralysis), speech disorders	Cerebrovascular diseases associated with ear symptoms (tinnitus, vertigo, hearing loss, and possibly secondary otalgia)
Mental/Psychiatric	Depression, anxiety, behavioral problems	Possibly resulting from social isolation related to hearing impairment

Physical Examination

Equipment Needed

- Centimeter ruler
- Penlight
- Otoscope with multiple specula of different sizes
- Pneumatic otoscope
- Tuning fork with 512 cps (cycles per second) frequency

Components of the Physical Examination

Inspection

Inspection always begins at the first contact and continues throughout the interview and physical examination.

Action	Rationale
1. Inspect the patient's general appearance, including the following:	
a. Note stability of the patient's gait when walking into room.	a. Unsteadiness of gait is common in vertigo but may be explained by other neurologic or musculoskeletal conditions.
b. Note speech patterns for loudness, appropriateness, and articulation.	b. Unusually loud intensity of speech is associated with sensorineural hearing loss, whereas unusually soft intensity is associated with conductive hearing loss. Inappropriate speech may indicate inability to hear questions or inability to hear that others in the room are speaking. Speech patterns may reflect moods of depression and anxiety. Dysarthria may indicate structural anomalies in the oropharynx that may be linked to otologic anomalies. It may also point to neurologic deficits as alternate explanations for ear symptoms.
c. Note apparent understanding of examiner's instructions and questions.	c. Inability to follow verbal instructions or answer appropriately may reflect hearing loss, apathy, depression, or inability caused by severe otalgia.
d. Observe the patient's head position during conversation.	d. Head position may indicate ear problems. In unilateral deafness, the head is rotated to turn the "good" ear toward the examiner. With severe otalgia, the patient's head may be bent laterally toward the painful ear. Minimization of head movements is common in vertigo.

Action	Rationale
e. Note facial expressions and body language.	e. Facial expressions and body language reflect pain and moods of depression, anger, frustration, and anxiety. Ear infection, otalgia, and vertigo are often disabling and are suggested by facial grimacing, crying, absence of excessive head movement, the need for balance support, and protective actions related to a painful ear. These can also indicate toxicity associated with infections.
f. Inspect for evidence of craniofacial and ear anomalies.	f. Congenital ear conditions are frequently associated with other craniofacial and otological anomalies. These include heterochromia of the irises, abnormal pigmentation of hair and skin, microtia, dimpling and skins tags near the external ear, low-set ears, cleft lip, facial asymmetry, hypoplasia of facial structures, hypertelorism, and microcephalyo.
2. Inspect the external ear. For external ear examination, patient should be seated with examiner either seated or standing at eye level. Each ear should be examined separately from the side of the patient, allowing good view with adequate direct lighting. A penlight maybe necessary for some inspection.	2. Optimal inspection of the external ear including the ridges and crevices of the pinna, the retroauricular areas, and the outer portions of the external canal can only be accomplished by close, eye-level examination using good lighting. Eye-level examination allows for detection of odors.
a. Observe for position, size, shape, and symmetry of pinnae.	a. Upper edge of pinna should be at or slightly above an imaginary line drawn from the outer canthus of the ipsilateral eye to the occiput; pinnae that are entirely below this line are referred to as low-set ears or excessively small ears (microtia) and maybe associated with other structural anomalies of the ear and congenital hearing loss. Pinnae typically become enlarged in older adults.
b. Observe skin of the ear and surrounding tissues.	b. Ulcerations, especially on the helix, may be sun-induced neoplasms, seborrheic keratoses, actinic keratoses, or keratoacanthomas. Nodules, with or without inflammation, on the pinna may be basal cell cancer, or sebaceous or pilar cysts. Tophi (nodules possibly with extruded white crystalline substance) maybe noted on the helix or antihelix in patients with gout. Firm, nontender nodules (keloids) may be noted on the lobes in African Americans following ear piercing. Deformities of the pinna (usually unilateral) may be the result of chondritis associated with recent or past trauma.

Action	Rationale
	Acute inflammation (edema, erythema, discoloration) may be associated with infections in the external canal or mastoid structures. Melanomas are common on the pinna and in the retroauricular area of the scalp.
c. Inspect the external canal. It may be necessary to pull the pinna out and back and either up (in adults) or down (in children). Observe for cerumen, drainage, foreign bodies, edema, erythema, scaliness, and tenderness. For any discharge, note color, odor, and consistency.	c. Otalgia may be explained by external otitis, which is manifested by erythema, purulent drainage, edema, and tenderness in the external canal. External otitis may also cause hearing loss (sudden) through swelling and occluding secretions in the canal. Foreign body insertions are common in children and may explain itching or sudden hearing loss, or serve as a nidus for infection. Impacted cerumen may explain hearing loss in adults, especially older adults who wear hearing aids. Scaly eruptions in the ear canal may indicate eczema or possibly fungal infections causing itching, and possibly otalgia and other symptoms. Noting the color, consistency, and odor of any discharge helps to identify specific diagnoses such as acute and chronic infections and trauma (see above under otorrhea).
3. Inspect the ear using an otoscope (**Figure 7-5**). For proper technique, see **Box 7-1**.	3. Otoscopic examination should be performed before any tests for hearing acuity are performed. This is to ensure patency of the ear canal and gross integrity of the tympanic membrane.

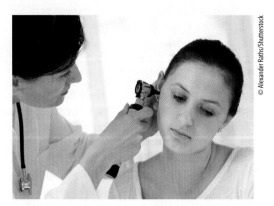

© Alexander Raths/Shutterstock

FIGURE 7-5 Inspecting the ear using an otoscope.

Action	Rationale
a. Inspect the deeper sections of external ear canal. Insert the otoscope about halfway into the depth of the canal and examine for cerumen, foreign bodies, points of injury from self-instrumentation (hematoma or lacerations), dermatological conditions (erythema, eczema, scaliness, fungal hyphae), tumors, blood, and other secretions.	a. The lining of the deeper sections of the ear canal may not be visible with external examination. Narrowing of the bony section of the canal without inflammation may be caused by exostoses of bone impinging on the lumen.

BOX 7-1   OTOSCOPIC EXAMINATION TECHNIQUE

For otoscopic examination, use the following technique:

1. Position yourself at eye level with the external ear canal.
2. Use a penlight to adequately visualize as much of the outer portion of the external ear canal as possible.
3. While illuminating the canal, gently pull the pinna into the position that best "straightens" the cartilaginous portion of the canal for easy insertion of the rigid ear speculum.
   - For older children and adults, this is generally upward, outward, and backward.
   - For children under age 3 years, the ear should be pulled downward, outward, and backward.
4. With the ear canal straightened and evaluated for tenderness, estimate the diameter to help in selection of the largest speculum that can comfortably fit.
5. Insert the speculum alone into the canal to assure its comfort before attaching it to the otoscope.
6. Attach the selected speculum to the otoscope and grasp the instrument firmly with the dominant hand, holding the instrument in an inverted position with the handle end of the instrument oriented to 12 o'clock.
7. Place the dorsal surface of the fingers of the dominant hand firmly against the patient's head directly above the ear and maintain this contact throughout the examination. This will prevent accidental insertion of the speculum too deeply into the ear canal, putting the patient at risk for injury to deeper structures should the patient's head suddenly move toward the examiner.
8. While pulling the pinna in the desired direction and without looking through the otoscope lens, look directly at the ear speculum and the ear canal while inserting the speculum to a depth of about 1 to 1.5 cm. This will allow more accurate and controlled insertion of the speculum.
9. Bring the eye into position to look through the instrument.
10. Examine the external canal and its contents (if any).
11. Attempt to visualize the tympanic membrane.
12. Upon completion of this static inspection of the tympanic membrane, use the bulb attachment of the pneumatic otoscope to gently apply small amounts of positive and negative pressure to detect movement of the tympanic membrane. The speculum must make a tight seal in the ear canal for this procedure. Movement is indicated by a change in shape of the cone of light reflex and is evidence of flexibility of the tympanic membrane.

Action	Rationale
b. Inspect the tympanic membrane. • Note color. A normal tympanic membrane is pearly (or pinkish) gray.	• Erythema is indicative of bacterial infection (otitis media), viral infection (bullous myringitis), trauma, and possibly mastoiditis. With otitis media, there is usually erythema with a loss of sheen and transparency. Injection (visible small blood vessels) can be noted normally at the periphery of the tympanic membrane and directly overlying the handle of the malleus, whereas injection in the center of the tympanic membrane is indicative of an inflammatory process (early or resolving acute otitis or chronic otitis). A yellow color also may indicate acute otitis media. Yellow, amber, or orange is associated with serous otitis. A bluish color to the tympanic membrane is indicative of blood in the middle ear associated with basilar skull fracture or tumors.

Action	Rationale

White patches on the tympanic membrane are caused by accumulations of collagen, hyaline, and/or calcifications associated with benign conditions like tympanosclerosis or resulting from chronic inflammation (chronic otitis media).

- Inspect for selected landmarks. Note the pars tensa, pars flaccida, the handle of the malleus, the umbo, and possibly the incus and the chorda tympani nerve.

- Notation of landmarks assures the examiner that the tympanic membrane is being viewed. Visualization of the bony landmarks (especially the incus) provides evidence for the transparency of the tympanic membrane.

  The prominence (or lack thereof) of the malleus allows conclusions about contour (see below).

- Inspect for contour. Normally the tympanic membrane is concave and oriented anteroinferiorly.

- Bulging is indicated by protrusion of the membrane outward into the external canal and is manifested by loss of clear visibility of the handle of the malleus. It is associated with fluid accumulations in the middle ear in association with otitis media, serous otitis, and temporal bone and basilar skull fracture. A bulging tympanic membrane is the most reliable indicator of acute otitis media. **Figure 7-6** illustrates acute otitis media.

  Retraction is indicated by exaggerated concavity and movement of the membrane into the middle ear and is manifested by accentuated visibility of the handle of the malleus. Retraction results from recurrent or unresolved otitis media leading to chronic otitis media, serous otitis, and eustachian tube dysfunction.

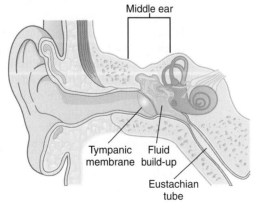

FIGURE 7-6A Acute otitis media.

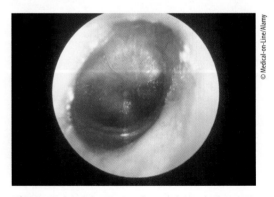

FIGURE 7-6B A bulging tympanic membrane is the most reliable indicator of acute otitis media.

Action	Rationale

- Examine the tympanic membrane for cone of light reflex. If present, it is noted in the anterior inferior quadrant of the membrane when using the otoscope.

- Inspect for transparency. Normally the tympanic membrane is semitransparent with several middle ear structures visible through it. These structures include the handle of the malleus, a portion of the incus bone, and a portion of the 7th cranial nerve (chorda tympani).

- Examine for integrity. Perforations are commonly noted in the pars flaccida area of the tympanic membrane but can also occur in the pars tensa. They can be central and involve a large surface area of the tympanic membrane or they can be located at the periphery. They can be single or multiple. **Figure 7-7** depicts a perforation.

- Inspect for movement. Manually changing the air pressure in the external canal by pneumatoscopy should cause the tympanic membrane to flex medially and laterally.

- Presence of a cone of light reflex is neither confirmatory nor disproving for any ear disease. Bending of the cone of light may indicate prominent bulging or retraction of the tympanic membrane.

- Loss of semi-transparency of the tympanic membrane (inability to visualize the malleus and incus) is noted in chronic scarring, which is associated with chronic otitis without perforation, tympanosclerosis, and repetitive perforations with healing.

  A transparent tympanic membrane can reveal air bubbles and air-fluid lines, associated with middle ear effusions in acute otitis media and serous otitis.

- Perforations of the tympanic membrane are noted in acute otitis media with effusions, chronic otitis media, acoustic trauma (sudden loud, high-frequency noises), barotrauma (sudden or repetitive changes in air pressure between the middle ear and the atmosphere), direct self-instrumentation, cholesteatomas, and trauma from foreign bodies.

- Absence of movement is associated with stiffness resulting from scarring and pressurized effusions. Conditions resulting in stiffness are otitis media, tympanosclerosis, and other scarring from chronic infections.

  Lack of flexibility causes conductive hearing loss.

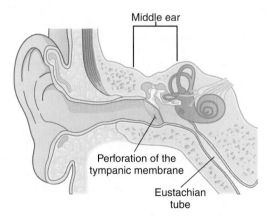

FIGURE 7-7A Perforation of the tympanic membrane.

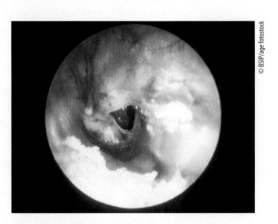

FIGURE 7-7B Perforation of the tympanic membrane.

Palpation

Action	Rationale
1. Carefully palpate each ear separately by pulling the pinna out and back and either up or down (**Figure 7-8**).	1. Tenderness with movement of the pinna suggests external otitis (bacterial, viral, or fungal), chondritis, hematomas from trauma, or infected epidermal cysts.

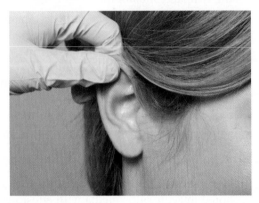

FIGURE 7-8 Palpating the ear.

Action	Rationale
2. Apply pressure to the tragus.	2. Tenderness with compression of the tragus is seen in external otitis.

Physical examination also includes hearing tests. See **Box 7-2** for descriptions and technique.

BOX 7-2   HEARING ACUITY TESTS

TUNING FORK TESTS
Tuning fork tests are designed to test the ability of the patient to hear pure tones.

Weber Test
This tests for adequacy of bone conduction. Holding it only by the stem, place the base of a 512-cps vibrating tuning fork firmly against the skull in the center of the forehead (or the nasal bridge or the front teeth in hearing impaired patients). Ask the patient to identify whether the tone is heard equally loud in both ears or louder in one ear or the other. Avoid suggestions as to a desired response to the question. If the tone intensity is not equal in both ears, ask in which ear the sound is loudest. The sound is said to lateralize to that ear.

The tone should be heard equally in both ears. Lateralization of the intensity of the tone to either side is abnormal and indicates either conductive hearing loss in the better-hearing ear or sensorineural hearing loss in the poorer-hearing ear.

Rinne Test
This tests for comparison of air conduction to bone conduction in each ear separately. Holding the 512-cps vibrating tuning fork only by its stem, apply the base of the stem first to the mastoid bone of one ear. After inquiring if the tone is heard, note the length of time that the sound is audible by asking the patient to signify when the tone is no longer heard. Without touching the tines of the tuning fork to alter its vibration, bring the end of the tines to a position about 1 inch from the same ear. Again ask if the tone is heard and again note the length of time that the sound is audible by asking the patient to signify when it is no longer heard. Compare the noted times for the bone-conducted sound and the air-conducted sound and determine which is longer. If the air conduction time is noted to be longer, note whether it is at least twice as long (a positive test). The test should then be repeated for the opposite ear.

A variation of the Rinne test is performed similarly, but instead of allowing the tuning fork to remain in place until the sound is no longer heard, the patient is simply asked whether the bone-conducted sound or the air-conducted sound is louder. If the air-conducted sound is louder than the bone-conducted sound in a given ear, the test is a positive Rinne.

BOX 7-2 HEARING ACUITY TESTS (*continued*)

A *positive* Rinne test is normal and is recorded when air conduction tone intensity is louder and/or heard longer than bone conduction tone intensity. A *negative* Rinne test is indicative of a conductive hearing loss in the affected ear and is manifested by bone conduction tone intensity being louder and/or heard longer than air conduction tone intensity. Sensorineural hearing loss in an affected ear is manifested by a positive Rinne test, but the intensity of both bone and air conduction is reduced, compared with normal intensity.

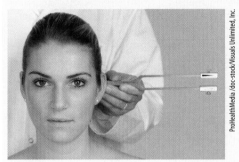

Rinne test.

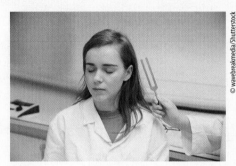

Rinne test.

Whisper Test

Used as a gross screening test for hearing acuity, the whisper test has several variations and tests the ability of the patient to hear and distinguish sounds in the vocal frequency range. To perform the test, mask your lips to prevent lipreading and stand either in front of or behind the patient. After an exhalation, whisper a series of words into each ear separately from a distance of about 2 feet. The words used consist of either one-syllable words, similar in vowel sound but with different consonant sounds (e.g., "hat," "bat," "cat") or words with two equally accented syllables (e.g., "baseball," "staircase," "daydream"). Some examiners use numbers ("nine-four," "three-seven") instead of words for the test. The ear not being tested is occluded by the patient's or the examiner's finger pressing inward on the tragus (some examiners require that the finger be wiggled back and forth during the test to mask any sounds being heard by the untested ear). Ask the patient to repeat the words making sure that the correct vowel and consonant sounds are repeated. A normal whisper test is correct repetition of at least 50% of the spoken words. If the patient fails to achieve this benchmark, repeat the test using successively louder whispers and finally full vocalization until the test is passed. Repeat the entire test on the opposite ear using a different series of words.

Normal hearing is indicated by correct repetition of one- and two-syllable speech sounds whispered into each ear separately. Failure to correctly identify different consonant sounds at least 50% of the time is suggestive of a hearing loss (either conductive or sensorineural) in the tested ear.

Diagnostic Reasoning

Based on findings in the health history and physical examination, the clinician should formulate his or her assessment and plan. For example, a patient may report symptoms that suggest many possible diagnoses; however, findings in the past medical history (PMI) and during the physical examination narrow the possible diagnoses down to one or two. Otalgia is a common chief complaint. **Table 7-1** illustrates differential diagnosis of common disorders associated with otalgia.

Table 7-1   Differential Diagnosis of Otalgia

Differential Diagnosis	Significant Findings in the Patient's History	Significant Findings in the Patient's Physical Examination	Diagnostic Tests
Acute otitis media	Pediatric patient, history of a recent URI, fever, exposure to smoke, tugging or pulling at the affected ear, irritability	Red, bulging tympanic membrane that is intact with no visible landmarks or light reflex	N/A
Chronic otitis media	Pediatric patient, repeated episodes of otitis media, hearing loss	Thick, immobile, retracted tympanic membrane or perforated tympanic membrane with drainage	N/A
Serous otitis	Pediatric patient, hearing loss	Retracted, immobile, tympanic membrane with effusion	Tympanogram
Trauma	History of recent trauma or penetration of the ear, direct self-instrumentation, or foreign body in the ear	Perforated tympanic membrane	N/A

Ear Assessment of Special Populations

Considerations for the Pregnant Patient

Note the following when assessing pregnant patients:

- Symptoms of ear congestion and fullness may occur secondary to the nasal and sinus congestions, commonly induced by pregnancy-related hormonal vascular dilatation in the head and neck (vasomotor rhinitis).
- Smoking during pregnancy results in a significant increase in ear infections in the newborn.
- Exposure to viral infections (e.g., rubella, cytomegalovirus) during pregnancy is associated with significant congenital ear and hearing abnormalities in the offspring.
- Maternal diabetes, Rh incompatibility, and toxemia of pregnancy are all associated with an increased incidence of congenital hearing loss in the offspring.
- Hearing acuity is impaired (usually conductive loss) as a result of edema of the tympanic membrane.
- Pregnancy is associated with an increased incidence of otosclerosis or acceleration of preexisting otosclerosis.

Considerations for the Neonatal Patient
General

Note the following when assessing a neonatal patient:

- The outer, middle, and inner ear in the embryo develops at the same time as other vital organ systems, including the kidney. Examining the ears gives clues as to other developmental abnormalities in the rest of the body, especially the kidneys.
- History taking is very important, including gestational age at birth, birth weight, and if hospitalized in a neonatal intensive care unit (NICU). There is concern that the high-frequency hearing loss in low-birthweight infants could be due to equipment noise in the intensive care environment.
- Smoking during pregnancy results in a significant increase in ear infections in the newborn.
- Exposure to viral infections (e.g., rubella, cytomegalovirus) during pregnancy is associated with significant congenital ear and hearing abnormalities in the offspring.
- Maternal diabetes, Rh incompatibility, and toxemia of pregnancy are all associated with an increased incidence of congenital hearing loss in the offspring.
- The ambient sound levels plus the use of ototoxic drugs, especially when used for more than 5 days, may have a negative effect on the development of hearing in the hospitalized preterm infant.
- Neonates discriminate a full spectrum of sounds but respond best to high-pitched sounds.

- Check gross hearing by ringing a small bell; the crying child will stop momentarily and the quiet child will blink and appear to attend to the sound.
- The neonate responds to a sudden sound by crying or by the startle or blink reflex and usually becomes quiet when spoken to in a calm and quiet manner.

Inspection

- Observe position of the ears. It is not unusual for infants to be born with one ear set slightly lower than the other. Low-set ears are associated with a number of congenital conditions including Down syndrome.
- Assess for small preauricular skin tags or dermal sinuses, which can be normal or can be associated with kidney or chromosomal abnormalities.

Considerations for the Pediatric Patient
General

- Remember, more than 75% of all children experience at least one episode of otitis media before the age of 3 years; otitis media accounts for 42% of antibiotic use in children. Many of these cases progress to chronic otitis media and its severe complications.
- Allow infants and young children to sit in their parent's lap; it makes the examination easier.
- Make a "game" of the examination; it helps gain cooperation of the examinee and the parent.
- Spend time getting acquainted with both the child and the parent prior to the examination, helping gain their confidence. Children develop an awareness and fearfulness of strangers around 1 year of age.
- Because toddlers and preschoolers can be frightened of examination equipment, explain the examination and allow the child to become acquainted with the equipment (**Figure 7-9**). This may allay some of their fears.

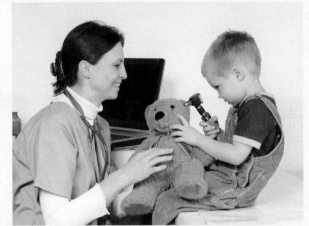

FIGURE 7-9 Allaying a toddler's fears before otoscopic examination.

- Note the following characteristics of pediatric patients:
  - Receptive speech is dependent on hearing, especially for the first 2 years of life. Children with frequent or chronic middle ear effusions can have disrupted language and social development.
  - Young children will often "play with their ears" when they teethe or as part of normal body curiosity. Ear tugging in the absence of fever or sleeping/feeding difficulties is generally not associated with acute infections.

Inspection

- Perform external inspection and all noninvasive portions of the examination before beginning procedures such as otoscopic examination.
- Note the position of the ear for otoscopic examination of small children. For children under age 3 years, pull the ear downward, outward, and backward.
- Note the following variations:
  - The eustachian tube is shorter in children compared with adults; this allows easier movement of fluid and microorganisms from the back of the nasopharynx to the middle ear.

- Crying will make the ear canal and tympanic membrane red by making radial and circumferential blood vessels in the tympanic membrane visible. The tympanic membrane is a vascular organ, so anything that produces vasodilation (fever, flushing, etc.) will cause the tympanic membrane to be red. Redness alone *does not* indicate the presence of infection.

Considerations for the Geriatric Patient

General

Note the following when assessing geriatric patients:

- Presbycusis is a common cause of hearing loss; approximately 30% to 40% of adults over age 65 years experience some degree of presbycusis.
- There is an increasing prevalence of tinnitus in all age groups until about 70 years of age.
- Vertigo increases with age; nonotological causes of vertigo in older adults are common and include neurological, psychological, and cardiovascular disorders.
- A common cause of hearing loss is cerumen impaction.
- Hearing loss may be associated with paranoia and agitation.
- Men have poorer hearing after age 40 years compared with women.

Inspection

- Note that the pinna becomes elongated and thickens on geriatric patients.
- Observe an increased amount and coarseness of hair growth in the cartilaginous portion of the external ear canal.
- Inspect for skin cancer; sun-induced skin cancer on the pinna is more common in older adults.

Case Study Review

Throughout this chapter, you have been introduced to JB. This section of the chapter pulls together her history and demonstrates documentation of her history and physical examination.

Chief Complaint

"My child is pulling at her right ear and cried all night."

Information Gathered During the Interview

JB is a 12-month-old female child who presents with a 5-day history of "cold" symptoms, including yellow/green nasal discharge, cough, and poor appetite. Last night, she developed a fever of 102 to 103°F, which was taken using the family's tympanic thermometer. She was very irritable and intermittently pulled at her right ear. Mrs. B, the child's mother, gave the child two doses of acetaminophen.

JB has had multiple upper respiratory infections (URIs), which were treated with antibiotics. She has experienced only one other problem with her ears. The earache occurred 2 months ago; however, she was not treated with antibiotics and recovered without incident. Her immunizations are up to date. JB has never been hospitalized for an illness. She appears to have a close relationship with mother; no evidence of child abuse visible. JB speaks single words, such as mama, dada, ba (for ball), and babbles sounds as though conversing—language development appropriate to age. Her birth was a normal vaginal delivery at 38 weeks after a normal pregnancy, with a weight of 7 lb, 8 oz and no visible birth defects. JB crawls without difficulty and pulls self up to examining table. Child has had the usual falls and head bumps from learning to stand and trying to walk—she has never lost consciousness or evidenced any significant head trauma.

JB takes a liquid multivitamin daily. Her mother is unaware of any exposure to ototoxic drugs during her pregnancy. There is no history of ototoxic drug use in the child. JB has four deciduous teeth in good condition. She may be allergic to amoxicillin (she developed a "rash" over body after treatment of URI several months ago).

JB lives with her parents and two siblings (sister age 4 and brother age 7); all are in good health. Father, age 35, is in good health; he has a history of "many ear infections" as a child and had "tubes" in his ears at age 18 months. Mother, age 30, is obese but in otherwise good health. Paternal grandmother, age 60, has diabetes, hypertension, and heart disease. Paternal grandfather died at age 65 in car accident; he did not have major health problems. Maternal grandmother, age 65, is obese and has hypertension and macular degeneration. Maternal grandfather, age 65, was diagnosed with otosclerosis at age 45; he does not have other health problems. JB's sister is in excellent health. Her brother has been diagnosed with attention-deficit/hyperactivity disorder, which is controlled with medication; his general health is excellent.

JB lives at home with parents in a single-family, middle-class dwelling with modern conveniences. Both parents work outside the home, and the family is covered by health insurance. JB spends most of the day at a day care center. Both parents smoke about a pack of cigarettes per day but report that they smoke outdoors to protect their children; they deny smoking in the car with children. JB continues to sleep with a bottle at night to "help her go to sleep." When child is not ill, she sleeps from 8:00 PM until 6:00 AM without waking. JB feeds herself with fingers. For the past 2 to 3 days, she has not been eating well. For the last 24 hours, she has been drinking poorly (using 2 to 3 diapers/24 hrs). JB's social interaction with family appears to be appropriate for a 12-month-old child.

Clues	Important Points
Age of the child	Middle ear infections are common at this age.
Five-day history of respiratory symptoms with additional complaints in the last 12 hours	Upper respiratory infections are often a prodrome to ear infections.
Pulling at right ear	Can be habit or a response to pain or other symptom; ear tugging plus eating and sleeping difficulties with fever are associated with acute infections.
Sleeping difficulties with fever	Middle ear infections interfere with sleep patterns.
Cough and fever (102°–103°F)	Suggestive of respiratory infectious process.
Acetaminophen therapy (two doses)	Consider effectiveness of antipyretic and analgesic medication for therapeutic planning.
Day care environment	Associated with crowding and transmission of infections.
Sleeps with a bottle	Possible retrograde regurgitarion of bottle feeding into the middle ear.
Parents smoke	Association between secondary cigarette smoke exposure and otitis media.

Name JB	Date 10-1-16	Time 0900
	DOB 10-1-15	Sex F

HISTORY

CC
"My child is pulling at her right ear and cried all night."

HPI
12-month-old child with 5-day history of upper respiratory infection; 12-hour history of fever, pulling at right ear, disrupted sleep, irritability and crying.

Medications
1. Multivitamins, daily

2. Acetaminophen syrup, ½ teaspoon every 4 hours for fever and pain × 2 doses

Allergies
Possibly amoxicillin—rash over body after last dose several months ago

PMI
Illnesses

Childhood immunizations up to date
Frequent upper respiratory infections
Otitis media—2 months ago

Hospitalizations/Surgeries

No past surgeries or trauma; has never received blood transfusion.

FH

One brother (age 7) with ADHD and one sister (age 4) in good health.
Father (age 35)—smokes 1 pk/day; otherwise good health; history as child having ear infections with "tubes."
Mother (age 30)—obese; good health; smokes 1 pk/day.
Maternal grandparents: Grandmother (65)—obese; hypertension; macular degeneration.
    Grandfather (65)—otosclerosis age 45; good health.
Paternal grandparents: Grandmother (60) diabetes mellitus type 2; hypertension; heart disease.
    Grandfather (deceased, car accident)—no significant health problems at time of death.

SH

Lives in single-family dwelling with modern conveniences with two siblings and both parents.
Both parents work and smoke cigarettes. Spends daytime at day care center. Speaks in single words and babbles appropriately for 12-month-old child. Goes to bed with bottle to "help her sleep."
When well, sleeps all night—8 pm–6 am. Feeds self finger foods.

ROS

General	Cardiovascular
Ill-appearing infant with fever.	No history of heart problems or defects.
Skin	**Respiratory**
Warm to touch; no rashes.	Rapid breathing; frequent crying. Coughing productive of white mucoid sputum.
Eyes	**Gastrointestinal**
Reaches for objects appropriately.	Eating poorly, especially last 12 hours.
Ears	**Genitourinary/Gynecological**
Pulling at right ear periodically.	2–3 wet diapers in 24 hours.
Nose/Mouth/Throat	**Musculoskeletal**
Nasal stuffiness, yellow-green discharge from nose.	Mother reports no major injuries.
Breast	**Neurological**
Mother denies any problems.	Mother denies any seizure disorder.

PHYSICAL EXAMINATION

Weight 20 lb	Temp 102.0 (Tympanic)	BP Not taken
Height 26 in	Pulse 160	Resp 40

General Appearance

12-month-old well-nourished Hispanic female in moderate distress sitting on mother's lap, crying occasionally. Well-groomed child clinging to mother; face flushed; irritable.

Skin

Clear, warm, dry, turgor—skin fold returns somewhat slowly to normal; no rashes.

HEENT

Head: Normal cephalic: no masses, no tenderness, no evidence of trauma; fontanels closed.
Head circumference 46 cm.
Eyes: PERRL, extraocular motion intact; sclera white, no nystagmus.
Ears: Symmetrical, well developed; no abnormalities noted; visibly upset when right ear manipulated.
Pinna: No evidence of eczema; no skin lesions.
Ear canal: No evidence of discharge, edema, or foreign body.
Hearing: Responds appropriately to normal intensity voice commands.
Mastoid: No tenderness, edema, or erythema bilaterally.
Tympanic membrane: Right—intact, bright red bulging tympanic membrane with no visible landmarks or light reflex; membrane opaque. Left—intact, notably prominent blood vessels at rim of nonbulging tympanic membrane; cone of light and landmarks visible and membrane transparent.

Pneumatoscopy: Right tympanic membrane reveals decreased mobility; left tympanic membrane mobile. Nares: Thick yellow-green mucus in both nares; turbinates erythematous and edematous. Oropharynx: Pharynx slightly inflamed; no lesions; tongue midline; four deciduous teeth in good condition; tonsils enlarged without exudates. Neck/Lymphatic: Neck supple; chin to chest without pain or discomfort. Cervical nodes: Right: enlarged 1–2 cm; mobile and nontender postauricular and posterior cervical nodes. Left: normal postauricular and posterior cervical nodes.
Cardiovascular Slight tachycardia (normal range age 12 months 90–150; mean 119). No murmurs detected.
Respiratory Breath sounds vesicular with no added sounds bilaterally; slightly increased respiratory rate; no sternal retraction or use of accessory muscles for breathing.
Gastrointestinal Abdomen soft, protuberant appropriate to age. No masses or tenderness detected. Umbilicus: no hernia.
Genitourinary Genitalia developmentally normal for age. Buttock and perineal area: skin clear, intact; no evidence of diaper rash.
Musculoskeletal Crawls on all four limbs appropriately. Pulls self up on examining table. Walks around objects for support. Picks up toys; muscle strength appropriate to age.
Neurological Hears spoken voice; responds to soft speech of examiner. Neurologically grossly intact appropriate for age.
Other
Lab Tests: None
Special Tests
Final Assessment Findings 1. Acute otitis media, right ear 2. Upper respiratory infection

Bibliography

Bagai, A., Thavendiranathan, P., & Detsky, A. S. (2006). Does this patient have hearing impairment? *Journal of the American Medical Association, 295,* 416.

Brunton, L., Chabner, B., & Knollman, B. (2011). *Goodman and Gilman's the pharmacological basis of therapeutics* (12th ed.). New York, NY: McGraw Hill Medical.

Carlson, L. (2002). Update on otitis media. *The American Journal for Nurse Practitioners, 6*(10), 9–14.

Carlson, L., & Marcy, S. M. (2004). Diagnosis and management of acute otitis media: Summary of the new clinical practice guideline. *Clinician Reviews: A Self-Study Supplement* (June), 2–13.

Chole, R. A., & Cook, G. B. (1988). The Rinne test for conductive deafness: A critical reappraisal. *Archives of Otolaryngology and Head and Neck Surgery, 114,* 399.

Cunningham, J., Cox, E. O., & The Committee on Practice and Ambulating Medicine and the Section in Otolaryngology and Bronchoesophagology. (2003). Hearing assessment in infants and children: Recommendations beyond neonatal screening. *Pediatrics, 111*(2), 436–440.

Dean, W. A., & Davison, M. (2002). Hearing loss in adults. *Clinician Reviews, 12*(6), 62–67. [Online.] Retrieved from www.medscape.com/viewarticle/439298.

Desai, H. (2002). Recurrent episodic vertigo. *Medscape Internal Medicine, 4*(2). [Online.] Retrieved from http://www.medscape.com/viewarticle/442820.

Meadows, C. (1999). Assessment of the auditory system. In W. J. Phipps, F. D. Monahan, J. K. Sands, J. F. Marek, & M. Neighbors (Eds.), *Medical-surgical nursing: Health and illness perspectives* (7th ed.). St. Louis, MO: Mosby.

Paul, B. C., & Roland, J. T., Jr. (2015). An abnormal audiogram. *Journal of the American Medical Association, 313,* 85.

Pirozzo, S., Papinczak, T., & Glasziou, P. (2003). Whispered voice test for screening for hearing impairment in adults and children: Systematic review. *British Medical Journal, 327,* 967.

Shuman, A. G., Li, X., Halpin, C. F., Rauch, S. D., & Telian, S. A. (2013). Tuning fork testing in sudden sensorineural hearing loss. *JAMA Internal Medicine, 173,* 706–707.

Uy, J., & Forciea, M.A. (2013). In the clinic. Hearing loss. *Annals of Internal Medicine, 158,* ITC4.

Yueh, B., Collins, M. P., Souza, P. E., Boyko, E. J., Loovis, C. F., Heagerty, P. J., . . . Hedrick, S. C. (2010). Long-term effectiveness of screening for hearing loss: The Screening For Auditory Impairment—Which Hearing Assessment Test (SAI-WHAT) randomized trial. *Journal of the American Geriatrics Society, 58,* 427–434.

Additional Resources

Auditory and Vestibular Pathways

http://thalamus.wustl.edu/course/audvest.html

This website provides anatomical and physiological background needed to understand the process of hearing.

Cranial Nerves

http://www.aan.com/familypractice/html/chp1p2.htm

This site provides information about the cranial nerves, including cranial nerve VIII, which is responsible for hearing.

Hearing, Ear Infections, and Deafness

http://www.nidcd.nih.gov/health/hearing/index.asp

This National Institute on Deafness and Other Communication Disorders site provides information on various ear disorders.

Chapter 8

Nose, Sinus, Mouth, and Throat Disorders

ADVANCED ASSESSMENT OF NOSE AND SINUS DISORDERS

Anatomy and Physiology Review of the Nose and Sinuses

The nose has four main functions:

- Acting as the primary site of inspiration and expiration
- Filtering, warming, and humidifying air
- Sensing smell (through stimulation of the olfactory receptors)
- Resonating speech sounds

The paranasal sinus has two major functions:

- Filtering, warming, and humidifying air
- Resonating speech sounds

External Nose

The external nose, or outer portion of the nose, is composed of bone and flexible cartilage with a mucous membrane lining. The upper one-third of the external nose is bone, while the lower two-thirds is flexible cartilage. Two nasal bones form the upper portion. These bones articulate with each other at the center and with the maxilla and frontal bones laterally. The external nose contains two external openings called nares or nostrils. The nares provide the entranceway for air into the nasal cavity. **Figure 8-1** depicts the external nose.

Internal Nose

The internal nose (**Figure 8-2**) extends from the anterior to the posterior nares, ultimately opening into the nasopharynx. It is composed of two nasal cavities separated by the nasal septum. Just inside each naris is a vestibule for each nasal cavity. Each cavity has three projections from the lateral wall called conchae, or turbinates. Cilia line the turbinates. In addition, the turbinates are highly vascular and are covered by mucous membrane. The vascular supply warms the incoming air. The mucous membrane lining increases the surface area in the nose and provides moisture. The turbinates use secreted mucus and ciliary action to filter the air by trapping dust and foreign particles. The collected debris is then moved via ciliary action to the throat, where it is swallowed. Beneath each turbinate is a meatus that allows drainage to enter from the sinuses.

Olfactory receptors are found on the mucosa in the upper part of the nasal cavity. Passing air stimulates these receptors, which trigger olfactory nerves to send a signal to the frontal lobe of the brain for interpretation.

Smell is considered a significant component of taste; the two are closely related. The sense of smell is tested by the stimulation of the olfactory nerve. Acute loss of smell and the related decreased ability to taste is most often transient and related to upper respiratory infections. Chronic loss of the sense of smell is poorly understood, and no standards exist as to a baseline assessment.

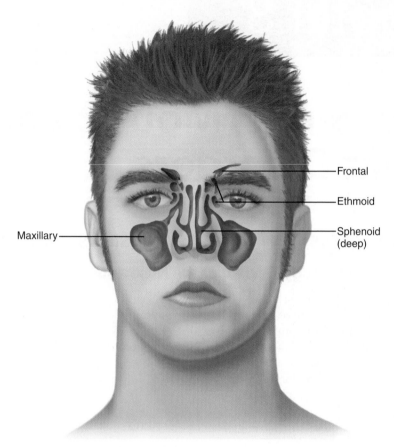

FIGURE 8-1 External nose.

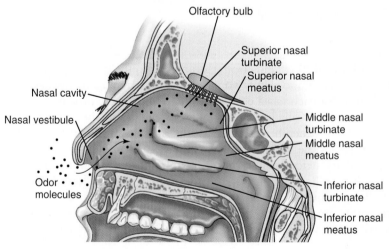

FIGURE 8-2 Lateral view of the internal nose.

Paranasal Sinuses

Four pairs of paranasal sinuses (air-filled cavities) are located on each side of the nasal cavity. They include the maxillary sinuses, located just below the orbit of the eye in the maxillary bone (cheek area); the frontal sinuses, located in the frontal bone just above the eyebrows; the ethmoidal sinuses, located in the ethmoid bone lying behind the eyes and nose; and the sphenoidal sinuses, located in the sphenoid bone lying behind the eyes and the nose. These air-filled cavities help to lighten the weight of the skull and provide resonance for speech.

Like the nasal cavity, each paranasal sinus is lined with cilia and mucous membrane that help to trap foreign particles and move them to the outside. The paranasal sinuses connect with the nasal cavity via the meatus. They are often the sites of infection because the opening into the nasal cavity can become easily blocked. The maxillary and frontal sinuses are accessible for indirect examination, whereas the ethmoidal and sphenoidal sinuses cannot be directly examined because they are smaller and located more deeply in the skull.

Health History

A detailed history of the present illness (HPI) and chief complaint (CC) is essential to the successful assessment of nasal complaints. Past medical history (PMI) and HPI, as well as social history (SH) and family history (FH), are also important. The review of systems (ROS) can contribute significant information as well.

Congestion and nasal discharge are common complaints causing a patient to seek medical care. Additionally, disorders related to the nose can affect other body systems. For example, appetite and nutritional status may be affected because smell is closely related to the sense of taste. Patients' eating patterns can become disrupted when taste and smell are disrupted. Additionally, nasal congestion may interfere with the patient's nutritional intake because he or she is too fatigued from labored breathing to eat. This decreased intake can lead to gastrointestinal problems, such as constipation or diarrhea, further contributing to nutritional problems.

Chief Complaint and History of Present Illness

"I can't breathe; I'm congested."

> CR is a 45-year-old Hispanic female. Ms. R says that she has experienced congestion, watery eyes, and fatigue for the last 3 days. Discharge has been clear. Ms. R states that she experiences these symptoms every spring.

Patients often present with the following common symptoms: congestion, sneezing, itching, rhinitis (allergic, vasomotor, and other), drainage, chronic discharge, nosebleed, and decreased senses of smell and taste.

Congestion

Onset	Was the onset sudden or gradual?
	Acute or gradual onset provides information as to the precipitating cause or associated illnesses.
Duration; pattern	How long has the patient experienced the congestion?
	This would provide information about whether the congestion is related to an acute or chronic condition.
	Does the congestion occur in the morning, during the day; at night while sleeping; or in certain areas, such as at home, at work, or at a friend's house?
	Congestion occurring in a specific environment may lead to the suspicion of a potential environmental allergen. Congestion lasting all day may suggest an acute infection.

Severity	How severe is the congestion? Does it interfere with work or disrupt sleep?
	The intensity of the symptoms helps determine the degree of intervention necessary.
Associated symptoms	Is the patient experiencing associated symptoms, such as productive cough, sneezing, or itching or watery eyes?
	A productive cough of clear discharge may be associated with allergic rhinitis. Sneezing or itching or watery eyes may be related to seasonal allergies.
Precipitating and aggravating factors	Ascertain if the symptoms occur with any activity or environmental event. Is the onset related to weather/seasonal changes?
	If the patient's congestion worsens at home, the likely cause may be an allergy to dust or pets.
	Seasonal symptoms suggest allergies related to pollen.
	Winter complaints may be related to mold or decreased humidity.
	Does bending over cause the patient any pain or pressure with the congestion?
	Increased pressure or pain when bending over associated with nasal congestion may suggest sinusitis.
Alleviating factors	What relieves the congestion? Ask about environmental factors.
	If the patient gets relief in an air-conditioned environment, the cause may be an allergy to pollens.
	Inquire about the use of decongestants, cough suppressants, or allergy medications, including the results. Inquire as to prescription, over-the-counter (OTC), and herbal treatments.
	Acetaminophen (Tylenol) or ibuprofen may help to relieve the signs and symptoms of an upper respiratory infection, such as pain. OTC decongestants such as pseudoephedrine or antihistamines such as diphenhydramine (Benadryl) and loratidine (Claritin) may be helpful in reducing the nasal congestion.
Other medications taken	Ask about other medications taken, especially the use of OTC nasal sprays.
	Nasal sprays, if used for more than 3 days, may lead to rebound congestion.
	Angiotensin-converting enzyme (ACE) inhibitors, beta blockers, and oral contraceptives may increase nasal congestion.

Nasal Discharge (Rhinorrhea)

Rhinorrhea is another common complaint. A careful history helps to determine its cause.

Duration; pattern; onset	How long has the patient been experiencing the symptom?
	This would provide information about whether the nasal discharge is related to an acute or chronic condition.
	Does the discharge occur in the morning, during the day, at night while sleeping, or in certain areas, such as at home, at work, or at a friend's house?
	Rhinorrhea occurring in a specific environment may lead to the suspicion of a potential environmental allergen. Rhinorrhea occurring in the morning may indicate allergic rhinitis, whereas rhinorrhea throughout the day may suggest an upper respiratory infection (URI) or cold.

Quality and severity	Ask the patient to describe the discharge, including color, quantity, consistency, and odor. *Copious, clear discharge is indicative of allergies, whereas a greenish or colored discharge most often indicates an infection. Allergy-related nasal discharge does not usually have an odor, whereas discharge related to an infection often has a foul odor. Unilateral discharge indicates an obstruction such as a foreign body, tumor, or polyp.*
Associated symptoms	Ask the patient about associated symptoms, including fever, sneezing, pain, and itchy or watery eyes. *Fever suggests an acute infection; sneezing may be associated with several problems, such as allergic rhinitis, cold, or upper respiratory infection. Pain, especially in the sinus area, suggests sinusitis. Itchy or watery eyes may indicate an allergy.*
Precipitating factors	Is the onset related to weather/seasonal changes or environmental issues? *Onset related to seasons suggests allergy to pollen.*
Alleviating factors	What alleviates the discharge? Ask about medication and other measures used. *OTC antihistamine medications may relieve allergy-mediated rhinorrhea.*
Other medications taken	Ask about additional medications. *Medication used intranasally, such as sprays or drops, may cause rhinorrhea.*

Bleeding

A careful history of this complaint, especially onset, amount, and precipitating factors, helps determine the cause.

Onset	Is the onset sudden or gradual? *Acute onset is most often related to trauma.*
Location	Is the bleeding unilateral or bilateral? *Unilateral bleeding is often associated with a sore or ulceration in the nares. Bilateral bleeding would most often originate in the vestibule or higher.*
Amount	How much is the patient bleeding? *Profuse or prolonged bleeding may be related to medications that have anticoagulant properties. Prescription anticoagulants, OTC pain medications, and some herbal medications such as ginkgo biloba may prolong bleeding.*
Duration; frequency	How long do the nosebleeds last and how frequently do they occur? *Copious and short-term bleeding is associated with trauma and is usually an isolated incident.* *Chronic bleeding may be related to drug therapies, chemotherapies, or a very dry environment and fragile nasal mucosa.*
Precipitating factors	Is the bleeding related to environmental changes or trauma? Does the patient have any nasal congestion or stuffiness, itching or irritation? *Environmental changes may lead to dryness of the mucous membranes and increased fragility of the blood vessels. Itching or irritation may cause the patient to rub or scratch the nose, leading to bleeding.*
Alleviating factors	What alleviates the bleeding? Is there difficulty stopping the bleeding? *Difficulty in stopping the bleeding may suggest a problem with coagulation or a blood disorder.*

Medications taken	Which medications is the patient taking?
	Assess if the patient is on any anticoagulation therapy or uses aspirin. Aspirin inhibits platelet aggregation, which can interfere with adequate clotting. Overuse of nasal sprays can lead to rebound congestion and subsequent increased fragility of the nasal capillaries.
	Herbal therapies may also contribute to the problem and should be assessed. Ginkgo biloba increases risk for bleeding related to antiplatelet activity.

Decreased Sense of Smell (and Taste)

Onset; duration	How long has the patient been experiencing a decreased sense of smell?
	Determination of the onset of the loss and its duration will help to determine if the loss is related to a chronic or acute condition.
Precipitating factors	Ascertain if the loss can be associated with a new medication, illness, or health issue.
	Both smell and taste decrease may be related to cold and influenza symptoms. Other causes are not generally known. Some mild loss may be associated with aging. Some medications may also be associated with changes in smell and taste.
Medications taken	Which medications does the patient take?
	Many medications have an aftertaste that masks taste sensations.

Sinus Pain and Pressure

Onset; duration; pattern	How long has the patient been experiencing the symptom?
	This helps determine whether the sinus pressure and pain is related to an acute or chronic condition.
	Does the pain or pressure occur in the morning, during the day, or at night while sleeping?
	This information would help provide clues to identify the possible cause. Sinus pain and pressure occurring in the morning that continues throughout the day may suggest a sinus infection.
Quality; severity; location	Ask the patient to describe the degree of pain or pressure, including the area where the pain and pressure are noted.
	The pain and pressure of sinusitis can range from mild to severe. The location of the pain or pressure can provide clues to which sinuses are affected. For example, pain over the cheeks and upper teeth suggests maxillary sinusitis, over the eyes indicates ethmoid sinusitis, over the eyebrows indicates frontal sinusitis, and behind the eyes suggests sphenoidal sinusitis.
Associated symptoms	Ask the patient about associated symptoms, including fever, sneezing, and nasal discharge (including its characteristics).
	Fever suggests an acute infection; sneezing may be associated with allergic sinusitis that results from seasonal allergies. Purulent nasal discharge is common in acute sinusitis. Allergic sinusitis is associated with a watery discharge. Increased pain or pressure with bending over or with touching the area suggests acute sinusitis.

Precipitating factors	Has the patient recently had a cold or bacterial infection? If the patient has allergies, has he recently experienced allergic rhinitis? Does the pressure or pain increase with specific activities, such as bending over or with touching the facial area?
	A URI may lead to acute sinusitis, either bacterial or viral in origin, depending on the causative organism. Persistent bacterial infections can lead to chronic sinusitis. Allergic sinusitis frequently occurs with allergic rhinitis.
Alleviating factors	What alleviates the pain or pressure? Ask about medication and other measures used.
	OTC analgesics such as acetaminophen and ibuprofen may help decrease the pain associated with sinusitis. OTC antihistamine medications may relieve the associated allergy-mediated congestion contributing to the pain and pressure. Heat or cold may help in alleviating the pain.

Past Medical History

> Ms. R has a history of seasonal allergies. She denies any history of asthma or eczema. She denies any nasal trauma and/or surgeries. She denies any recent colds or flu-like episodes. She reports that she sees a dentist regularly and her teeth are in good condition.

The past medical history includes detailed information about any nasal trauma and/or surgeries. Also, inquire about the history of upper respiratory infections and allergies; describe this history in detail.

Past health conditions or surgeries	Ask about past health conditions, including allergies, influenza, and colds as well as any chronic respiratory problems such as polyps, sinusitis, or septal deviation or surgeries.
	Allergies are often associated with a history of eczema and asthma, which present with nasal symptoms. Signs and symptoms of congestion, discharge, or decreased smell and taste may linger for 1 to 2 weeks after influenza or an upper respiratory infection.
	Surgeries may result in obstruction secondary to scar tissue formation.
Trauma	Ask about past trauma.
	Trauma may result in obstruction.
Polyps	Does the patient have a history of polyps?
	They are often found in patients with chronic allergies. Polyps are obstructive.
Dental history	Inquire about dental history.
	Extensive dental care, such as surgeries or tooth extractions, may modify the structure of the nasal passages and the mouth.

Family History

> Ms. R's parents are alive and well. She has a 42-year-old sister. Ms. R denies a family history of asthma, cancer, or eczema. Her parents and sister suffer from seasonal (spring and fall) allergies.

A family history is important in identifying possible clues to the underlying cause of the patient's complaints. Certain conditions such as allergies often have a familial component. Additionally, conditions such as polyps and cancer may be genetically determined.

Age of living relatives	Include the relationship and health of parents, brothers, sisters, and children.
Deaths	Include the relationship of the deceased to the patient and the cause of death (specifically illnesses that affect the nose, such as cancer of the nose or sinuses).
Chronic diseases	Ask about chronic diseases in the family; include relationship of the patient to the family member with the disease and how long that family member has had the disease. Focus on diseases manifesting with nasal symptoms that may be familial or genetic, such as eczema and asthma, or environmental, such as air quality and chemical exposure. *Patients with seasonal allergic rhinitis often have positive family histories.*
Allergies	Ask about allergies. *Patients with a family history of allergies are at risk for allergic signs and symptoms.*

Social History

Ms. R denies any use of cigarettes or secondhand exposure. She lives alone, in an air-conditioned new home. Ms. R has a pet dog. She denies any air travel. She is a computer programmer and enjoys reading and cooking in her spare time. Her alcohol intake is infrequent and she denies using any recreational drugs.

The social history helps in determining if the environment contributes to the symptoms. Air travel or altitude changes can cause vasomotor rhinitis. Home, occupational, and recreational environments can adversely affect nasal and sinus functioning.

Family	Ask the patient to describe the current family unit and any related nasal morbidities.
Occupation	Ask the patient about her work environment. *Exposure to toxins, chemicals, or allergens contributes to nasal problems.* Inquire about the patient's living environment, type of heating and air conditioning, and the frequency filters are changed. *Filters can harbor microorganisms, increasing the patient's risk for infection. Additionally, the filters harbor pollutants and allergens that if not changed frequently can exacerbate a patient's allergies.*
Hobbies	Ask about hobbies. *Some hobbies have increased particulate matter that can be irritating to the nasal mucosa and the throat, such as model building and woodworking. Sewing of materials with permanent-press finishes can also cause irritation.*
Pets	Determine if the patient owns pets. If she does, where does the pet sleep and is it an indoor or outdoor pet? *Pet dander is a frequent allergy trigger with associated nasal symptoms.*

Use of tobacco	Information to obtain includes type of tobacco used (cigarettes, cigars, pipes, smokeless), duration and amount (pack-years = number of years of smoking times number of packs smoked per day), age started; and the extent of smoking by others at home or at work.
	Use of tobacco products and exposure to secondhand smoke are closely associated with cancer, including that of the nose and sinuses.
Use of alcohol	Does the patient drink alcohol? How much? Which type (e.g., wine, beer, liquor)?
Use of recreational drugs	Ask about recreational drug use, including type and amount.
	Recreational drugs such as cocaine via snorting can lead to perforation of the nasal septum. Repeated use of cocaine via snorting also may lead to chronic rhinitis.

Review of Systems

Many nose diseases and disorders have manifestations in systems other than the nose. A comprehensive review of systems should be performed whenever possible; however, due to time and other constraints, the provider may be able to perform only a focused review of systems. During a focused review of systems, the provider targets questioning to the systems in which nasal problems are most likely to have manifestations. Following is a summary of common manifestations of nasal problems.

System	Symptom or Sign	Possible Associated Diseases/Disorders
General	Fever	Common cold, upper respiratory infection, sinusitis
Skin	Eczema or allergic reactions/hypersensitivity reactions; darkened areas (allergic shiners) under eyes; frequent wiping of the nose (with observable crease across nose, termed allergic salute)	Allergic rhinitis
	Bruising or breaks in the skin around the nose area	Nasal trauma/fracture of the nose
	Soreness or pain at nares with complaints of irritation and cracks at site from frequent wiping of nasal discharge	Common cold, upper respiratory infection, allergic rhinitis
Eyes	Itchy, watery eyes	Allergic rhinitis
Ears	Popping, ringing, or fullness in the ears	Common cold, upper respiratory infection
Respiratory system	Shortness of breath, wheezing, cough (productive or nonproductive)	Allergic rhinitis, upper respiratory infection, asthma

Physical Examination

Equipment Needed

- Penlight or other light source
- Otoscope
- Nasal speculum or largest ear speculum available
- Gloves

Components of Physical Examination

The examination of the nose depends primarily on inspection and palpation of the external nose and inspection of the internal nose. Inspection, palpation, and percussion of the sinuses and, if necessary, transillumination are performed when assessing the nose. Good lighting is essential. Gloves are to be worn when there will be contact with the mucous membranes.

Inspection

Action	Rationale
1. Inspect the external nose for overall shape, symmetry, and edema. Inspect the nares for symmetry; check for patency by occluding one naris and having patient breathe in and out through the other naris.	1. The nose should appear smooth and symmetrical in shape. Asymmetry may indicate past fractures and possible deviation.
2. Inspect the skin around the nose for lesions, color, and irregularities.	2. The nose should be similar in color to the rest of the face and free of lesions. The nose is a risk site for skin cancer, which appears as lesions. The presence of broken capillaries may be related to alcohol use. The presence of a lateral nasal crease is often associated with chronic allergies.
3. Inspect the sinus areas for edema.	3. Normally, the sinuses should appear flat without evidence of puffiness or swelling. Swelling noted in the sinus area may be accompanied by swelling under or around the eyes or eyebrows, suggesting possible sinus infection.
4. Observe the nares for discharge or drainage. If discharge is present, inspect for color, consistency, amount, odor, and presence of blood.	4. The character of the discharge helps identify the cause. For example, clear watery discharge suggests allergic rhinitis, whereas purulent discharge suggests infection.
5. Inspect the nasal cavity (**Figure 8-3**). Ask the patient to blow his or her nose. Have the patient tilt his or her head backward. Use your nondominant hand and fingers to stabilize the patient's head in this position. With your thumb, apply slight upward pressure to the tip of the nose and shine the light of the otoscope into the nose. If needed, use a nasal speculum to gently open the naris.	5. Blowing the nose clears the nasal cavity of any drainage or particles that could interfere with inspection. This positioning facilitates inspection of internal structures. Adequate illumination is needed for accurate inspection. A nasal speculum opens the naris, providing for better inspection.

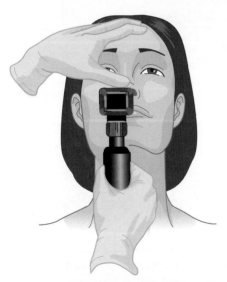

FIGURE 8-3 Positioning and technique for inspecting internal nose.

Action	Rationale
a. Assess the nasal cavity for patency and the nasal septum for continuity.	a. The nasal cavity should be patent and free of any blockage or obstruction. The nasal septum should be continuous without any deviations or perforations. The ability to inhale and exhale through one nostril while the other is closed indicates patency of the nonoccluded side. Inability to do so suggests an obstruction due to swelling, congestion, polyps, or a foreign body.

b. Assess the turbinates for color, texture, and discharge. Inspect the color of the mucous membranes.	b. The turbinates should appear dark pink, moist, and without any lesions or swelling. Typically discharge is absent. The mucous membranes should appear dark pink and moist without any drainage.
	
	    Pale, boggy turbinates are suggestive of allergies.
	
	    Erythematous, swollen turbinates are often seen in infections.

c. Note any masses, lesions, or polyps.	c. The nasal cavity should be clear and open without any evidence of masses, lesions, or polyps. Lesions may be associated with cocaine use, trauma, chronic infection, or chronic nose picking. Polyps may be noted in patients with allergies.

Palpation and Percussion

Action	Rationale
1. Palpate the bridge and soft tissues of the nose (**Figure 8-4**).	1. The bridge of the nose should feel firm, whereas the soft tissue should yield to the touch. Tenderness on palpation would suggest infection.

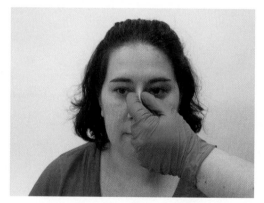

FIGURE 8-4 Palpating the bridge and soft tissues of the nose.

Action	Rationale
2. Palpate the sinuses. Place your thumbs on the patient's forehead at the orbital ridge (eyebrow) and press upward on the eyebrow to palpate the frontal sinuses. Then move your thumbs to each side of the patient's cheeks and apply gentle pressure upward just below the cheekbones, on the maxillary area. Note any evidence of a crackling sensation during palpation. **Figure 8-5** illustrates palpation of the sinuses.	2. The sinuses should be nontender bilaterally. Tenderness on palpation may indicate allergic rhinitis or sinus infection. Crackling (crepitus) suggests accumulation of a large amount of exudates.

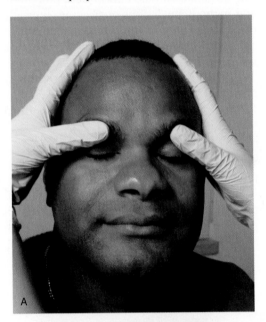

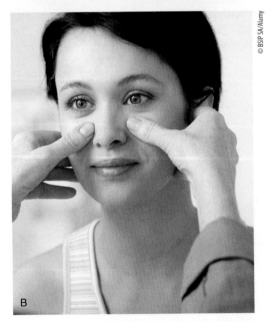

© BSIP SA/Alamy

FIGURE 8-5 Palpating the sinuses. A. Frontal. B. Maxillary.

Action	Rationale

3. Percuss the sinuses. Lightly tap over the frontal and maxillary sinuses for tenderness. **Figure 8-6** illustrates percussion of the sinuses.

3. The sinuses should be resonant on percussion and tenderness should be absent. Tenderness or dullness on percussion may indicate allergic rhinitis or sinus infection.

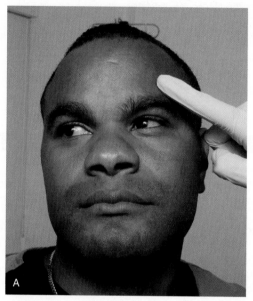

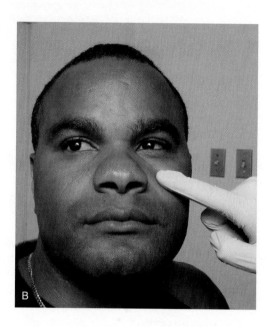

FIGURE 8-6 Percussing the sinuses. A. Frontal. B. Maxillary.

4. If tenderness is noted on palpation and percussion of the sinuses, transilluminate the sinuses to gather additional information.

   a. Darken the room. To transilluminate the frontal sinuses, shine a strong, narrow stream of light closely under the eyebrow. Use your other hand to shield the light. Compare the glow of the light through the sinuses bilaterally.

   b. Transilluminate the maxillary sinuses by shining the light directly over the maxillary sinus (cheekbone area). Have the patient open her mouth; look for the glow of light on the hard palate. Compare the glow of light for each side.

4. Transillumination helps to determine if the sinuses are filled with air or fluid.

   a. Normally, when sinuses are air filled, the light is seen as a red glow. If this is absent, then the sinuses are most likely filled with fluid or purulent drainage.

   b. Normally, when sinuses are air filled, the light is seen as a red glow. If this is absent, then the sinuses are most likely filled with fluid or purulent drainage.

Diagnostic Reasoning

Based on findings in the health history and physical examination, the clinician should formulate the assessment and plan. For example, a patient may report symptoms that suggest many possible diagnoses; however, findings in the past medical history and during the physical examination might narrow the possible diagnoses down to one or two. Congestion is a common chief complaint. **Table 8-1** illustrates differential diagnosis of common disorders associated with congestion.

Diagnostic tests may help examiners with diagnosis. **Box 8-1** describes common laboratory and other tests used to diagnose disorders of the nose.

Table 8-1   Differential Diagnosis of Congestion

Differential Diagnosis	Significant Findings in the Patient's History	Significant Findings in the Patient's Physical Examination	Diagnostic Tests
Foreign body	Patient aged 3 to 5 years old	Unilateral redness, swelling and edema, cloudy or colored discharge, compromised patency of one naris	N/A
Allergic rhinitis	Patient and family history of seasonal allergies, eczema, or asthma	Bilateral clear discharge, boggy nasal mucosa, allergic shiners, nasal crease	Radioallergosorbent or intradermal sensitivity testing, nasal smear for eosinophilia
Sinusitis	Dull ache over the cheeks and above the eyes that increases when the patient bends over	Thick green to dark yellow discharge (which may have an odor), absence of red glow upon transillumination	Sinus films

BOX 8-1   COMMON LABORATORY AND DIAGNOSTIC STUDIES USED TO DIAGNOSE NOSE DISORDERS

ALLERGY STUDIES
- The radioallergosorbent test (RAST) is a blood assay of the IgE antibodies. It can identify specific allergens that are causing symptoms. It does not involve exposure to the allergens and, therefore, does not risk anaphylaxis.
- Intradermal sensitivity studies involve the introduction of specific suspected allergens under the skin and evaluation of the response. These cause a local allergic reaction that can be uncomfortable. This type of testing identifies specific allergens.
- Eosinophil counts are accomplished by the submission of a mucus smear from the nasal passage. This test is useful in gauging the degree of allergy reaction but lacks specificity of allergens.

OTHER TESTS
- The thyroid-stimulating hormone (TSH) test determines the level of TSH and is useful in determining thyroid function, which may have an effect on congestion.
- Coagulation studies may be useful in determining the origins of chronic nosebleeds.
- Radiographic examinations of the sinus and the nasal passages produce an image of the nasal structures and any physical deviations, tumors, or other impediments.
- Ultrasound of the facial sinuses determines the extent of fluids accumulating in the sinus cavities.

Nose and Sinus Assessment of Special Populations

Considerations for the Pregnant Patient
- Changes in hormones may have effects on the nasal mucosa and result in increased congestion.
- Increased circulation fluid volume may contribute to congestion.
- Increased vascularity due to changing hormones may contribute to nosebleeds.

Considerations for the Neonatal Patient
General

Recognize physiological differences in neonates:
- Newborns (and infants) are normally nose breathers. They sneeze to clear the air passage, which is considered normal.
- Newborns have no way of clearing the nasal mucosa of discharge, and the use of a nasal syringe can be used to clear mucus.
- Increased discharge and congestion can interfere with the newborn's ability to nurse and sleep.

Inspection

- Assess flaring of the nares. It is an indication of concern and requires a thorough respiratory assessment.
- Check nasal patency by closing the mouth and occluding one nostril at a time; note any difficulty or distress. If choanal atresia (blockage of the posterior nares) is suspected, insert a small catheter (10 to 12 Fr) into the nasal cavity and into the nasopharynx. Normally, the catheter should pass freely without any resistance. Repeat the test on the opposite nostril.

Considerations for the Pediatric Patient

Inspection

- Assess for a foreign body. Young children may have inserted various small items in the nose. These foreign bodies range from peanuts and raisins to doll shoes and toy soldiers.
- Assess for nasal flaring in the infant or young child. This often indicates respiratory distress.
- Do not use a nasal speculum to inspect the nasal cavity. Instead, push the tip of the nose upward and use a light to visualize the internal nose structures.

Palpation

Do not palpate the sinuses of infants and young children because the sinuses are not fully developed and, therefore, not palpable. The frontal sinuses fully mature at approximately the age of 6 years.

Considerations for the Geriatric Patient

Note the following physiological changes:

- Older adults may have decreased hydration and ability to maintain tissue integrity, which will increase the fragility of the mucosa.
- Many older adults are on anticoagulant therapy that can increase bleeding.

Case Study Review

Throughout the first half of this chapter, you have been introduced to Ms. R. This section of the chapter pulls together her history and demonstrates the documentation of her history and physical examination.

Chief Complaint

"I can't breathe; I'm congested."

Information Gathered During the Interview

Ms. R is a 45-year-old Hispanic female. Ms. R says that she has experienced congestion, watery eyes, and fatigue for the last 3 days. Discharge has been clear. She states that she experiences these symptoms every spring.

Ms. R has a history of seasonal allergies. She denies any history of asthma or eczema. She denies any nasal trauma and or surgeries. She denies any recent colds or flu-like episodes. She reports that she sees a dentist regularly and her teeth are in good condition.

Ms. R's parents are alive and well (A&W). She has a 42-year-old sister. Ms. R denies a family history of asthma, cancer, or eczema. Her parents and sister suffer from seasonal (spring and fall) allergies.

Ms. R denies any use of cigarettes or secondhand exposure. She lives alone in an air-conditioned new home. Ms. R has a pet dog. She denies any air travel. She is a computer programmer and enjoys reading and cooking in her spare time. Her alcohol intake is infrequent and she denies using any recreational drugs.

Clues	Important Points
Seasonal cycle	Common allergies are mold and pollen, which are related to seasonal changes.

Clear, watery discharge; watery eyes; congestion; and fatigue	Clear discharge is most often an allergic response, green is seen in bacterial infections, and white is seen in viral infections. Watery eyes, congestion, and fatigue are associated symptoms of allergies.
Patient relates a history of allergies and family history of allergies	Allergies often have a familial component.

Name CR	Date 10/03/15	Time 0900
	DOB 08/04/70	Sex F

HISTORY

CC
"I can't breathe; I'm congested."

HPI
45-year-old, Hispanic female with a 3-day history of nasal congestion with moderate clear discharge, watery eyes, and fatigue for the last 3 days.

Medications
Ms. R denies using any prescription medications. Takes an over-the-counter multivitamin. She denies using any herbal supplements. She occasionally uses a popular cold-and-sinus remedy with some relief and an occasional Tylenol for headaches. She denies using OC or HRT.

Allergies
NKA

PMI
Illnesses
No history eczema or asthma. Has experienced mild seasonal allergies over the past several years.

Surgeries
None

FH
Parents A&W, both suffer from spring and fall allergy symptoms; sister (42) A&W.

SH
Computer programmer. Does not smoke. Has pet dog. Reports no recent air travel. Alcohol intake is infrequent. Denies any recreational drugs. Home is air conditioned.

ROS

General	Cardiovascular
Alert and oriented, no distress noted.	Denies any problems.
Skin	Respiratory
Warm and dry, no rashes.	Denies any SOB or wheezing. Occasional cough.
Eyes	Gastrointestinal
Wears glasses for distance.	No problems noted.
Ears	Genitourinary/Gynecological
Denies any hearing loss, itching, or congestion.	No problems noted.
Nose/Mouth/Throat	Musculoskeletal
See HPI.	Denies any problems.
Breast	Neurological
No problems noted; does BSE.	No problems noted.

PHYSICAL EXAMINATION

Weight 164 lb	Temp 98.6	BP 135/72
Height 5'4"	Pulse 84	Resp 14

General Appearance
45-year-old Hispanic female in no apparent distress. Slightly overweight, neat appearance, alert and cooperative.

Skin
Light tan, warm to the touch, no rashes noted.

HEENT
Normal cephalic. External ear, ear canal, and TM normal. Eyes have mild bilateral injection, no exudate, and mild bilateral shiners. Nose has bilateral boggy turbinates; scant clear discharge noted. Frontal and maxillary sinuses are nontender with pressure. Transillumination is normal. Mouth and throat normal, no adenopathy.

Cardiovascular
Heart rate is regular without murmurs.

Respiratory
Breathing is regular and nonlabored. All lung fields are clear to auscultation.

Gastrointestinal
Not examined.

Genitourinary
Not examined.

Musculoskeletal
Patient moves with ease and is able to get on and off the examination table without assistance. Gait normal.

Neurological
CN I–XII grossly intact.

Other

Lab Tests
None at this time. Pt should be offered allergy testing, either RAST or skin sensitivity test, if the allergies are significant enough and interfere with her lifestyle or work.

Special Tests
None indicated.

Final Assessment Findings
Allergic rhinitis related to seasonal allergies.

ADVANCED ASSESSMENT OF MOUTH AND THROAT DISORDERS

Anatomy and Physiology Review of the Mouth and Oropharynx

The mouth has the following primary functions:

- Aiding in the production of sounds necessary for speech
- Helping with intake of nutrients and initial steps of digestion via mastication, salivary secretion, and swallowing
- Providing taste sensation via the taste buds
- Acting as an additional passageway for air entry

The oropharynx is responsible for three functions:

- Passing food into the esophagus
- Producing speech through resonation and articulation
- Acting as an airway

Mouth

The upper and lower jaw forms the structural foundation of the mouth, or oral cavity. **Figure 8-7** depicts the oral cavity. The lips and cheeks form the outer boundary of the oral cavity. The lips act as the frontal boundary, providing the entranceway for the mouth and acting as sensory structures for

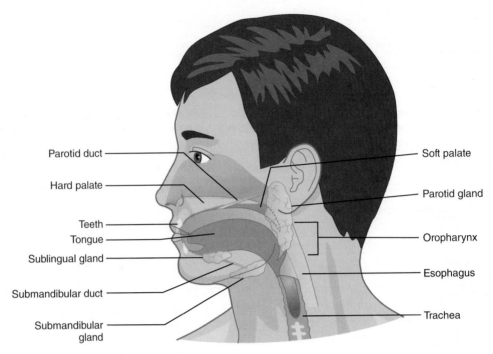

Parotid duct

Hard palate

Teeth

Tongue

Sublingual gland

Submandibular duct

Submandibular gland

Soft palate

Parotid gland

Oropharynx

Esophagus

Trachea

FIGURE 8-7 Lateral view of the oral cavity.

temperature and texture. The cheeks act as the lateral boundaries for the oral cavity and are covered by mucous membrane.

Within the oral cavity are the following structures: hard and soft palate, teeth, tongue, gums, salivary glands, and tonsils. The palate divides the nasal and oral cavities and forms the roof of the mouth. The hard palate is located in the front of the mouth and the soft, or fleshy, palate lies in the back. Extending off the center back of the soft palate is the uvula, which moves via innervation by the glossopharyngeal nerve. Above the soft palate, high in the nasopharynx, lie the pharyngeal tonsils (small masses of lymphoid tissue).

The teeth (32 in the adult) are situated in the mucous membrane–covered gums (gingivae). Each tooth consists of a root (which is implanted in the gum) and a top visible enamel portion (crown). The teeth are responsible for breaking up food into smaller particles to aid in digestion.

The three major salivary glands are the parotid, submandibular, and sublingual glands. The parotid glands, located in the cheek area below and in front of the ears, secrete saliva via Stensen's ducts. These ducts are found in the cheek, at about the area of the second molar. The submandibular glands are located in the floor of the oral cavity, secreting saliva into the mouth via Wharton's ducts. These ducts are located on either side of the frenulum of the tongue. The sublingual glands are found under the tongue, providing saliva via several ducts located in the floor of the mouth, posterior to Wharton's ducts. These glands, along with many other salivatory glands, secrete saliva, which mixes with masticated food to form a bolus. The saliva also helps to maintain oral hygiene by removing and destroying bacteria that can lead to dental caries.

The tongue lies at the floor of the mouth and is attached posteriorly to the mandible and hyoid bones. A small fold of tissue called the frenulum connects the anterior portion of the tongue to the floor of the mouth. At the base of the tongue lie the linguinal tonsils. The tongue is covered by mucous membrane. On the upper surface, the mucous membrane has projections, called papillae. The papillae located on the apex (front) and sides of the tongue contain the taste buds. The extrinsic muscles of the tongue cause the tongue to move in different directions; the intrinsic muscles change the shape of the tongue. Together these movements aid in chewing, propelling the food bolus to the oropharynx, and swallowing.

The mouth and tongue are significantly affected by several cranial nerves (CN). CN IX and X are associated with swallowing, rise of the palate, and the gag reflex. CN V, VII, X, and XII modulate the voice and speech and CN XII the tongue. The tonsils are located in the oral cavity and the pharynx.

Oropharynx

The oropharynx is continuous with the oral cavity, joining with the nasopharynx, and extending to the laryngopharynx. The palatine tonsils are located on both sides of the oropharynx, just posterior to the arches of the soft palate. The oropharynx grasps food and moves it toward the esophagus. It also aids in speech through resonance and articulation. Speech sounds are formed as the size and shape of the oropharynx change. Along with the nasopharynx, the oropharynx serves as an airway.

Health History

The mouth and throat play major roles in digestion and respiratory function. Problems affecting these areas can impact the patient's ability to function, such as obtaining adequate nutrition and performing activities of daily living. The health history can offer clues to possible risk factors for disorders such as cancer of the mouth, tongue, or throat, providing valuable information from which to develop a teaching plan for prevention.

Chief Complaint and History of Present Illness

"My throat hurts."

> HL, a 29-year-old Caucasian male, states that he has had a sore throat for 2 days. He has not noticed being feverish. Mr. L reports that he has experienced a mild runny nose. He has an occasional cough but denies any sputum with the cough. He denies any earache and/or eye irritation. He has a son in day care who is being treated for pharyngitis. Mr. L is taking acetaminophen with some relief.

The history of present illness should focus on the duration of the complaint, the associated symptoms, any alleviating practices, and the intensity of the symptoms. Common symptoms related to the mouth and throat include sore throat, dysphagia, toothache, bleeding gums, halitosis, and lesions.

Sore Throat

Onset	Was the onset sudden or gradual?
	Sore throats caused by bacterial infections usually occur abruptly and may be related to others living in the house who have similar signs and symptoms.
	Viral-related signs and symptoms are often more gradual in onset and linger over time. They may be related to a post-bacterial infection.
Duration; frequency	How long has the patient experienced the sore throat? How often does he or she have a sore throat?
	Scratchy throat that is experienced in the morning and that quickly resolves may be related to mouth breathing or a low-humidity environment.
Quality; severity	Describe the nature and severity of the sore throat.
	Sore throats associated with bacterial infections are described as very sore and may interfere with swallowing.
	Sore throats associated with viruses are often less painful. The sore throat associated with allergies is often described as irritated, scratchy, or itchy.

Associated symptoms	Ask about associated symptoms, including fever, hoarseness, difficulty swallowing, or rash.
	Fever may indicate an acute infection. Hoarseness may suggest an upper respiratory infection or allergy, or be due to smoking, inhalation of irritants, or overuse of the voice. Difficulty swallowing may be associated with a viral or bacterial infection. Patients with group A beta-hemolytic Streptococcus infection (GABHS) may also have a rough, fine, red rash on the abdomen and arms.
Precipitating factors	Is the sore throat brought on by any environmental or other changes?
	Allergy-related sore throats occur seasonally or as a result of contact with pets or other allergens.
Alleviating factors	What alleviates the pain?
	If gargles and over-the-counter (OTC) pain relievers alleviate symptoms, it may indicate the sore throat is related to an inflammatory response due to a possible infection.
	If the use of sinus medication relieves the pain, it may indicate allergy-related discomfort.
Other medications taken	Which medications is the patient currently taking?
	Dry mouth is a side effect of many medications, which causes the patient to breathe through the mouth and thus dry the throat, leading to throat pain and altered taste.

Dysphagia (Difficulty Swallowing)

Onset	Was the onset sudden or gradual?
	Dysphagia caused by bacterial infections usually occurs abruptly in conjunction with the sore throat.
	Viral-related signs and symptoms are often more gradual in onset and linger over time. They may be related to a post-bacterial infection.
Duration; frequency	How long has the patient experienced the dysphagia? How often does he or she have dysphagia?
	Dysphagia associated primarily with a sore throat suggests that the problem is related to inflammation and swelling of the area. Dysphagia lasting for a prolonged period of time or in the absence of pain may indicate a neurologic disorder, anxiety, esophageal disorder, or cancer of the mouth or throat.
Quality; severity	Describe the nature and severity of the dysphagia.
	Dysphagia related to bacterial infection of the throat can be severe, whereas that associated with a virus may be less severe.
Associated symptoms	Ask about associated symptoms including vomiting, regurgitation, weight loss, anorexia, hoarseness, dyspnea, or a cough.
	Dysphagia is the most common symptom associated with esophageal disorders and may be the only symptom. Dysphagia associated with vomiting, regurgitation, and weight loss suggests esophageal problems and may lead to dehydration and nutritional problems. Dysphagia associated with dyspnea or a cough may suggest airway obstruction or laryngeal cancer.

Precipitating and aggravating factors	Is the dysphagia associated with solids or liquids? Is the dysphagia different with different temperatures of food, such as cold, warm, or lukewarm foods? Does spicy food affect it?
	Dysphagia involving solids and liquids may be associated with achalasia, chronic pharyngitis, spasms of the esophagus, or a neuromuscular disorder. Dysphagia involving solids that progresses to involve liquids may indicate a neuromuscular disorder such as amyotrophic lateral sclerosis or progressive systemic sclerosis. Spicy foods may exacerbate the irritation, commonly with a sore throat. Warm or cold foods may irritate or soothe the inflamed mucosa of a sore throat.
Alleviating factors	What, if anything, alleviates the difficulty swallowing? Does the problem disappear after swallowing several times, drinking water, or changing position?
	Swallowing several times provides saliva that adds moisture to an irritated, dry, sore throat. Dysphagia relieved by position changes or drinking water suggests an esophageal condition such as esophageal spasm.
Other medications taken	Which medications is the patient currently taking?
	Some medications can irritate mucous membranes or dry out secretions.

Bleeding Gums

Onset	When did you first notice your gums bleeding?
	This information provides clues to possible causes and whether the problem is related to an acute or chronic condition.
Severity; frequency	How much and how often do the gums bleed?
	Profuse bleeding with mouth care may indicate an underlying blood disorder involving coagulation, such as aplastic anemia or hemophilia, or the use of certain drugs, such as warfarin or heparin. Nutritional deficiencies, such as vitamin C and vitamin K deficiencies, also are associated with bleeding gums.
Precipitating factors	Is the bleeding related to dental care or hormonal changes?
	Bleeding may occur related to the hormonal changes of puberty or pregnancy; it is a normal physiologic change in the first or second trimester.
	Gingival bleeding, most commonly oozing, associated with dental hygiene may be related to trauma from too vigorous tooth brushing or gingivitis.
Associated symptoms	Ask about associated symptoms, including gum pain, inflammation, and unpleasant taste.
	Gums that are bright red, swollen, and painful are associated with gingivitis.
	An unpleasant taste in the mouth accompanying bleeding may indicate periodontal disease.
Medications taken	Ask about medications taken, including OTC drugs such as aspirin or nonsteroidal anti-inflammatory drugs (NSAIDs) and herbal supplements.
	Oral contraceptives and hormonal replacement therapy may increase the risk for bleeding gums.
	Anticoagulant therapy, such as with heparin or warfarin, or drugs that can affect platelet aggregation, such as aspirin or NSAIDs, may increase the risk for bleeding. Some herbal supplements, such as ginkgo biloba, also can decrease clotting time.

Halitosis

Quality	Ask the patient to describe the odor.
	The sweet breath of diabetes mellitus is described as fruity. A large bowel obstruction may be associated with a fecal breath odor. A musty, sweet, or mousy (new-mown hay) odor indicates hepatic encephalopathy.
	The breath of a patient with kidney failure is often musty or has an ammonia odor (end-stage renal disease).
	A musty breath odor also may accompany a common cold or chronic sinusitis.
	Certain foods, such as garlic or onions, may create a characteristic odor.
Associated symptoms	Ask about associated symptoms, including dental caries, gingival bleeding, or facial pain; sore throat, postnasal drip, or dry hacking cough; polyuria, polyphagia, and polydipsia; and blood in the stool or emesis.
	Halitosis with dental caries and gingival bleeding may suggest periodontal disease. Sore throat, postnasal dripping, or cough accompanying halitosis may suggest sinusitis. Polyuria, polyphagia, and polydipsia suggest hyperglycemia. Blood in the stool or emesis with fecal breath odor would indicate a possible bowel obstruction. Infection in the mouth and upper respiratory area may also be a cause. Halitosis that has associated epigastric pain may be related to reflux. Exudative pharyngitis, which may have pain that increases with swallowing, has a characteristic fetid odor.
Precipitating factors	Ask about dental care, use of tobacco, and other possible factors such as a history of diabetes or renal disease.
	Poor dental hygiene is the most frequent cause of halitosis. Tobacco use may also be a cause.
	Dry mouth as a result of medication and/or radiation therapy may contribute to poor breath.
Alleviating factors	What alleviates halitosis?
	Most benign halitosis is relieved by dental hygiene and/or diet modification.
Medications taken	Which medications is the patient taking, including any herbal remedies?
	Many medications affect taste and may affect breath. For example, salicylates may cause fruity breath odor. Use of garlic capsules may cause halitosis.

Toothache

Onset	Was the onset sudden or gradual?
	If the patient has periods of sensitivity and if the tooth pain is increasing in frequency and intensity, there may be a recent history of loss of filling, trauma, or lack of dental attention.
	In patients between the ages of 15 and 25 who have good dental care, pain that occurs gradually but is continuous may be caused by eruption of wisdom teeth.
Location; radiation	Describe the location of the pain. Does it radiate?
	Tooth decay is the most frequent cause of tooth pain. As the decay progresses, the pain increases and becomes constant. The pain may radiate to the gums, jaw, and facial structures.

Associated symptoms	Ask about associated symptoms including discoloration of the teeth, exudate from the surrounding gums, halitosis, and edema.
	Discoloration, exudates, halitosis, and edema may indicate periodontal disease and subsequent infection.
	Facial swelling or asymmetry may indicate decay and an infectious process in the tooth or gum.
Precipitating and aggravating factors	What precipitates or aggravates the pain?
	Eating cold food may increase pain, suggesting tooth sensitivity. Eating hot or cold food may also precipitate tooth pain.
	If the patient has periods of sensitivity and if the tooth pain is increasing in frequency and intensity, loss of filling, trauma, or lack of dental attention may be the cause.
	Pain caused by wisdom teeth eruption (in the upper or lower posterior mouth) may increase with opening and closing of the jaw.

Mouth Ulcerations

Onset	Was the onset sudden or gradual? Do the ulcerations occur seasonally or do they tend to recur?
	Canker sores occur most often in the winter and spring, come on suddenly, and can recur.
Quality; character; severity	Describe the sores, including color, location, and exudate. How painful are they?
	The patient with herpetic lesions will often report a period of tingling before eruption. Herpetic lesions are usually located in the perioral area, and the sores crust over after about a day.
	Canker sores are often located inside the mouth and oral mucosa. Impetigo has a honey-color exudate that continues for several days. It is usually around the nose and mouth and may spread to the cheeks. Soft, elevated plaques on the buccal mucosa, tongue, and possibly the palate, gums, and floor of the mouth indicate candidal infection. These plaques can be wiped away.
	A white lesion that cannot be removed by rubbing may occur from chronic denture irritation, or from smoking (cigarettes or pipe). It also may indicate cellular dysplasia or early squamous cell cancer. Cheilosis (cracking or fissures in the corners of the mouth) is usually annoying but not extremely painful. It may be related to nutritional deficiencies or malclosure of the mouth, which results in skin maceration.
Precipitating factors	Do the sores appear after eating certain foods? Is the patient properly nourished? Has the patient been ill? Does the patient use tobacco products? Has the patient experienced any recent trauma to the mouth?
	Eating raw pineapple or other highly acidic, enzymatic, or very hot foods may cause mouth ulcers.
	Multiple vitamin deficiencies may result in cheilosis.
	Herpes flares may follow the onset of an illness or a period of stress. Oral cancer is usually related to use of tobacco.
	Trauma is the most common cause of mouth lesions; for example, orthodontic equipment rubbing on the oral mucosa can lead to ulceration.

| Medications taken | Ask the patient about any medications being used, including OTC medications and herbal remedies. |
| | *Allergic reactions to numerous medications, such as penicillin, sulfonamides, aspirin, and barbiturates, commonly result in the development of oral ulcers. Inhaled steroid medications can lead to candidiasis. Mouth ulcers are a common side effect of chemotherapeutic agents.* |

Past Medical History

> Mr. L had a tonsillectomy as a preschool child. He reports experiencing one to two upper respiratory infections each year. He denies any chronic illnesses, such as diabetes. Mr. L has no known allergies. He has regular dental care. He denies any recent mouth trauma.

The past medical history includes detailed information about any mouth trauma and/or surgeries. Also, inquire about the history of upper respiratory infections and allergies; describe this history in detail.

Past health conditions or surgeries	Ask about health conditions, including diabetes, cardiovascular disease, allergies, upper respiratory infections (URIs), and sexually transmitted diseases (STDs).
	Due to the microvascular complications of diabetes, it is necessary to have a thorough oral assessment of the mouth and gums.
	Cardiovascular disease contributes to gum disease. Some cardiovascular medications (phenytoin and nifedipine) may predispose the patient to gum disease. Allergies involving nasal congestion may cause the patient to breathe through the mouth, which dries out the oral cavity and increases the patient's risk for irritation and the development of ulcerations. Postnasal dripping associated with allergies and sinusitis can lead to sore throat.
	A history of URIs and chronic sinusitis can lead to halitosis.
	Genital STDs may lead to oral STDs.
	Ask about past surgeries, specifically those involving the mouth and throat. Note dates and outcomes.
Dental history	Ask about dental care and problems.
	Dental problems and treatments may have a significant impact on the oral environment.
	The use of fluoride and sealants can help to prevent dental caries. Gingivitis, if not treated, can lead to periodontitis and loss of teeth. Lost or missing teeth can cause malocclusion and problems with chewing.
Traumas or injuries to the mouth or throat	Ask about any history of trauma to the mouth, including any broken or lost teeth, and the throat.
	Trauma or injury to the mouth requiring treatment may provide clues to current problems. For example, if a prosthetic tooth was used, inflammation and pain may be related to the prosthesis becoming loose or malpositioned.
Eating disorders	Does the patient have a history of eating disorder(s)?
	Bulimic patients may have microscopic cracks and enamel erosion on the backs of the front teeth from the gastric acid in vomit.

Family History

> Mr. L's family history is positive for seasonal allergies and negative for eczema and asthma. His mother is alive and has mild hypertension and diabetes that are controlled by diet and oral medications. His father died of a stroke at age 67. Mr. L has two older brothers, both of whom are in good health.

Some diseases, such as cancer, run in families.

Age of living relatives	Include the relationship and health of parents, brothers, sisters, and children. *Children in daycare centers or school are exposed to a plethora of respiratory illness. They transmit illness to family members.*
Deaths	Include the relationship of the deceased to the patient and the cause of death (specifically illnesses that affect the mouth or throat). *Family information is important because there is a genetic predisposition for oral cancer.*
Chronic diseases/ disorders	Ask about chronic diseases or disorders in the family; include the relationship of the patient to the family member. Focus on diseases that affect the mouth and throat that may be familial or genetic. *Risk of oral cancer is increased with a family history of oral cancer.*
Genetic defects	Is there a history of genetic or birth defects? *Cleft disorders may be isolated or associated with complex syndromes. Cleft disorders are most often diagnosed at birth and are best treated by a team that specializes in facial anomalies. These disorders' effects on nose and mouth function are specific to the actual cleft and the associated syndromes and the repair processes. The patient's care is usually managed by a specialty team. A detailed history is the best determinant of the cleft effects on the nose and mouth.*

Social History

> Mr. L is divorced. He has a 4-year-old son who is in a daycare program and visits on the weekend. Mr. L smokes one pack of cigarettes per day. He denies any drug use or oral sexual activity. He works in an investment firm. He lives in a modern townhouse.

Family	Ask the patient to describe the current family unit. *Children attending daycare programs and school-age children have exposure to multiple acute and chronic diseases that may be shared with the family.*
Occupation	Ask about the patient's occupation and level of stress. *The degree of stress may foster poor health habits, such as poor dental hygiene and care, and the use of tobacco as a means for stress reduction. Working in crowded areas fosters disease transmission.*
Use of tobacco	Information to obtain includes type of tobacco used (cigarettes, cigars, pipes, smokeless); duration and amount (pack-years = number of years of smoking times number of packs smoked per day); age started; efforts to quit smoking, with factors influencing success or failure; and the extent of smoking by others at home or at work. *Smoking causes vasoconstriction and may affect the gums and oral mucosa. Tobacco is a carcinogen, and the use of oral tobacco products is related to increased risk of oral cancers.*

Use of alcohol	Does the patient drink alcohol? If so, which type and how much does he drink?
	Use of alcohol can predispose the patient to oral cancer and halitosis.
Use of recreational drugs	Does the patient use recreational drugs? If so, which type, how much, and how often?
	Smoking marijuana causes many of the same health problems as cigarette smoking.
Piercing	Does the patient have any oral piercings?
	Tongue piercing may cause microscopic enamel cracks related to the constant abrasion from the jewelry.
Sexual practices	Ask the patient to describe his sexual history.
	Participation in oral sex, multiple sexual partners, and participation in unprotected sexual intercourse increase the risk for sexually transmitted diseases, including herpes simplex and gonorrhea.

Review of Systems

Many oral diseases and disorders have manifestations in systems or parts other than the mouth or throat. A comprehensive review of systems should be performed whenever possible; however, due to time and other types of constraints, the provider may be able to perform only a focused review of systems. During a focused review of systems, the provider targets questioning to the systems in which oral or throat problems are most likely to have manifestations. Following is a summary of common manifestations of oral and throat problems.

System	Symptom or Sign	Possible Associated Diseases/Disorders
General	Fever	Pharyngitis, herpangina, peritonsillar abscess, herpes simplex
Ear	Pain	Pharyngitis
Nose	Congestion	Viral pharyngitis
Gastrointestinal	Heartburn	Gastroesophageal reflux disease (GERD)
	Anorexia, abdominal pain	Herpangina
Respiratory	Cough	GERD, viral pharyngitis
	Difficulty breathing	Epiglottitis, peritonsillar abscess

Physical Examination

Equipment Needed

- Gloves
- Light source, otoscope, or penlight
- Tongue depressor
- Gauze

Components of the Physical Examination

Physical examination of the mouth and throat involves inspection and palpation. Wear gloves when there will be contact with the patient's mucous membranes.

Inspection

The assessment of the mouth is primarily based on the use of inspection. Good lighting is essential; a penlight or otoscope may be used.

Action	Rationale

1. Have the patient sit with head held erect and at the examiner's eye level.
 	
   Ask the patient a question. As he or she speaks, observe movement of the mouth and lips and note any asymmetry.
	1. The patient should speak clearly with symmetrical movement of the mouth and lips.
	
	   Asymmetry may suggest a problem involving the cranial nerves that innervate the mouth and lips. Ill-fitting dentures or loss of teeth may interfere with the clarity of the patient's speech. Asymmetry of the mouth is most often associated with a neurologic deficit such as stroke, nerve inflammation, or trauma.

2. Inspect the lips for symmetry, color, edema, and lesions.	2. The lips should be symmetrical, pink, and free of lesions.
	
	   Lesions on the lip border are often associated with herpes simplex.
	
	   Cracks at the corners of the mouth are associated with multivitamin deficiencies.
	
	   Pallor around the lips is associated with anemia or shock; bluish coloring (cyanosis) indicates hypoxemia. Reddish color around the lips may indicate chronic obstructive pulmonary disease (COPD) with polycythemia or carbon monoxide poisoning.
	
	   Edema of the lip area may suggest an acute infection, either localized or systemic. It also may be associated with a severe allergic reaction, such as anaphylaxis.

3. Ask the patient to remove any dental appliances and open his or her mouth wide. Note odor.	3. Dental appliances may interfere with visualization of the mouth. The patient's mouth should be free of any strange or unusual odors.
	
	   A sweet, fruity odor may suggest diabetic ketoacidosis. A large bowel obstruction may be associated with a fecal breath odor. A musty, sweet, or mousy (new-mown hay) odor suggests hepatic encephalopathy.
	
	   The breath of a patient with kidney failure is often musty or has an ammonia-like odor (end-stage renal disease).
	
	   A musty breath odor also may accompany a common cold or chronic sinusitis.
	
	   Certain foods, such as garlic or onions, may create a characteristic odor. Poor dental hygiene measures may lead to a foul odor.

4. Using a bright light and tongue depressor (**Figure 8-8**), inspect the buccal mucosa and gums for color, ulcerations, lesions, or trauma.	4. The buccal mucosa and gums should be pink, smooth, and free of lesions or trauma.

Action

Observe for the parotid gland openings (Stensen's ducts), located on the inside of the cheeks, across from the second molars.

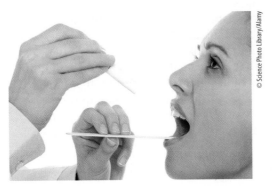

FIGURE 8-8 Using a penlight and tongue depressor to facilitate inspection of the oral cavity.

Rationale

Stensen's ducts should be apparent and without redness or swelling; saliva from the ducts should be visible.

White patches, called leukoplakia (**Figure 8-9**), in this area may suggest oral cancers. Leukoplakia is considered a precancerous lesion.

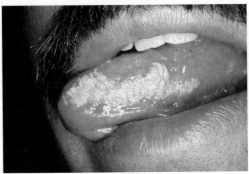

FIGURE 8-9 Leukoplakia.

White, cheesy, curd-like patches that can be scraped off, leaving a reddened mucosa and bleeding, suggest a candidal infection (**Figure 8-10**). Brown patches indicate canker sores.

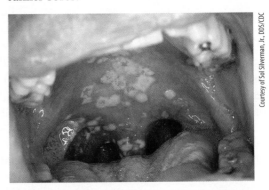

FIGURE 8-10 Acute pseudomembranous candidiasis.

Reddened, swollen gums that bleed easily indicate gingivitis or a vitamin deficiency. Gingival hyperplasia is commonly found in pregnancy and during puberty. A bluish-black or gray-white line along the gum line suggests lead poisoning.

Lack of visible saliva at Stensen's ducts may suggest a blockage.

5. Inspect the tongue. Have the patient stick out his or her tongue.

   a. Note the color.

5. The tongue should be midline in the floor of the mouth. Ability to stick out the tongue indicates intact CN XII function.

   a. There is variance in the color and textures of the normal tongue.

      The tongue typically is pink and moist with papillae present; fissures may be present.

Action   **Rationale**

Absence of papillae with a reddish shiny tongue suggests a nutritional deficiency such as niacin or vitamin B12. An enlarged tongue might indicate hypothyroidism or Down syndrome.

b. Are there any lesions or masses?

b. The tongue should be smooth, shiny, and pink in color without any visible lesions.

Lesions in the mouth are highly suggestive of cancer, especially on the underside of the tongue.

c. Ask the patient to raise his or her tongue to touch the roof of the mouth, and inspect the underside for color, texture, and any signs of redness, irritation, or lesions.

Also note the frenulum and observe for the openings of Wharton's ducts, which are located on either side of the frenulum.

c. The patient should be able to move the tongue upward toward the roof of the mouth. Inability to do so indicates a possible problem with CN XII. The frenulum should appear midline and saliva or moistness should be visible in the area of the ducts. A short frenulum may limit the patient's ability to move the tongue.

d. Inspect the sides of the tongue. Wearing gloves, use a gauze pad to move the tongue from one side to the other. Inspect for color, texture, and any evidence of lesions or ulcerations.

d. The sides of the tongue should be pink and moist, without any evidence of lesions.

Recurrent or long-standing ulcers or lesions or leukoplakia may suggest cancer. Canker sores may be noted on the side of the tongue.

6. Observe position, color, and number of teeth. Inspect for caries or other signs of disease.

6. The teeth should appear white and evenly spaced.

The back of the front teeth in bulimic patients may show areas of enamel loss.

Areas that appear brown, chalky white, or discolored may indicate dental caries.

Yellow to brownish coloring of teeth may be seen in patients who smoke, drink large amounts of tea or coffee, or who ingest excessive amounts of fluoride.

7. Have the patient tilt his or her head back slightly and open the mouth wide. Shine a light on the roof of the mouth. Inspect the hard and soft palate for color and appearance.

7. The hard palate should appear pale; the soft palate should appear pink, moist, soft, smooth, and movable.

A yellowish palate may suggest jaundice; white patches or plaques indicate a candidal infection. Dark purple lesions, either flat or raised, suggest Kaposi's sarcoma of the mouth.

8. Ask the patient to say "ah." Observe the movement of the uvula.

8. The uvula should rise symmetrically.

Asymmetrical movement or lack of movement of the uvula suggests a neurologic problem, such as cerebrovascular accident or dysfunction of CN IX and CN X.

9. Using a tongue depressor to depress the tongue, inspect the posterior throat.
    a. Note the presence and size of tonsils and any exudate.

9. Use of the tongue blade enhances visualization.

   a. Tonsils are largest in the young and tend to shrink with age. Many adults had routine tonsillectomies as children. Tonsils may be absent or present. Exudate should be absent.

Action	Rationale
	Reddened, enlarged tonsils with patches of white or yellow exudates indicate tonsillitis. The presence of exudates is most often associated with bacterial infection.
b. Note the color of and presence of lesions on the posterior wall of the throat.	b. The posterior wall of the throat should appear pink, moist, and without any exudates or lesions.
	Yellow or white exudate accompanied by a reddened posterior wall suggests pharyngitis. Yellow mucus appearing on the posterior throat may be associated with postnasal drainage from the sinuses.

Palpation

Action	Rationale
1. Palpation of the lips is not routinely performed; however, it is recommended for patients with cosmetic augmentation.	1. Substances injected to enhance the lips can move and cause asymmetry. They may also mask lesions or masses.
2. Palpate the gums for tenderness and firmness and any evidence of bleeding.	2. Normal gums are not tender and do not bleed with palpation.
	Complaints of tenderness, pain, or bleeding suggest an infection or periodontal disease.

3. Using a gauze pad to secure the tongue and gloves on the hands, palpate the tongue for texture and consistency (**Figure 8-11**).

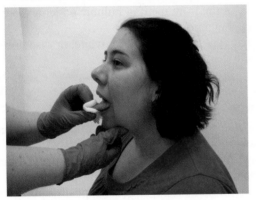

FIGURE 8-11 Palpating the tongue.

Action	Rationale
a. Note any masses or lesions.	a. The tongue should be firm but pliable without any masses or lesions. Lesions of the tongue may suggest cancer.
b. Assess the strength of the tongue by asking the patient to press the tip of the tongue against the inner cheek while you apply pressure with your fingers on the outer surface of the cheek.	b. Typically the tongue should offer strong resistance to external pressure. Difficulty with resisting the pressure may indicate a problem with CN XII or a short frenulum that limits tongue movement.

Action	Rationale
4. Using the finger pads, palpate the lymph nodes in the neck area: front of the ear under the patient's chin (preauricular); behind the ear (postauricular); behind the ear at the posterior base of the skull (occipital); at the angle of the mandible anteriorly just below the ear (tonsillar); below the chin approximately in the middle of the jaw (submandibular); and just behind the tip of the mandible (submental). Palpate each area bilaterally using a circular motion. Assess the nodes for size, shape, mobility, consistency, and tenderness, comparing findings bilaterally.	4. The lymph nodes should be nonpalpable. However, occasionally some nodes may be palpable and, if so, should be soft, mobile, and nontender. Usually these are not significant. Lymph nodes that are tender suggest inflammation. For example, an enlarged postauricular lymph node may be associated with an ear infection; an enlarged tonsillar node may be indicative of pharyngitis or tonsillitis; enlarged submental or submandibular nodes may indicate an inflammation of the gums or oral cavity. Lymph nodes that are hard or fixed may indicate a malignancy. Lymph nodes are enlarged overall (lymphadenopathy), an immunodeficiency may be the underlying cause.
5. Assess the patient's ability to taste. Apply sweet and salty substances to the sides and tip of the patient's tongue.	5. The patient should be able to accurately state which substance is sweet and which is salty. Diminished taste sensation or absence of ability to discriminate tastes suggests a nutritional deficiency, such as zinc, or a problem with CN VII. Some medications may alter the patient's taste sensation.

Diagnostic Reasoning

Based on findings in the health history and physical examination, the clinician should formulate the assessment and plan. For example, a patient may report symptoms that suggest many possible diagnoses; however, findings in the past medical history and during the physical examination might narrow the possible diagnoses down to one or two. Sore throat is a common chief complaint. **Table 8-2** illustrates differential diagnosis of common disorders associated with sore throat.

Table 8-2 Differential Diagnosis of Sore Throat			
Differential Diagnosis	Significant Findings in the Patient's History	Significant Findings in the Patient's Physical Examination	Diagnostic Tests
Irritation related to postnasal drip	Seasonal allergies (most often in the spring or fall), mild to moderate pain that increases when lying down	Clear nasal discharge that drains to the posterior throat, congestion, boggy nasal turbinates	N/A
Bacterial pharyngitis, tonsillitis	Acute onset, history of families or colleagues who have been ill, most often presents in the winter or early spring, few systemic symptoms	Erythema of the pharynx or tonsils with white to yellow exudate, fever of 101°F or greater	Culture and sensitivity Quick beta strep
Viral pharyngitis, tonsillitis	Rapid onset, systemic symptoms, cough, rhinorrhea, conjunctivitis	Rare exudate	None

Mouth and Throat Assessment of Special Populations

Considerations for the Pregnant Patient

- Inspect carefully for dental caries, as pregnant patients may be at risk for dental caries related to the increased nutritional demands of pregnancy.
- Note any gingival hyperplasia or bleeding—a common finding associated with pregnancy.

Considerations for the Neonatal Patient

- Inspect for white patches associated with thrush, which is common in newborns.
- Inspect the palate of a newborn; it should be intact.
- Inspect for cleft lip, which can range from a small notch in the upper lip to a total separation of the lip and facial structures up to the floor of the nasal cavity, and cleft palate, which involves an opening in the hard or soft palate or both, usually at the midline.
- Be aware of possible small, round, shiny, well-circumscribed cysts on the palate of the newborn. These cysts, called Epstein's pearls, are an insignificant finding and typically disappear spontaneously in approximately 1 week.
- Observe for small white epithelial pearls on the gums, an insignificant and benign finding that can occur in some newborns.
- Expect to find an increase in mucus in the mouth of newborns delivered by cesarean section.
- When assessing the tongue of a newborn, be aware that the tongue usually appears large and prominent, but short, with the frenulum attached very close to the tip of the tongue.

Considerations for the Pediatric Patient

- Allow the child to sit in the parent's lap during the physical examination; this facilitates cooperation and reduces the child's anxiety (**Figure 8-12**).
- Inspect teeth carefully. Assess for the eruption of teeth and tooth loss and adult tooth formation and eruption.
- Although teething patterns vary, expect the first deciduous tooth to be present at approximately 6 months of age and to find all 20 deciduous teeth present by the age of 3 years.

Considerations for the Geriatric Patient

- Older adults often experience problems associated with loss of teeth, necessitating the use of dentures; periodontal disease; changes in taste; dental caries; and dry mouth due to decreased saliva production, which can compromise their nutritional status.

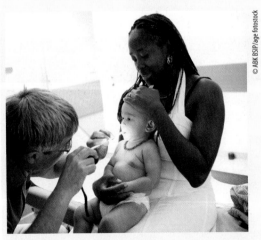

© ABK BSIP/age fotostock

FIGURE 8-12 Allow the pediatric patient to sit on mother's lap to facilitate inspection.

- Assess patients with a history of tobacco use for oral cancers, as they have an increased risk.
- As patients age, many complain of the loss of taste. Some resources document that taste does slightly diminish with age, but the use of drug therapies may be the primary cause of altered taste. Patients on cardiovascular drug therapies may also experience gingival hyperplasia.
- Inspect for varicose veins on the underside of the tongue, a possible normal finding in elderly patients.
- Expect the oral mucosa to be somewhat drier and more fragile in the elderly patient due to age-related changes in the lining of the salivary glands.

Case Study Review 2

Throughout the second half of this chapter, you have been introduced to Mr. L. This section of the chapter pulls together his history and demonstrates the documentation of his history and physical examination.

Chief Complaint

"My throat hurts."

Information Gathered During the Interview

HL, a 29-year-old Caucasian male, states that he has had a sore throat for 2 days. He has not noticed being feverish. Mr. L has noted that he is experiencing a mild runny nose and some cough but denies any sputum with the cough. He denies any earache and/or eye irritation. He has a son in a daycare program who is being treated for pharyngitis. Mr. L is taking acetaminophen with some relief.

Mr. L had a tonsillectomy as a preschool child. He reports experiencing one to two upper respiratory infections each year. He denies any chronic illnesses, such as diabetes. He has no known allergies. He has regular dental care. He denies any recent mouth trauma.

Mr. L's family history is positive for seasonal allergies and negative for eczema and asthma. His mother is alive and has mild hypertension and diabetes that are controlled by diet and oral medications. His father died of a stroke at age 67. Mr. L has two older brothers, both of whom are in good health.

Mr. L is divorced. He has a 4-year-old son who is in a daycare program and visits on the weekend. Mr. L smokes one pack of cigarettes per day. He denies any drug use or oral sexual activity. He works in an investment firm. He lives in a modern townhouse.

Clues	Important Points
Child in day care	Children often transmit bacterial and viral upper respiratory infections.
Does not have fever or persistent cough	Usually fever is associated with bacterial infections. Nonproductive cough is associated with viral infections.
Smokes one pack of filtered cigarettes per day	Smoking causes inflammation and irritation to the mucosa. A chronic nonproductive cough is associated with smoking.

Name HL		Date 07/02/15	Time 1615
		DOB 10/03/86	Sex M
HISTORY			
CC "My throat hurts."			

HPI
2-day history of sore throat that Tylenol helps. Denies fever; has mild clear discharge and occasional nonproductive cough. Denies any earache or eye irritation.

Medications
Occasional Tylenol for headaches.

Allergies
Mild seasonal allergies; no reported drug allergies.

PMI
Illnesses
1–2 mild URIs per year. Denies any mouth trauma; sees a dentist regularly. Denies any chronic illnesses.

Hospitalizations/Surgeries
Tonsillectomy as a preschooler.

FH
Positive for mild, seasonal allergies; negative for eczema and asthma. Mother with well-controlled DM and mild HTN. Father died of a stroke at age 67.

SH
Works in an investment firm; divorced; smokes 1 pack of filtered cigarettes per day. Denies any recreational drug use. Denies any oral sexual activity. Son in day care with moderate amount of URIs.

ROS

General	Cardiovascular
Alert and oriented, no distress.	Denies any SOB, chest pain, or exercise intolerance.
Skin	Respiratory
Denies any changes in skin or rashes; uses sun screen.	Occasional nonproductive cough.
Eyes	Gastrointestinal
Wears contact lenses; no other problems.	Denies any problems.
Ears	Genitourinary/Gynecological
Denies any hearing loss, congestion, or itching.	No problems noted.
Nose/Mouth/Throat	Musculoskeletal
Sore throat, mild nasal discharge.	Denies any problems.
Breast	Neurological
Negative.	Denies any problems.

PHYSICAL EXAMINATION

Weight 210 lb	Temp 98.6	BP 142/89
Height 6'	Pulse 76	Resp 12

General Appearance
Alert and oriented, no distress.

Skin
Warm and dry, no rashes.

HEENT
Normal cephalic. External ear, ear canal, and TM normal. Eyes have mild bilateral injection; no exudate.
Nose: Normal turbinates; scant clear discharge noted. Frontal and maxillary sinuses are nontender with pressure; translumination is normal. Mouth normal, posterior throat mild erythema, no exudate, no adenopathy.

Cardiovascular
Heart rate is normal; no murmurs are appreciated.

Respiratory
Lungs are clear to auscultation to all lobes.

Gastrointestinal
Not examined.
Genitourinary
Not examined.
Musculoskeletal
Gait normal; able to get up and down from the examination table without difficulty.
Neurological
CN I–XII grossly intact.
Other
Lab Tests
Beta strep if the son is positive.
Special Tests
None.
Final Assessment Findings
Throat irritation related to smoking.

Bibliography

Baroody, F. (1998). Epidemiology and pathogenesis/immunology of rhinosinusitis. *Infectious Medicine, 15*(10F), 6–15.

Cohen, B., & Wood, D. (2000). *Memmler's the human body in health and disease* (9th ed.). Philadelphia, PA: Lippincott Williams & Wilkins.

Copstead, L., & Banasik, J. (2000). *Pathophysiology: Biological and behavioral perspectives* (2nd ed.). Philadelphia, PA: W. B. Saunders.

Ferri, F. (2015). *Ferri's clinical advisor: Instant diagnosis and treatment.* St. Louis, MO: Mosby.

Guyton, A., & Hall, J. (2001). *Textbook of medical physiology* (10th ed.). St. Louis, MO: Elsevier.

Hay, W., Hayward, A., Levin, M., & Sondheimer, J. M. (2003). *Current pediatric diagnosis and treatment* (16th ed.). New York, NY: McGraw-Hill.

Jones, G. (2003). Emergency care of the person with minor injury and minor illness. In G. Jones, R. Endacott, & R. Crouch. (Eds.), *Emergency nursing care: Principles and practice* (pp. 135–152). London, UK: Greenwich Medical Media.

Madler, B. (2002). Chronic cough: Evaluation and management. *Journal of the American Academy of Nurse Practitioners, 14*(6), 261–268.

Mastin, T. (2003). Recognizing and treating non-infectious rhinitis. *Journal of the American Academy of Nurse Practitioners, 15*(9), 398–409.

Out, P. S. (1927). Nose and throat observations in examination of patients with bronchial asthma. *Journal of the American Medical Association, 89*(11), 868–869.

Pray, W. (2000). Acute sinusitis and treatment strategies. *U.S. Pharmacist, 25*(12). Retrieved from http://www.medscape.com/viewarticle/407637.

Rambur, B. (2002). Pregnancy rhinitis and rhinitis medicamentosa. *Journal of the American Academy of Nurse Practitioners, 14*(12), 527–530.

Tichenor, W. (1999). Sinusitis: A practical guide for physicians. *Medscape General Medicine, 1*(1). Retrieved from http://www.medscape.com/viewarticle/408707.

Uphold, C., & Graham, M. (2013). *Clinical guidelines in family practice* (5th ed.). Gainesville, FL: Barmarrae Books.

Wilson, W. R., Nadol, J., & Randolph, G. (2002). *The clinical handbook of ear, nose, and throat disorders*. Nashville, TN: Parthenon.

Winder, J. (1999). Nasal polyposis: Rationale for treatment with topical intranasal corti-costeroids. *Medscape General Medicine, 1*(3). Retrieved from http://www.medscape.com/viewarticle/408724.

Wynne, A., & Woo, T. (2011). *Pharmacotherapeutics for nurse practitioner prescribers*. Philadelphia, PA: F.A. Davis.

Chapter 9

Respiratory Disorders

Anatomy and Physiology Review of the Respiratory System

The respiratory system consists of those organs that deliver oxygen to all body cells through the circulatory system. It is responsible for the following functions:

- Aiding in the removal of carbon dioxide
- Helping regulate acid–base balance in tissues
- Protecting the body against inhaled disease-causing organisms and toxic substances
- Housing the cells that detect smell
- Assisting in the production of sounds for speech

If respiratory function is interrupted for more than a few minutes, serious, irreversible damage to tissues occurs.

Respiration

The respiratory and circulatory systems work together to deliver oxygen to cells and remove carbon dioxide in a two-phase process called respiration. The first phase of respiration begins with inhalation, which draws oxygen from the external environment into the lungs. The oxygen travels through blood vessels to the heart, which pumps the oxygen-rich blood to the systemic circulation on into body cells. At the cellular level, oxygen is used in a separate energy-producing process (cellular respiration), which produces carbon dioxide as an end product. The second phase of respiration begins with the movement of carbon dioxide from the cells into the systemic circulation, which carries it to the heart, preventing the lethal buildup of this waste product in body tissues. The heart pumps the carbon dioxide–laden blood to the lungs. Exhalation removes carbon dioxide from the body, thus completing the respiration cycle.

Respiratory Tract

The upper respiratory tract consists of the nose and the pharynx, or throat. The lower respiratory tract includes the larynx; the trachea, which splits into two main branches called bronchi; tiny branches of the bronchi called bronchioles; and the lungs. **Figure 9-1** illustrates the components of the respiratory tract. The nose, pharynx, larynx, trachea, bronchi, and bronchioles conduct air in and out of the lungs.

Breathing is controlled by the nervous system and involves controlled spontaneous flow of air in and out of the lungs. It is initiated by the brain stem, which is part of the respiratory center. The brain stem sends simultaneous signals to the diaphragm and rib muscles. The diaphragm lies under the lungs and appears as a large, dome-shaped muscle that, when stimulated by a nervous impulse, flattens and moves downward. This movement of the diaphragm expands the lung cavity, allowing more volume to enter into the lungs.

When the rib muscles are stimulated by nervous stimuli, they also contract, pulling the rib cage up and out. This movement allows expansion of the thoracic cavity and more volume. The increased volume of the thoracic cavity causes air to enter into the lungs.

When the nervous stimulation ceases (it is brief), the diaphragm and rib muscles relax and exhalation occurs. Under normal conditions, the respiratory center transmits impulses at a rate of 12 to 20 per minute, resulting in 12 to 20 breaths per minute.

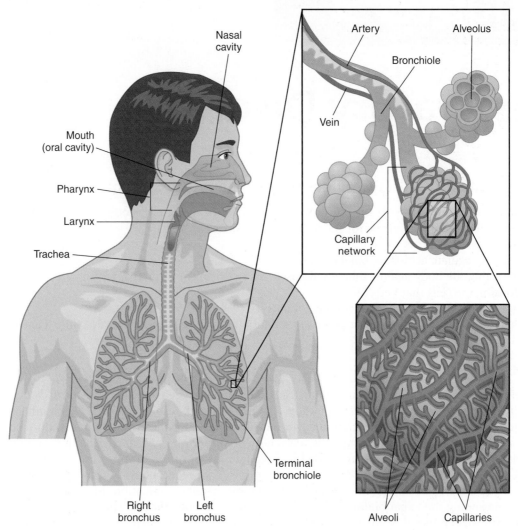

FIGURE 9-1 Respiratory system.

In cases of brain injury, stimulation of the brain stem may be impaired and the cerebral cortex may take over. If exhalation does not occur, carbon dioxide accumulates in the blood, which, in turn, causes the blood to become more acidic. The blood is monitored by chemoreceptors, located in the vasculature of the neck and the brain stem. If acid builds up in the blood, the chemoreceptors in the carotid arteries send signals to the brain stem, which overrides the signals from the cerebral cortex, causing exhalation and breathing. The exhalation expels the carbon dioxide and brings the blood acid level back to normal.

A person can exert limited control over inhalation volume. To prevent overinflation of the lungs, stretch receptors measure lung volume. When volume reaches an unsafe threshold, the stretch receptors send signals to the respiratory center, which shuts down the muscles of inhalation and reduces the intake of air.

Health History

Chief Complaint and History of Present Illness

"My cough is getting worse, and now my chest hurts."

Mr. V is a 58-year-old man who presents with a 2-day history of left-sided pleuritic chest pain, dyspnea, orthopnea, intermittent fever and chills, and a cough productive of yellow sputum, which became brown yesterday. The pleuritic chest pain radiates to the proximal left upper quadrant (LUQ) during coughing. He has not experienced nausea but did have one episode of emesis yesterday. He also states that this morning he experienced rhinorrhea and a sore throat, which have now resolved.

A thorough health history helps the examiner narrow diagnoses. The healthcare provider should ask detailed questions focusing on the history of present illness (HPI).

Cough

Cough is a common symptom of a pulmonary problem. It usually is preceded by a deep inspiration. Causes may be related to localized or more general problems in any area of the respiratory tract. Although a cough may be a voluntary action, it is usually a spontaneous response to an irritant, such as a foreign body, an infectious agent, or a tumor/mass of any sort that would compress the respiratory tree. Coughing may also indicate anxiety.

Onset	Was the onset sudden or gradual?
	An acute onset, particularly with fever, suggests infection. In the absence of fever, a foreign body or inhaled irritants are possible causes.
Duration	How long has the patient had the cough?
Pattern	Is the cough occasional, regular, or paroxysmal? Has the cough changed over time?
	A paroxysmal cough is often heard in tuberculosis.
	Is the cough related to the time of day?
	Cough occurring in the evenings is suggestive of stress.
Quality	Is the cough dry, moist, wet, hacking, hoarse, barking, whooping, bubbling, productive, or nonproductive?
	A moist cough may be caused by infection and can be accompanied by sputum production.
	A dry cough can have a variety of causes—such as cardiac problems, use of angiotensin-converting enzyme (ACE) inhibitors, allergies, or human immunodeficiency virus (HIV) infection—which may be indicated by the quality of its sound.
	A dry cough may sound brassy if it is caused by compression of the respiratory tree, as by a tumor, or hoarse if it is caused by croup.
	Pertussis produces an inspiratory whoop at the end of a paroxysm of coughing.
Pitch and loudness	Is the cough loud and high pitched or soft and relatively low pitched?
	High-pitched coughs usually indicate constriction of airway, whereas low-pitched coughs indicate presence of secretions or inflammatory conditions.
Severity	Does the cough tire the patient, disrupt sleep or conversation, or cause chest pain?
	The patient's response illustrates how severe the cough is and how it disrupts activities of daily living. As the level of disruption increases, the severity of the underlying disease increases.
Sputum production	Is the cough productive? Assess duration, frequency, and occurrence with activity or at certain times of day.

	Exercise or early morning may produce more sputum or stimulate the bronchus and result in constriction or irritation. Ask about amount, color (clear, mucoid, purulent, blood-tinged, mostly blood), and odor. (See also Sputum Production later in this section.)
	Blood-tinged sputum is usually present with pneumonia or active tuberculosis. Green sputum indicates production of neutrophils, seen with acute bronchitis.
Precipitating factors	Is the cough related to weather, activities (e.g., exercise), talking, or taking deep breaths?
	Precipitating factors can provide clues to the type of disease. For example, a cough related to exercise suggests exertional asthma as the cause.
	Is the cough influenced by posture?
	A cough occurring soon after a person has reclined or assumed an erect position may be related to nasal drip or pooling of secretions in the upper airway.
Associated symptoms	Important associated symptoms to assess include shortness of breath, chest pain or tightness with breathing, fever, coryza, congestion, noisy respirations, hoarseness, gagging, choking, and stress.
	A fever indicates probable bacterial infection.
Alleviating factors	What lessens or worsens symptoms? Has the patient taken any prescription or nonprescription drugs? Is the patient using a vaporizer? How effective was treatment?
Other medications taken	Is the patient taking any other prescription or nonprescription medications?
	Other drugs can cause a reaction which can affect cough.

Chest Pain

Chest pain may occur with various systemic disorders, including those related to the cardiovascular, respiratory, and endocrine systems. A thorough history will help determine the cause.

Onset	Is the chest pain sudden or gradual?
Duration	How long has the patient had chest pain?
Precipitating factors	Has the patient experienced a recent trauma or upper respiratory infection?
	Chest pain caused by trauma to the rib cage often mimics cardiac pain; thus the examiner will need to address this area specifically during physical assessment to narrow the focus and determine an accurate diagnosis. Trauma to the chest will cause the patient to have chest pain with inspiration, whereas cardiac chest pain is not associated with inspiration.
Associated symptoms	Important associated symptoms to assess include shallow breathing, fever, uneven chest expansion, coughing, anxiety about being able to breathe, and radiation of pain to neck or arms.
	Chest pain associated with fever suggests an infectious process, such as pleuritis or costochondritis.
Alleviating and aggravating factors	What lessens or worsens the patient's symptoms? Has the patient used heat, splinting, or pain medication?
	Has the treatment been effective?
Other medications taken	Ask about prescription or nonprescription medications.

Sputum Production

Production of sputum is generally associated with cough. When sputum production occurs in more than small amounts and with any degree of regularity, it suggests the presence of disease.

Onset	Is the onset sudden or gradual?
	If the onset is acute (sudden), infection is most probable.
Duration; frequency	How often does it occur? How frequent is the production of sputum?
	Chronicity indicates the possibility of some significant anatomic change (e.g., tumor, cavitation, bronchiectasis).
	Intermittent production is associated with chronic infectious disease.
Amount	How much sputum is produced?
	Slight amounts are associated with chronic infectious disease and pulmonary carcinoma.
Color; presence of blood	Describe the color. Is there blood in the sputum?
	Bacterial infection causes yellow, green, rust (blood mixed with yellow sputum), clear, or transparent sputum. The sputum may be purulent, blood streaked, mucoid, or viscid.
	Viral infection is often associated with mucoid or viscid sputum. It may also be blood streaked, although this is not common.
	Chronic infectious disease may occasionally cause sputum mixed with large amounts of blood.
	A pulmonary carcinoma produces blood-streaked sputum, which occurs as the tumor invades the tissue.
	A pulmonary infarction produces a large amount of blood in the sputum, which may be clotted. This is due to ischemia and necrosis of the infarcted area.
	Likewise, a large amount of blood in the sputum is seen in tuberculosis, due to invasion of the infected tissue.
	It is important to determine whether blood in sputum is associated with a nosebleed (note the color of the blood and its quantity). Nosebleeds tend to produce copious, bright red blood.
Odor	Ask the patient about odor of breath and sputum.
	Streptococci infections and fecal impactions may cause odor to the patient's breath or sputum.

Dyspnea (Shortness of Breath)

Determine whether the patient has difficult and labored breathing with shortness of breath, which is commonly observed with pulmonary or cardiac pathology. Dyspnea increases with the severity of the underlying condition.

Onset	Is the dyspnea sudden or gradual? Did the patient experience a gagging or choking incident a few days before onset?
	Aspiration (choking) can cause aspiration pneumonia, which produces dyspnea due to constriction of the airway.
Duration	How long has the patient had shortness of breath?
Pattern; precipitating factors	Is it present even when the patient is resting? Which position is most comfortable? How many pillows does the patient use when sleeping? Does it occur at a certain time of day? Does it occur when eating? Does it occur only

	when the patient is walking? Is it necessary to stop and rest when climbing stairs? Do other activities of daily living (ADLs) provoke dyspnea?
	Orthopnea is a shortness of breath that begins or increases when the patient lies down; the patient may need to sleep on more than one pillow.
	When dyspnea increases in the upright posture, it is referred to as platypnea. This is seen in patients with emphysema or chronic bronchitis and asthma.
	Paroxysmal nocturnal dyspnea (PND) is the sudden onset of shortness of breath after a period of sleep; sitting upright is helpful. PND is seen often in patients with congestive heart failure or pulmonary hypertension.
Severity	To what extent does the dyspnea limit the patient's activity? Is there fatigue with breathing? Is it harder to inhale or exhale? Does the patient have anxiety about being able to breathe?
Associated symptoms	Important associated symptoms to assess include pain or discomfort (including the relationship to a specific point in respiratory exertion and location), cough, diaphoresis, and ankle edema.
	Ankle edema suggests congestive heart failure as a possible main origin of disease.
	Presence of pain can lead the examiner to suspect pleuritis or cardiac pericarditis.

Abnormal Respiratory Rate

Tachypnea is a rapid, persistent respiratory rate of 25 or more respirations per minute. Tachypnea is seen with hyperventilatory states. Bradypnea is a slow respiration rate (fewer than 12 breaths per minute) often seen in patients with neurological disease such as agonal breathing or Kussmaul's breathing. Hyperpnea is breathing that is deeper and more rapid than is normal at rest. Hyperpnea is also seen with neurological pathology.

Onset	Is the onset sudden or gradual? Is the respiratory rate persistent?
	Rapid, shallow breathing (tachypnea) may occur during hyperventilation or as a response to anxiety or anticipation.
Respiratory rate	How frequent are respirations?
	A respiratory rate slower than 12 respirations per minute may indicate neurological or electrolyte disturbance, infection, or a response to protect against the pain of pleurisy.
	Central nervous system and metabolic disease may cause rapid, deep breathing (hyperpnea).
Respiratory rhythm/breathing patterns	Note any variations in respiratory rhythm/breathing pattern.
	Table 9-1 discusses and illustrates various breathing patterns.
	It may be difficult to determine abnormalities unless they are quite obvious.
Associated symptoms	Ask about associated symptoms.
	Tachypnea is often a symptom of splinting from pain of a broken rib or pleurisy.
	Massive liver enlargement due to hepatitis or cirrhosis and abdominal ascites may prevent descent of the diaphragm and produce tachypnea.
	Bradypnea may indicate cardiorespiratory fitness but most often is due to metabolic or neurological disease such as spinal cord injury.

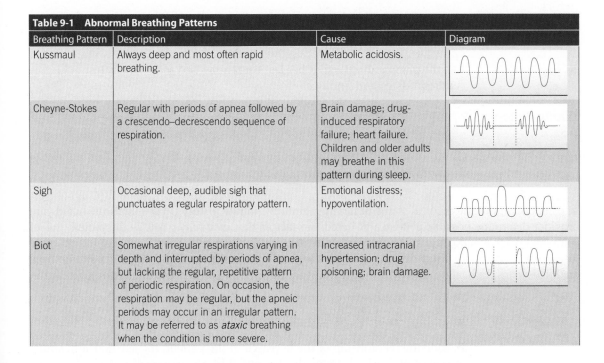

Breathing Pattern	Description	Cause	Diagram
Kussmaul	Always deep and most often rapid breathing.	Metabolic acidosis.	
Cheyne-Stokes	Regular with periods of apnea followed by a crescendo–decrescendo sequence of respiration.	Brain damage; drug-induced respiratory failure; heart failure. Children and older adults may breathe in this pattern during sleep.	
Sigh	Occasional deep, audible sigh that punctuates a regular respiratory pattern.	Emotional distress; hypoventilation.	
Biot	Somewhat irregular respirations varying in depth and interrupted by periods of apnea, but lacking the regular, repetitive pattern of periodic respiration. On occasion, the respiration may be regular, but the apneic periods may occur in an irregular pattern. It may be referred to as *ataxic* breathing when the condition is more severe.	Increased intracranial hypertension; drug poisoning; brain damage.	

Table 9-1   Abnormal Breathing Patterns

Past Medical History

Mr. V has had asthma since childhood, which is under good control despite the fact that he ran out of his albuterol inhaler and has not been using it for some time. He denies a history of past surgeries or trauma. He states he has had the influenza shot and the pneumonia vaccine.

The healthcare provider should ask detailed questions focusing on all past medical history/illnesses (PMI), traumatic events, and elective surgeries. This information will provide critical information that will aid in the formulation of a detailed plan of care.

Past health conditions or surgeries	Has the patient had any thoracic trauma or surgery? Has patient been hospitalized for pulmonary disorders? Record pertinent dates. *Information could suggest a relationship to the current chief complaint or to possible complications or progression of disease (e.g., scar tissue, contractures, or surgery for cancer).* Does the patient have a chronic pulmonary disease, such as tuberculosis (ask about date of diagnosis, treatment, and compliance to medication regimen), bronchitis, emphysema, bronchiectasis, asthma, cystic fibrosis, allergies, atopic dermatitis, recurrent spitting up and choking, recurrent pneumonia, or possible gastroesophageal reflux? *A chronic pulmonary disease compromises treatment of the present illness.* Does the patient have any other chronic diseases? *Cardiac diseases, cancer, and blood dyscrasias could significantly compromise respiratory system function by decreasing oxygen-carrying capacity.*
Use of oxygen or ventilation-assist devices	Is the patient using oxygen or a ventilation-assist device? Assess for possible dependence on oxygen or need for continued use of oxygen. *Use may suggest underlying progressing disease or pathology or progression of the illness state.*

Immunization history	Ask the patient about history of annual influenza immunization and history of pneumococcal vaccination.
Diagnostic tests	Ask the patient about his or her last chest x-ray and tuberculosis test. Ascertain dates and findings.

Family History

Both of Mr. V's parents are alive. His father (age 82) has been diagnosed with hypertension (HTN). His family history is negative for coronary artery disease, asthma, diabetes, and cancer.

Information about the medical status of family members—family history (FH)—helps the healthcare provider determine possible genetic and hereditary factors that may play a role in the patient's chief complaint (CC). A genogram may be important to include if family members who are alive have chronic diseases (e.g., coronary artery disease, hypertension) and to note the cause of death of those who have died. This helps the healthcare provider determine specific screening procedures to plan for patient care.

Age of living relatives	Include the relationship and health status. Do relatives have any respiratory conditions, such as asthma?
Deaths	Include the relationship of the deceased to the patient, the age at death, and the cause of death. Examine deaths caused by respiratory disorders.
Chronic diseases	Ask about chronic diseases in the family. Include the relationship of family member with the chronic disease and how long the family member has had the disease. Explore respiratory diseases. *A family history of asthma increases the patient's risk for asthma.*
	Include familial genetic disorders and congenital birth defects. Include any genetic diseases (e.g., any congenital heart deformities).

Social History

Mr. V denies tobacco or drug use. He reports alcohol use, two glasses of wine on Friday evenings when dining out. Mr. V is a salesman with a book company and has never been married.

In taking the social history (SH), the provider should determine the patient's ability to interact with others in healthy ways. Therefore, in addition to inquiring about hobbies and social interactions, determine the patient's use of alcohol, and ask directly about use of tobacco and illegal drug use. Ask the patient about exposure to environmental air toxins or air contaminants, such as asbestos or secondhand smoke.

Family	Ask the patient to describe the family unit. How many in the family? Are they alive and well? Do they have any respiratory diseases?
Occupation	Ask about current and past positions; nature of work; extent of physical and emotional effort and stress; environmental hazards; exposure to chemicals, animals, vapors, dust, pulmonary irritants (e.g., asbestos), and allergens; use of protective devices; and exposure to respiratory infections, influenza, and tuberculosis.
Housing	Ask about the patient's residence, including geographical location, possible allergens, type of heating, use of air conditioning and humidifier, and ventilation. Ask about the effects of weather on respiratory efforts and occurrence of infections.

Diet/nutritional status	Ask about weight loss or obesity over past few months. Is the patient having difficulty swallowing? *Exposure to certain foods, such as those prepared with MSG, may cause inflammatory asthma.*
Travel	Ask patient about travel history, including travel outside of the normal geographical location or out-of-country trips. **Box 9-1** discusses diseases commonly related to travel. *Overseas travel and the intake of unclean water and food products increase the risk of exposure to organisms and certain diseases.*
Activity/exercise intolerance	Ask about any change in the ability to carry on activities of daily living, immobilization or marked sedentary habits, and alteration in living habits or activities as a result of respiratory symptoms. *A sedentary lifestyle increases a patient's risk for respiratory problems.*
Hobbies	Ask about the patient's hobbies. Specifically, do those hobbies include owning birds, such as pigeons or parrots; woodworking; welding; or other hobbies with possibilities of noxious exposure?
Tobacco use	Information to obtain includes type of tobacco used (cigarettes, cigars, pipes, smokeless); duration and amount (pack-years = number of years of smoking times number of packs smoked per day); age started; efforts to quit smoking, with factors influencing success or failure; and the extent of smoking by others at home or at work.

BOX 9-1   DISEASES RELATED TO TRAVEL

- African sleeping sickness (African trypanosomiasis)
- AIDS/HIV
- Altitude illness
- Amebiasis
- Bovine spongiform encephalopathy (BSE; "mad cow disease") and new-variant Creutzfeldt–Jakob disease (nvCJD)
- *Campylobacter* infections
- Chagas' disease (American trypanosomiasis)
- Cholera
- Coccidioidomycosis
- Cryptosporidiosis (*Cryptosporidium* infection)
- Cyclosporiasis (*Cyclospora* infection)
- Dengue fever
- Diarrhea
- Diphtheria, tetanus, and pertussis
- Encephalitis
- *Escherichia coli* (*E. coli*)
- Filariasis
- Giardiasis (*Giardia* infection)
- Hantavirus
- Head lice (pediculosis)
- Hepatitis
- Histoplasmosis
- Influenza (flu)
- Leishmaniasis (*Leishmania* infection)
- Leptospirosis
- Lyme disease
- Malaria
- Measles, mumps, and rubella (MMR)
- Meningitis
- Norovirus infection (Norwalk/Norwalk-like virus infection)
- Onchocerciasis (river blindness)
- Plague
- Poliomyelitis
- Rabies
- Rickettsial infections
- Rotavirus
- Salmonellosis (*Salmonella* infection)
- Scabies
- Schistosomiasis
- Sexually transmitted diseases (STDs)
- Shigellosis (*Shigella* infection)
- Smallpox
- Tuberculosis (TB)
- Typhoid fever
- Typhus fevers (see rickettsial infections)
- Varicella (chickenpox)
- *Vibrio parahaemolyticus*
- Viral hemorrhagic fevers (e.g., Ebola, Lassa, Marburg, Rift Valley)
- West Nile virus
- Yellow fever

	Smoking increases the patient's risk for many respiratory disorders, including bronchitis, lung cancer, and chronic obstructive pulmonary disease.
Use of alcohol	Does the patient drink alcohol? How much? Which type (e.g., wine, beer, liquor)? What time of the day? How long has he or she been drinking? See the CAGE assessment.
Use of illegal street drugs	Does the patient use illegal drugs? How much? Which type (e.g., ecstasy, PCP, cocaine, heroin)? What time of the day does he or she use them? How often? By self or with others? Question patient on his or her use of marijuana, making note if patient states it is prescription medical marijuana. Obtain copy of prescription to document administration directives.

Review of Systems

Many respiratory diseases and disorders have manifestations in systems other than the respiratory system. A comprehensive review of systems should be performed whenever possible; however, due to time and other types of constraints, the provider may be able to perform only a focused review of systems. During a focused review of systems, the provider targets questioning to the systems in which respiratory problems are most likely to have manifestations. The following table summarizes common manifestations of respiratory problems.

System	Symptom or Sign	Possible Associated Diseases/Disorders
General	Fever, chills	Pneumonia, viral upper respiratory infection, bronchitis, pleuritic
	Weakness, weight loss, fatigue	Tuberculosis, lung cancer
Skin	Pallor, cyanosis	Hypoxia, aspiration pneumonia
Cardiovascular	Rhythm disturbances, chest pains	Chronic obstructive pulmonary disease, bronchiolitis, pneumonia, tuberculosis, pleuritic, pleural effusion
Gastrointestinal	Cough when eating	Asthma
	Poor feeding in infants	Pneumonia
	Anorexia	Tuberculosis
Neurological	Headache, mental status changes (decreased level of consciousness), anxiety	Acute bronchitis, emphysema, acute asthma attack

Physical Examination

Equipment Needed

- A magic marker or eyeliner (silver is good for dark skin); make sure it washes off and does not stain the skin
- A tape or ruler marked in centimeters
- Stethoscope with bell and diaphragm (you may want to use a smaller-diameter diaphragm when examining children)
- Draping for the patient's privacy

Components of the Physical Examination

Respiratory assessment involves examination of the chest and lungs through inspection, palpation, percussion, and auscultation. None of these techniques by themselves will provide adequate information for accurate diagnosis of a disease process. Auscultation of the lungs without inspection and palpation of the chest will inhibit the chance to interpret findings in the most accurate way. Dullness on percussion, for example, is found with both pleural effusion and lobar pneumonia; however, breath sounds are absent in pleural effusion and may be present in pneumonia. On palpation, you will often find the tactile fremitus is absent when an effusion exists, but it is increased with lobar pneumonia. The differentiation of these conditions is established with a complete physical examination.

Inspection

Action	Rationale
1. Place the patient in an upright position. If possible, do so without supporting the patient, so you can see the effort it takes to maintain that position and inspect breathing patterns. Remove clothing to better visualize the chest area.	1, 2, 3, 4. These activities may accentuate findings that are subtle and otherwise difficult to detect, such as minimal pulsations or retractions or the presence of deformity (e.g., minimal pectus excavatum).
2. Make sure the room and stethoscope are warm and a gooseneck lamp is available to highlight chest movement.	
3. Position the patient so that the gooseneck lamp can be positioned to shine at different angles.	
4. If the patient is unable to leave the bed due to his or her condition, raise and lower the bed as needed. Also, ensure room for maneuvering around the bed.	
5. Inspect the general appearance.	5.
a. Inspect the skin, noting whether pallor is present.	a. Skin color can tell the examiner if circulation is adequate. Pallor or cyanosis can indicate low oxygenation or hypoxemia.
b. Inspect the face and mouth. • Observe the lips for cyanosis and pursing.	• Pursing of the lips is associated with increased expiratory effort. As cyanosis is a latent sign of hypoxia, when cyanosis is visible, the hypoxic condition has progressed to a dangerous level.
• Smell the patient's breath.	• Infection present in the respiratory system may make the patient's breath malodorous. Metabolic conditions, such as diabetes, may give the patient's breath a fruity odor.
• Observe the nares for flaring.	• Nasal flaring during inspiration is a common sign of air hunger, particularly when the alveoli are considerably involved.
c. Observe the fingers for clubbing.	c. Clubbing of fingers is commonly noted in patients with chronic fibrotic changes in the lungs. Other chronic problems involving the lungs, such as asthma and emphysema, are not associated with clubbing.
6. Inspect the thorax.	
a. Determine the shape and symmetry of the thorax (anterior and posterior). **Figure 9-2** illustrates thoracic landmarks.	a. Location of the landmarks allows for proper documentation. The rib cage should be obvious, with the clavicles apparent superiorly, and the sternum flat. The chest is not symmetrical, but each side can be used to compare with the other. **Figure 9-3** illustrates configurations of the thorax, including abnormal findings. The anteroposterior (AP) diameter of the chest is normally less than the transverse diameter, often by as much as half.

Action   **Rationale**

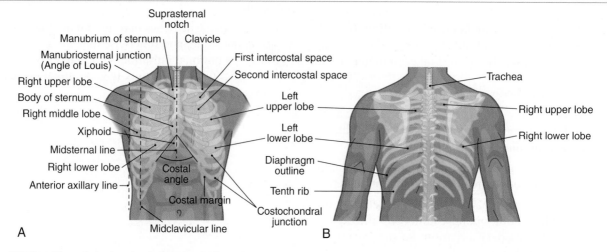

FIGURE 9-2 Thoracic landmarks. A. Anterior. B. Posterior.

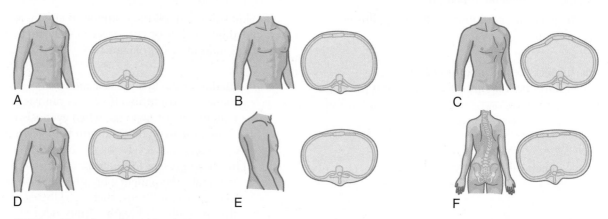

FIGURE 9-3   Thoracic configurations. A. Normal thoracic configuration. B. Barrel chest. C. Pectus carinatum. D. Pectus excavatum. E. Kyphosis. F. Scoliosis.

Barrel chest (**Figure 9-3B**) associated with chronic asthma, emphysema, or cystic fibrosis results from the patient's long-term compromised respiration. The ribs are horizontal, the vertebral spine will appear kyphotic, and the sternal angle more prominent. The trachea may be posteriorly displaced as a result of the compromised breathing patterns.

Pectus carinatum (pigeon chest), where the sternum protrudes, and pectus excavatum (funnel chest), where the lower sternum above the xiphoid process is indented, may be clues to respiratory or cardiac disorder (**Figures 9-3C and D**).

Also note any deviation of the spine. It may be deviated either posteriorly (kyphosis) or laterally (scoliosis) (**Figures 9-3E and F**).

Action	Rationale
b. Note whether there are supernumerary nipples.	**b.** Supernumerary nipples (SNs) are a congenital abnormality, particularly found in Caucasian patients. They are defined as presence of nipples and/or related tissue in addition to the two nipples normally appearing on the anterior chest wall. SNs are located along the embryonic milk line. (The embryonic milk line extends bilaterally from a point slightly beyond the axilla on the arm, down the chest and the abdomen toward the groin, and ends at the proximal inner side of the thigh.) SNs can appear complete with breast tissue and ducts and are then referred to as polymastia, or they can appear partially with some breast tissue involved.
c. Look for any superficial venous patterns over the chest.	**c.** Venous patterns over the chest may be a sign of heart disorders, vascular obstruction, or disease. They are caused by thoracic pressure.
d. Determine the presence of fat or prominence of bony areas.	**d.** Underlying fat and relative prominence of the ribs provide information as to nutritional state.
e. Establish the respiratory rate. To avoid anticipatory response that could mislead you, do not let the patient know that you are counting respirations. Count respirations while palpating the pulse.	**e.** The respiratory rate should be 12–20 respirations per minute; the ratio of respirations to heart rate is approximately 1:4. Respiratory rates higher than 20 respirations per minute need evaluation to determine respiratory distress, obstruction, anxiety, and pain. Respiratory rates can vary when the patient is awake or asleep. When counting respiratory rate, make sure the patient is as comfortable as possible.
f. Determine the pattern of respiration and pay close attention to how the chest moves when the patient breathes (e.g., paradoxical movement). Note any variations in rhythm and determine if patient is breathing too shallowly or too laboriously.	**f.** The chest should expand symmetrically. Paradoxical breathing suggests pneumothorax.
g. Inspect the patient's breathing patterns when he or she inspires and expires. Check for use of accessory muscles.	**g.** Visualization of the chest wall will help to isolate chest wall deformities. When chest asymmetry is noted, it can often be associated with unequal expansion and respiratory compromise caused by a collapsed lung or limitation of expansion caused by extrapleural air, fluid, or a mass. Bulging of the chest wall can be an indication of pulmonary compromise; it is a reaction of the ribs and intercostal spaces to the compromise. A prolonged expiratory phase could be due to obstruction or compression of the bronchiole due to a tumor, aneurysm, or enlarged heart. In this case, the costal angle widens beyond 90 degrees.

Action	Rationale
	Retractions may suggest an obstruction in the respiratory tract. As intrathoracic pressure becomes negative, the pulmonary musculature retracts in an effort to overcome the obstruction. The severity of the retraction depends on the extent and level of the pulmonary obstruction. A high pulmonary obstruction (e.g., with tracheal or laryngeal involvement) will result in breathing that is characterized by stridor, and the chest wall seems to retract in at the sternum. An obstructed airway due to a foreign body in one or the other of the bronchi (usually the right because of its wider orifice and more straight anatomical structure) will result in unilateral retraction. Retraction of the lower chest is seen in patients with asthma or bronchiolitis. These clues suggest obstruction or compression of air through the bronchus or bronchioles.

Palpation

Action	Rationale
1. Palpate the thoracic muscles and rib cage, noticing any pulsations, tenderness, masses, lesions, bulges or depressions, or unusual movement. Pay special attention to patient posture or positioning.	1. Bilateral symmetry should be noted. Sternum and xiphoid process are inflexible and should be stationary. Thoracic spine should be straight and even. Look for kyphosis or lordosis (see Figure 9-3), which can severely compromise respiratory function.
2. Palpate for crackles and rubs (**Figure 9-4**). Save any areas of pain for last. Watch the patient's face for indication of tenderness. Use gentle dipping movements to test muscle tone. Move from region to region without breaking contact with the skin.	2. Localized rigidity is usually organic disease. A rigid appearance suggests anxiety, inflammation, and pain. **Crepitus** is a "rice crispy" feeling that can be palpated and auscultated. Presence of air in the subcutaneous tissue is most often due to a leak somewhere in the respiratory system or due to infection. It may be localized (e.g., over the suprasternal notch and the base of the neck) or cover a wider area of the thorax, usually anteriorly and toward the axilla. If palpation reveals coarse vibrations (usually felt upon on inspiration), the healthcare provider should suspect a pleural friction rub, due to inflammation of the pleural tissue, which rubs against the lung fields. It sounds similar to rubbing of fingers together.

Action   **Rationale**

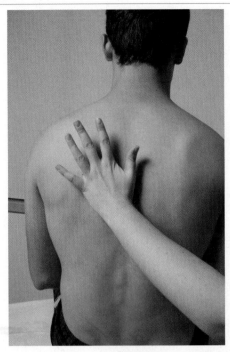

FIGURE 9-4 Palpating for crackles and rubs.

3. Evaluate thoracic expansion.

    First, evaluate the posterior aspect of the patient's chest. Stand behind the patient and place your thumbs along the spinal processes at the level of the tenth rib, with your palms lightly in contact with the posterolateral surfaces. Watch your thumbs move during the patient's inspiration and expiration (see **Figure 9-5**).

    The same process is done anteriorly by facing the patient and placing thumbs along the costal margin and the xiphoid process. With your palms touching the anterolateral chest, watch thumbs move as the patient breathes. Note symmetry.

4. Evaluate tactile fremitus.

    Determine the presence of tactile fremitus, which is the palpable vibration of the chest wall that results from speech or other verbalizations. Fremitus is best felt posteriorly at the second or third intercostal space, usually at the level where the bronchi separate. Variability exists due to the intensity of the pitch of the patient's voice and the structure and thickness of his chest wall.

    Figure 9-6 illustrates locations to palpate for tactile fremitus. The healthcare provider needs to avoid the patient's scapulae, which can obscure fremitus. Ask the patient to recite a number such as "99" or say the word "mine" while you are

3. A loss of symmetry in the movement of the thumbs should alert the provider to a lung expansion problem. It may indicate a collapsed lung.

4. Decreased or absent fremitus may be caused by bronchial obstruction, pneumothorax, emphysema, consolidation, infection, or edema.

    Increased tactile fremitus is described as a harsher or louder vibration. It occurs when there is pulmonary fluid, a mass/tumor in the lungs (consolidation), or copious but nonobstructive bronchial secretions.

Action   **Rationale**

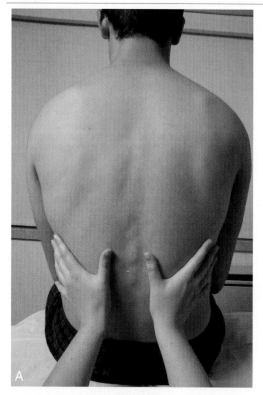 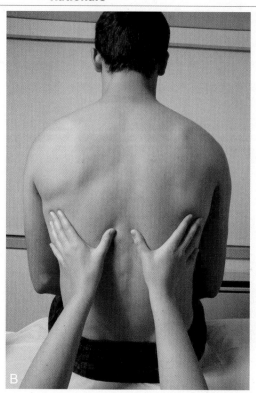

FIGURE 9-5   Evaluating thoracic expansion. A. Initial hand positioning. B. Movement upon inspiration.

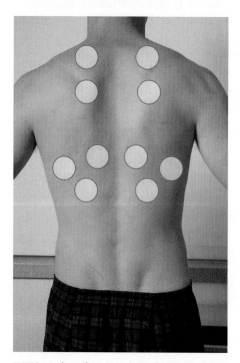

FIGURE 9-6   Locations to palpate for tactile fremitus.

Action   **Rationale**

systematically palpating the posterior chest with
the palmar surfaces of the fingers or with the ulnar
aspects of the hand. Use a light but firm touch
when establishing contact. Compare both sides
of the patient's posterior chest, simultaneously
and symmetrically, or use one hand and quickly
alternate between the two sides (this is more
difficult to do). **Figure 9-7** illustrates palpating for
tactile fremitus.

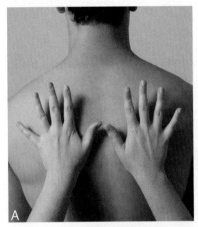 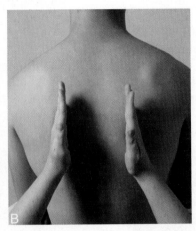

FIGURE 9-7 Palpating for tactile fremitus. A. Using the palmar surface of the hands.
B. Using the ulnar aspect of the hands.

5. Determine the position of the trachea.
   Palpate the trachea by placing the index finger
on the side of the trachea (in the suprasternal
notch) and moving it gently, side to side,
along the upper edges of each clavicle and in
the spaces above to the inner borders of the
sternocleidomastoid muscles (**Figure 9-8**).

5. A small deviation to the right side is considered
normal. But when the deviation is significant, it
could be due to problems within the chest such
as atelectasis, thyroid hypertrophy, pulmonary
consolidation or fibrosis, pleural effusion, tension
pneumothorax, a tumor, or nodal enlargements
on the contralateral side, or it may be pulled by a
tumor on the side to which it deviates.

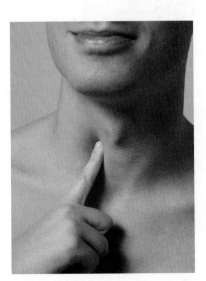

FIGURE 9-8 Determining the position of the trachea.

Palpation

Action	Rationale
1. Percuss the chest. The chest may be percussed directly or indirectly.	**1.** Percussion tones are heard over the entire chest. They can also be heard in the abdomen.

2. Compare all areas bilaterally, using one side as the control for the other. Percuss over the intercostal spaces at the positions described in this section, moving systematically from superior to inferior and medial to lateral. **Figure 9-9** illustrates locations to percuss.
    Ask the patient to bend his or her head forward and fold his or her arms in front of the chest, as illustrated in **Figure 9-10**.
    Next, ask the patient to raise his or her arms over the head and percuss the lateral and anterior chest areas.
	2. Resonance should be heard over all areas of the posterior lungs.
	    If the healthcare provider hears hyperresonance sounds, this can be associated with hyperinflation states such as emphysema, pneumothorax, or asthma.
	    Dullness or flat sounds are often associated with pneumothorax, infection, or asthma.
	    This moves the scapulae laterally, exposing more of the posterior chest, and allows the healthcare provider to percuss more of the lung fields.

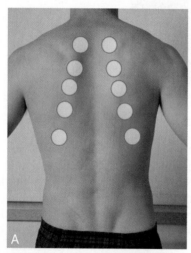
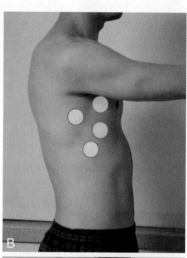
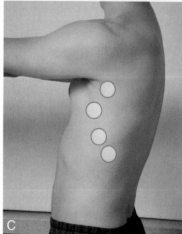
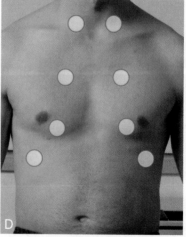
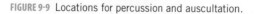

FIGURE 9-9 Locations for percussion and auscultation.

Action   **Rationale**

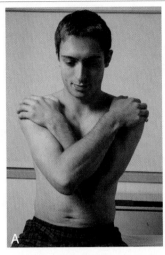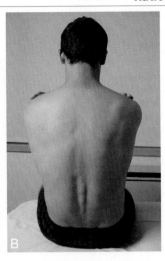

FIGURE 9-10 Positioning for percussion.

3. Determine the diaphragmatic excursion
   (**Figure 9-11**). Keep in mind that the diaphragm
   is higher on the right side than on the left side
   due to the anatomical location of the liver. Ask
   the patient to take in a deep breath and hold it.
   Percuss along the scapular line starting from the
   second or third intercostal space until you locate
   the border of the liver, noting a change in sound
   from resonance to dullness. Mark this location
   with a marking pencil (at the scapular line).

3. Excursion distance is usually 3–5 cm in length.
   When diaphragmatic excursion descent is limited,
   it suggests conditions such as emphysema, ascites,
   or tumors, or it may be due to severe pain, such
   as that experienced from a fractured rib or torn
   muscle.

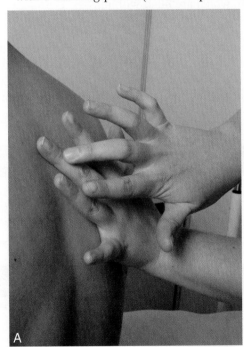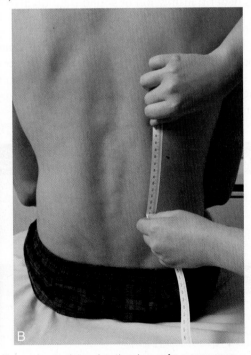

FIGURE 9-11 Determining diaphragmatic excursion. A. Percussing to determine the change from resonance
to dullness. B. Measuring the excursion distance.

Action   **Rationale**

Allow the patient to relax and breathe normally for a few minutes and then repeat the procedure on the other side. Ask the patient to take several breaths and then to exhale as much air as possible. Once he or she has, ask the patient to stop breathing so that you can determine where the diaphragm is after full expiration. Percuss from the marked point upward and make a mark at the point where the sound changes from dullness to resonance. Allow the patient to breathe normally. Repeat on the other side. Measure the distance (in centimeters) between the marks on each side.

Auscultation
Breath Sounds

Breath sounds are made by the flow of air through the respiratory tree. They are characterized by pitch, intensity, quality, and relative duration of their inspiratory and expiratory phases and are classified as vesicular, bronchovesicular, and bronchial (tubular). **Table 9-2** discusses the classification of breath sounds.

Amphoric breath sounds are abnormal sounds heard with consolidation or a tension pneumothorax; they are hollow, low-pitched sounds. Cavernous breath sounds are an empty tympanic sound heard over a fibrotic lesion/cavity.

When fluid or exudate has accumulated in the pleural space (such as is seen with empyema), when the lungs are hyperinflated, or when breathing is shallow from splinting for pain, the breath sounds are typically more difficult to hear or are, in many cases, absent. In disease where consolidation of tissue is present (as with pneumonia), the breath sounds are easier to hear because the consolidation promotes better transmission of sound than do alveoli, which are filled with air.

Adventitious Breath Sounds

Most of the abnormal breath sounds heard during lung auscultation are "extra" or adventitious sounds to the normal breath sounds. These sounds include crackles (formerly called rales), rhonchi, wheezes, and friction rubs (**Table 9-3**). Crackles are discontinuous sounds in that they are often heard at the beginning or end of inspiration; rhonchi and wheezes are continuous in that they are heard continuously throughout the respiratory cycle.

Table 9-2   Classification of Breath Sounds

Breath Sound	Location	Description
Vesicular	Heard over healthy lung tissue.	Low in pitch and intensity
Bronchovesicular	Heard over the major bronchi; abnormal if heard over the peripheral lung base.	Moderate in pitch and intensity
Bronchial	Heard over the trachea; abnormal if heard over the peripheral lung base.	High in pitch and intensity

Table 9-3   Adventitious Breath Sounds

Breath Sound	Description	Cause	Auscultation Tips
Crackles (fine, medium, coarse)	Heard more often during inspiration, crackles are fine, high or low pitched, short in duration, coarse, and last a few milliseconds. Sibilant crackles are high-pitched sounds; sonorous crackles are low-pitched sounds. When the crackles	Caused by air flowing by fluid.	Ask the patient to open the mouth when he or she inhales.

Table 9-3 Adventitious Breath Sounds (*continued*)

Breath Sound	Description	Cause	Auscultation Tips
	occur high in the respiratory tree, they have a dry quality; when they occur low in the respiratory tree, they have a wet quality.		
Rhonchi	Originating in larger airways, rhonchi are low-pitched sounds that are more likely to be prolonged and continuous than crackles. The more sibilant, higher-pitched rhonchi arise from the smaller bronchi, as in asthma; the more sonorous lower-pitched rhonchi arise from larger bronchi, as in tracheobronchitis.	Caused by air passing over a solid or thick secretion.	It may be difficult to distinguish between crackles and rhonchi. In general, rhonchi tend to disappear after coughing, whereas crackles do not. If such sounds are present, listen to several deep breaths before and after cough.
Wheezes	Heard during inspiration or expiration, wheezes are continuous, high-pitched, musical sounds.	Caused by air flowing through constricted passageways. They are usually heard bilaterally in a bronchospasm of asthma or acute bronchitis. If they are heard unilaterally, are localized, or stridor, they are most likely caused by a foreign body obstruction; if the wheeze is consistent, a tumor or abscess is compressing a part of the airway.	Stridor is often louder over the neck than over the chest wall.
Friction rub	Friction rubs occur most commonly outside the airways and are dry, crackling, rubbing, low-pitched sounds that are heard in both inhalation and exhalation.	Caused by inflammation of the pleural or pericardial tissue, as in pericarditis or pleurisy.	The friction rub will disappear when the breath is held, which stops the "rub." (When the rub is cardiac in origin, the sound will not disappear.)
Mediastinal crunches (Hamman's sign)	Mediastinal crunches are loud, wet, crackling sounds heard at the end of expiration. The sounds are synchronous with the heartbeat and asynchronous with respiration.	Mediastinal emphysema.	Ask the patient to lean to the left or lie down on his or her left side to magnify the sound.
Succession splashes	Succession splashes are loud, wet sounds similar to "splashes" heard in the pleural cavity or within the lungs.	Caused by presence of air and fluid in the pleural cavity or within the lungs.	With the patient sitting, place the stethoscope over the lung fields and place a hand on the patient's shoulder and shake the shoulder. The movement will cause the fluid to splash from side to side.

Action	Rationale
1. If the patient is able to sit upright, have him or her breathe slowly and deeply through the mouth.	1. This allows the examiner to better hear intensity, pitch, quality, and duration of sounds.
2. Use the diaphragm of the stethoscope to listen to the lungs. Place the diaphragm of the stethoscope on the skin. Avoid extraneous movement while breath sounds are evaluated.	2. The diaphragm transmits high-pitched sound better.
3. Auscultate the thorax. *(See Figure 9-9 for locations to auscultate.)*	
a. Auscultate the posterior thoracic cage. Ask the patient to sit as for percussion, with head bent forward and arms folded in front of the chest to widen the posterior chest area. Then, have the patient raise his or her arms overhead for auscultating the lateral chest. Next, have the patient sit with the shoulders back for auscultation of the anterior chest.	a. Using the same sequence with each examination ensures that the examination covers all lung fields. It allows the examiner to determine which organs are underneath the area auscultated and identify great vessel involvement through presence of abnormal breath sounds. For example, diminished sounds could indicate a collapsed lung area.

Action	Rationale
b. Systematically auscultate with the patient supine, sitting, and decubitus. Make sure to compare sounds from side to side, and from apex to base, at specific short intervals.	**b.** The sounds of the middle lobe of the right lung and lower lobe on the left are best heard in the respective axillae. Abnormalities in these areas would isolate atelectasis or consolidation.

Diagnostic Reasoning

Based on findings in the health history and physical examination, the clinician should formulate the assessment and plan. For example, a patient may report symptoms that suggest many possible diagnoses; however, findings in the past medical history and during the physical examination might narrow the possible diagnoses down to one or two. Cough is a common chief complaint. **Table 9-4** illustrates differential diagnosis of common disorders associated with coughing.

Table 9-4 Differential Diagnosis of Cough			
Differential Diagnoses	Significant Findings in the Patient's History	Significant Findings in the Patient's Physical Examination	Diagnostic Tests
Bronchitis (acute, chronic)	Cough, fever with chills, muscle aches, nasal congestion, sore throat, sputum production, history of smoking.	Normal breath sounds or diffuse crackles/rhonchi, injected pharynx, mild dyspnea.	Chest x-ray (to rule out pneumonia), oxygen saturation, sputum culture. CXR, cultures, and PFTs are done only with clinical indications, certain comorbidities or increased risk.
Pneumonia*	Signs and symptoms vary a great deal (depending on the organism involved) but may include cough with sputum production, fever, pleuritic chest pain.	Flushed appearance; confusion; crackles over the affected lung, rhonchi, diminished breath sounds, or pleural friction; dullness on percussion over the affected lung, decreased tactile and vocal fremitus, grunting, nasal flaring, tachypnea.	Chest x-ray, sputum culture, complete blood count (CBC), bronchoscopy.
Tuberculosis	History of exposure, cough with or without sputum, fatigue, fever, night sweats, anorexia, pleuritic chest pain.	Crackles on auscultation, tachypnea, decreased breath sounds.	Tuberculin skin test (purified protein derivative [PPD] or Mantoux), sputum culture, chest x-ray, bone x-ray, and other tests to determine extent of disease.

*Due to high mortality and morbidity, it is important to diagnose pneumonia correctly, recognize any complications or underlying conditions, and treat the patient appropriately.

Respiratory Assessment of Special Populations

Considerations for the Pregnant Patient

While taking the history, note the following:

- Weeks of gestation or estimated date of conception (EDC)
- Presence of multiple fetuses, polyhydramnios, or other conditions in which a larger uterus displaces the diaphragm upward
- Exercise type and energy expenditure

Recognize the following physiological changes:

- Pregnant women experience both structural and ventilatory changes.
- Dyspnea is common in pregnancy and is usually a result of normal physiologic changes.
- The costal angle (approximately 68 degrees before pregnancy) increases to about 103 degrees in the third trimester.
- There is an increase of 100 to 200 mL in vital capacity, which is the amount of air that can be expelled at the normal rate of exhalation after a maximum inspiration.
- The tidal volume—the amount of air inhaled and exhaled during normal breathing—increases 40%, along with minute ventilation.
- Overall, the pregnant woman increases her ventilation by breathing more deeply, not more frequently.

Considerations for the Neonatal Patient
General

- While taking the history, note the following:
  - Premature birth
  - Ventilation assistance, if any, and duration of that assistance
  - Respiratory distress syndrome
  - Bronchopulmonary dysplasia
  - Transient tachypnea
- A newborn's Apgar scores at 1 and 5 minutes after birth tell you a great deal about the infant's respiratory effort. A newborn whose respirations are inadequate but who is otherwise normal may initially score 1 or even 0 on heart rate, muscle tone, response to a catheter, and color. Depressed respiration often has its origins in the maternal environment during labor, such as sedation or compromised blood supply to the child, or it may result from mechanical obstruction due to mucus.
- The newborn's lung function is particularly susceptible to a number of environmental factors. The pattern of respirations will vary with room temperature, feeding, and sleep. In the first few hours after birth, the respiratory effort can be depressed by the passive transfer of drugs given to the mother before delivery.
- Approach examination of the chest and lungs of the newborn in a sequence similar to that of adults.

Inspection

- Try to conduct inspection without disturbing the newborn.
- Inspect for retraction at the supraclavicular notch and contraction of the sternocleidomastoid muscles; they should be considered significant signs of respiratory distress.
- Inspect for respiratory grunting, during which the infant tries to expel trapped air or fetal lung fluid while trying to retain air and increase oxygen levels. When persistent, it is a cause for concern. It indicates the presence of respiratory constriction and obstruction.
- Inspect for flaring of the nares, another indicator of respiratory distress at this, or any, age.
- Inspect the thoracic cage, noting its size and shape. Measure the chest circumference, which in the healthy full-term newborn is usually in the range of 30 to 36 cm, sometimes 2 to 3 cm smaller than the head circumference. The difference between the two increases with prematurity. An infant with intrauterine growth retardation will have a relatively smaller chest circumference compared with the head; the infant of a mother with poorly controlled diabetes will have a relatively large chest circumference. As a rough measure, the distance between the nipples is approximately one-fourth the circumference of the chest.
- Observe the nipples for symmetry in size and for the presence of swelling and discharge. A healthcare provider might observe supernumerary nipples, ordinarily not fully developed, along a line drawn from the primary nipple. In Caucasian children, but not as often in African American children, SNs may be associated with a variety of congenital abnormalities.
- Note that cyanosis of the hands and feet (acrocyanosis) is common in the newborn and can persist for several days in a cool environment without causing concern.
- Count the respiratory rate for 1 minute (see **Table 9-5**). The expected rate varies from 30 to 80 respirations per minute, although a rate of 80 respirations per minute is not uncommon. Infants delivered by cesarean section generally have a more rapid rate than those delivered vaginally. If the room temperature is very warm or cool, a noticeable variation in the rate occurs, most often tachypnea but sometimes bradypnea.
- Note the regularity of respiration. Infants are obligate nose breathers. It sometimes seems that they would prefer respiratory distress to opening their mouths to breathe. The more premature an infant at birth, the more likely some irregularity in respiratory pattern will be present. Periodic breathing—a sequence of relatively vigorous respiratory efforts

Table 9-5 Normal Neonatal and Pediatric Respiratory Rates	
Age	Respirations per Minute
Newborn to 1 year	30–80
1 to 3 years	20–40
3 to 6 years	20–30
6 to 10 years	16–20
10 to 17 years	16–20
17 years	12–20

followed by apnea lasting as long as 10 to 15 seconds—is common. Periodic breathing is cause for concern if the apneic episodes tend to be prolonged and the infant becomes centrally cyanotic (i.e., cyanotic about the mouth, face, and torso). The persistence of periodic breathing episodes in preterm infants is relative to gestational age of the baby, with apneic periods diminishing in frequency as the infant approaches term status. In the term infant, periodic breathing should wane a few hours after birth.

- Observe chest expansion. Newborns rely primarily on the diaphragm for their respiratory effort, only gradually adding the intercostal muscles (whereas infants quite commonly use their abdominal muscles as well). If the chest expansion is asymmetrical, suspect some compromise of one of the lungs (e.g., pneumothorax or diaphragmatic hernia).

Palpation

- Palpate the rib cage and sternum, noting loss of symmetry, unusual masses, or crepitus. Crepitus around a fractured clavicle (with no evidence of pain) is common after a difficult forceps delivery.
- Note that the newborn's xiphoid process is more mobile and prominent than that of an older child or adult. It has a sharp inferior tip that moves slightly back and forth under your finger.

Percussion

- Percussion is usually unreliable in the neonate. The examiner's fingers may be too large for the baby's chest, particularly the premature infant.
- With either direct or indirect percussion, it is easy to miss the dullness of underlying consolidation. If you sense some loss of resonance, attach to it as much importance as you would frank dullness in the adolescent or adult.

Auscultation

- Localization of breath sounds is difficult, particularly in the very small chest of the preterm newborn. Breath sounds are easily transmitted from one segment of the auscultatory area to another; therefore, the absence of sounds in any given area may be difficult to detect. Sometimes it helps to listen to both sides of the chest simultaneously using a double-belled stethoscope.
- It is not uncommon to hear crackles and rhonchi immediately after birth because fetal fluid has not been completely cleared. Whenever auscultatory findings are asymmetrical, a problem should be suspected (e.g., aspiration of meconium).
- Gurgling from the intestinal tract, slight movement, and mucus in the upper airway may all contribute to adventitious sounds, making evaluation of the newborn difficult. If gastrointestinal gurgling sounds are constantly heard in the chest, suspect diaphragmatic hernia, but wide transmissions of these sounds can sometimes be deceptive.
- Stridor is a high-pitched, piercing sound, most often heard during inspiration. It is a result of destruction somewhere high in the respiratory tree. A compelling sound at any age, it cannot be dismissed as inconsequential, particularly when inspiration (I) may be three or four times longer than expiration (E), giving an I/E ratio of 3:1 or 4:1. If stridor is accompanied by a cough, hoarseness, and retraction, it signifies a serious problem in the trachea or larynx: a floppy epiglottis; congenital defects; croup; or edematous response

to infection, allergens, smoke, chemicals, or aspirated foreign body. Newborns who have a narrow tracheal lumen readily respond with stridor to its compression by a tumor, abscess, or double aortic arch.

Considerations for the Pediatric Patient
General
During the history, question the patient's parent about the following:

- Possible aspiration of a small object, toy, or food
- Possible ingestion of kerosene or other hydrocarbon
- Inadequate weight gain (good indication of exercise intolerance)
- Apneic episodes; use of apnea monitoring
- Sudden infant death in sibling
- For infants: difficulty feeding (increased perspiration, cyanosis, tiring quickly, disinterest in feeding)

Inspection
- Inspect for "roundness" of the chest. If the "roundness" of the young child's chest persists past the second year of life, there is the possibility of a chronic obstructive pulmonary problem, such as cystic fibrosis. The persistence of a barrel chest at the age of 5 or 6 years suggests underlying problems.
- Inspect thoracic muscles. Children use thoracic (intercostal) musculature for respiration by the age of 6 or 7 years. In young children, obvious intercostal exertion (retractions) on breathing suggests some pulmonary or airway problem.

Auscultation
- Because children younger than 5 or 6 years of age may not be able to give enough of an expiration to satisfy the healthcare provider (particularly when subtle wheezing is suspected), ask them to "blow out" a flashlight or to blow away a bit of tissue in the provider's hand to bring out otherwise difficult-to-hear end-expiratory sounds.
- Ask the child to run around; it is easier to hear the breath sounds when the child breathes more deeply after running.
- Note physiologic differences. Because children's chests are thinner and ordinarily more resonant than adults' chests, the intrathoracic sounds are easier to hear, and hyperresonance is common in young children.
- Because of the thin chest wall, the breath sounds of the young may sound louder, harsher, and more bronchial than those of the adult.
- Bronchovesicular breath sounds may be heard throughout the chest.
- Seize the opportunity a crying child presents. A sob is frequently followed by a deep breath. The sob itself allows evaluation of vocal resonance and permits you to feel for tactile fremitus; use the whole hand—both palm and fingers—gently. The crying child may pause occasionally, and the heart sounds may be heard. These pauses may be a bit prolonged as the breath is held, giving you the chance to distinguish a murmur from a breath sound.

Considerations for the Geriatric Patient
General
- The examination procedure for older adults is the same as that for younger adults, although there may be variations in some expected findings. Older patients have more difficulty breathing deeply and holding their breath than younger patients, and they may tire more quickly, even when well. The pace and demands of examination should, therefore, be adapted to individual need. Most pathologic pulmonary conditions in the elderly occur in the lung bases; examine these first before fatigue sets in.
- Because older adults are at risk for chronic respiratory diseases (lung cancer, chronic bronchitis, emphysema, and tuberculosis), pay particular attention to the following:
  - Smoking history
  - Cough, dyspnea on exertion, breathlessness

- Fatigue
- Weight change
- Fever, night sweats
- Exposure to and frequency of respiratory infections, history of pneumococcal vaccination, and annual influenza immunization
- Effects of weather on respiratory efforts
- Immobilization or reduced activity
- Difficulty swallowing
- Alteration in daily living habits or activities as a result of chief complaint

Inspection

- Observe expansion. Chest expansion is often decreased in older patients. The patient may be less able to use the respiratory muscles because of muscle weakness, general physical disability, or a sedentary lifestyle. Calcification of the rib articulations may also interfere with chest expansion, requiring use of accessory muscles. Bony prominences are marked, and there is loss of subcutaneous tissue.
- Inspect the spine and configuration of the thorax. The dorsal curve of the thoracic spine is pronounced (kyphosis), with flattening of the lumbar curve. The anteroposterior diameter of the chest is increased in relation to the lateral diameter.

Auscultation

- Some older patients may display hyperresonance as a result of increased distensibility of the lungs.
- This finding must be evaluated in the context of the presence or absence of other symptoms.

Case Study Review

Chief Complaint

"My cough is getting worse, and now it hurts."

Information Gathered During the Interview

Mr. V is a 58-year-old man who presents with a 2-day history of left-sided pleuritic chest pain, dyspnea, orthopnea, intermittent fever and chills, and a cough productive of yellow sputum, which became brown yesterday. The pleuritic chest pain radiates to the proximal left upper quadrant (LUQ) during coughing. He has not experienced nausea but did have one episode of emesis yesterday. He also experienced rhinorrhea and a sore throat this morning, which have now resolved.

Mr. V has had asthma since childhood, which has been under good control despite the fact that he ran out of his albuterol inhaler and has not been using it for some time. He does not have a history of past surgeries or trauma. He denies ever having received a blood transfusion.

Both of Mr. V's parents are alive. His father has been diagnosed with hypertension (HTN). His family history is negative for coronary artery disease, asthma, diabetes, and cancer. Mr. V denies tobacco or drug use. He reports alcohol use, two glasses of wine on Friday evenings when dining out. Mr. V is a salesman with a book company and has never been married.

Clues	Important Points
Two-day history of chief complaint	Symptoms are worse (2 days) with increasing shortness of breath, fever, and chills.
Left-sided pleuritic chest pain, which radiates to the left upper quadrant (LUQ) during coughing	The pain is associated with bacterial origin of infection, such as pneumonia. It compromises breathing patterns.
Dyspnea/orthopnea	Compromised breathing patterns suggest emergent care.
Intermittent fever and chills	Fever suggests bacterial or viral origin of infection.
Productive cough; yellow sputum, which became brown	Reddish-brown sputum suggests bacterial origin of infection.

Emesis	Check for dehydration or possible second diagnosis: gallbladder disease.
Rhinorrhea, sore throat	Supports cold, flu diagnosis.
Decreased breath sounds over left lobe of lung	Supports pneumonia diagnosis.

Name CV	Date 9/15/16	Time 0940
	DOB 7/10/58	Sex M

HISTORY

CC
"My cough is getting worse, and now it hurts."

HPI
59-year-old male presents with 2-day history of left-sided, pleuritic chest pain that radiates to LUQ during coughing, dyspnea, orthopnea, fever and chills, cough w/yellow sputum that became brown yesterday, not experiencing nausea but had one episode of emesis yesterday, rhinorrhea and sore throat this morning which have resolved.

Medications
Albuterol: 2 puffs prn for chest tightness, last dose—3 mo ago.

Allergies
NKA, patient suspects seasonal allergies to mountain cedar.

PMI
Illnesses.
Asthma since childhood, received the flu vaccine.

Hospitalizations/Surgeries
Denies history of surgery, trauma, or blood transfusion.

FH
Positive for HTN, negative for CAD, diabetes, and cancer.

SH
Denies tobacco or drug use, reports alcohol use (2 glasses of wine on Fridays), salesman, never been married.

ROS

General	Cardiovascular
Fever and chills.	Left-sided pleuritic chest pain.
Skin	Respiratory
Denies any changes, including changes to pallor.	See HPI.
Eyes	Gastrointestinal
No changes in vision.	Denies nausea, 1 episode of emesis yesterday.
Ears	Genitourinary/Gynecological
Denies pain and other symptoms.	Negative history.
Nose/Mouth/Throat	Musculoskeletal
Rhinorrhea and sore throat, which have resolved.	Negative history.
Breast	Neurological
Denies problems.	Negative history.

PHYSICAL EXAMINATION

Weight 180 lb.	Temp 99.4	BP 100/60
Height 6 ft.	Pulse 120	Resp 24

General Appearance
58-year-old, Asian American male in apparent respiratory distress. Pleasant, well groomed.

Skin
Warm, dry, no color change.

HEENT
Normal cephalic; pupil response normal; corneal reflexes intact; hearing normal; nose without discharge, obstruction, or deviation; oropharynx clear w/o obvious mucosal lesions.

| Cardiovascular |
| Tachycardia; no murmurs appreciated. |

| Respiratory |
| Right side clear to auscultation. The left upper lobe is clear to auscultation with significantly decreased breath sounds. E-to-A changes in the left lower lobe and across the middle of the right lung field. Rhonchi noted in right lower lobe. |

| Gastrointestinal |
| Normal bowel sounds; soft; tympany except at border of the LUQ near the site of the patient's chest pain, where consolidation is noted. |

| Genitourinary |
| Not examined. |

| Musculoskeletal |
| Strengths 4–5/5 throughout and symmetrical. Pulses are 1+ bilaterally. |

| Neurological |
| Alert and oriented 3; CN II–XII intact; deep tendon reflexes 2+; Babinski negative. |

| Other |

| Lab Tests |
| Sputum Gram stain: many WBCs, few epithelial cells, moderate gram-positive cocci in chains and pairs. |
| Sputum and blood cultures pending. |

Na 142 mEq/mL	Hgb 14.2 g/dL	Ca 8.2 mEq/L
K 3.7 mEq/mL	Hct 42%	Mg 1.3 mEq/L
Cl 99 mEq/ml	WBC 14.7 ¥ 10^3/mm^3	Phos 2.7 mg/dL
CO2 20 mEq/L	72% Neutrophils	CPK 256 IU/L
BUN 7 mg/dL	12% Bands	
SCr 0.9 mg/dL	14% Lymphs	
Glu 126 mg/dL	2% Monocytes	

| UA: Cloudy urine; SG 1.018, pH 5.0, protein > 300 mg/dL, trace ketones, moderate blood, 2 WBCs/hpf, 4 RBCs/hpf, no bacteria isolated. |

| Special Tests |
| Chest x-ray: Consolidation on inferior segments of left lower lobe, as well as superior segment of left lower lobe. Other lung fields clear. Heart, normal size. |

| Final Assessment Findings |
| 1. Left lower lobe pneumonia, probably pneumococcal. |
| 2. Urine (+) for protein and ketones with elevated CPK of uncertain etiology. |

Bibliography

American Academy of Family Physicians. (n.d.). Diagnosis and management of acute bronchitis. Retrieved from http://www.aafp.org/afp/2002/0515/p2039.htm.

Collins, R. D. (2012). *Algorithmic diagnosis of symptoms and signs. Cost-effective approach* (3rd ed.). Philadelphia, PA: Lippincott Williams & Wilkins.

Considine, J. (2005). The role of nurses in preventing adverse events related to respiratory dysfunction: Literature review. *Journal of Advanced Nursing, 49*, 624–633.

DeGowin, R., & Brown, D. (2014). *DeGowin's diagnostic examination* (10th ed.). Philadelphia, PA: McGraw-Hill.

Dunphy, L. M., & Winland-Brown, J. E. (2015). *Primary care: The art and science of advanced practice nursing* (4th ed.). Philadelphia, PA: F. A. Davis.

Hogan, J. (2006). Why don't nurses monitor the respiratory rates of patients? *British Journal of Nursing, 15*, 489–492.

Knutson, D., & Braun, C. (2002). Diagnosis and management of acute bronchitis. *American Family Physician, 65*(10), 2039–2045.

Metlay, J., Kapoor, W. N., & Fine, M. J. (1997). Does this patient have community-acquired pneumonia? Diagnosing pneumonia by history and physical examination. *Journal of the American Medical Association, 278*(17), 1440–1445.

Myers, K. A., & Farquhar, D. R. E. (2001). Does this patient have clubbing? The rational clinical examination. *Journal of the American Medical Association, 286*, 341–347.

National Heart, Lung, and Blood Institute, National Asthma Education and Prevention Program. (2007). *Expert panel report 3: Guidelines for the Diagnosis and Management of Asthma.* Washington, DC: U.S. Department of Health & Human Services. Retrieved from http://www .nhlbi.nih.gov/health-pro/guidelines/current/asthma-guidelines.

Noble, J. (Ed.). (2001). *Textbook of primary care medicine* (3rd ed.). St. Louis, MO: Mosby.

Ouelette, D. R. (n.d.). Pulmonary embolism. *Medscape.* Retrieved from http://emedicine.medscape .com/article/300901-overview.

Ralston, S. L., Lieberthal, A. S., Meissner, H. C., Alverson, B. K., Baley, J. E., Gadomski, A. M., . . . American Academy of Pediatrics. (2014). Clinical practice guideline: the diagnosis, management, and prevention of bronchiolitis. *Pediatrics, 134*(5), 1474–1502.

Rojas, M., Granados Rugeles, C., & Charry-Anzola, L. (2009). Oxygen therapy for lower respiratory tract infections in children between 3 months and 15 years of age. *Cochrane Database of Systematic Reviews*, CD005975.

Ryu, J. H., Olson, E. J., & Pellikka, P. A. (1998). Clinical recognition of pulmonary embolism: Problem of unrecognized and asymptomatic cases. *Mayo Clinic Proceedings, 73*, 873–879.

United States Public Health Service. (1998). *Putting prevention into practice: Clinician's handbook of preventive services* (2nd ed.). Maclean, VA: International Medical Publishers.

Vestbo, J., Hurd, S. S., Agusti, A. G., Jones, P. W., Vogelmeier, C., Anzueto, A., . . . Rodriguez-Roisin, R. (2013). Global strategy for the diagnosis, management, and prevention of chronic obstructive pulmonary disease: GOLD executive summary. *American Journal of Respiratory Critical Care Medicine, 187*(4), 347–365.

Chapter 10

Cardiovascular Disorders

Anatomy and Physiology Review of the Cardiovascular System

The cardiovascular system is composed of the heart and a closed system of vessels including the arteries, veins, and capillaries. The blood is continuously pumped by the heart through the vessels and returned to the central circulation. The cardiovascular system is responsible for the following functions:

- Maintaining homeostasis
- Providing a means of exchanging nutrient-rich blood for waste products
- Oxygenating tissue throughout the body

Heart

The heart is a hollow muscular organ that is situated between the lungs in the middle of the mediastinum and enclosed within the pericardium. It lies obliquely in the chest, behind the body of the sternum, just left of the midline, and above the diaphragm. The heart is conical in shape and approximately the size of a clenched fist. It rhythmically pumps 5 to 6 liters of blood per minute throughout the body.

There are four chambers of the heart: the upper two chambers are referred to as the right and left atria; the lower two chambers are the right and left ventricles (**Figure 10-1**). The atria are thin-walled, low-pressure chambers that receive blood from the venae cavae and pulmonary arteries and pump blood into the respective ventricle. The ventricles—thick muscular-walled chambers—pump blood from the atria to the lungs and throughout the body via the aorta. The right atrium and right ventricle constitute the right side of the heart. The left atrium and left ventricle are collectively known as the left side of the heart. A blood-tight partition, the cardiac septum, divides the right and left sides of the heart. The right ventricle forms the anterior and inferior surfaces of the heart, whereas the left ventricle constitutes the posterior and anterolateral aspects of the heart.

The heart consists of three layers of cardiac muscle: epicardium, myocardium, and endocardium. The epicardium is the thin, outermost protective layer of the heart. The myocardium, the thick muscular middle layer, includes spontaneously contracting cardiac muscle fibers, which allow the heart to contract. Thus it is responsible for pumping blood through the heart. The innermost layer of the heart, the endocardium, lines the inner cavities and covers the valves within the heart. The pericardium is a fibrous fluid-filled sac that surrounds the heart and serves to limit heart motion and provide a barrier to infection.

Cardiac valves are flap-like structures that permit the flow of blood in only one direction. There are two types of cardiac valves: atrioventricular (AV) valves and semilunar valves. The two AV valves, tricuspid and mitral, prevent the backflow of blood into the atria during ventricular contraction. The tricuspid valve, located between the right atrium and right ventricle, consists of three somewhat triangular cusps. The mitral valve is located between the left atrium and left ventricle and is formed by only two cusps. The triscupid and mitral valves open when the ventricles relax, permitting blood to enter the ventricles from the atria.

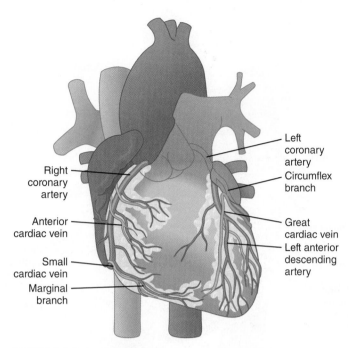

FIGURE 10-1 Anterior view of the heart.

The semilunar valves, each of which has three cusps, are the pulmonic and aortic valves. The semilunar valves open during ventricular contraction, allowing the forward flow of blood into the pulmonary artery and aorta. During ventricular relaxation, the valves close, preventing the backflow of blood into the ventricles. The pulmonic valve is positioned between the right ventricle and the pulmonary artery. The aortic valve is located between the left ventricle and the aorta. **Figure 10-2** illustrates the valves.

The broader upper portion of the heart is known as the base. The base includes not only the superior portion of the heart, but also the great vessels (aorta, pulmonary vessels, and venae cavae) that supply blood to the right and left atrium. The inferior narrower tip of the heart is referred to as the apex.

Arteries and Veins

Arteries are tough, tensile, and less distensible than veins. The tough and tensile walls protect the arteries against damage as the arterial pressure increases after ventricular contraction. Arteries become smaller and smaller as they get farther from the heart. At their smallest point, arteries become capillaries. Capillaries deliver oxygen and nutrients and remove waste products from the cardiac cells. Capillaries become larger as they leave each cell and become veins. Thus the blood travels from the arteries, through the capillaries to the cardiac cells, and then to the veins. Because the blood travels through veins at a lower pressure, the walls are thinner and require valves to maintain unidirectional blood flow. In general, veins can serve as a reservoir for blood and significantly increase blood volume when needed.

The coronary arteries supply oxygen- and nutrient-rich blood to the myocardium; coronary veins return the blood to the general circulation. The right and left coronary arteries arise at the base of the aorta directly above the aortic valve. The right coronary artery supplies blood to the right atrium and right ventricle in most patients. It is also the usual blood supply for the sinoatrial (SA) and atrioventricular (AV) nodes. The left coronary artery divides into two large arteries, the left anterior descending (LAD) and the circumflex (CFX). The LAD runs between the ventricles on the anterior aspect of the heart and, therefore, supplies blood to the anterior wall. The CFX runs

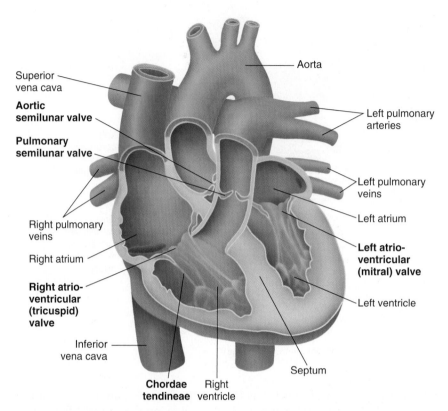

FIGURE 10-2 Valves of the heart.

between the left atrium and left ventricle to supply blood to the lateral wall of the heart. **Figure 10-3** depicts the coronary arteries.

Cardiac Cycle

The cardiac cycle involves two phases as the heart contracts and relaxes rhythmically: systole and diastole. Systole refers to the contraction of the ventricles as blood is ejected from the right ventricle into the pulmonary arteries and from the left ventricle into the aorta. Diastole refers to the passive filling of the ventricles followed by contraction of the atria, thereby moving blood from the atria to the ventricles.

During systole, ventricular contraction raises the pressure inside of the ventricles, forcing the AV valves to close shut. The closure of the AV valves creates the first heart tone, S_1. It is the characteristic "lub" in "lub-dub." At the same time, the aortic and pulmonic valves open, allowing the ejection of blood from the ventricles into the respective arteries. The opening of valves is silent, so it does not contribute to audible heart tones.

When the ventricles are almost empty, the pressure in the arteries is higher than that of the ventricles, forcing the semilunar valves closed. The closures of the aortic and pulmonic valves contribute to the second heart sound, S_2. It is the characteristic "dub" in "lub-dub." S_3 is related to diastolic motion and rapid filling of the ventricles in early diastole. S_4 is related to atrial contraction in late diastole to ensure the ejection of remaining blood.

The heart has an intrinsic electrical conduction system, depicted in **Figure 10-4**, that allows for ventricular contractility in the absence of external stimuli (automaticity of the heart). The electrical impulse stimulates each myocardial contraction (depolarization) that occurs during the cardiac cycle. The impulse originates in the SA node, which is located in the wall of the right atrium and is often referred to as the natural pacemaker of the heart. The SA node sends impulses automatically at a rate of 60 to 100 beats per minute. The impulse travels through both

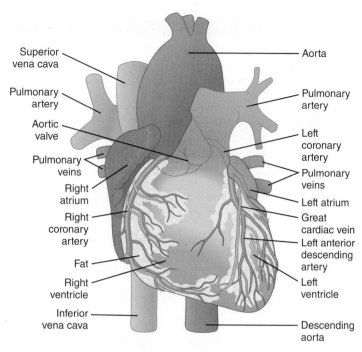

FIGURE 10-3 Anterior view of the coronary arteries.

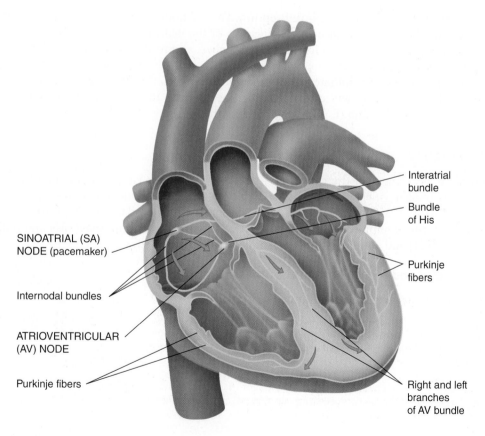

FIGURE 10-4 Cardiac conduction system.

BOX 10-1   ELECTROCARDIOGRAMS

An electrocardiogram (ECG) records electrical activity as it travels through the cardiac muscle fibers. It records two phases of myocardial contraction and relaxation, known as depolarization and repolarization. *Depolarization* is the spread of the stimulus through the cardiac muscle, whereas *repolarization* is the return of the stimulated cardiac muscle to a resting state. The ECG records electrical changes in the heart; it does not record myocardial contraction. However, myocardial contraction usually occurs immediately after electrical depolarization.

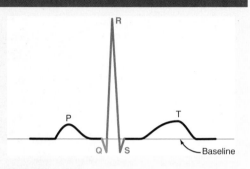

Normal waveform.

Reproduced from *12 Lead ECG: The Art of Interpretation*, courtesy of Tomas B. Garcia, MD.

An ECG records electrical activity as waveforms: P wave, PR interval, QRS complex, ST segment, T wave, and U wave (occasionally).

- The P wave represents the wave of depolarization spreading from the sinoatrial (SA) node throughout the atria.
- The PR interval represents the time between the onset of atrial depolarization and ventricular depolarization.
- The QRS complex represents ventricular depolarization, as the electrical stimulus spreads through the ventricles.
- The ST segment is the time at which the entire ventricle is depolarized.
- The T wave represents ventricular repolarization, or the return of the ventricular myocardium to its resting potential.
- The U wave, although not always present, represents the final phase of ventricular repolarization.

atria to the AV node, located in the atrial septum. The AV node slows the impulse down to allow complete contraction of the atria before activation of the ventricles. The impulse then travels to the bundle of His, to the right and left bundle branches, and to the Purkinje fibers located in the ventricular myocardium.

Ventricular contraction is initiated from the endocardium to the epicardium and from the apex to the base. The electrical activity can be recorded as it travels through the conduction system by means of an electrocardiogram (ECG), which is described in **Box 10-1**.

Health History

A noninvasive assessment of the cardiovascular system provides easily attainable, valuable, and cost-effective data on a patient's cardiac status. Exploring the patient's history of present illness (HPI), past medical history (PMI), a detailed review of systems (ROS), and data obtained from any hemodynamic monitoring equipment will help guide the clinician to a prompt diagnosis and treatment. Family history (FH) and social history (SH) should also be reviewed.

Chief Complaint and History of Present Illness

"I have a stabbing pain in my chest that will not go away."

Mr. S is a 69-year-old Caucasian male who presents with a 5-year history of coronary artery disease (CAD) with exertional angina. His angina is usually relieved once the activity ceases, but occasionally sublingual nitroglycerin is required to relieve his chest pain. These traditional methods have proved ineffective for the past day. On a scale of 1 to 10, his pain has increased in intensity from 3 to 6. The pain is substernal with radiation down his left arm. It is associated with diaphoresis and nausea. The patient is not currently experiencing any dyspnea, orthopnea, syncope, palpitations, or cough.

Chest Pain

Onset and duration	Is the onset sudden or gradual? How long does the pain last?
Quality	Describe the pain. Is it burning, crushing, knifelike, aching, pressure, sharp, or dull?
Location	Where is the pain (e.g., sternal, back, scapula)? Does it radiate to the arms, neck, jaws, or teeth?
Severity	Have the patient rank the pain on a scale of 1 to 10. Does it interfere with the patient's activities of daily living (ADLs) or interfere with or disrupt his or her sleep?
Aggravating and alleviating factors	What aggravates the pain (e.g., physical exertion, eating, coughing, emotional experiences)? What alleviates the pain (e.g., rest)? *This information may offer some clues to the cause and offer possibilities for differential diagnoses, such as musculoskeletal pain, pleural pain, or gastrointestinal disease.* Which medications, including prescription, over-the-counter, herbals, and alternative therapies, has the patient tried? *It is important to ask the patient if she or he has seen a healthcare professional previously for this problem and to obtain the prescribed treatment to determine its effectiveness.*
Use of alcohol or recreational drugs	Is there a history of alcohol or drug use? *It is important to ask (especially a young adult or adolescent) about recreational drug use, particularly cocaine, because it can cause spasm of the coronary arteries.*
Associated symptoms	Important associated symptoms to assess include anxiety, dyspnea, nausea, vomiting, diaphoresis, faintness, clamminess, and pallor.

Table 10-1 describes common types of chest pain. Complaints of chest discomfort are often vague and difficult to diagnose. Explore associated symptoms, including their quality and location. It is important to consider differential diagnoses prior to instituting invasive diagnostic testing.

It is important to remember that 23% of patients will not have classic chest pain but could be having an active cardiovascular event. This patient population includes the elderly, patients with diabetes, and women.

Table 10-1	Characteristics of Common Types of Chest Pain
Type	**Characteristics of Pain**
Anginal	Classically substernal; precipitated by exertion, emotional experiences, and food consumption; relieved by rest and medications (such as nitroglycerin); frequently accompanied by diaphoresis, nausea, and vomiting.
Stable	Occurring in repetitive pattern; precipitated by similar exertional demands; duration is greater than 30 seconds to a few minutes; resolves with rest or typical medication regimens.
Unstable	Occurring in escalating, crescendo pattern; duration is greater than stable type but usually less than 20 minutes; takes longer to resolve and often requires intravenous nitrates.
Pleural	Occurring with respiration and coughing; described as a sharp pain that is alleviated when breath is held.
Gastrointestinal	Substernal burning; radiates occasionally to the upper chest; intensified in flat positions; relieved with antacids and sometimes food consumption.
Musculoskeletal	Precipitated by twisting and bending movements; long lasting or chronic; frequently arises with focal pain points.

Palpitations

Palpitations and rhythm disturbances are common events and can cause weakness and syncope. It is important to determine the type and nature of the disturbance. **Figure 10-5** depicts ECG strips of common arrhythmias.

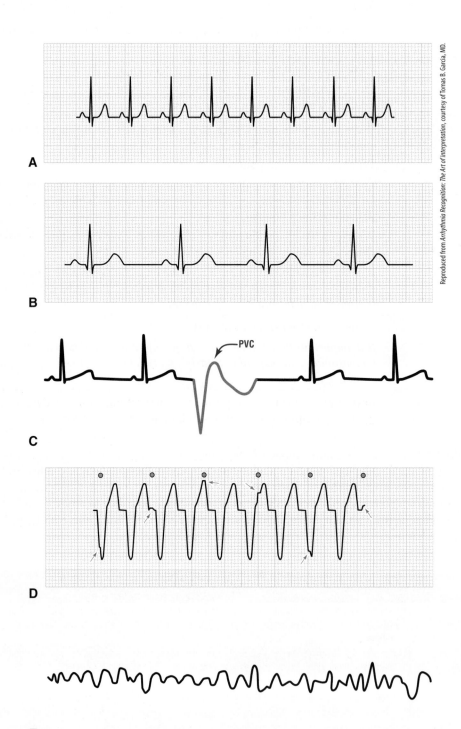

Reproduced from *Arrhythmia Recognition: The Art of Interpretation*, courtesy of Tomas B. Garcia, MD.

FIGURE 10-5 ECG strips depicting common arrhythmias. A. Sinus tachycardia. B. Sinus bradycardia. C. Premature ventricular contraction. D. Ventricular tachycardia. E. Ventricular fibrillation.

Onset and duration	Is the onset sudden or gradual? How long do the palpitations last?
Quality	Are the palpitations regular or irregular?
	Are the palpitations continuous or intermittent?
Aggravating and alleviating factors	What aggravates the palpitations (e.g., anxiety, physical exertion, recreational drug use)?
	What alleviates the palpitations (e.g., coughing or bearing down)?
Associated symptoms	Are the palpitations associated with dyspnea, chest pain, blurred vision, dizziness, or feelings of faintness?

Dyspnea

Dyspnea (shortness of breath) is a common complaint with both cardiac and respiratory conditions. Dyspnea may be associated with myocardial ischemia or infarction, congestive heart failure, or pulmonary disorders.

Onset and duration	Is it sudden or gradual?
	How long does it last?
Aggravating and alleviating factors	What aggravates and alleviates the dyspnea? Ask the patient if it is aggravated by physical or emotional stress and, if so, how much. Does it occur with walking on flat surfaces or with going up inclines? Does the patient use pillows to sleep at night to aid breathing?
	These factors help indicate exercise tolerance and ventricular function and possibly suggest cardiac failure.
Associated symptoms	Is the dyspnea associated with chest pain? Do you have a cough? Is it productive or nonproductive?
	This information helps determine the dyspnea's systemic cause.

Syncope

If a patient presents with a syncopal episode, a cardiovascular event must always be ruled out as a possible cause.

Onset	Is it sudden or gradual?
Associated symptoms	Does the patient experience associated symptoms (e.g., chest pain, palpitations, dyspnea)?
	Syncope with chest pain may be associated with myocardial ischemia or gastrointestinal disorders. Palpitations are indicative of atrial fibrillation or other arrhythmias.
Precipitating factors	What provokes the episode (e.g., sudden changes in position—orthostatic hypotension—or exertion)?

Fatigue

Onset and duration	Is the fatigue transient or persistent?
Quality	Does it interfere with activities of daily living? Does it interfere with job performance? Is bedtime earlier than usual?
Associated symptoms	Is the fatigue associated with angina, dyspnea, or palpitations?
	Is it associated with physical or emotional stress? Fatigue, in conjunction with other symptoms, may be associated with myocardial disease.

Edema

Onset and duration	Is it present in the morning? Does it appear or worsen as the day progresses? How long does it last?
Associated symptoms	Important associated symptoms to assess include dyspnea, diaphoresis, orthopnea, and varicosities.
	Edema with dyspnea and orthopnea may suggest pulmonary congestion indicative of congestive heart failure. Increased hydrostatic pressure due to increased intravenous volume results in edema, causing varicose veins.
	Patients may also complain of "indigestion" or nausea before or during a cardiac event.
	Triscupid and mitral valves open when the ventricles relax, permitting blood to enter the ventricles from the atria.
Alleviating and aggravating factors	What lessens or worsens symptoms (e.g., elevation, compresses, massage therapy, heat)?
	Which medications is the patient taking (including prescription, over-the-counter, herbals, and alternative therapies)?

Leg Cramps and Pain

Onset and duration	What provokes the pain or cramps? Does it occur with activity or at rest? Is there pain with dorsiflexion or plantarflexion of the foot?
	Is the onset of pain acute or chronic?
Quality	Describe the pain/cramping (e.g., burning, aching, or "charley horse").
Associated symptoms	Are there skin changes on the leg, including temperature changes, color changes, loss of hair, redness, and sores?
	These are all indicators of peripheral vascular disease. Atherosclerosis of the peripheral vasculature is a reliable indicator of coronary artery disease (CAD).
	Has the patient had surgery or been immobile recently?
	Immobility and recent surgery increase the risk of deep vein thrombosis. Symptoms of deep vein thrombosis include tenderness and warmth over the deep calf veins, swelling with minimal ankle edema, and unexplained fever.
	Diagnosis of peripheral vascular disease and deep vein thrombosis can be made with Doppler flow studies.

Past Medical History

A detailed exploration of the patient's past medical history assists in divulging prior disease states or lifestyle factors that could increase risk for cardiovascular disorders.

> Mr. S has a 5-year history of left anterior descending (LAD) CAD, which was diagnosed by cardiac catheterization. At that time, a stent was placed to return optimal flow through the artery. In addition, Mr. S was diagnosed with hypertension 20 years ago. He denies a history of diabetes or hypercholesterolemia. There is no history of past surgeries, childhood illnesses, or recent traumas. Mr. S is experiencing extreme fatigue and is unable to engage in daily activities.

Past trauma or surgery	Ask about past traumas and surgeries—specifically, about those related to the cardiovascular system. Has the patient been previously hospitalized for any cardiac disorders?
	Such incidents may relate to the current chief complaint or to the possibility of advancement or complications of existing cardiovascular diseases.

Presence of chronic cardiac disease	Inquire about known CAD or congestive heart failure.
	The presence of diseases such as atherosclerosis, including carotid artery disease and peripheral vascular disease, increases the probability of coexisting CAD and could complicate treatment.
Presence of other chronic diseases	Is there a diagnosis of other chronic diseases?
	Diseases such as hypertension, obesity, diabetes mellitus, and hyperlipidemia significantly increase the risk of developing cardiovascular disorders.
	Thyroid disorders and anemias may have underlying cardiovascular manifestations that would impair cardiac function.
Activity or exercise intolerance	Determine if the patient is easily fatigued.
	Also inquire about exercise and any recent intolerance to the exercise regimen.
	Fatigue could be a symptom of cardiovascular failure or compromise.
	A sedentary lifestyle increases the risk of cardiovascular disorders.
Childhood illnesses	Inquire about known congenital disorders, such as murmurs.
	Ask specifically about rheumatic fever, which can lead to valvular damage.

Family History

Mr. S's parents are deceased. His mother died of lung cancer at the age of 70. His father had a history of hypertension (HTN), CAD, and diabetes mellitus; he died of a myocardial infarction at the age of 65. Mr. S's brother is 65 years old, living, and has a history of CAD.

Age of living relatives	Include relationship and health of immediate relatives.
Deaths	Include relationship, age, and cause of death. Were there any sudden deaths, particularly in young and middle-aged relatives?
Chronic diseases	Is there any history of chronic disease (e.g., CAD, HTN, diabetes)? How long has the family member had the illness? What is his or her relationship to the patient?
Genetic defects	Include any family genetic disorders and congenital birth defects (e.g., congenital heart defects, ventricular septal defect). What is the affected family member's relationship to the patient?

Social History

Mr. S is a retired airplane pilot. His wife is deceased and he lives alone. He has three adult children, who visit him several times during the week. Mr. S walks 1 mile each day but has been unable to do so recently due to his chief complaint. The patient has a history of smoking one pack of cigarettes per day for the past 25 years. He reports consuming about three beers each weekend. He denies recreational drug use.

Family	Ask the patient to describe the current family unit.
Occupation	Inquire about the nature of the patient's work to determine physical exertion and stress. (It is also important to inquire about coping mechanisms.)
Leisure activities	Does the patient have hobbies? Do they allow the patient to relax?

Exercise	Which type (e.g., run, walk, cycle)? How many times per week? How long is the exercise each time?
Tobacco use	Which type (chewing tobacco, pipe, cigarettes, or cigars)? Age when started? Age when stopped (if at all)? How many attempts have been made to quit smoking? How often is the patient around others who smoke? How much (pack-years = numbers of years of smoking × number of packs smoked per day)?
Alcohol use	Which type of alcohol does the patient drink (e.g., liquor, beer)? At what age did the patient start drinking? How much is consumed? How often does the patient drink?
Use of recreational drugs	Does the patient use recreational drugs? How much? How often? Which type of drugs (cocaine, heroin, prescription)?

Review of Systems

Many cardiovascular diseases and disorders have manifestations in systems other than the cardiovascular system. A comprehensive review of systems should be performed whenever possible; however, due to time and other types of constraints, the provider may be able to perform only a focused review of systems. During a focused review of systems, the provider targets questioning at the systems in which cardiovascular problems are most likely to have manifestations. Following is a summary of common manifestations of cardiovascular problems.

System	Symptom or Sign	Possible Associated Diseases/Disorders
General/constitutional	Fatigue, weight loss or gain, disrupted sleep patterns	Coronary artery disease, infective endocarditis, congestive heart failure (CHF), acquired valvular disease. Fatigue may also be associated with anemia or thyroid disorders. The cardiac possibilities become part of the differential diagnosis.
	Fever, chills	Infective endocarditis, pericarditis
Skin	Pigmentation or texture change, hair loss, temparture change, edema	Peripheral vascular disease, deep vein thrombosis
	Clammy skin	Myocardial infarction (MI)
Eyes	Blurred vision, double vision, decreased visual acuity, vertigo, headache (onset, duration, location, precipitating factors)	Hypertension
Respiratory	Cough (productive or nonproductive), pain related to respiration, dyspnea, or orthopnea, auscultated crackles or wheezes	CHF, endocarditis, acquired valvular disease
Gastrointenstinal	Nausea, vomiting, anorexia	CHF, MI
Musculoskeletal	Joint pain	Infective endocarditis

Physical Examination

Equipment Needed

- Marking pencil
- Centimeter ruler or tape measure
- Stethoscope with bell and diaphragm
- Drapes
- Sphygmomanometer with appropriate-size cuff

Components of the Physical Examination

Information obtained from examinations of other systems will have a considerable impact on decisions made about the cardiovascular system. For example, crackles noted on the pulmonary exam and engorgement of the liver or spleen noted during the abdominal examination may help diagnose a patient with right-sided heart failure. A focused review of systems in combination with a thorough physical assessment will aid prompt diagnosis and treatment. Examination of the cardiovascular system includes inspection, palpation, percussion, and auscultation, and measuring blood pressure. Throughout the examination, it is important to provide appropriate draping.

Inspection

Action	Rationale
1. Ensure that the temperature of the room is comfortable and the atmosphere is quiet.	1. A comfortable atmosphere facilitates examination.
2. Ask the patient to remove his or her clothing from the waist up and sit in the upright position.	2. This helps the clinician to visualize abnormalities that would otherwise not be noticed.
3. Provide the patient with a drape; remove the drape as each area of the chest is visualized.	3. Draping allows for modesty.
4. Try to ensure a bright tangential light source is present.	4. The light source allows shadows to emphasize underlying cardiac movement.
5. Inspect the patient's general appearance, including weight in proportion to height.	5. Obesity is a risk factor for cardiac disease.
6. Inspect the face.	
a. Inspect the skin and lips.	a. Each may appear pale, indicating anemia, or cyanotic, indicating decreased oxygen saturation. A bluish discoloration of the lips, skin, and mucous membranes indicates a decreased oxygen saturation of circulating hemoglobin. This is referred to as central cyanosis. It may be due to impaired pulmonary function, right-to-left cardiac shunting, or hypoxia.

b. Examine the eyes.
    • Inspect for color, lesions, and protrusion.
    • Use an ophthalmoscope to perform a fundoscopic exam to visualize changes in retinal blood vessels. (This portion of the exam should be performed with the lights dimmed.)
	b. Xanthelasmas (flat, slightly raised, irregularly shaped yellow lesions on the periorbital tissue) often indicate abnormal lipid metabolism.
	
	    Exophthalmos (protrusion of the eyeballs) may indicate hyperthyroidism; however, it may also indicate increased periorbital edema, suggesting congestive heart failure.
	
	    Arcus senilis is a thin, lightly colored, circumferential ring around the iris. When seen in patients younger than 40 years old, it suggests a lipid disorder, often hyperlipidemia. It is an expected finding in patients older than 60 years of age.
	
	    Retinal blood vessels provide a wealth of information about the severity and extent of hypertensive vascular changes in other vessels within the body.

Action	Rationale
7. Inspect the skin and nail beds.	7. Peripheral cyanosis, often seen in the nail beds or extremities, results from a localized reduction in blood flow due to vascular disease or decreased cardiac output. Clubbing of the nail beds is often the result of chronic hypoxia; however, clubbing is seen with congenital heart defects, especially those with a left-to-right shunt.
8. Note the presence of edema, hair distribution, and temperature changes on bilateral extremities.	8. Although edema may be the result of pathological dysfunctions of any body system, it is an important indicator of cardiac function. As a result of poor left ventricular function, cardiac output is decreased. This results in compromised renal blood flow with subsequent retention of fluid. This increased intravascular volume can precipitate peripheral edema. Abnormal hair distribution accompanied by a change in skin color and temperature may indicate peripheral vascular disease.
9. Inspect the chest wall.	
a. Ask the patient to lie in the supine position. The healthcare provider should move around both sides of the bed to completely visualize the chest wall. A tangential light source may be used to visualize subtle abnormalities of the chest wall.	a. The clinician can visualize abnormalities of the chest wall (e.g., pectus excavatum, pectus carinatum, barrel chest). These are structural deformities and are not indicators of cardiovascular disease.
b. Locate the apical pulse. It should be visualized in most adults just lateral to the left midclavicular line at the fifth intercostal space (ICS). This is often referred to as the *point of maximal impulse* (PMI).	b. The apical impulse is the only normal pulsation visualized on the chest wall; if present, it should be noted for intensity, size, and location. In some cases, the apical impulse is not visible. It may be due to obesity, large breasts, or heavy musculature. In other cases, it may indicate pathological conditions.
10. Evaluate jugular venous pressure. **Figure 10-6** illustrates the location of jugular veins. **Box 10-2** describes the waveforms of jugular venous pressure (JVP). Have the patient lie supine with the head elevated at a 45-degree angle. Adjust the height of the bed until the tangential light illuminates the neck veins above the sternal angle. Use a centimeter ruler to measure the vertical distance between the angle of Louis and the highest level of jugular venous pulsation. Add 5 cm to this measurement because the right atrium is 5 cm below the sternal angle. **Figure 10-7** depicts technique for measuring JVP.	10. Because the jugular veins empty directly into the superior vena cava, they are often a good indicator for activity on the right side of the heart. The level at which the internal jugular vein pulsates is used to estimate right atrial pressure. The normal jugular venous pressure is less than 8 cm H_2O. With a jugular venous pressure greater than 8 cm H_2O, right ventricle and tricuspid valve function should be further evaluated. The ability to obtain accurate measurements may be compromised with a pulse greater than 100.

Action	**Rationale**

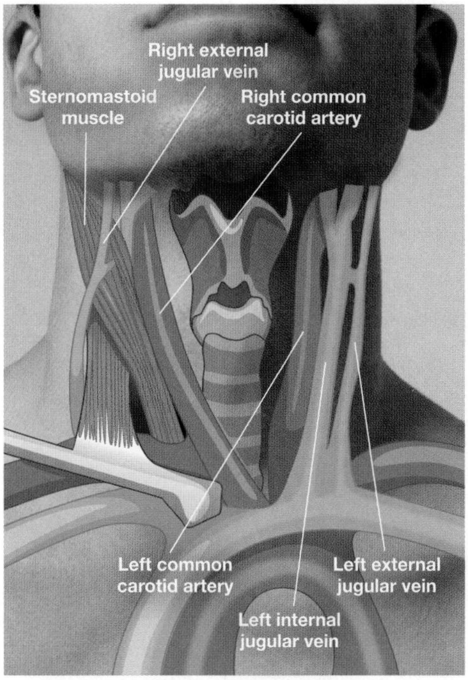

FIGURE 10-6 Jugular veins.

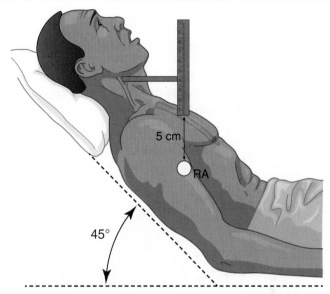

FIGURE 10-7 Measuring jugular venous pressure.

BOX 10-2   WAVEFORMS OF JUGULAR VENOUS PRESSURE

The activity on the right side of the heart is transmitted back through the jugular veins as a visible, not palpable, pulse. Five identified wave components are noted: three positive waveforms accompanied by two descending slopes.

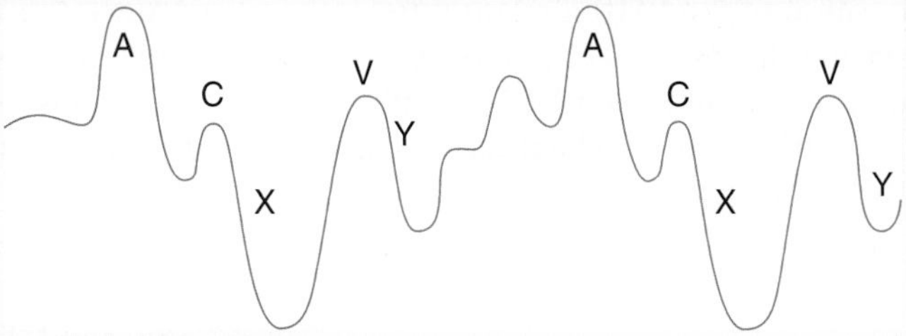

Jugular venous pulse waveform.

A WAVE

The A wave is the first wave visualized on inspection and represents venous pressure at the time of right atrial contraction just prior to the closure of the tricuspid valve. Large A waves may be the result of right atrial contraction against a partially obstructed tricuspid valve orifice, as seen in tricuspid stenosis. They may also be seen with decreased right ventricular compliance, as in cardiomyopathy or cor pulmonale.

C WAVE

The C wave is a transmitted impulse from the vigorous backward push produced by closure of the tricuspid valve during systole.

X DESCENT

The downward X slope is the result of passive atrial filling.

V WAVE

The V wave is the second wave visualized and reflects the increasing volume and pressure in the right atrium as a result of right ventricular contraction against a closed tricuspid valve. Prominent V waves often indicate tricuspid regurgitation or primary right heart failure.

Y DESCENT

The Y descent following the V wave is the result of an open tricuspid valve and rapid ventricular filling.

Palpation

Action	Rationale
1. Have the patient lie supine while you palpate the precordium, the area of the chest wall that covers the heart. The base of the fingers on the palmar side and the lateral aspect of the palm are the most sensitive to pressure and vibrations. Gently place the base of four fingers on the chest and allow the cardiac movements to raise your hand.	1. Palpation allows the clinician to use touch to evaluate for abnormalities, such as dextrocardia, ventricular hypertrophy, heave, lift, or thrill.
2. Palpate the apical pulse (point of maximal impulse; PMI), as in **Figure 10-8**.	

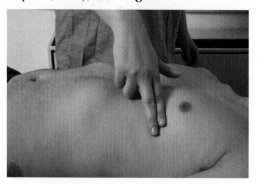

FIGURE 10-8 Palpating the apical pulse.

Action	Rationale
a. Note the location of the PMI in relation to the midclavicular line and sternal border. As previously mentioned, the PMI is usually located lateral to the left midclavicular line at the fifth intercostal space.	a. A deviation of the PMI to the right or left would suggest displacement with underlying disease. Also consider that obesity, large breasts, and heavy musculature may hinder palpation.
b. Note the size.	b. The PMI should be palpated within a 1-cm radius. Anything larger than 1 cm is considered abnormal. For example, lateral displacement combined with an enlarged apical impulse may suggest left ventricular hypertrophy.
c. Note the intensity.	c. The impulse should be gentle and brief. A *heave* or *lift* is more diffuse and vigorous than expected. A lift around the left sternal border may indicate right ventricular hypertrophy. A *thrill* is felt as a palpable vibration and associated with loud murmurs, usually grade IV. It generally indicates disruption of blood flow (related to a defect in one of the semilunar valves). Palpation of a thrill in the aortic area may indicate aortic stenosis or hypertension.
d. Determine the apical pulse rate and regularity.	d. A normal heart should beat rhythmically at a rate of 60 to 100 beats per minute. If the rate increases during inspiration and decreases during expiration, it is referred to as respiratory sinus arrhythmia. This is an expected finding in children.

Action **Rationale**

3. With the patient in the supine position, use the fingertips to palpate the carotid pulse in the lower half of the neck (see **Figure 10-9**). The fingertips are very sensitive to pressure. The carotid pulse must be palpated below the level of the carotid bodies, which, if stimulated, may decrease heart rate.

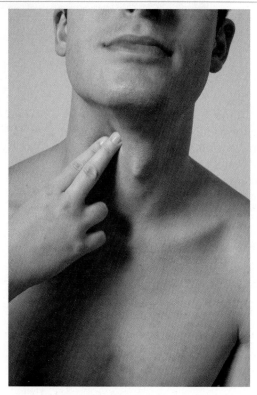

FIGURE 10-9 Palpating the carotid pulse.

a. Palpate each carotid artery with gentle pressure and independently of one another; compare findings. *Never palpate both carotid arteries simultaneously.*

a. Even gentle pressure may cause complete occlusion in the pressure of plaque or arteriosclerosis, compromising cerebral blood flow. Therefore, only one carotid artery at a time should be palpated.

b. While palpating the carotid artery, place the other hand on the precordium. Note that the carotid pulse and S1 are synchronous.

b. Unequal pulsation may suggest carotid obstruction.

4. Maintaining the patient in the supine position, bilaterally palpate the six other major arterial vessels: brachial, radial, ulnar, popliteal, dorsalis pedis, and posterior tibial arteries. Note the pulse for presence, equality, and volume.

4. The extremity pulses are evaluated individually but compared bilaterally. Pulse volume should be symmetrical bilaterally. Pulses are graded on a scale of 0 to 4 based on the amplitude:

+4 Bounding
+3 Full, increased
+2 Expected (faintly palpable, weak and thready)
+0 Absent

An absent pulse may indicate obstruction of distal blood flow. Absence of a peripheral pulse must be confirmed by absence of a Doppler signal. A diminished pulse may indicate poor perfusion peripherally. In the presence of edema, pulses may have diminished amplitude.

Table 10–2	Assessing Pitting Edema		
Scale	Description	Depth of Indentation	Return to Baseline
4+	Severe	8 mm	2–5 minutes
3+	Moderate	6 mm	1–2 minutes
2+	Mild	4 mm	10–15 seconds
1+	Trace	2 mm	Disappears rapidly

Action	Rationale
5. Note the capillary refill time to evaluate the arterial circulation of the extremity. Compress the nail bed to produce blanching. When the pressure is released, there should be a return of blood flow and nail color in less than 3 seconds.	5. If the return of nail color is prolonged, arterial insufficiency is considered.
6. Note pitting edema of the extremities. Pitting edema is the result of an impression on the skin once the finger is removed.	6. As noted earlier, edema may be the result of pathologic dysfunctions of any body system; however, edema is an important indicator of cardiac function. For example, during right-sided heart failure, there is an increased fluid volume, leading to an increase in hydrostatic pressure within the vascular space. This results in edema of the dependent parts of the body. Pitting edema may be the result of heart failure, renal insufficiency, liver failure, or venous insufficiency with venous stasis. Pitting edema is graded on a scale of 1+ to 4+, as described in **Table 10-2**. If bilateral, pitting edema may indicate congestive heart failure. If unilateral, consider major venous occlusion. If edema occurs without pitting, suspect arterial disease and occlusion.
7. Evaluate the extremities for thrombophlebitis.	7. Thrombophlebitis predisposes a patient to pulmonary emboli and chronic venous insufficiency. With deep vein thrombosis (DVT), pressing the calves against the tibia may elicit pain, tenderness, and increased firmness in the muscle. Notice any heat, unexplained fever, or tachycardia.

Percussion

Percussion is a less reliable assessment tool than inspection and palpation when locating the PMI. Information obtained about hypertrophy of the right or left ventricle would best be determined by other methods of assessment. A chest x-ray will provide the examiner with a detailed picture of the heart borders as well as information on the pulmonary and skeletal system.

Action	Rationale
1. Percuss the borders of the heart. Begin tapping at the anterior axillary line, moving medially, along the intercostal space towards the sternum. On the left, the loss of resonance to dullness will be heard near the PMI at the apex of the heart. Remember, the PMI is usually located just lateral to the left midclavicular line at the fifth intercostal space.	1. An unexpected change from resonance to dullness may indicate ventricular hypertrophy due to obesity, pregnancy, heavy musculature, or pathological conditions.

Auscultation

Action	Rationale
1. Make sure the patient is warm and as relaxed as possible prior to auscultation. As with inspection, ensure a quiet environment.	1. Comfort is important. In addition, chills, shaking, and background noise make it difficult to hear low-frequency heart sounds.
2. Have the patient sit upright leaning slightly forward, disrobed above the waist (**Figure 10-10**). Place a warm stethoscope directly on the skin and auscultate all five auscultatory areas first with the diaphragm, and then with the bell.	2. The diaphragm is better at transmitting high-pitched murmurs, whereas the bell transmits lower pitched filling sounds more effectively.

Figure 10-11 illustrates the five traditional auscultatory areas: aortic valve, pulmonic valve, second pulmonic, tricuspid, and mitral or apical areas.

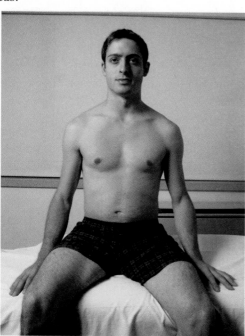

FIGURE 10-10 Initial position for auscultation.

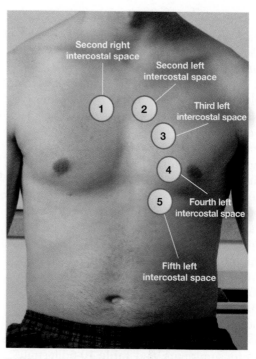

FIGURE 10-11 Five traditional auscultatory areas. 1. Aortic valve area. 2. Pulmonic valve area. 3. Second pulmonic valve area. 4. Tricuspid area. 5. Mitral area (PMI).

3. If the patient's condition allows, also perform auscultation in supine and left lateral recumbent positions, illustrated in **Figure 10-12**. Patients with dextrocardia should be examined in the right lateral recumbent position due to the right rotation of the heart.	3. Changing the patient's position allows the examiner to hear various sounds. For example, high-pitched murmurs are more easily heard in the upright position. Low-pitched diastolic filling sounds are more commonly heard in the left lateral recumbent position.

Action   **Rationale**

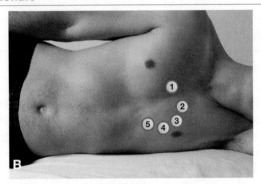

FIGURE 10-12 Additional positions for auscultation with traditional auscultation sites. A. Supine position. B. Left lateral recumbent position.

Patients with dextrocardia should be examined in the right lateral recumbent position due to the right rotation of the heart.

4. It is important to remember to move slowly and methodically as you examine the auscultatory areas rather than moving quickly from one area to the next.

   a. Isolate each component of the cardiac cycle at all sites but do not limit yourself to the five auscultatory areas. Allow your stethoscope to follow the heart sounds. Take the time to notice subtle differences in intensity, pitch, location, radiation, duration, and timing.

   b. Identify heart sounds. **Box 10-3** describes heart sounds. Extra heart sounds are categorized by their location in the cardiac cycle. **Table 10-3** describes extracardiac sounds. Assess for murmurs, which are classified according to their timing, intensity, pattern, location, and radiation. (**Table 10-4** describes various murmurs, and **Table 10-5** illustrates classification.)

4. By moving too quickly, you may miss abnormalities.

   a. These distinctions provide important clinical clues to potential abnormalities, such as murmurs or valvular dysfunction.

   b. The presence of extra heart sounds is suggestive of cardiac abnormalities and warrants further investigation.

   Murmurs are audible sounds caused by vibrations from turbulent blood flow through the heart and great vessels. They are attributed to high flow rates through normal or abnormal valves, forward motion of blood through constricted valves or a dilated chamber, and regurgitation from incompetent valves, septal defects, or patent ductus arteriosus. Significant murmurs are most commonly caused by anatomic disorders of the valves. Many murmurs are benign, particularly in young children, adolescents, and young athletes. They are caused by vigorous systolic blood flow from large heart chambers to smaller blood vessels. Diastolic murmurs are always significant and are indicative of underlying cardiac disease.

BOX 10-3   HEART SOUNDS

The four basic heart sounds are S_1, S_2, S_3, and S_4. S_1 marks the onset of systole, whereas S_2 signals the beginning of diastole. S_1 and S_2 are the distinct "lub-dub" sounds and should be isolated individually during auscultation, because variations can offer significant diagnostic clues. S_3 and S_4 are sometimes classified as extracardiac sounds, but their presence is not necessarily indicative of a pathologic condition. S_3 and S_4 must be assessed in relation to patient history and other sounds and events in the cardiac cycle.

S_1

S_1 is the first heart sound. It results from closure of the mitral and tricuspid valves. The intensity is loudest over the mitral area or apex, and it is best heard with the diaphragm of the stethoscope. Conditions that increase intensity include increased blood viscosity and stenosis of the mitral valve. Intensity is decreased by deposits of fat (from obesity) or fluid (from pericardial fluid accumulation), systemic or pulmonary hypertension, and fibrosis or calcification of the mitral valve. The last condition can result from rheumatic fever. Although S_1 is usually heard as one sound, splitting is possible from asynchronous contraction of the left and right ventricles. Splitting of S_1 is best heard in the tricuspid area.

S_2

S_2 is the second heart sound. It results from closure of the aortic and pulmonic valves. S_2 is heard best over the base of the heart at the aortic area with the diaphragm of the stethoscope. Because right ventricular systolic ejection time is longer than left ventricular systolic ejection time, the pulmonic valve closes slightly later than the aortic valve. This asynchrony of valve closure, referred to as physiologic splitting, is an expected finding. It is best heard at the peak of inspiration over the pulmonic area.

Abnormal splitting of S_2 can also occur. If there is delayed emptying of the right ventricle, the split will widen from a delay in pulmonic valve closure. This condition occurs with right bundle branch block, but can also occur from stenosis of the pulmonic valve. Paradoxic splitting occurs from left bundle branch block, which results from delayed closure of the aortic valve. This is also called a reverse split and occurs during expiration. Fixed splitting is not affected by respiration and is characteristic of an atrial septal defect. Conditions that increase intensity of S_2 include systemic and pulmonary hypertension, exercise, mitral stenosis, and congestive heart failure. Decreasing intensity of S_2 is associated with shocklike states with arterial hypotension, aortic or pulmonic stenosis, and deposits of fat or fluid overlying the heart.

S_3

S_3 is an early diastolic sound that results from passive flow of blood from the atria. This sound is low pitched and is best heard with the bell of the stethoscope with the patient in the left lateral recumbent position. Increasing venous return by asking the patient to raise his or her legs may make the sound easier to hear. The rhythm of the cardiac cycle with an audible S_3 resembles that of "Ken-tuc-ky." S_3 is also referred to as ventricular gallop or a protosystolic gallop.

Although this sound is normal in children and young adults, it is an indicator of systolic dysfunction after age 40, representing abnormal early filling of the ventricles. S_3 will increase in intensity if filling pressure is increased or if the ventricles are noncompliant. S_3 closely follows S_2 and, therefore, makes it difficult to differentiate an S_3 from a physiologic S_2. It is important to remember that S_3 is a single sound unaffected by the respiratory cycle best heard at the apex, whereas S_2 varies with respiration and is best heard over the pulmonic area.

S_4

S_4 is a late diastolic sound immediately preceding S_1; it is best heard with the bell at the apex or mitral area with the patient in the left lateral recumbent position. The rhythm of the cardiac cycle with an audible S_4 resembles that of "Tenn-es-see." S_4 is also referred to as an atrial gallop or a presystolic gallop.

An S_4 sound is characteristic of diastolic dysfunction, representing a noncompliant ventricle that resists expansion. Associated conditions include hypertension, coronary artery disease, high-output states such as pregnancy, recent myocardial infarction, and aortic stenosis. S_4 requires atrial contraction against a noncompliant ventricle to produce sound; therefore, it is not audible in atrial fibrillation or any rhythm with atrioventricular (AV) dissociation.

Table 10-3   Extracardiac Sounds

Sound	Location/Characteristics	Associated Conditions
Systolic Ejection Clicks		
Mitral ejection click	■ Best heard at the apex ■ Most common ejection sound	Mitral valve prolapse; mitral regurgitation (if the click is accompanied by a soft blowing murmur)
Aortic ejection click	■ Heard at both the base and the apex (but is usually louder at the apex) ■ Does not change with respiration	Ascending aortic aneurysm; coarctation of the aorta; hypertension with aortic dilation, aortic stenosis; obstruction of the aorta
Pulmonary ejection click	■ Heard at the base in the pulmonic area ■ Changes markedly with respiration ■ Decreases in intensity with inspiration (and may disappear) ■ Increases in intensity during expiration	Pulmonic stenosis; pulmonary hypertension; idiopathic dilatation of the pulmonary artery; hyperthyroidism
Diastolic Sounds		
Opening snap of the mitral valve	■ Best heard just inside the apex ■ Radiates toward the base ■ Sharper and higher pitched than ventricular filling sounds	Mitral stenosis (found in more than 90% of the cases)
Opening snap of the tricuspid valve	■ Difficult to differentiate from the louder opening snap of the mitral valve ■ Often submerged by the mitral snap	Occasionally heard with atrial septal defects, but otherwise has limited diagnostic value
Other Sounds		
Pericardial friction rub	■ Best heard over the left sternal border in the upright position with the patient leaning slightly forward ■ High pitched, scratchy ■ Not eliminated by breath holding (unlike the pleural friction rub)	Uremic pericarditis with underlying hypertension and air in the mediastinum; myocardial infarction (however, it is evident the first week and lasts only a few hours)
Mediastinal crunch	■ Random crunching or grating sounds, indirectly related to the cardiac and respiratory cycle ■ Also referred to as Hamman's sign	Cardiac surgery may cause it to occur

Table 10-4   Types of Murmurs

Type	Timing in Cardiac Cycle	Location/Radiation/Comments
Systolic Murmurs		
Mitral regurgitation	Holosystolic	■ Best heard at the apex to left sternal border ■ Radiates to the midaxilla and occasionally to the left lower thorax ■ Not affected by respiration
Tricuspid regurgitation	Holosystolic	■ Best heard at the parasternal border at the level of the third and fifth intercostal space (ICS) ■ Intensifies with respiration
Ventricular septal defect	Holosystolic	■ Best heard at the left sternal border at the level of the third to fifth ICS ■ May radiate to the parasternal border
Aortic stenosis	Midsystolic	■ Classically best heard at the second ICS, but occasionally audible at the lower sternal border in the third and fourth ICS and the apex ■ Radiates to the carotid arteries
Pulmonary stenosis	Midsystolic	■ Best heard at the second left ICS ■ May radiate to the carotid arteries, with the left side greater than the right
Diastolic Murmurs		
Mitral stenosis	Early diastole	■ Best heard at the mitral area ■ Usually does not radiate
Tricuspid regurgitation	Diastolic	■ Best heard at the tricuspid area or epigastrium ■ Little radiation
Aortic regurgitation	Present through the first third of diastole	■ Best heard at the aortic area of the base of the heart ■ Unchanged by respiration
Pulmonic regurgitation	Diastolic	■ Best heard at the pulmonic area ■ No radiation

Table 10-5 Classification of Murmurs	
Characteristic	Description
Timing	Early, mid, late, holosystolic, diastolic, or continuous
Intensity	Grade I—Very faint; barely audible in a quiet room Grade II—Soft but audible in a quiet room Grade III—Moderately loud without accompanying thrill Grade IV—Loud and easily heard, associated with a thrill Grade V—Very loud, with an easily palpable thrill Grade VI—Very loud, with a visible and palpable thrill; can be heard with the stethoscope fully off of the chest
Pattern	Crescendo, decrescendo, or crescendo/decrescendo (also referred to as diamond shaped)
Location	Described in relation to anatomic landmarks in the area of greatest intensity; for example, it may be described as best heard in the aortic, mitral, pulmonic, or tricuspid areas
Radiation	Described in terms of where else the murmur is heard (the site farthest from the greatest intensity at which sound can still be heard)

Diagnostic Reasoning

Based on findings in the health history and physical examination, the clinician should formulate his assessment and plan. For example, a patient may report symptoms that suggest many possible diagnoses; however, findings in the past medical history and during the physical examination narrow the possible diagnoses down to one or two. Chest pain is a common chief complaint (CC). **Table 10-6** illustrates differential diagnosis of some common disorders associated with chest pain.

Box 10-4 describes common diagnostic tests for problems related to the cardiovascular system.

Table 10-6 Differential Diagnosis of Chest Pain			
Differential Diagnoses	Significant Findings in the Patient's History	Significant Findings in the Patient's Physical Examination	Diagnostic Tests
Myocardial infarction	Sudden onset of angina; intense heaviness, crushing or squeezing chest pain that radiates to the arm, shoulder, or neck; nausea; fatigue; exercise intolerance	Diaphoresis; dyspnea; anxiety; bradycardia or tachycardia; palpitations	12-lead ECG, echocardiogram, cardiac catheterization, cardiac isoenzymes (CK-MB), troponin I
Aortic dissection	Sudden onset of tearing chest pain that radiates to the shoulders or back; history of hypertension	Hypertension; aortic diastolic murmur	Echocardiogram; CT scan
Pericarditis	Variable onset of sharp pain that radiates to the arm, shoulder, back, or neck; pain worsens with coughing; fever	Tachycardia; pericardial friction rub	ECG; WBC; chest x-ray

Note: CT, computed tomography; ECG, electrocardiogram; WBC, white blood cell count.

BOX 10-4   DIAGNOSTIC TESTS

Many tests may be ordered to confirm a diagnosis of chest pain of cardiovascular origin. The following tests may provide useful diagnostic information:

ELECTROCARDIOGRAM (ECG)
A 12-lead ECG provides a three-dimensional picture of the electrical activity within the heart. It can provide a wealth of information about the cardiac status and serve as a basis for which other diagnostic tests may be ordered.

ECHOCARDIOGRAM (EKG)
An echocardiogram (also called an echo) is a type of ultrasound test that uses high-pitched sound waves sent through a device called a transducer. The device picks up echoes of the sound waves as they bounce off different parts of the heart. These echoes are turned into moving pictures of the heart that can be seen on a video screen. Look for the cause of abnormal heart sounds (murmurs or clicks), an enlarged heart, unexplained chest pains, shortness of breath, or irregular heartbeats.

(continues)

BOX 10-4   DIAGNOSTIC TESTS (*continued*)

The echocardiogram serves the following functions:
- Checks the thickness and movement of the heart wall.
- Looks at the heart valves and checks how well they work.
- Determines how well an artificial heart valve is working.
- Measures the size and shape of the heart's chambers.
- Checks the ability of the heart chambers to pump blood (cardiac performance). During an echocardiogram, the clinician can calculate how much blood the heart is pumping during each heartbeat (ejection fraction).

ULTRASOUND OF ABDOMEN
The ultrasound of the abdomen is considered the appropriate diagnostic tool in older adults with strong history or presenting symptoms of aneurysm.

CHEST X-RAY
Chest x-rays are a noninvasive and cost-effective method of visualizing cardiac anatomy. The heart and the great vessels are moderately dense and, therefore, should appear as gray areas on the film. They may also help rule out possibility of pulmonary pathology.

HEMATOLOGIC STUDIES
Hematologic studies (ABG, CBC, chemistry panel, lipid panel, coagulation studies, CK-MB, and troponin I) analyze the amount of various components and characteristics of the blood (carbon dioxide, oxygen, red blood cells, electrolytes, serum lipid levels, and serum clotting times). CK-MB isoenzyme provides information about damaged myocardial tissue. Troponin I levels, however, are better diagnostic markers for the diagnosis of myocardial infarction.

CARDIAC CATHETERIZATION
Depending on the results of diagnostic tests, the patient may need emergent invasive procedures or surgery to prevent further myocardial damage. Cardiac catheterization is an invasive hemodynamic procedure that can provide in-depth information about coronary artery blood flow. It also allows the use of balloons and stents to return optimal blood flow through the arteries.

Cardiovascular Assessment of Special Populations

Considerations for the Pregnant Patient

Remember that pregnancy is associated with significant changes in the cardiovascular system:
- Maternal blood volume increases approximately 1600 mL with a single gestation and 2000 mL with a multiple gestation.
- The increase in blood volume begins during the first trimester and plateaus at approximately 30 weeks.
- By term of a single pregnancy, blood volume increases by approximately 50% above prepregnant volume.
- Blood volume returns to prepregnancy levels 3 to 4 weeks after delivery.
- Maternal heart rate increases as early as 7 weeks of gestation.
- By term, the heart rate increases approximately 20% above prepregnant rate. This increase is compensatory to accommodate for the increase in blood volume.
- Maternal cardiac output is increased at approximately 10 weeks' gestation and peaks at 50% over prepregnant levels by 25 to 32 weeks' gestation.
- Maternal blood pressure slightly decreases during the first trimester, reaches its lowest point during the second trimester, and approaches prepregnant levels during the last 2 months of pregnancy.
- Techniques for inspection, palpation, percussion, and auscultation are consistent with the nonpregnant patient. However, when the patient is in the supine position, aortocaval syndrome may be present, necessitating left uterine displacement.
- Aortocaval syndrome can occur as early as 13 to 16 weeks' gestation due to compression of the great vessels from the weight of the fetus.

■ Percussion of the apex of the heart may reveal a left lateral displacement. This is an expected finding in the pregnant patient.

Considerations for the Neonatal Patient
General Considerations
■ Note that the examination of the cardiac status of the newborn can be challenging due to immediate changes from fetal to pulmonic circulation.
■ Examine the heart within the first 24 hours of life and again when the neonate is 2 to 3 days old.
■ Measure blood pressure (a routine measurement on all newborns); assess in all four extremities if a cardiac anomaly is suspected. Blood pressure that is markedly higher in the arms than in the legs is indicative of coarctation of the aorta.
■ Perform a thorough cardiac examination, including assessment of skin, lungs, and liver.

Inspection
Inspect the skin carefully. Skin and mucous membranes should be pink. Cyanosis at birth may be indicative of transposition of the great vessels, tetralogy of Fallot, severe septal defects, or pulmonic stenosis. Acrocyanosis (cyanosis of the hands and feet) is an expected finding and will usually diminish several hours after birth.

Palpation
■ Count apical pulse for 1 full minute.
■ Know variations in anatomy. The heart lies more horizontally in the chest with the apex to the left of the nipple line; as a consequence, the apical impulse may be higher and more medially located between the fourth and fifth intercostal spaces. Displacement of the apical impulse may indicate pneumothorax (shifts the apical impulse to the opposite side of the pneumothorax), dextrocardia (apical impulse displaced to the right), or a diaphragmatic hernia. Because diaphragmatic hernias are more common on the left, the apical impulse will usually be displaced to the right.
■ Note that pulse rate is variable and influenced by physical activity, crying, and wakefulness.
■ Palpate the liver. An enlarged, firm liver indicates right-sided heart failure and unlike adults, this will precede pulmonary congestion.

Auscultation
■ Note heart tones. The vitality of heart tones is a key measure of cardiac function in the infant. Diminished vitality may be the only apparent clue that an infant is in heart failure.
■ Know variations. Splitting of S_2 is common in neonates, occurring a few hours after birth.
■ Assess for tachycardia. Tachycardia that is comparatively fixed is indicative of underlying cardiac concerns.
■ Sinus tachycardia is common in response to stressors such as anxiety, pain, fever, hypoxia, hypercapnia, or hypovolemia.
■ Unlike in adults, cardiac output in neonates is more dependent on heart rate than on stroke volume. Tachycardia is a typical physiologic response to a decrease in cardiac output.
■ Carefully auscultate for murmurs. Ninety percent are transient and caused by transition from fetal to pulmonic circulation. These murmurs are commonly grade I or II in intensity and are not associated with other signs and symptoms. Significant murmurs indicate patent ductus arteriosus, pulmonic or aortic stenosis, or small septal defects.

Considerations for Pediatric Patients
Include a comprehensive evaluation of pulses, blood pressure, respiratory function, and general physical growth and development. (See **Table 10-7** for normal blood pressures for children.)

Table 10-7	Normal Blood Pressures in Children	
Age	Systolic (mmHg)	Diastolic (mmHg)
Birth (12 hours, < 1000 g)	39–59	16–36
Birth (12 hours, 3 kg)	50–70	25–45
Newborn (96 hours)	60–90	20–60
6 months	87–105	53–66
2 years	95–105	53–66
7 years	97–112	57–71
15 years	112–128	66–80

Table 10-8	Normal Heart Rates in Children	
Age	Awake Rate*	Sleeping Rate*
Newborn to 3 months	85–205	80–160
3 months to 2 years	100–190	75–160
2 years to 10 years	60–140	60–90
> 10 years	60–100	50–90

*Rate described in beats per minute.

Inspection

Upon examination of a child with known heart disease, observe carefully for developmental delays, clubbing, and cyanosis.

Palpation

Note location of the apical pulse. By age 8, the apical pulse is felt at the fifth intercostal space at the midclavicular line.

Auscultation

Note variations in normal findings for pediatric patients:

- Sinus arrhythmia, a heart rate that is faster on inspiration and slower on expiration, is an expected finding in children.
- S_3 is a normal finding in children and young adults and is best heard with the bell at the apex or mitral area.
- Children's heart rates vary more than adults, with greater fluctuation to any stressors by as much as 10 to 20 beats per minute. (See **Table 10-8** for normal heart rates in children.)

Considerations for Geriatric Patients

- Know that advancing age is accompanied by physiologic changes in the cardiovascular system.
- Follow the same examination procedure as for younger adults; make some age-related modifications for assessing cardiovascular function in the older patient.
- Remember to slow down the pace of the examination for the older patient. Some patients may become short of breath while changing positions or even unable to assume certain positions due to a lack of comfort.
- Evaluate and record blood pressure in both the right and left arms, if possible. If there is a large difference between the two obtained measurements, the higher blood pressure should be considered the most reliable. Systolic pressure rises with increasing age due to a loss of elasticity of the vessels. Diastolic pressure is less affected by age and either remains the same or decreases.
- Assess for hypertension. Hypertension in the older population is defined as a systolic pressure greater than 140 mmHg and diastolic pressure greater than 90 mmHg.
- Assess for abdominal aneurysm through inspection, palpation, and auscultation of the abdominal aortic, renal, and iliac arteries. Abdominal aortic aneurysm (AAA) is a relatively common and often fatal condition that primarily affects older patients. Aortic aneurysms

were the primary cause of 9863 deaths in 2014 and a contributing cause in more than 17,215 deaths in the United States in 2009 (Centers for Disease Contol & Prevention, 2016). About two-thirds of people who have an aortic dissection are male. The U.S. Preventive Services Task Force recommends that men between the ages 65 and 75 years who have ever smoked should get an ultrasound screening for abdominal aortic aneurysms, even if they have no symptoms. With an aging population, the incidence and prevalence of AAA, as well as that of femoral, iliac, and popliteal aneurysms, are certain to rise. It is important to understand which patients are at risk for the development of AAA and how to appropriately evaluate a patient who has been diagnosed with an aneurysm. The common iliac arteries may be aneurysmal and palpable in the lower abdominal quadrants. Patients should be examined for the presence of femoral and popliteal pulses and possible aneurysmal dilatation. The presence of a prominent popliteal or femoral artery pulse warrants an abdominal ultrasound to rule out an AAA and a lower extremity arterial ultrasound to rule out peripheral artery aneurysm.

Inspection

Note age-related changes during inspection:

- On inspection of the aging thorax, a greater anterior–posterior diameter with possible kyphosis may be noted. (This may make palpation of the PMI more difficult.)
- Multiple superficial vessels in the neck, forehead, and extremities will appear more prominent and tortuous.
- Inspection of the abdomen for pulsations should be a part of the cardiovascular assessment of older adults.

Palpation

Peripheral pulses may be difficult to palpate in the older patient. Good perfusion of the peripheral extremities can be noted by capillary refill, pain, sensation of touch, and temperature.

During palpation of the abdomen, press down deeply in the midline above the umbilicus. The aortic pulsation is easily felt on most individuals. A well-defined, pulsatile mass, greater than 3 cm across, suggests an aortic aneurysm. The common iliac arteries also may be aneurysmal and palpable in the lower abdominal quadrants. Patients should be examined for the presence of femoral and popliteal pulses and possible aneurysmal dilatation. The presence of a prominent popliteal or femoral artery pulse warrants an abdominal ultrasound to rule out an AAA and a lower extremity arterial ultrasound to rule out peripheral artery aneurysm.

Auscultation

Know age-related changes to normal findings:

- The endocardium thickens. The valves of the heart become sclerotic and compromised by fibrosis, contributing to audible murmurs.
- The myocardium increases in collagen formation, contributing to the stiffness of the aging heart. This leads to a decrease in myocardial compliance, evidenced by decreasing stroke volume and cardiac output.
- Resting heart rate decreases with age, due to an increase in the vagal tone of the heart.
- Advancing age produces changes in the ECG. Ectopic beats may or may not be normal; further investigation of an arrhythmia is necessary.
- S_4 is more commonly auscultated while completing a cardiovascular assessment on an older patient. This is due to the increased rigidity of the ventricular wall and may be associated with hypertrophy or ischemia.
- The likelihood of aneurysm increases with age. Auscultation of aortic, renal, iliac, and femoral arteries for bruits and thrills should be performed.

Case Study Review

Throughout this chapter, you have been introduced to Mr. S. This section of the chapter pulls together his history and demonstrates documentation of his history and physical examination.

Chief Complaint

"I have a stabbing pain in my chest that will not go away."

Information Gathered During the Interview

Mr. S is a 69-year-old Caucasian male who presents with a 5-year history of coronary artery disease (CAD) with exertional angina. His angina is usually relieved once the activity ceases, but occasionally sublingual nitroglycerin is required to relieve his chest pain. These traditional methods have proved ineffective for the past day. On a scale of 1 to 10, his pain has increased in intensity from 3 to 6. The pain is substernal with radiation down his left arm. It is associated with diaphoresis and nausea. The patient is not currently experiencing any dyspnea, orthopnea, syncope, palpitations, or cough.

Mr. S has a 5-year history of left anterior descending (LAD) CAD, which was diagnosed by cardiac catheterization. At that time, a stent was placed to return optimal flow through the artery. In addition, Mr. S was diagnosed with hypertension 20 years ago. He denies a history of diabetes or hypercholesterolemia. There is no history of past surgeries, childhood illnesses, or recent traumas. The patient is experiencing extreme fatigue and is unable to engage in daily activities.

Mr. S's parents are deceased. His mother died of lung cancer at the age of 70. His father had a history of hypertension, CAD, and diabetes mellitus; he died of myocardial infarction at the age of 65. His brother is 65 years old, living, and has a history of CAD. Mr. S is a retired airplane pilot. His wife is deceased and he lives alone. He has three adult children, who visit him several times during the week. He walks 1 mile each day but has been unable to do so recently due to his chief complaint. Mr. S has a history of smoking one pack of cigarettes per day for the past 25 years. He reports consuming about three beers each weekend. He denies recreational drug use.

Clues	Important Points
5-year history of CAD	There is probable progression of the disease process.
1-day history of chief complaint	Chest pain is unrelieved by the patient's traditional therapy; warrants emergency diagnostic tests and treatment.
Quality of the chest pain	The intensity of the pain has doubled from 3 to 6.
Traditional therapy is now ineffective	Given the patient's history, chest pain unrelieved by traditional methods is highly suggestive of angina that has become unstable.
Substernal pain	This is a classic location for angina.
Radiation of chest pain	Angina may radiate to the extremities, neck, or jaw. This supports a diagnosis of unstable angina with possible myocardial infarction (MI).
Diaphoresis	Diaphoresis is commonly associated with angina and supports symptoms associated with an MI.
Nausea	Nausea is commonly associated with angina and supports symptoms associated with an MI.

Name KS	Date 1/13/15	Time 1400
	DOB 12/17/45	Sex M

HISTORY

CC

"I have a stabbing pain in my chest that will not go away."

HPI

5-year history of CAD, with exertional angina. Angina is usually relieved once the activity ceases, but occasionally sublingual nitroglycerin is required to relieve his chest pain. These traditional methods have proved ineffective for the past day. On a scale of 1 to 10, pain has increased from 3 to 6. Pain is substernal with radiation down his left arm and associated with diaphoresis and nausea. No dyspnea, orthopnea, syncope, palpitations, or cough.

Medications

ASA: 81 mg daily to prevent clot formation; last dose this AM.

Nitroglycerin sublingual: used this AM × 3 with no relief.

Metoprolol: 25 mg BID for hypertension; last dose this AM.

Multivitamin: 1 tablet QAM for vitamin supplementation; last dose this AM.

Nicotine patch: 21 mg QAM to help quit smoking; changed patch this AM.

*For acute exacerbations of chest pain in the primary care office the following, if available, may be administered while awaiting ambulance transport:

Oxygen 2 L per nasal canula

2 tablets ASA 325 mg

Nitroglycerin sublinqual, repeat every 5 minutes to a maximum of 3 tablets.

Allergies

NKA

PMI
Illnesses

5-year history of LAD CAD diagnosed by cardiac catheterization. Stent placed at time of dx. Positive history of HTN (diagnosed 20 years ago). Negative history of diabetes or hypercholesterolemia. No childhood illnesses.

Hospitalizations/Surgeries

Negative history of past surgeries or trauma.

FH

Parents are deceased. Positive history of lung cancer (mother) and hypertension, CAD, and diabetes mellitus (father). His brother is 65 years old, living, and has a history of CAD.

SH

Retired airplane pilot. Wife is deceased and he lives alone. Has 3 adult children who visit often. Walks 1 mile each day, but his CC prevented him recently. History of smoking 1 pack of cigarettes per day for the past 25 yrs. Reports consuming about 3 beers each weekend. Denies recreational drug use.

ROS

General	Cardiovascular
Fatigue, inability to perform ADL.	Chest pain (see HPI); denies syncope, palpations.
Skin	Respiratory
Clammy, pale.	Quit smoking 2 weeks ago; denies cough, dyspnea, and orthopnea.
Eyes	Gastrointestinal
Farsighted, wears glasses.	Nausea.
Ears	Genitourinary/Gynecological
Some hearing loss; no recent change.	Denies difficulty urinating.
Nose/Mouth/Throat	Musculoskeletal
Denies changes.	Denies changes.
Breast	Neurological
Denies changes.	Denies changes.

PHYSICAL EXAMINATION

Weight 242 lb	Temp 98.7	BP 145/92
Height 5'10"	Pulse 63	Resp 20

General Appearance

Overweight, Caucasian male lying in bed complaining of chest discomfort. Appears mildly anxious.

Skin

Normal turgor, slightly pale and clammy.

HEENT

Pupils, equal and reactive to light; ears and nose are clear and free of discharge.

Cardiovascular

S_1 and S_2 audible and regular. No evidence of splitting, murmurs, or extracardiac sounds appreciated. Lower extremity pulses 1 + bilaterally; upper extremity pulses 2 + bilaterally. No carotid bruits noted.

Respiratory
Lungs clear to auscultation bilaterally.

Gastrointestinal
Bowel sounds present in 4 quadrants. Abdomen is large but soft and nontender to palpation.

Genitourinary
Not examined.

Musculoskeletal
Strength 3–4/5 throughout and symmetrical.

Neurological
Alert and oriented × 3, CN II–XII intact, DTRs 2+, Babinski (−).

Other

Lab Tests
ABG—PH: 7.38; PO_2: 71; PCO_2: 37; HCO_3: 23
CBC—Hct: 40%; Hgb: 13.7 g/dL; RBC: 5 mm³; WBC: 7.2 × 10³/mm³; P1t: 225,000/mm³
Chem—Na: 141 mEq/mL; K: 4.8 mEq/mL; Ca: 8.6 mEq/mL; Cl: 100 mEq/mL
Mg: 1.7 mEq/mL; Phos: 3.8 mg/dL; BUN: 8 mg/dL; Cr: 0.8 mg/dL; Glu: 118 mg/dL
Lipid—Total: 222 mg/dL; Trigly: 400 mg/dL; LDL: 145 mg/dL; HDL: 22 mg/dL
Coagulation studies—PT: 11.5 sec; INR: 1.1; PTT: 65 sec
CK-MB: > 5%
Troponin I: Elevated

Special Tests
ECG: 12-lead ECG shows ST-segment elevation in leads V1–V4 and T-wave inversion in leads I and aVL.
Chest x-ray: Lungs are clear with mild fibrotic changes associated with aging. Heart is slightly enlarged.

Final Assessment Findings
1. Elevated lipid panel indicating hypercholesterolemia.
2. Elevated cardiac enzymes and troponin I, indicating myocardial infarction.
3. ECG suggest anterior wall MI.
4. Referred for emergent cardiac catheterization.

Bibliography

Centers for Disease Control & Prevention. (2016). Aortic aneurysm fact sheet. Retrieved from http://www.cdc.gov/dhdsp/data_statistics/fact_sheets/fs_aortic_aneurysm.htm.

Frich, J., Malterud, K., & Fugelli, P. (2006). Women at risk of coronary heart disease experience barriers to diagnosis and treatment: A qualitative interview study. *Scandinavian Journal of Primary Health Care, 24,* 38–43.

Khan, N. A., Rahim, S. A., Anand, S. S., Simel, D. L., & Panju, A. (2006). Does the clinical examination predict lower extremity peripheral arterial disease? *Journal of the American Medical Association, 295*(5), 536–546.

Klabunde, R. E. (2011). *Cardiovascular physiology concepts.* Philadelphia, PA: Lippincott Williams & Wilkins.

Mangione, S., Nieman, L. Z., Gracely, E., & Kaye, D. (1993). The teaching and practice of cardiac auscultation during internal medicine and cardiology training: Nationwide survey. *Annals of Internal Medicine, 119,* 47–54.

Meininger, J. C. (1997). Primary prevention of cardiovascular disease risk factors: Review and implications for population-based practice. *Advanced Practice Nurse Quarterly, 3*(2), 70–79.

Perloff, J. K. (2010). *Physical examination of the heart and circulation* (4th ed.). Philadelphia, PA: WB Saunders.

Upchurch, G. R., Jr., & Schaub, T. A. (2006). Abdominal aortic aneurysm. *American Family Physician, 73*(7), 1998–1204. http://www.aafp.org/afp/2006/0401/p1198.html.

Wells, P. S., Owen, C., Doucette, S., Fergusson, D., & Tran, H. (2006). Does this patient have deep vein thrombosis? *Journal of the American Medical Association, 295*(2), 199–207.

Chapter 11

Gastrointestinal Disorders

Anatomy and Physiology Review of the Gastrointestinal System

The gastrointestinal system is the largest endocrine organ in the body, secreting numerous hormones that control secretions, mobility, and blood flow in the digestive tract. It secretes hormones and enzymes responsible for the following functions:

- Digestion of proteins
- Digestion of carbohydrates
- Digestion of fats
- Breakdown of hepatic glycogen to glucose
- Breakdown of adipose tissue to triglyceride
- Breakdown of gluconeogenesis from amino acids
- Production of insulin, which stimulates glucose use by tissues

Gastrointestinal Tract

The gastrointestinal tract consists of the mouth, oropharynx, esophagus, and the organs of the abdominal cavity (**Figure 11-1**). In the abdominal cavity, there are both solid and hollow organs. The solid organs maintain their shape, whereas the shape of the hollow organs depends on their content. The solid organs include the liver, spleen, pancreas, adrenal glands, kidneys, and ovaries. The hollow organs include the stomach, gallbladder, small intestines, colon, bladder, and uterus.

For convenience in describing the abdomen, the abdominal wall is divided into four quadrants by two imaginary lines: a vertical line drawn from the xiphoid process to the symphysis pubis and a horizontal line drawn crossing through the umbilicus (**Figure 11-2**). See **Box 11-1** for a list of each quadrant's contents.

Visualization of each organ as it is auscultated or palpated through the abdominal wall is important.

Digestion

Food passes from the mouth and pharynx through the esophagus to the stomach, where it mixes with gastric secretions. After the masticated food mass mixes with gastric juices in the stomach, it empties into the duodenum by peristalsis. Digestion mostly occurs in the stomach and the duodenum. Peristalsis begins around the middle of the stomach and moves toward the pylorus. It also occurs in the jejunum and the ileum; however, it is not forceful unless an obstruction is present.

The pancreas has both endocrine and exocrine secretions that are important for digestion and the absorption of glucose by the cells. Bile secreted by the liver aids fat digestion and absorption in the intestine. The ducts from the pancreas and the liver open into the duodenum. The terminal part of the ileum, the cecum, and the appendix are part of the ascending colon. The large intestine consists of ascending, transverse, and descending colon; the rectum; and the anal canal.

Most reabsorption of water occurs in the ascending colon. Feces form in the descending and sigmoid colon and reside in the rectum before evacuation.

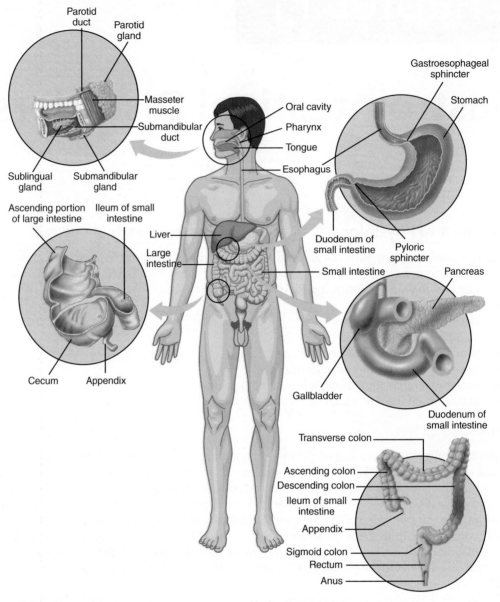

FIGURE 11-1 Gastrointestinal tract.

Health History

Health history must include symptoms related to the gastrointestinal system, such as those associated with eating and bowel habits or function. It should incorporate the chief complaint (CC), history of present illness (HPI), past medical history (PMI), surgeries, and exposures to toxic materials.

Chief Complaint and History of Present Illness

"I have a pain in my abdomen."

Mrs. J is a 49-year-old obese, Caucasian woman with a 3-day history of intermittent epigastric and right upper quadrant pain (RUQ), which has increased in intensity over the last 4 hours. Currently, she is experiencing nausea and has vomited. Although she has not taken her temperature, she says she feels warm. She denies chills or an upper respiratory infection.

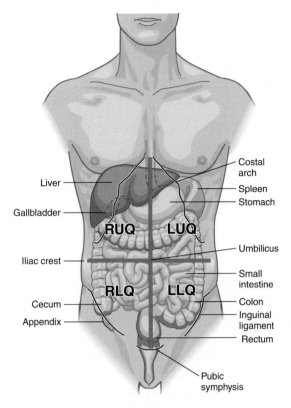

FIGURE 11-2 Abdominal quadrants.

BOX 11-1   ABDOMINAL ORGANS WITHIN QUADRANTS

RIGHT UPPER QUADRANT (RUQ)	LEFT UPPER QUADRANT (LUQ)
Liver (right lobe)	Stomach
Gallbladder	Liver (left lobe)
Duodenum	Spleen
Pancreas (head)	Pancreas (body)
Right kidney (upper pole)	Left adrenal gland
Right adrenal gland	Left kidney (upper pole)
Hepatic flexure of colon	Splenic flexure of colon
Ascending colon (part)	Transverse colon (part)
Transverse colon (part)	Descending colon (part)
Stomach (pylorus)	
RIGHT LOWER QUADRANT (RLQ)	**LEFT LOWER QUADRANT (LLQ)**
Right kidney (lower pole)	Left kidney (lower pole)
Cecum	Descending colon (part)
Appendix	Sigmoid colon
Ascending colon (part)	Left ovary
Right ovary	Left fallopian tube
Right fallopian tube	Uterus, if enlarged (otherwise, the uterus is midline LLQ and RLQ)
Right ureter	Left ureter
Right spermatic cord	Left spermatic cord

Abdominal Pain

Most abdominal disease presents with pain.

Onset	Is the pain sudden or gradual?
	Sudden, severe pain awakening a patient from sleep may be associated with acute perforation, inflammation, or torsion of an abdominal organ.
Location	Describe the location and radiation of pain. The location of pain at its onset, as well as its localization and radiation, are clues to the cause of pain.
	Table 11-1 provides the location and descriptions of abdominal pain associated with various gastrointestinal disorders.
Duration	How long has the patient experienced pain? How long does the pain last?
Frequency of occurrence; regularity	Does the pain occur at certain times? Describe the occurrences.
Precipitating factors	Are there things that cause the pain, such as eating certain foods, alcohol intake, smoking, drug use, or stress?
	With gastroesophageal reflux disease (GERD), pain occurs 30 to 60 minutes after eating.
Associated symptoms	Important associated symptoms to assess include anorexia, weight loss, fatigue, fever, flatulence, belching, and bloating.
	Projectile vomiting occurs with head injury, cranial lesion, or pyloric obstruction.
	Fever occurs with viral syndrome and appendicitis.
	Diaphoresis, dizziness, and chest pain occur with myocardial ischemia/infarction.
	Pyloric stenosis creates blockages that cause vomiting, an eagerness to eat again, and weight loss.
Alleviating factors	What lessens or worsens symptoms?
	Which treatments and/or medications has the patient taken/tried?

Table 11-1 Locations and Descriptions of Pain Associated with Gastrointestinal Disease	
Gastrointestinal Disease	**Location and Description of Pain**
Appendicitis	Periumbilical or epigastric pain. Starts as colicky, then localizes to RLQ.
Cholecystitis	Severe epigastric or RUQ pain that is referred to the shoulder.
Diverticulitis	Epigastric pain that radiates to the left side of the abdomen, especially after eating.
Intestinal obstruction	Severe, abrupt, spasm-like pain that is referred to umbilicus and epigastrium. Described as "gripping."
Leaking abdominal aneurysm	Steady, throbbing, midline pain over aneurysm that may radiate to back or flank. Described as "tearing."
Pancreatitis	Acute, excruciating, LUQ, umbilical or epigastric pain that may be referred to the flank and left shoulder. Pain may be so severe that fainting occurs.
Perforated gastric or duodenal ulcer	Abrupt, RLQ pain that may refer to shoulder. Described as "burning."
Rupture of abdominal organ	Pain is felt "all over the abdomen" with no localization.
Biliary stones	Intense pain in the RUQ. Described as "cramping."

Abbreviations: LUQ, left upper quadrant; RLQ, right lower quadrant; RUQ, right upper quadrant.

Nausea and Vomiting

Occurrence of nausea without vomiting	Do you have nausea without vomiting?
	Nausea without vomiting is a common symptom in patients with hepatocellular disease, pregnancy, and metastatic disease.
Relationship between nausea and/or vomiting and pain	Is the nausea and/or vomiting associated with abdominal pain?
	Did the nausea precede the pain?
	The relationship between vomiting and abdominal pain is important.
	In acute appendicitis, pain precedes vomiting by a few hours.
Changes in stool	Is there constipation, diarrhea, loss of appetite, or change in the color of stools?
	Changes in the stool could suggest the cause of nausea and vomiting.
Quality of vomitus	What is the color of the vomitus?
	The color of vomitus may assist in determining the cause.
	Acute gastritis causes the patient to vomit stomach contents.
	Biliary conditions cause greenish-yellow vomitus fluid.
	Is there any unusual or foul odor to the vomitus?
	Intestinal obstruction causes the vomit to be bilious material followed by fecal-smelling fluid.
Frequency of occurrence	How often do you vomit?
	Toxins cause persistent vomiting.
Relationship of vomiting to eating	Is vomiting related to eating? If yes, how soon after eating do you vomit? Do you vomit only after eating certain foods?
	Vomiting related to food can give a clue to cause.
	Vomiting caused by eating fatty foods can be related to gallbladder disease.
Associated symptoms	Important associated symptoms to assess include fever, vertigo, and headache.
	Fever may point to a localized abdominal condition, such as acute cholecystitis or acute appendicitis. Inner ear disease such as Ménière's disease and labyrinthitis may cause vomiting.
	Migraine, concussion, cerebral tumor or other space-occupying lesions, meningitis, and subarachnoid hemorrhage are associated with nausea and vomiting.
Alleviating factors	What lessens or worsens symptoms?
	Which treatments and/or medications has the patient taken/tried? Any over-the-counter medications used?
	Many drugs, such as digitalis, aspirin, nonsteroidal antiinflammatory agents, antihypertensive agents, and antibiotics, may cause gastric irritation or gastritis.
Use of alcohol, recreational drugs	Is there a history of alcohol or recreational drug use?
	Alcohol may cause gastric irritation or gastritis.

Past Medical History

> Mrs. J has not had any gastrointestinal surgery or trauma, peptic ulcer disease, or lipid abnormalities. She does not take any medications, except birth control pills and an occasional aspirin for headache. Childhood illnesses include measles, mumps, rubella, and varicella.

Past health conditions or surgeries	Ask about past health conditions. Has the patient had any surgeries? Previous surgeries could have an effect on nutritional status. *Esophageal resection is associated with fat malabsorption, abnormal swallowing, and obstruction.* *Stomach resection is associated with dumping syndrome, anemia, delayed emptying, and malabsorption. Pancreatic resection is associated with insufficient secretion of insulin, glucagon, and pancreatic digestive enzymes.* *Small bowel resection is associated with steatorrhea, fat malabsorption, anemia (vitamin B12 malabsorption), and short bowel syndrome.*
Recent hospitalization or gastrointestinal illness	Assess if there is a current diagnosis of peptic ulcer, gastrointestinal hemorrhage, liver or pancreatic disease, or abdominal trauma. *Any of these conditions could result in nutrition and vitamin deficiencies.*
Food and bowel patterns	Ask about eating patterns, appetite, excessive hunger or thirst, swallowing difficulties, heartburn, food intolerances, excessive belching, and bowel patterns to help define the etiology. *Bowel patterns, stool characteristics, frequency of bowel movements, stool consistency, constipation or diarrhea, bloody stools, black tarry stools, rectal bleeding, or hemorrhoids can give clues to diagnosis.*
Medications	Ask about use of enemas, antacids, medications with gastrointestinal side effects (i.e., cardiac drugs), and medications that interfere with absorption. How frequently does she take aspirin?

Family History

Information about the patient's family—family history (FH)—may describe genetic factors and provide evidence of the patient's social network.

> Mrs. J's parents died in an accident when her father was 65 and her mother was 63. She has a sister, age 50, and brother, age 54; both are living and well. She has two grown children who live in the area. Both are well. She denies any history of cancer.

Age of living relatives	Include relationship and health of parents, brothers, sisters, and children.
Deaths	Include relationship, age, and cause of death.
Chronic diseases	Ask about chronic diseases in the family. Include the relationship to the family member with disease and how long the family member has had the disease.
Genetic defects	Include any family genetic disorders; include any congenital birth defects. *Cystic fibrosis often presents as gastrointestinal symptoms; thus knowledge of a family history of cystic fibrosis would be important.*

Social History

In taking the social history (SH), the healthcare provider should ask the questions that follow.

> Mrs. J is a teacher who lives with her husband. She has two grown sons who live in the community. She denies the use of alcohol, tobacco, or recreational drugs. She enjoys working in her garden and visiting friends and family.

Family	Ask the patient to describe the current family unit.
Occupation	Ask about past positions, volunteer activity, and community activities.
	If the patient is retired, ask how long he or she has been retired and how he or she is adjusting.
	Has he or she had exposure to toxic substances?
Leisure activities	List hobbies, exercise, and travel.
Use of tobacco	Include type of tobacco used, duration, and amount (pack-years = number of years of smoking × number of packs smoked per day).
Use of alcohol	Does the patient drink alcohol? How much? Which kind (wine, beer, liquor)? When? How frequently?
Use of recreational drugs	Does this patient use recreational drugs? How much? How frequently? When? Which type (cocaine, heroin, PCP, ecstasy)?

Review of Systems

Many gastrointestinal diseases and disorders have manifestations in systems other than the gastrointestinal system. A comprehensive review of systems (ROS) should be performed whenever possible; however, due to time and other types of constraints, the provider may be able to perform only a focused review of systems. During a focused review of systems, the provider targets questioning at the systems in which gastrointestinal problems are most likely to have manifestations. Following is a summary of common manifestations of gastrointestinal problems.

System	Symptom or Sign	Possible Associated Disease/Disorders
General/ constitutional	Weight loss or gain	Ulcerative colitis, gallbladder cancer, pancreatic cancer
	Exercise intolerance, fatigue	Liver carcinoma
Vital signs	Tachycardia, low blood pressure, increased temperature	Fluid and electrolyte imbalance
Eyes	Headaches (inquire about location, time of onset, duration, precipitating factors); vertigo; lightheadedness; injury; vision problems, including double vision, tearing, blind spots, pain	Fluid and electrolyte imbalance
Mouth/throat	Dental difficulties, gingival bleeding, dentures, neck stiffness, pain, tenderness, masses in thyroid or other areas	Malnutrition, fluid and electrolyte imbalances, gastroesophageal reflux disease (GERD)
Skin	Rash, itching, pigmentation changes, moisture or dryness, texture, changes in hair growth or loss, nail changes, jaundice	Hepatitis, cirrhosis, liver carcinoma, gallbladder cancer, pancreatic cancer
Respiratory	Pain (ask about location, quality, relation to respiration), shortness of breath, wheezing, stridor, cough (ask about time of day; if productive, ask about amount in tablespoons or cups per day and color of sputum), hemoptysis, respiratory infections, tuberculosis (or exposure to tuberculosis), fever or night sweats	Respiratory system irregularities will demonstrate the degree of gastrointestinal pathology, as is the case with gastrointestinal bleeding and subsequent loss of red blood cells (RBCs), which decreases the circulating oxygen-carrying ability
Musculoskeletal	Pain, swelling, redness, or heat of muscles or joints; limitation of motion; muscular weakness; atrophy; cramps	Fluid and electrolyte disorders
Endocrine	Polydipsia, polyuria, asthenia, hormone therapy, growth, secondary sexual development, intolerance to heat or cold	Fluid and electrolyte disorders

Physical Examination

Equipment Needed

- Tongue blade
- Stethoscope
- Gloves
- Lubricant
- Hemoccult developer
- Magic marker
- Tape or ruler marked in centimeters
- Covering for the patient

Components of the Physical Examination

In the physical examination of the abdomen, the usual sequence of inspection, palpation, percussion, and auscultation is modified. Auscultation should occur immediately after inspection. Auscultation provides information about bowel mobility and vascular integrity. Percussion provides information about the size and density of abdominal organs and the location of air, fluid, and masses. Palpation uses light and touch to determine size and tension of the abdominal organs.

Inspection

Action	Rationale
1. Position the patient so that she or he is lying comfortably on an exam table or bed. Drape the patient with a sheet to expose the abdomen. You should stand on the patient's right side. 2. Make sure the room is warm.	1. 2. Providing a comfortable position for the patient will help complete the exam for a patient with abdominal pain. Standing on the patient's right side enables the examiner to easily determine liver span. Also, most examiners are right handed.
3. Inspect general appearance, including the face, hands, and skin.	3. The general appearance of the patient often furnishes valuable information as to the nature of the condition.
a. Inspect the face. • Inspect for temporal wasting. • Inspect the skin around the mouth and oral mucosa. • Smell the patient's breath.	 • Temporal wasting may indicate a nutritional deficit. • Melanin deposits around the oral cavity are indicative of Peutz–Jeghers syndrome (**Figure 11-3**), which is associated with benign intestinal polyps. The polyps may bleed, cause intussusception, or cause obstruction, but they are usually not malignant. • Mouth odors are often associated with gastrointestinal disease (see **Table 11-2**).

Table 11-2 Mouth Odors and Associated Gastrointestinal Disease	
Gastrointestinal Disease/Disorder	Description of Mouth Odor
Neoplasm of esophagus or stomach	Severe bad breath
Peptic ulcers	Acid breath
Hepatic failure	Sickly sweet odor
Esophageal diverticulum	Odor of decay
Severe bowel obstruction	Odor of feces
Cirrhosis with portal shunting	Odor of rotten eggs and garlic

Action   **Rationale**

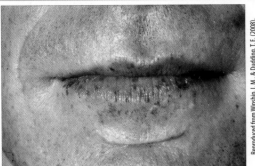

FIGURE 11-3 Melanin deposits around the oral cavity are indicative of Peutz–Jeghers syndrome.

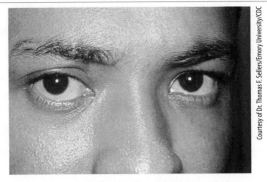

FIGURE 11-4 Jaundice, as seen in the conjunctiva.

b. Inspect the skin.
  - Inspect the skin and conjunctiva for jaundice. Use natural light, if possible, because incandescent light can mask the existence of jaundice.

  - Observe the skin for color and scars; note any rashes or lesions.

  - Assess for spider angiomas.

- **Figure 11-4** depicts a patient with jaundice, which is usually first noted in the conjunctiva of the eyes. Jaundice becomes apparent when serum bilirubin level in adults exceeds 2.5 mg/dL and 6.0 mg/dL in neonates. Hyperbilirubinemia can also result in intense generalized pruritus.

- The presence of scars could lead the examiner to identify a history of past surgeries or trauma that could create the presence of adhesions.

- **Figure 11-5** depicts spider angiomas, which are dilated cutaneous blood vessels usually found above the umbilicus. These lesions are commonly associated with liver disease, pregnancy, and malnutrition. The angiomas advance and regress with the severity of liver disease. They typically appear between the second and fifth months of pregnancy and disappear within days of delivery.

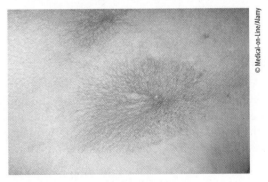

FIGURE 11-5 Spider angiomas, which are commonly associated with liver disease, pregnancy, and malnutrition.

Action	Rationale

c. Inspect hands and nails.
  • Assess for palmar erythema, a reddening of the palms of the hands, that usually accompanies spider angiomas.
  • An increase in the size of the lunula ("half and half" nails) is observed in patients with cirrhosis.	

4. Inspect the abdomen. Good lighting is essential.	

a. Observe the patient's exposed abdomen from the foot of the bed for peristalsis, asymmetry, and abdominal distention.	a. Peristalsis in intestinal obstruction may be visible from the foot of bed.
	    Asymmetry caused by hepatomegaly or splenomegaly may also be apparent on inspection.
	    Abdominal distention is the most common manifestation of gastrointestinal disorders. The most common causes include fat, flatus, feces, fluid, and fibroid tumor.

b. Observe the patient's umbilicus.	b. Normally the umbilicus is located within 1 cm of the midpoint between the xiphoid and the symphysis pubis. Deviations of more than 1 cm should lead to thorough palpation.
c. Measure the abdominal girth, if appropriate.	c. Abdominal girth is an important measurement of patients with increasing or decreasing abdominal distention.
d. Assess skin of abdomen, observing color, scars, rashes, or lesions.	d. Periumbilical ecchymosis (Cullen's sign) is the classic sign of ruptured ectopic pregnancy and acute necrotizing pancreatitis. It appears as bluish discoloration around the umbilicus caused by intraperitoneal bleeding. Flank ecchymosis (Grey–Turner's sign) indicates either an intra-abdominal or retroperitoneal hemorrhage, or injury due to pancreatitis. This appears as discoloration of the lower abdomen and back.

Auscultation

Action	Rationale
1. Auscultate the abdomen. Warm your stethoscope by rubbing with the palm of your hand. Lightly rest the chest piece of the stethoscope in each of the four quadrants of the abdomen. Assess for sounds for 2 to 5 minutes in each quadrant.	1. Normal sounds in the small intestine are high pitched and gurgling. Colonic sounds are low pitched and have a rumbling quality. Bowel sounds normally occur at a rate of 5 to 35 per minute. Bowel sounds may be very loud, indicating hyperperistalsis. Increased sounds may be heard with diarrhea or early intestinal obstruction. Bowel obstructions produce high-pitched tinkles and rushes. Absence or decreased bowel sounds may be due to paralytic ileus, peritonitis, or acute abdomen.

Action   **Rationale**

2. Auscultate for vascular sounds. Place the stethoscope on the arteries of the abdomen.

   a. Auscultate for bruits. Bruits are vascular sounds resembling heart murmurs. **Figure 11-6** depicts the sites to auscultate for bruits.

        a. A bruit with both systolic and diastolic components is associated with turbulence of partially obstructed arterial blood flow. Systolic bruits in the epigastric area are normal.

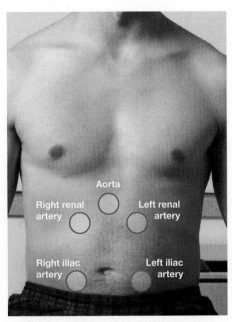

FIGURE 11-6 Locations to auscultate for bruits.

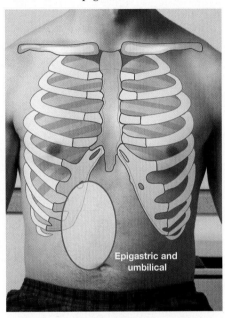

FIGURE 11-7 Location to auscultate for venous hum.

   b. Auscultate for venous hums. **Figure 11-7** illustrates the location for listening for venous hums.

        b. Venous hums are rare. They sound like continuous humming and indicate increased collateral circulation between the portal and venous system.

   c. Auscultate for friction rubs (**Figure 11-8**).

        c. Friction rubs are also rare. Rubs sound like rubbing sandpaper. Friction rubs over the liver can be heard in hepatoma and cholangiocarcinoma. Rubs are also heard after liver biopsy, and can be heard in viral hepatitis, alcoholic hepatitis, and cholecystitis.

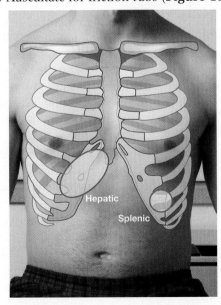

FIGURE 11-8 Locations to auscultate for friction rubs.

Percussion

Action	Rationale

1. Percuss the abdomen. The patient should be supine.

   a. Percuss all quadrants for dullness. Mark the point at which the percussion becomes dull.

   a. Percussion sound changes to dull over solid organs. Dullness is normal over the liver and spleen (**Figure 11-9**) but is abnormal in the middle of the abdominal area, which should be tympanic. Dullness is also heard over fluid. It is useful to determine the amount of free fluid present in the abdominal cavity.

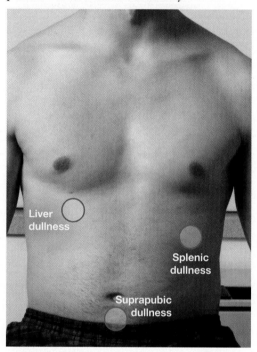

FIGURE 11-9 Normal sites for dullness.

   b. Percuss for tympany.

   b. Tympany is the predominant percussion sound over the stomach and small intestines. When a patient inspires, the tympanic sound turns into a dull sound depending on the abdominal anatomy. High-pitched tympanic sounds lead the examiner to suspect distention. Widespread dullness indicates organ enlargement or the presence of an abdominal mass.

   c. Percuss for hyperresonance. **Figure 11-10** depicts the normal location of hyperresonance.

   c. Hyperresonance should be present only around the umbilicus. Its presence elsewhere could indicate distended vasculature, aneurysms, or varicosities.

2. Percuss the liver. **Figure 11-11** illustrates the direction of liver percussion. Begin liver percussion at the abdomen just below the umbilicus at the right midclavicular line in an area of tympany. Percuss upward until dullness is heard.

2. The estimated size of the liver can be determined with percussion. Normally, lower liver border dullness is heard at the costal margin or slightly below it. To determine the upper border of the liver, begin percussion from an area of lung resonance

Action	Rationale

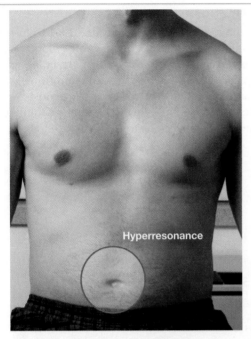

FIGURE 11-10 Location of hyperresonance.

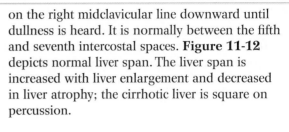

on the right midclavicular line downward until dullness is heard. It is normally between the fifth and seventh intercostal spaces. **Figure 11-12** depicts normal liver span. The liver span is increased with liver enlargement and decreased in liver atrophy; the cirrhotic liver is square on percussion.

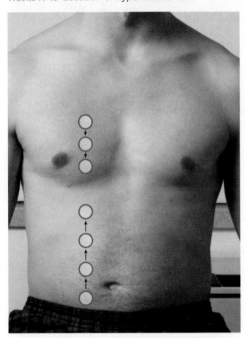

FIGURE 11-11 Direction of liver percussion.

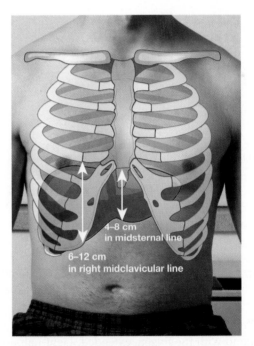

FIGURE 11-12 Normal liver span.

3. Percuss the spleen. The size of the spleen is difficult to determine because it normally is hidden within the rib cage against the posterior lateral wall in the abdomen.

3. Splenic dullness may be heard from the 6th to the 10th ribs. Normal percussion sound can be either resonance or tympanic. As the spleen enlarges, the tip moves downward and toward the midline. If the percussion sound is dull, splenomegaly

Action

Have the patient lie in a supine position and breathe normally. Percuss in the lowest intercostal space in the left anterior axillary line, beginning at an area of lung resonance. **Figure 11-13** illustrates percussion of a normal spleen.

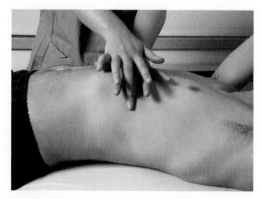

FIGURE 11-13 Percussion of a normal spleen.

4. Percuss for bladder volume.

Rationale

is diagnosed as present. **Figure 11-14** illustrates an enlarged spleen. Considerable enlargement may occur before it is palpable. An enlarged spleen is associated with such conditions as portal hypertension, thrombosis, stenosis, deformed splenic vein, cysts, tumors, trauma, and mononucleosis infection.

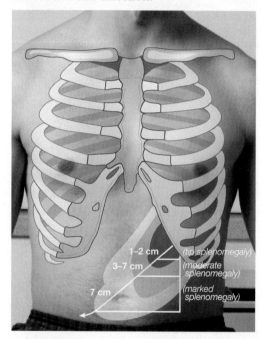

1–2 cm   (tip splenomegaly)
3–7 cm   (moderate splenomegaly)
7 cm   (marked splenomegaly)

FIGURE 11-14 Degrees of splenomegaly.

4. Percussion of the suprapubic area can detect the dullness of bladder volume. The volume in the bladder must be about 400 to 600 mL before dullness is noted.

Palpation

Action

1. Palpate the abdomen. Make sure that your hands are warm, and begin with light palpation of the four quadrants. Palpate any area of pain last.

   a. Perform light palpation. Use the palm of your hand with the fingers extended. Light palpation is done in all four quadrants using the pads of the fingers. Using a light motion, depress the abdomen 1 cm.

   If you touch the area of maximal pain, the abdominal muscles will tighten, and the examination will be more difficult. Always examine the areas where the patient describes his or her pain last or the patient will be tense for the rest of the exam.

Rationale

a. Light palpation helps the examiner to assess areas of tenderness or areas where the patient might have pain.

Action	Rationale

b. Perform moderate palpation. Palpate exerting moderate pressure using the same hand position as for light palpation.

b. Moderate palpation will allow the examiner to assess deeper structures beneath the skin for muscle irregularities, presence of hernias, or other muscle structural changes.

c. Perform deep palpation. Use the palmar surface of your extended fingers, pressing deeply and evenly into the abdominal wall. Palpate all four quadrants, moving the fingers over the abdominal contents. **Figure 11-15** illustrates light and deep palpation.

c. Deep palpation may elicit tenderness in the healthy person over the cecum, sigmoid colon, and aorta, and near the xiphoid process. Muscle rigidity or involuntary guarding with abdominal distention suggests peritonitis. Rigidity may be absent with infection in the posterior abdomen or pelvis. This can occur in perforation of a gastric or duodenal ulcer. As peritonitis progresses, muscles' rigidity becomes less to absent.

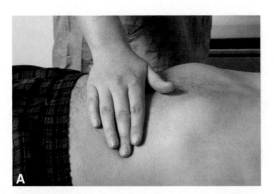
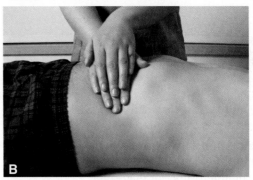

FIGURE 11-15 Degrees of palpation. A. Light. B. Deep.

2. Assess for presence of ascites. Use the fluid wave test. With the patient's hand placed vertically in the middle of his abdomen, place your hands on each side of the patient's abdomen and tap one side while palpating the other side **(Figure 11-16)**.

2. If ascites is present, the examiner will feel the fluid shifting from side to side.

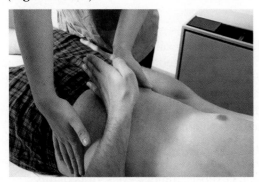

FIGURE 11-16 Performing a fluid wave test.

3. Palpate for rebound tenderness. Elicit rebound tenderness by deeply palpating the abdomen and then suddenly releasing the pressure **(Figure 11-17)**.

3. Rebound tenderness is defined as pain that increases when deep palpation ends. It usually indicates peritoneal irritation; if the rebound tenderness is present in the RLQ (McBurney's point), it suggests that the patient has appendicitis.

Action   **Rationale**

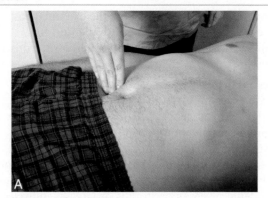

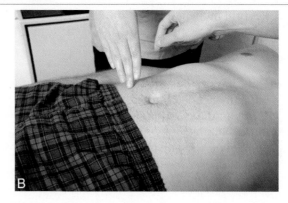

FIGURE 11-17 Palpating for rebound tenderness.

    RLQ pain (positive iliopsoas muscle test) indicates iliopsoas muscle irritation due to inflamed or perforated appendix.

4. Palpate for inspiratory arrest (Murphy's sign). Palpate below the right costal margin. Ask the patient to take a deep breath. If the patient stops breathing mid inspiration because of pain, the sign is positive.

4. Murphy's sign is seen with acute cholecystitis but may also be present with hepatitis or hepatomegaly.

5. Palpate for McBurney's sign. McBurney's sign is tenderness and rigidity from the umbilicus to the right anterosuperior iliac spine.

5. McBurney's sign is frequently seen in appendicitis.

6. Perform the obturator test. The obturator test is a good way to assess for ruptured appendix or pelvic infection. With this test, the patient is placed in a supine position and his or her right leg is flexed at the hip and knee. Place a hand just above the patient's knee with your other hand at the ankle. Then rotate the patient's leg internally and externally. **Figure 11-18** illustrates performing the obturator test.

6. If the patient feels pain in the hypogastric area, then the appendix may be ruptured or the patient has a pelvic infection.

7. Palpate for abdominal aortic aneurysm. The aorta bifurcates at the level of the umbilicus. Palpate for aortic aneurysm in the epigastric area. Place each hand on either side of the aorta and estimate the diameter of the aorta (**Figure 11-19**). A diameter of 3 cm or greater is considered positive.

7. This allows the examiner to check for aortic pulsations or determine the width of the aorta, which helps determine irregularities of the aorta. It is important to check for pulsations before palpating the aorta. Palpating an aortic aneurysm increases the risk for rupture of the aneurysm.

8. Palpate the liver (**Figure 11-20**). Place one hand on the other hand below the right anterior costal margin and then ask the patient to take a deep breath. The liver should come down to meet the fingers as you press down.

8. Palpation of the liver will determine areas of tenderness, presence of masses or enlarged liver span, cirrhosis, tumors, cysts, or hepatitis.

9. Palpate the spleen. Use the same technique as noted previously to palpate the spleen. **Figure 11-21** illustrates palpation of the spleen. Always percuss the spleen before you palpate

9. Palpation increases the risk of rupturing the spleen, especially if it is enlarged.

Action	Rationale

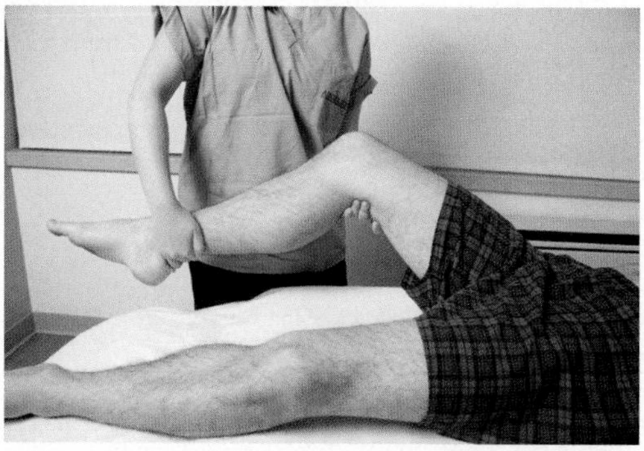

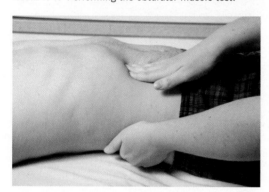

FIGURE 11-18 Performing the obturator muscle test.

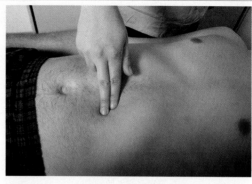

FIGURE 11-19 Palpating for abdominal aortic aneurysm.

FIGURE 11-20 Palpating the liver.

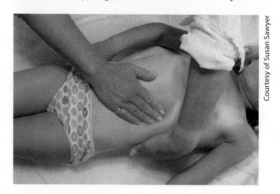

FIGURE 11-21 Palpating the spleen.

Courtesy of Susan Sawyer

Remember that a pelvic examination should be performed on females complaining of abdominal pain. A rectal examination should be performed on both males and females who present with abdominal pain.

Diagnostic Reasoning

Based on findings in the health history and physical examination, the clinician should formulate his or her assessment and plan. For example, a patient may report symptoms that suggest many possible diagnoses; however, findings in the past medical history and during the physical examination might narrow the possible diagnoses down to one or two. Abdominal pain is a common chief complaint. **Table 11-3** highlights the differential diagnosis of common disorders associated with pain in the epigastrium.

Table 11-3 Differential Diagnosis of Epigastric Pain			
Differential Diagnoses	Significant Findings in the Patient's History	Significant Findings in the Patient's Physical Examination	Diagnostic Tests
Cholecystitis/ cholelithiasis	Pain that has the following characteristics: ■ Located in the epigastrium or RUQ ■ Radiating to the right scapular region or back ■ Severe, dull, or boring, and constant (not colicky)	Vital signs reflecting the degree of illness, fever (may be absent, especially in elderly patients), epigastric or RUQ tenderness, fullness in the RUQ, Murphy's sign (an inspiratory pause on palpation of the right upper	WBC, comprehensive metabolic panel, ultrasound, nuclear medicine studies, endoscopic retrograde cholangiopancreatography

(continues)

Table 11-3 Differential Diagnosis of Epigastric Pain *(continued)*			
Differential Diagnoses	Significant Findings in the Patient's History	Significant Findings in the Patient's Physical Examination	Diagnostic Tests
	▪ Causing patients to move around to seek relief from the pain ▪ Developing hours after a meal ▪ Occurring frequently at night, awakening the patient from sleep. Associated symptoms include nausea, vomiting, pleuritic pain, and fever.	quadrant), guarding during palpation, jaundice (found in less than 20% of patients), sepsis *Note: Most uncomplicated cholecystitis does not display these peritoneal signs, so search for other complications (e.g., perforation, gangrene) or other sources of pain.*	
Peptic ulcer disease	Abdominal pain with the following characteristics: ▪ Located in the epigastrium to left upper quadrant ▪ Described as burning ▪ Possibly radiating to the back ▪ Occurring 1 to 5 hours after meals ▪ Relieved by food, antacids (duodenal), or vomiting (gastric) ▪ Following a daily pattern specific to the patient	Mild epigastric tenderness, normal bowel sounds, and signs of peritonitis or gastrointestinal bleeding (e.g., fever and pain)	CBC (to evaluate acute or chronic blood loss), chest x-ray, upper gastrointestinal endoscopy
Pancreatitis	Pain located in the epigastrium or upper right quadrant that may radiate to the back, recent surgeries and invasive procedures (i.e., endoscopic retrograde cholangiopancreatography), family history of hypertriglyceridemia, history of biliary colic and binge alcohol consumption, nausea and/ or vomiting	Fever; tachycardia; tachypnea; hypotension; abdominal tenderness, distention, guarding, and rigidity; mild jaundice; diminished or absent bowel sounds; basilar rales upon lung auscultation; Grey-Turner's sign (bluish discoloration of the flanks); and Cullen's sign (bluish discoloration of the periumbilical area)	CBC, amylase levels (preferably the amylase P, which is more specific to pancreatic pathology), CT scan

Abbreviations: CBC, complete blood count; CT, computed tomography; RUQ, right upper quadrant; WBC, white blood cell count.

Gastrointestinal Assessment of Special Populations

Considerations for the Pregnant Patient

Note the following variations:

▪ More than 50% of pregnant women experience gastrointestinal symptoms.
▪ Morning sickness, which is nausea with or without vomiting, is common in the first trimester. High human chorionic gonadotropin (hCG) and estrogen levels are thought to be the cause.
▪ Pregnant women are sensitive to odors and may have altered taste.
▪ Heartburn is a common symptom in pregnancy. It is thought to be caused by the relaxation of the gastroesophageal sphincter by progesterone. In the third trimester, heartburn is thought to be caused by pushing upward of the uterus.
▪ Digestion is delayed due to a decrease in gastric mobility and a decrease in gastric acid secretion.

Considerations for the Neonatal Patient

Inspection

▪ Check patency of the gastrointestinal tract, which is confirmed by the passage of meconium within the first 24 hours. Failure to pass meconium within 24 hours merits evaluation to rule out cystic fibrosis.

- Note that, because of the immature development of the abdominal muscles, the abdomen of a newborn is protuberant.
- Inspect the umbilical cord. The normal umbilical cord contains two ventrally located thick-walled arteries and one dorsally placed thin-walled vein. Newborns with a single artery often have congenital renal abnormalities.
- Inspect for umbilical hernias. They are common in African American infants. An umbilical hernia in a non–African American infant may be indicative of hypothyroidism. (Umbilical hernias should spontaneously resolve by 5 years of age.)
- Inspect for jaundice. Newborn jaundice is of special concern if it develops in the first 24 hours of life, if there is an ABO incompatibility between infant and mother, or if the mother is Coombs positive.

Percussion
- Percuss the liver span by using the adult technique.
- Note normal percussion sounds: tympany over the intestines and dullness over the liver, feces, and full bladder.

Palpation
- Palpate the liver. The liver edge may be felt as far as 1 cm below the right costal margin. A liver edge more than 2 cm below the right costal margin suggests hepatomegaly.
- Palpate the spleen. During the first month of life, the spleen is palpable 1 cm below the left costal margin.

Considerations for the Pediatric Patient
General
Note the following:
- Intussusception is an acute abdominal condition caused by telescoping of the large intestine. It is the most common cause of acute abdomen for children younger than 2 years of age. Peak incidence is 3 to 12 months of age. There is increased incidence following rotavirus infection. Intussusception is most common in the upper right quadrant. Children will present with tense abdomens, vomiting, and colicky pain. The classic finding of intussusception is red currant jelly stools, which result from hematochezia. However, only 10% of children with intussusception will have this symptom.
- Level of consciousness is the most reliable indicator of dehydration. Children will not have changes in their vital signs until they are moderately to severely dehydrated. Also important to note is the urine output; amounts of less than 2 cc/kg/hr are indicative of dehydration. This translates into no urine production for more than 8 hours.

Inspection
- Aortic pulsation is commonly seen in lean children.
- Inspect inguinal nodes. Positive inguinal nodes are often found in preschool to school-age children. They are most noticeable in children with cuts or scrapes of the lower extremities.

Auscultation
- Have children who are ticklish hold the stethoscope head during auscultation.

Palpation
- Hold the hips and knees in a flexed position to palpate the abdomen of an infant.
- In infants with pyloric stenosis, note that large peristaltic waves may be seen moving from left to right in the upper abdomen. An olive-shaped mass may be palpable in the epigastrium. Infants with pyloric stenosis are normal until 2–3 weeks of age. They present with irritability, poor weight gain, and a history of projectile vomiting after each feeding. Most children will not have flat or scaphoid abdomens until they are 4 to 5 years old.

- Have children who are ticklish place their hands over yours during palpation; it may make them more comfortable.
- Palpate the liver and spleen. At 6 months of age, the estimated liver span varies from 2.5 to 3 cm. At 1 year of age, the liver span is approximately 3 cm.
- To palpate the kidneys, place your left hand under the right side of the child's back and lift upward. At the same time, place your right hand in the right upper quadrant and palpate for the right kidney. Reverse hands to palpate the left kidney.

Considerations for the Geriatric Patient

Note the following physiological changes:

- There is alteration in secretion, mobility, and absorption in the elderly due to atrophy of the gastrointestinal mucosa, with a reduction in the number of stomach and intestinal glands.
- Diverticulosis is thought to occur due to the changes in elastic tissue and colonic pressure.
- Pancreatic atrophy is common.
- Decreased hepatic mass, hepatic blood flow, and microchromosomal enzyme activity also occur. These changes result in an increased half-life of lipid-soluble drugs.
- Constipation becomes a problem with aging, along with hemorrhoids.
- Weakening of the cardiac sphincter—a muscle that regulates the flow of food from the esophagus into the stomach—can lead to esophageal reflux, which causes "heartburn."

Case Study Review

Throughout this chapter, you have been introduced to Mrs. J. This section of the chapter pulls together her history and demonstrates the documentation of her history and physical examination.

Chief Complaint

"I have a pain in my abdomen."

Information Gathered During the Interview

Mrs. J is a 49-year-old obese, Caucasian woman with a 3-day history of intermittent epigastric and right upper quadrant pain, which has increased in intensity over the last 4 hours. Currently, she is experiencing nausea and has vomited. She says she feels warm, although she has not taken her temperature. She denies chills or upper respiratory infection. In addition to the abdominal pain, Mrs. J reports loss of appetite due to nausea. During the past few years, fatty foods have given her indigestion, but she has not had nausea until this present illness. She generally has a bowel movement daily, which is normal color, and she has never had blood in her stools.

Her childhood illnesses include measles, mumps, rubella, and varicella. She did not have rheumatic fever, scarlet fever, or polio. There is no history of gastrointestinal surgery, peptic ulcer disease, lipid abnormalities, or abdominal trauma. Mrs. J has never received a blood transfusion.

Mrs. J's parents died in an accident when her father was 65 and her mother was 63. She has a sister, age 50, and brother, age 54, both living and well. She has two grown children living in the area. Both are well. She denies any family history of cancer. Mrs. J is a teacher. She denies the use of alcohol, tobacco, or recreational drugs. She enjoys working in her garden and visiting friends and family. She has not traveled recently.

Clues	Important Points
Right upper quadrant (RUQ) pain	Pain in the RUQ is associated with liver or biliary problems. The patient needs to specifically describe pain in the abdomen. Pain in the RUQ with nausea and vomiting is a common presenting symptom of cholecystitis. The examiner needs to determine if there is radiation of the pain and obtain a clear description of type. Remember that an extra-abdominal condition, such as pneumonia, can cause RUQ pain.
Obese female	Common characteristics of a cholecystitis patient are the "four F's": *female*, over *40* years old, *fair* complexion, *fat* or overweight.
Nausea and vomiting	Nausea and vomiting are often present with abdominal pain. They are reported with cholecystitis, appendicitis, pancreatitis, and peritonitis.
Fever	Fever suggests an inflammatory process.

Name LJ	Date 10/1/16	Time 0900
	DOB 7/12/66	Sex F

HISTORY

CC

"I have pain in my abdomen."

HPI

50-year old woman with a 3-day history of intermittent epigastric and RUQ pain, which increased over the last 4 hr; experiencing nausea and vomiting; feels feverish.

Medications

1. Birth control pills (unknown name), one per day by mouth
2. ASA, 650 mg as needed for headaches

Allergies

NKA

PMI
Illnesses

Childhood illnesses include measles, mumps, rubella, and chickenpox. No history of rheumatic fever, scarlet fever, or polio. No history of peptic ulcer disease and lipid abnormalities.

Hospitalizations/Surgeries

No past surgeries or trauma; has never received a blood transfusion.

FH

Parents deceased (car accident); sister (50) and brother (54) living and well; has two grown children.

SH

Is a teacher. Lives with husband. Denies use of alcohol and recreational drugs. No recent travel.

ROS

General	Cardiovascular
Fever.	Denies chest pain.
Skin	**Respiratory**
No changes in color.	Denies cough or SOB.
Eyes	**Gastrointestinal**
Wears reading glasses.	RUQ pain; nausea and vomiting; loss of appetite.
Ears	**Genitourinary/Gynecological**
No history of hearing loss.	No changes in function.
Nose/Mouth/Throat	**Musculoskeletal**
No problems identified.	Denies any h/o fractures, arthritis, osteoporosis, amputations, or trauma.
Breast	**Neurological**
Denies history of cancer.	Denies history of seizures or strokes.

PHYSICAL EXAMINATION

Weight 165 lb	Temp 100.2	BP 126/84
Height 63 in	Pulse 100	Resp 14

General Appearance

49-year-old Caucasian female in mild distress; 30 lb overweight; well-groomed, alert, and cooperative.

Skin

Normal turgor and color (no jaundice); warm to the touch.

HEENT

Head: Normocephalic, without signs of trauma. Eyes: Uses reading glasses. No nystagmus or other symptoms. Ears: Clear, no infection. Nose and oropharynx are clear and normal.

Cardiovascular

Tachycardia, S1 and S2 are normal, no S3 or S4. No murmurs appreciated.

Respiratory			
No cough; normal breathing pattern; breath sounds vesicular with no added sounds.			

Gastrointestinal			
RUQ tender on palpation. Positive Murphy's sign. No abdominal bruits present. Guarding noted in epigastrium and RUQ. Bowel sounds heard in 4 quadrants.			

Genitourinary			
No flank tenderness; urine is clear.			

Musculoskeletal			
Strength 4/5 throughout and symmetrical. Pulses present and symmetrical.			

Neurological			
Alert and oriented × 3. Cranial nerves II–XII intact. Deep tendon reflexes 2+; plantar reflexes down.			

OTHER

Lab Tests

Na	139 mEq/L	Hgb 14.6 g/dL	Ca 8.9 mg/dL
K	4.0 mEq/L	Hct 43.8%	mg 2.0 mg/dL
Cl	107 mEq/L	WBC 11,000 cu/mm	Phos 2.7 mg/L
CO_2	20 mEq/L	Total bilirubin 0.9 mg/dL	Amylase 60 m/mL
Bun	8 mg/dL	Ast 25 m/L	Lipase 12 m/L
Scr	0.9 mg/dL	Alt 14 m/L	Troponin 0.3 ng/mL
Glu	110 mg/dL	Alk phos 100 m/L	

UA: Clear urine; SG 1.030; no protein, RBCs, WBCs, or casts; no bilirubin

Special Tests

Ultrasound: Evaluation of the liver reveals a smooth capsule. No masses are identified.

Common bile duct is mildly dilated with a few gallstones but no clear evidence of choledocholithiasis.

The gallbladder is filled with sludge and the wall is slightly thickened; suggestive of cholecystitis.

Chest x-ray: No tracheal deviation can be seen. Lungs are clear. Heart, mediastinum, and diaphragm show no abnormalities.

EKG: Sinus tachycardia.

Final Assessment Findings

Cholecystitis

Bibliography

Bagshaw, E. (1999). Abdominal pain protocol: Right upper quadrant pain. *Lippincott's Primary Care Practice, 3*(5), 486–492.

Barkun, A. N., Bardou, M., Kuipers, E. J., Sung, J., Hunt, R. H., Martel, M., . . . International Consensus Upper Gastrointestinal Bleeding Conference Group. (2010). International consensus recommendations on the management of patients with nonvariceal upper gastrointestinal bleeding. *Annals of Internal Medicine, 152*, 101–113.

Bickley, L. S. (2016). The abdomen. In *Bates' guide to physical exam and history taking* (12th ed., 449–508). Philadelphia, PA: Lippincott Williams & Wilkins.

Collins, R. D. (2003). *Algorithmic diagnosis of symptoms and signs: Cost-effective approach*. Philadelphia, PA: Lippincott Williams & Wilkins.

Dunphy, L. M., & Winland-Brown, J. E. (2001). *Primary care: The art and science of advanced practice nursing*. Philadelphia, PA: F. A. Davis.

Fink, H. A., Lederle, F. A., Roth, C. S., Bowles, C., Nelson, D. B., & Haas, M. A. (2000). The accuracy of physical examination to detect abdominal aortic aneurysm. *Archives of Internal Medicine, 160*, 833–836.

Green, P. H. R., & Cellier, C. (2007). Celiac disease. *New England Journal of Medicine, 357*(17), 1731–1743.

Johnson, C. (2001). Upper abdominal pain: Gallbladder. *British Medical Journal, 323*(7322), 1170–1173.

Kelso, L., & Marcelo, K. (1997). Nontraumatic abdominal pain. *Clinical Issues: Advanced Practice in Acute and Critical Care, 8*(3), 437–448.

Kerlikowske, K., Smith-Bindman, R., Ljung, B., & Grady, D. (2003). Evaluation of abnormal mammography results and palpable breast abnormalities. *Annals of Internal Medicine, 139,* 274–284.

Kinney, M., Dunbar, S. B., Brooks-Brunn, J., Molter, N., & Vitello-Cicciu, J. (1998). *AACN clinical reference for critical care nursing.* St. Louis, MO: Mosby.

McNamara, R., & Dean, A. J. (2011). Approach to acute abdominal pain. *Emergency Medicine Clinics of North America, 29,* 159–173.

Noble, J. (Ed.). (2001). *Textbook of primary care medicine* (3rd ed.). St. Louis, MO: Mosby.

Orient, J. (2000). *Sapira's art and science of bedside diagnosis.* Philadelphia, PA: Lippincott Williams & Wilkins.

Ross, A., & LeLeiko, N. S. (2010). Acute abdominal pain. *Pediatric Reviews, 31*(4), 135–144.

Trowbridge, R. L., Rutkowski, N. K., & Shojania, K. G. (2003). Does this patient have acute cholecystitis? *Journal of the American Medical Association, 289*(1), 80–86.

U.S. Public Health Services. (1998). *Putting prevention into practice: Clinician's handbook of preventive services* (2nd ed.). Maclean, VA: International Medical Publishers.

Chapter 12

Male Genitourinary Disorders

Anatomy and Physiology Review of the Male Genitourinary System

The male genitourinary system is responsible for many functions in the body, including the following:

- Contributing to the reproduction process
- Removing and filtering waste products in the body
- Maintaining volume states and fluid composition in the body, accomplished through reabsorption and secretion of various substances in the kidneys
- Assisting in the regulation of acid–base balance of the body by secretion of hydrogen ions
- Regulating blood pressure
- Producing erythropoietin and vitamin D

Male Genitalia

The male genitalia consist of the penis, testicles, epididymides, scrotum, vas deferens, seminal vesicles, and prostate gland (see **Figure 12-1**).

The penis has two functions in the male. First, the penis provides for the passage of urine by way of the urethra. The urethra extends through the entire length of the penis to the end of the urethral opening. Second, the penis serves as the canal for the flow of semen when the penis is erect.

The penis consists of the shaft, glans, corona, and prepuce. The skin of the penis usually has no hair and is darker than the rest of the male's body. The shaft of the penis contains three areas of cylindrical tissues; when they become engorged with blood, the penile tissue becomes erect. The two larger and upper parts of the cylindrical tissue are called the corpora cavernosa penis. The smaller and lower part of the cylindrical tissue is called the corpus spongiosum urethra because it contains the urethra. The distal part of the corpus spongiosum overlaps the end of the two corpora cavernosa to form a slightly larger structure called the glans penis. The glans penis is surrounded by the foreskin or prepuce, a folded-over skin tissue that is loosely fitted. A circumcision may be performed at birth to remove the foreskin. The junction of the glans penis and the shaft of the penis forms the corona.

The scrotum is a pouch covered with skin that is suspended from the perineal region and located at the base of the penis. Internally, a septum divides the scrotum into two sacs. Each sac contains a testicle, epididymis, and portion of the spermatic cord. The left side of the scrotum usually lies lower than the right side because the left spermatic cord is longer. The cremasteric muscle—the muscle layer of the scrotum—allows the scrotum to relax or contract.

The testicles mainly function to produce sperm and to secrete testosterone. The testicles are small ovoid glands that are slightly flattened from each side. They measure about 4 to 5 cm in length and weigh about 10 to 15 grams. The testicles are suspended by attachment to scrotal tissue and the spermatic cords. The tunica albuginea, a dense white fibrous capsule, encases each testis. It sends out partitions that radiate throughout the testis, dividing it into 200 or more cone-shaped lobules. Each lobule of the testis contains one to three tiny, coiled seminiferous tubules and numerous interstitial cells, called the cells of Leydig. The cells of Leydig secrete testosterone, which is the hormone responsible for the male changes that occur during puberty. Usually, puberty begins

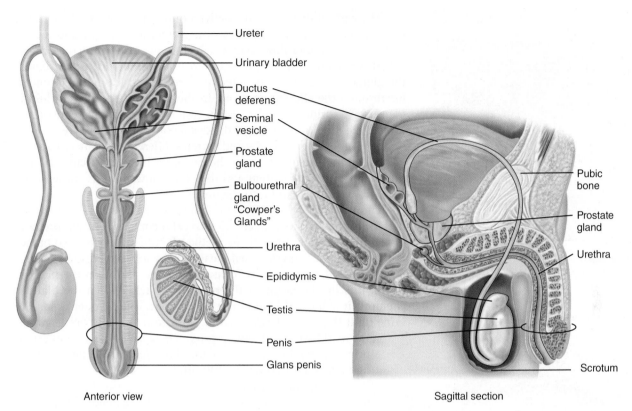

Ureter

Urinary bladder

Ductus deferens

Seminal vesicle

Prostate gland

Bulbourethral gland "Cowper's Glands"

Urethra

Epididymis

Testis

Penis

Glans penis

Pubic bone

Prostate gland

Urethra

Scrotum

Anterior view

Sagittal section

FIGURE 12-1 Male pelvic structures.

between the ages of 9 and 13. Testosterone stimulates the testicles to enlarge, the penis to increase in size, the pubic hair to grow, and the secondary sex characteristics to appear. The secondary sex characteristics include facial hair, body hair, muscle development, and voice changes.

The epididymis curves over the posterolateral surface of each testicle. This creates a visible bulge on the surface of the scrotum. In some men, the epididymis is located toward the front. Sperm matures in the epididymis.

The vas deferens serves as a place where sperm is stored and as a pathway for the sperm. It starts at the lower end of the epididymis and extends through the spermatic cord and travels through the inguinal canal. The vas deferens ends in the abdominal cavity, where it lies on the fundus of the bladder.

The seminal vesicles are a pair of sac-like glands located on the lower posterior portion of the bladder in front of the rectum. Secretions from the seminal vesicles help to form the seminal fluid. Each vas deferens joins to the corresponding seminal vesicle to form the ejaculatory duct.

The prostate gland, located just below the urinary bladder, is a walnut-shaped organ that surrounds the urethra in the male. It produces a thin, milky, alkaline fluid that combines with fluid from the seminal vesicles to enhance sperm activity during ejaculation.

Urinary System

The urinary system consists of two kidneys, two ureters, the urethra, and the bladder.

The kidneys are located in the retroperitoneal space of the upper abdomen, with the right kidney usually lying slightly lower than the left (**Figure 12-2**). They extend from the vertebral level of T12 to L3. The peritoneal fat layer protects the kidneys. Each kidney is composed of the renal medulla, which is the outer portion of the kidney, and the renal cortex, which is the inner portion of the kidney. The renal cortex contains nephrons, which are considered the functioning units of the kidney. Each kidney has more than 1 million functioning nephrons.

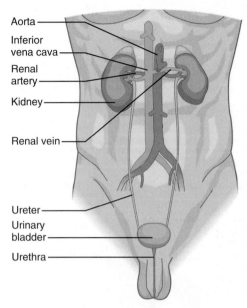

Aorta

Inferior
vena cava

Renal
artery

Kidney

Renal vein

Ureter

Urinary
bladder

Urethra

FIGURE 12-2 Kidneys.

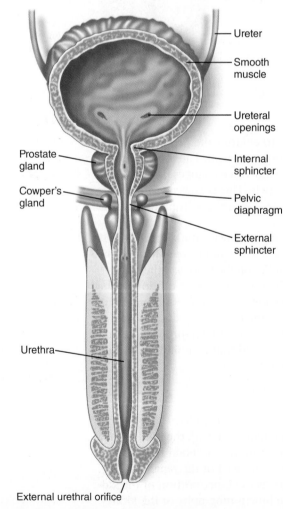

Ureter

Smooth
muscle

Ureteral
openings

Prostate
gland

Internal
sphincter

Cowper's
gland

Pelvic
diaphragm

External
sphincter

Urethra

External urethral orifice

FIGURE 12-3 Bladder and urethra.

The end-product of all the activity of the nephrons in the kidneys is urine. Each nephron consists of a glomerulus system and a tube system. The glomerulus system, which is enclosed in a membrane called Bowman's capsule, filters fluid from the blood. Blood enters the glomerulus through the afferent arteriole and leaves the glomerulus through the efferent arteriole. In the tube system, filtered fluid is converted to urine. The tube system contains the proximal convoluted tubule, the loop of Henle, and the distal convoluted tubule. Each part of the tubule system absorbs and secretes different substances to assist in maintaining homeostasis in the body. Each nephron empties into the collecting tubule system and then fluid flows into the base of the pelvis of the kidney and into the ureters.

The ureters carry urine from the kidneys to the bladder. There are two ureters; each is approximately 25.5 to 30.5 cm long. The left ureter is longer than the right ureter because the left kidney is positioned higher in the body. Urine travels down the ureters by way of peristaltic action.

The bladder is normally located in the pelvis. When the bladder is full, it is displaced under the peritoneal cavity; when the bladder is empty, it is located behind the pelvic bone. The bladder holds the urine until there is a desire to void. This desire usually occurs when the bladder is filled with approximately 500 mL to 1000 mL of urine. Generally, in children and the elderly, the capacity of the bladder is approximately 200 mL less.

The urethra is a small duct that carries urine from the bladder to the outside of the body. The urethra extends through the length of the penis and is surrounded by the prostate gland (**Figure 12-3**). If the gland becomes enlarged, it can hinder elimination of urine.

While the primary functions of the urinary system are removing and filtering waste products in the body, maintaining volume states, and regulating the acid–base balance, it has two additional important functions. First, the kidneys assist in the regulation of the blood pressure through the renin–angiotensin system. Renin is produced and secreted by the juxtaglomerular cells, located in the afferent arteriole. Renin starts the transformation of angioten-sinogen to angiotensin I, and because of this process, the kidneys are also considered part of the endocrine system. Second, erythropoietin and vitamin D are formed by the kidneys. Erythropoietin is necessary for the formation of red blood cells, and vitamin D is essential in calcium and phosphorus metabolism. Red blood cell production and calcium and phosphorus metabolism are abnormal in kidney disease.

Health History

As presented in the introductory chapters, obtaining detailed information related to current symptoms (i.e., history of present illness [HPI]) from the patient is very important to determine the genitourinary problem.

Chief Complaint and History of Present Illness

"It hurts when I urinate, and I go to the bathroom a lot."

PJ is a 78-year-old Caucasian male who presents with a 4-day history of pain with urination. Mr. J describes his urine as a little cloudy in appearance with a foul odor. He complains of going to the bathroom frequently and urinating only a small amount each time. He denies fever, chills, vomiting, or night sweats. He does complain of needing to urinate more during the night.

Common chief complaints (CCs) related to the male genitourinary system include dysuria, frequency or urgency, polyuria, hematuria, nocturia, urinary incontinence, penile discharge, pain in the genital region, and lesions. Dysuria, urgency, and penile discharge are discussed in detail here.

Polyuria is the voiding of at least 2500 mL of urine a day. Possible causes of polyuria include diabetes insipidus; diabetes mellitus; the use of diuretic medications; and psychological, neurologic, or certain renal disorders, such as pyelonephritis or postobstructive uropathy. Hematuria is the presence of abnormal amounts of red blood cells (RBCs) in the urine. Normal urine specimens do not have detectable amounts of blood in the urine. Gross hematuria, which is obvious on inspection of the urine, may cause the urine to become brown or shades of red, including bright red, depending on the amount of blood in the urine and the concentration of the urine. Nocturia is defined as the need to void frequently during the night. Nocturia may suggest a urinary tract infection (UTI), a prostate problem, polyuria, or fluid overload in the body (occurring with conditions such as venous insufficiency, heart failure, nephrotic syndrome, and hepatic cirrhosis with ascites). Urinary incontinence is the involuntary release of urine from the bladder. It can be a small or large amount. Urinary incontinence may be the result of a UTI, weak bladder muscles, bladder tumors, and various neurologic dysfunctions.

Pain in the genital region is also a common complaint. Possible causes of testicular pain include epididymitis, orchitis, and testicular torsion. Perineal pain may be the result of acute or chronic prostatitis. Lower abdominal pain is often related to genitourinary disorders, such as urolithiasis and prostate cancer.

Dysuria

Dysuria, or painful urination, usually suggests a lower UTI. Asking questions related to the timing of the pain during urination may be helpful in providing a differential diagnosis.

Onset	Did the dysuria occur suddenly, or was it a gradual progression of pain?
	Gradual onset of pain would support a more chronic problem.
Duration	How long has the patient had the painful urination or burning sensation (some patients describe dysuria as a burning sensation)?
Frequency of occurrence, regularity	Has the patient experienced pain with urination in the past? If so, how many times? Does the pain accompany each instance of urination?
	When does the pain occur: just before urination, at the beginning, during the entire urination, or at the end of urination?
	Pain occurring just before urination may suggest bladder irritation. Pain occurring at the beginning of urination may suggest a bladder outlet obstruction or gonococcal urethritis. Pain occurring at the end of urination may suggest a bladder spasm. Pain occurring through the entire process of urination may suggest pyelonephrosis.
Severity	As the dysuria affecting the patient's lifestyle and activities of daily living? Assess the severity of the pain by using a pain scale—for example, 0 to 10 (with 0 equal to no pain and 10 equal to the worst pain ever experienced). Remember, pain is subjective.
	Severe pain may suggest kidney trauma or kidney stone.

Associated symptoms	Is the patient experiencing pain in any other areas of the body? Does the pain seem to radiate to other areas of body, such as the back, suprapubic area, scrotal area, or abdomen?
	Pain in the lower back may suggest cystitis or pyelonephritis.
	Ask about other symptoms associated with the dysuria, including hematuria, urgency, penile discharge, chills, fever, nausea, vomiting, shortness of breath, and changes to the color or odor of urine.
	Pyelonephrosis often also presents with fever, chills, night sweats, and/or hematuria. A UTI often presents with frequency, nocturia, and suprapubic pain.
	Urine is normally clear and straw colored. Any change in the color of the urine may suggest problems with the urinary system or give clues to other problems with the body such as liver, heart, or endocrine problems. For example, urine that is very clear and diluted in appearance may suggest diabetes insipidus or the use of diuretic therapy. Complaints of burning, dysuria, and foul-smelling urine are common with kidney infections.
Alleviating factors	How has the patient tried to obtain relief from the dysuria? Has he taken any prescription or nonprescription drugs or tried any home remedies such as drinking cranberry juice? How effective was the treatment?

Urinary Frequency and Urgency

Urinary frequency refers to voiding at frequent intervals. Urinary urgency is a feeling or an exaggerated sense of needing to urinate, even when there may not be any urine in the bladder. Urinary frequency and urgency usually occur when there is inflammation or irritation in the bladder, which may cause a decrease in bladder capacity. Urinary frequency also may occur with urethral stricture, prostate problems, and neurologic disorders.

Onset	Was the onset sudden or gradual?
Frequency	How often is the patient going to the bathroom?
Amount	How much urine does the patient think he voids each time?
Quality	Does the patient try to force the urine completely out of the bladder?
	Is there always a sensation of fullness in the bladder? Does the patient feel pressure with urination?
	Is the patient able to make it to the bathroom? What is the daily intake of fluid?
	The patient's response to the questions will help to identify if this is a chronic or an acute problem. In addition, the knowledge of the patient's fluid intake will assist in the diagnosis of dehydration versus kidney failure.
Associated symptoms	Ask about associated symptoms, such as dysuria, pain, and fever.
	Urethritis may present with the additional symptoms of dysuria and pain.
	Prostatitis may present with dysuria, perineal pain, fever, and chills.

Penile Discharge

Onset	Was the onset acute or gradual?
Quality	Ask the patient to describe the discharge, including color and consistency.
	Gonococcal urethritis presents with a thick, greenish discharge. Chlamydia presents with scant mucoid discharge.

Associated symptoms	Ask the patient about associated symptoms, including pain, pruritus, dysuria, swelling, fever, and lesions.
	Balanitis presents with pain and prepuce swelling. Urethritis may present with edema, dysuria, and pruritus.
	Epididymitis often presents with scrotal pain and edema; with severe infection, the patient may present with fever.
Sexual history	Ask the patient to describe his sexual history, including the number of partners and use of contraceptives. What is the patient's sexual preference? How many sex partners has the patient had? Does the patient have any concerns about sexual performance? Is the patient single or married?
	Sexual history can provide clues about diagnoses, such as sexually transmitted diseases.

Past Medical History

> Mr. J had a urinary tract infection 4 weeks ago. He was treated with Bactrim. Mr. J is no longer sexually active. He has hypertension, which is treated with medication. He denies any history of past surgeries or trauma.

The healthcare provider asks detailed questions about all past medical illness/history (PMI).

Presence of recurring genitourinary problems	Has the patient experienced the genitourinary problems in the past? If so, has the severity or pattern changed?
Sexual history	Ask the patient to describe his sexual history (see "Past Medical History").
	Sexual history can provide clues about diagnoses, such as sexually transmitted diseases.
	Does the patient have any problems with sexual function?
	Priapism is a painful condition of prolonged penile erections. In many cases, priapism is idiopathic; however, it may be observed in patients with leukemia or hemoglobinopathies.
	Peyronie's disease is a disorder of unknown cause that occurs when there is a fibrous band in the corpus cavernosum. Generally, it affects one side of the corpus cavernosum, and it causes the penis to deviate to one side during erection. Depending on the extent of the fibrous band, erections can be painful.
Past health conditions or surgeries	Does the patient have any chronic diseases?
	Many chronic diseases manifest with genitourinary symptoms.
	Type 2 diabetes mellitus may cause polyuria or urinary tract disorders.
	Ask the patient about past surgeries. Ask about past trauma, especially to the abdominal and genital regions.
Self-examination	Does the patient perform self-examination of penis and scrotum for any masses, drainage, lesions, sores, and rashes?

Family History

Mr. J reports that his father had hypertension and coronary artery disease and died of a heart attack at the age of 60. His mother died at the age of 84 of old age. Mr. J has one younger brother, age 70, who has hypertension. Mr. J has two adult children. His daughter is 48 and his son is 45. Both are alive and well.

A family history (FH) often reveals clues to diagnosis. Certain disorders tend to occur in families.

Age of living relatives	Include the relationship and health of parents, siblings, and children.
Deaths	Include the relationship of the deceased person to the patient and the cause of death (specifically disorders that affect the genitourinary system, such as testicular cancer).
Chronic diseases	Ask about chronic diseases in the family; include the relationship of the patient to the family member with the disease. Focus on genitourinary disorders or disorders that have genitourinary manifestations. Is there a family history of renal disease, such as polycystic disease, renal insufficiency, acute renal failure, chronic renal failure, chronic dialysis, kidney stones, renal tubular acidosis, or renal or bladder carcinoma? Have any family members had prostate, testicular, or penile cancer? Ask about a family history of inguinal or femoral hernias. Also ask about infertility. *Some diseases, such as cancers, tend to occur in families.*
Genetic defects	Is there a history of congenital birth defects?

Social History

Mr. J is married and lives with his wife on the second floor of a four-story apartment building. There is an elevator to his apartment. Mr. J worked as a carpenter for 35 years. He retired at the age of 60. Mr. J denies smoking, use of alcohol, and use of recreational drugs.

A patient's social history (SH) often helps narrow the diagnosis.

Family	Ask the patient to describe the current family unit.
Occupation	Which type of employment? Is there any risk of trauma or injury to the suprapubic or genitalia area?
Exercise	Does the patient exercise? Does the patient wear some type of protective or supportive device during exercise and during sport activities?
Use of tobacco	Ask about tobacco use, including types, amounts, duration of use, and exposure to secondary smoke. *Nicotine is a vasoconstrictor and may contribute to urinary problems.*
Use of alcohol	Does the patient drink alcohol? If so, which type and how much does he drink? *Alcohol use may be associated with dysuria. It may also negatively impact sexual performance.*
Use of recreational drugs	Is the patient using recreational drugs? If so, which drugs and how much? *Many recreational drugs impact sexual performance.*

Review of Systems

Many genitourinary diseases/disorders have manifestations in systems other than the genitourinary system. A comprehensive review of systems (ROS) should be performed whenever possible; however, due to time and other types of constraints, the provider may be able to perform only a focused review of systems. During a focused review of systems, the provider targets questioning at the systems in which genitourinary problems are most likely to have manifestations. Following is a summary of common manifestations of male genitourinary problems.

System	Symptom or Sign	Possible Associated Diseases/Disorders
General	Fever	Acute bacterial pyelonephritis, renal cell carcinoma, urolithiasis, nephrolithiasis, acute prostatitis, epididymitis, syphilis
	Weight loss	Renal cell carcinoma, prostate cancer
Skin	Rash on palms	Syphilis
Respiratory	Cough	Testicular cancer
Gastrointestinal	Nausea or vomiting	Acute bacterial pyelonephritis, urolithiasis, prostate cancer, testicular cancer, epididymitis
	Anorexia	Acute glomerulonephritis
Musculoskeletal	Body aches	Acute prostatitis
	Lower extremity edema	Bladder cancer, prostate cancer, testicular cancer

Physical Examination

Equipment Needed

- Gloves
- Gown
- Draping
- Flashlight

Components of Urinary Examination

For this examination, it is helpful if the patient is wearing a gown so that the abdomen and back can be exposed as needed. Remember to provide appropriate draping. Examination of the urinary system includes inspection, palpation, percussion, and auscultation. Inspection, palpation, and percussion are discussed in this section. Auscultation of the urinary system only includes listening for bruits in the abdominal area. A bruit that radiates laterally in the epigastric region may suggest renal artery stenosis.

Inspection

Action	Rationale
1. Position the patient in a comfortable sitting upright position on the examination table or on the side of the hospital bed. Provide proper covering for the patient, but expose the chest and back areas. If the patient is unable to sit upright, you can position him on his left side.	1. This position allows for adequate inspection of the back and chest area.
2. Inspect the chest and back area for any skin discoloration or scars.	2. Skin discoloration or scars may suggest renal disease or problems.
3. Inspect the flank areas of the patient.	3. In a normal adult, the flank areas are symmetrical. Flank areas that are full or asymmetrical suggest renal disease.

Percussion and Palpation

Action	Rationale

1. Percuss the kidneys. Ask the patient to sit upright. Expose the patient's back; drape as needed.
 	
   To use the indirect method, place the palmar surface of one hand against the costovertebral angle. Using the other hand, make a fist and use the ulnar surface to strike the first hand (**Figure 12-4**).
 	
   To use the direct method, make a fist and use the ulnar surface to strike the costovertebral angle directly.
 	
   Whichever method you use, strike the costovertebral angle with enough force to cause the patient to receive a painless jolt. Observe patient for any pain or discomfort in this area.
	1. The patient should not experience any tenderness or pain.
	
	   Pain and tenderness may indicate glomerulonephritis or glomerulonephrosis.

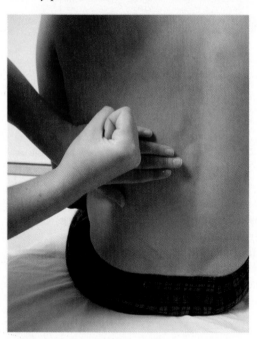

FIGURE 12-4 Percussing the kidneys using the indirect method.

Action	Rationale

2. Palpate the kidneys. Ask the patient to lie in a supine position. Expose the patient's abdomen, draping as appropriate.
   a. To palpate the left kidney: Stand on the patient's right side. Reach across the patient with your left arm and place your hand behind the patient's left flank area. Then, lift the left flank area with your left hand and palpate deeply with the palmar surface of your right hand (**Figure 12-5**).
	a. This will displace the kidney anteriorly. Normally, the left kidney is not palpable.
	   A tender, painful kidney indicates an infection.
	   An enlarged kidney may indicate hydronephrosis or polycystic disease.

Action   **Rationale**

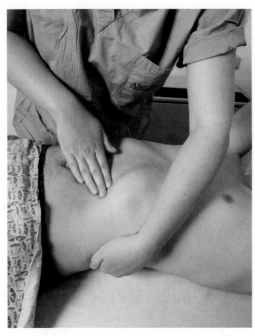

FIGURE 12-5 Palpating the left kidney.

b. To palpate the right kidney: Remain on the patient's right side and lift the right flank area with your left hand. Use your right hand to palpate deeply.

3. Percuss for bladder volume (**Figure 12-6**).

b. The right kidney is more often palpable. The kidney should feel firm, smooth, and solid. Chronic renal disease may cause the kidney to feel soft.

3. Percussion of the suprapubic area can detect the dullness of bladder volume. The volume in the bladder must be about 400 to 600 mL before dullness is noted. A distended bladder may also be detected during percussion.

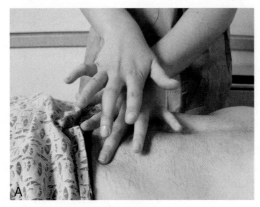
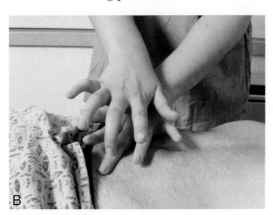

FIGURE 12-6 Percussing the bladder.

Action	Rationale
4. Palpate the bladder.	4. The bladder is not usually palpable unless it is distended. A full bladder may be palpated as a smooth and round mass in the lower abdomen.

Components of the Genitalia Examination

Assessment of the genitalia can be uncomfortable for patients and may cause a high level of anxiety. The healthcare provider needs to provide an environment that is comfortable for the patient. In addition, the healthcare provider needs to provide a private area for the patient during the interview process and the physical examination.

Ensure that the room is a comfortable temperature and that privacy can be maintained. For the examination, the patient should be undressed, wearing a gown, and draped appropriately. Examination includes inspection and palpation. Some males may feel uncomfortable with a female healthcare provider during this part of the examination. The patient needs to be reassured and made to feel comfortable during the examination.

Inspection and Palpation of the Penis and Scrotum

Generally, inspection and palpation of the genital area are performed together to provide flow and a sense of comfort for the patient. The patient should be in the supine position on the examination table or standing. Ensure that there is adequate lighting for the examination. The healthcare provider should be seated during the examination.

Action	Rationale
1. Inspect and note the distribution of the pubic hair.	1. Pubic hair is coarser than scalp hair. Normally, there is no hair on the penis. There may be a distribution of hair around the scrotum extending to the anal orifice. Small brown lice may be seen at the base of the hair with pubic lice (pediculosis) infestation (**Figure 12-7**). 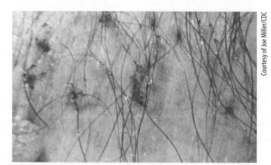 FIGURE 12-7 Pubic lice.
2. Inspect the penis for any lesions, sores, rashes, or masses. If the patient is uncircumcised, retract the foreskin to examine the glans penis.	2. The penis should appear smooth and without lesions. If the patient is uncircumcised, the foreskin should retract easily. There may be a white, cheesy smegma seen over the glans penis; this is a normal finding. Paraphimosis occurs when the foreskin of the male becomes retracted behind the glans penis and cannot be retracted back over the penis. This condition is usually congenital, but it also can occur as a result of infrequent retracting of the foreskin for cleaning. It may also be caused by recurrent infections of the glans penis and foreskin.

Action   **Rationale**

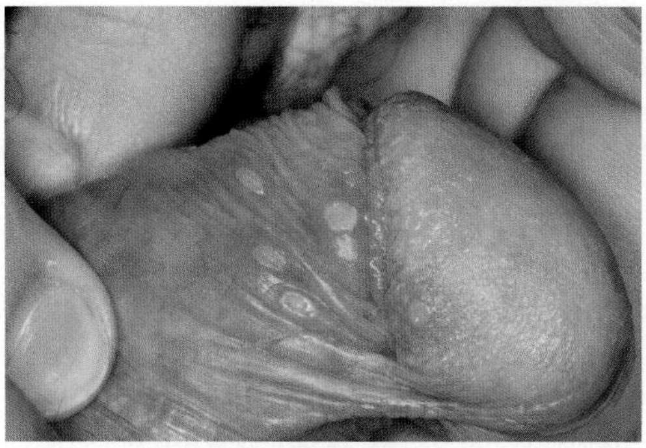

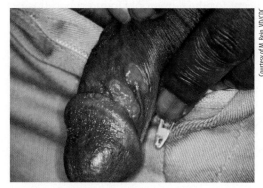

FIGURE 12-8 Herpes simplex virus.

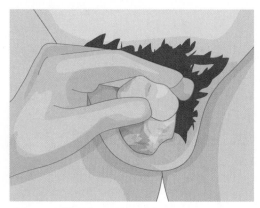

FIGURE 12-9 Primary syphilis.

The presence of a rash, lesion, or sore may suggest the presence of a sexually transmitted disease. Herpes simplex presents as group of vesicles on an erythematous base that become eroded (**Figure 12-8**). Syphilis usually presents with a single chancre (**Figure 12-9**). Genital warts (condyloma acuminatum), caused by a papovavirus, are soft and red in appearance. The lesions can occur on the glans penis, on the shaft of the penis, and within the urethra. The lesions may change from a malignant lesion to squamous cell carcinoma. Lesions of lymphogranuloma venereum appear as painless erosions at or near the coronal sulcus. Molluscum contagiosum (caused by a poxvirus) presents with pearly gray, smooth, dome-shaped lesions. The lesions are usually located on the glans penis.

3. Inspect the urinary meatus for any drainage. Note the position of the urinary meatus. Press the glans penis between the gloved thumb and the forefinger (**Figure 12-10**), and observe for the color of the opening and for any drainage.

3. The urinary meatus should be located on the ventral surface from the tip of the glans penis. The opening should appear pink or dark brown, or slightly darker than the skin color. The presence of a discharge may suggest an infection. A yellow or green discharge suggests gonococcal urethritis. A scant, thin, mucoid discharge suggests nongonococcal urethritis.

FIGURE 12-10 Examining the urinary meatus.

4. Palpate the shaft of the penis. Note any tenderness or induration.

4. The shaft of the penis should feel smooth and semi-firm. (The penis may become erect during the examination. Ensure the patient that this is a normal response).

Action	Rationale
5. Inspect the scrotum for lesions, rashes, color changes, or edema.	5. The scrotum is more deeply pigmented than the rest of the body. An edematous, elevated scrotum may be the result of testicular torsion, which is an abnormal twisting of the spermatic cord **(Figure 12-11)**
	The scrotum appears asymmetrical because the left testicle is lower than the right testicle. The spermatic cord is longer on the left side. Edema may be caused by a hydrocele, which is a collection of fluid in the space of the tunica vaginalis testis or along the spermatic cord **(Figure 12-12)**.
	Normally, there are no lesions on the scrotum, except for the commonly found sebaceous cysts.

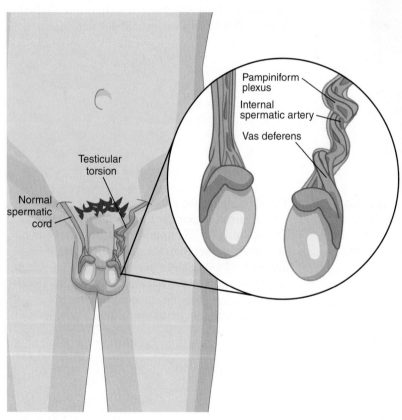

FIGURE 12-11 Testicular torsion.

Action   **Rationale**

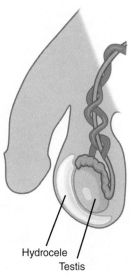

Hydrocele

Testis

FIGURE 12-12 Hydrocele.

6. Gently palpate the testes for masses or tenderness using the thumb and the first two fingers.

7. Palpate each epididymis, located on the posterolateral surface of the testes.

8. Palpate each spermatic cord along the length of the cord from the epididymis up to the external inguinal ring. **Figure 12-13** illustrates palpation of the spermatic cord.

6. The testes should feel oval, smooth, and rubbery. The testes should move freely when palpated. They are sensitive to gentle pressure, but not tender. If a mass is felt in the scrotal area, assess for tenderness. A firm, painless, smooth mass may indicate testicular cancer. If the mass is distal or proximal to the testis, place your finger over it; note whether the mass is reducible and if you can auscultate bowel sounds over the mass. If you can auscultate bowel sounds, this may indicate a herniation of the intestines into the scrotal area. This requires immediate surgical attention.

7. The epididymis should feel discrete and smooth. The epididymis feels softer than the testes.

8. The spermatic cords should feel smooth and nontender. If palpation elicits pain and tenderness, this may indicate a varicocele, a mass of dilated and tortuous varicose veins in the spermatic cord (**Figure 12-14**).

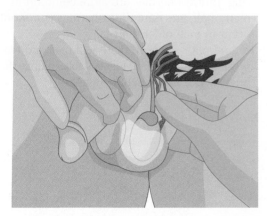

FIGURE 12-13 Palpating the spermatic cord.

Action	**Rationale**

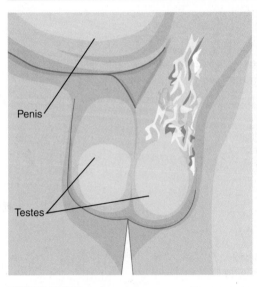 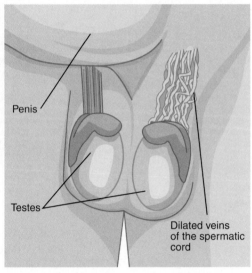

FIGURE 12-14 Varicocele.

9. If you note any swelling or mass in the scrotal area, transilluminate the area. Dim the lights and shine a flashlight from behind the scrotal contents.

9. The normal scrotum and epididymis will appear as dark masses with regular borders on transillumination. The testes appear with small areas of transilluminated space around the testes and larger transilluminated space superior to the testes.

    Serous fluid will transilluminate with a red glow. Tissue and blood will not transilluminate.

10. Assess for inguinal hernias.
   a. Inspect the inguinal area for a bulge. Ask the patient to bear down.

   a. A bulge seen when the patient bears down suggests an inguinal hernia. The most common hernia occurring in males is the inguinal hernia. An inguinal hernia can be direct or indirect. A direct inguinal hernia occurs when the hernial sac enters the inguinal canal through its posterior wall. An indirect inguinal hernia (**Figure 12-15**) occurs when the hernial sac enters the internal inguinal ring. Indirect hernias are more common in men of all ages, and direct hernias commonly occur in men older than 40.

   b. Ask the patient to relax, and then palpate the inguinal area for a hernia by placing the gloved finger into the lower part of the scrotum and follow along the vas deferens into the inguinal canal (**Figure 12-16**).

     Ask the patient to cough. (Use the index finger or middle finger to palpate for a hernia in an adult male; use the little finger to palpate for a hernia in a child.)

   b. If a hernia is present, there will be a sudden presence of abdominal viscus felt against the finger when the patient coughs.

Action   **Rationale**

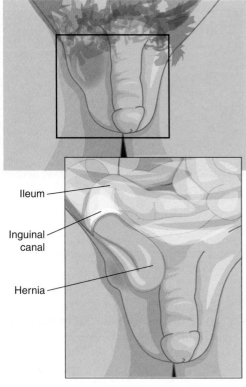

Ileum

Inguinal
canal

Hernia

FIGURE 12-15 Indirect inguinal hernia.

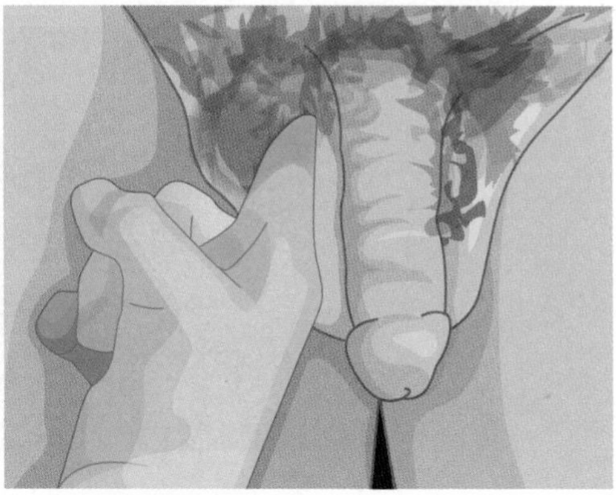

FIGURE 12-16 Palpating for a hernia.

11. Stroke the inner thigh with a blunt instrument, such as the handle of a reflex hammer. Observe for the testicle and scrotum to rise on the stroked side.

11. This is the cremasteric reflex, assessed to determine the normal reflex response in this area. The absence of this response may indicate a testicular torsion.

Encourage male patients to perform self-examination of the genital area each month to assess for lumps, bumps, discharges, rashes, lesions, and sores. **Box 12-1** describes the technique for self-examination.

BOX 12-1   GUIDELINES FOR GENITAL SELF-EXAMINATION

A male should be encouraged to start self-examinations beginning at the age of 13. The main focus of the self-examination is the assessment of the testes for any masses. Generally, a testicular tumor has no early symptoms. The patient should, however, examine the whole region. Instructions to patients should include the following points:
- The best time to perform genital self-examination is during a shower or bath.
- Examine the skin in the pubic area for any sores and blisters.
- Hold your penis in your hand and examine the tip of the penis for any drainage.
- If you are not circumcised, retract the foreskin and examine the glans penis.
- Inspect and feel the tip of the penis and the entire head of the penis in a clockwise manner.
- Inspect and feel the entire shaft of the penis for bumps, lumps, sores, and blisters (**Figure A**).
- Examine and feel the scrotum for any sores, blisters, and lumps. Gently feel each testicle; note any swelling or soreness (**Figure B**).
- Report any abnormal findings (sores, bumps, drainage, pain) to your healthcare provider.

(continues)

BOX 12-1   GUIDELINES FOR GENITAL SELF-EXAMINATION *(continued)*

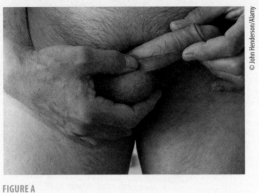

FIGURE A

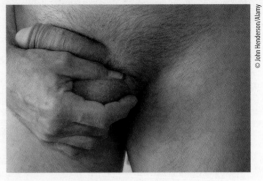

FIGURE B

Palpation of the Prostate Gland
Palpation of the prostate gland is usually done when performing a rectal examination.

Action	Rationale
1. Ask the patient to stand next to the examination table, lean forward, and rest his upper body comfortably on the table. Help him to position himself with his hips flexed and his toes pointed toward each other. If the patient cannot stand, have the patient lie in the left lateral position.	1. This position allows the buttocks to flatten and the deters gluteal muscles to contract.
2. Insert a lubricated gloved finger gently into the anal canal. Your finger should be moving in the direction of the umbilicus. You will feel the prostate gland on the anterior wall. Palpate the prostate gland with the pad of the index finger. Note the size, contour, consistency, and mobility of the prostate gland.	2. The prostate gland should feel firm, rubbery, smooth, and slightly movable. It should be about the size of a walnut. Palpation should not be painful for the patient. The prostate gland should not protrude into the rectal lumen. Prostatitis often presents with a painful, swollen prostate. In acute prostatitis, the prostate may feel warm to the touch. Benign prostatic hyperplasia presents with smooth, firm enlargement of the prostate gland. The classification of prostate enlargement is graded according to the protrusion of the prostate gland into the rectum (**Table 12-1**). Palpation may reveal a hard nodule in patients with prostate cancer.

Table 12-1 Grading of Prostate Enlargement	
Grade	Degree of Protrusion
I	1 to 2 cm
II	2 to 3 cm
III	3 to 4 cm
IV	> 4 cm

Action	Rationale
3. Stroke the prostate gland from the distal to the proximal areas.	3. This motion may force secretions through the urethral opening. Any secretion that appears through the opening should be examined and cultures obtained.

Box 12-2 describes laboratory and special tests useful in diagnosing male genitourinary disorders.

BOX 12-2   DIAGNOSTIC TESTS

The diagnostic examination should include tests that will assist and aid in confirming a diagnosis.

- **Blood tests:** These tests include a basic metabolic panel (BMP; sodium, potassium, chloride, carbon dioxide, glucose, blood urea nitrogen, creatinine); serum osmolality; renal panel (includes BMP, phosphorus, and calcium levels); and complete blood count
- **Routine urinalysis:** This analysis tests the pH of the urine, its specific gravity, its sodium level, and urine osmolality. The normal pH of the urine can vary from 4.5 to 8. The normal range of specific gravity for urine is 1.003 to 1.025. Normally, there is no detectable amount of occult blood in the urine. Positive results for nitrite in the urine indicate bacteriuria. Leukocyte esterase detects the esterase that is released from the white cells in the urine. A significant amount of white cells in the urine may indicate a UTI.
- **Urine for culture and sensitivity:** Urine cultures can identify specific bacteria. The presence of a significant amount of bacteria may indicate a UTI. Generally, a bacteria count greater than 100,000 per milliliter indicates an infection.
- **24-hour collection for protein and creatinine:** Proteinuria is an increased amount of protein detected in the urine. Increased amounts of protein in the urine may suggest kidney problems.
- **Intravenous pyelography (IVP):** This test provides an assessment of the kidneys, ureters, and bladder.
- **Fractional excretion of Na$^+$ (FE$_{Na+}$) level:** FE$_{Na+}$ levels can assist in determining the renal status of the patient. Renal problems can be classified as prerenal, renal, or postrenal. Some examples of their causes are provided here:

Prerenal FE$_{Na+}$ < 1	Renal FE$_{Na+}$ > 1	Postrenal FE$_{Na+}$ < 1
Hypovolemia	Glomerular disease	Urethral obstruction
Impaired cardiac function	Tubulointerstitial nephritis	Bladder neck obstruction
Bacteremia	Acute tubular necrosis	Prostatic hypertrophy
Antihypertensive drugs, including ACE inhibitors	Renal artery occlusion	Bladder carcinoma
Heart failure	Acute vasculitis	Bladder infection
Myocardial infarction	Malignant hypertension	Kidney stones
Pericardial tamponade	Atheroembolic disease	Bilateral obstruction of ureters
Acute pulmonary embolism	Drug toxicity	Hematoma
Surgical operations	Renal cortical necrosis	Pelvic abscess

- **Glomerular filtration rate (GFR):** Estimation of the GFR is the most commonly used method to assess the severity of renal impairment.
- **Prostate-specific antigen (PSA) test:** PSA is a glycoprotein that is specific to the prostate gland. An enlarged prostate can cause the PSA levels to be elevated. The use of PSA tests as a screening tool to detect prostate cancer remains controversial. However, the current recommendation is to use PSA tests along with digital rectal examination (DRE) for prostate cancer screening in high-risk men older than the age of 50, and for men older than the age of 40 at even higher risk, such as those with a family history of prostate cancer or African Americans.

Diagnostic Reasoning

Based on findings in the health history and physical examination, the clinician should formulate her or his assessment and plan. For example, a patient may report symptoms that suggest many possible diagnoses; however, findings in the past medical history and during the physical examination might narrow the possible diagnoses down to one or two. Dysuria is a common chief complaint. **Table 12-2** illustrates the differential diagnosis of common disorders associated with dysuria.

Table 12-2 Differential Diagnosis of Dysuria			
Differential Diagnoses	Significant Findings in the Patient's History	Significant Findings in the Patient's Physical Examination	Diagnostic Tests
Urinary tract infection	Dysuria, frequency urgency, nocturia	Suprapubic tenderness	Urinalysis
Prostatitis	Dysuria, frequency, nocturia, hematuria, chills, fever	Palpation of the prostate reveals a tender, swollen prostate	Urine culture and sensitivity of divided specimens
Epididymitis	Dysuria, frequency, scrotal pain, fever, nausea	Edema, redness, and tenderness of the scrotum	Gram's stain, culture

Genitourinary Assessment of Special Populations

Considerations for the Neonatal Patient
General

Note the following:
- A newborn's first void of urine should occur during the first 24 hours of birth.
- Urine in a newborn is colorless and usually odorless.
- A persistent diaper rash in a newborn and/or infant may be a sign that a UTI is present.
- Determine whether the mother used sex hormones or birth control pills during pregnancy. This may be a clue to further examine the neonate for birth defects.

Inspection
- Assess if the newborn is circumcised and determine whether there were any problems during or from the procedure.
- In the uncircumcised patient, determine whether the foreskin is retractable.
- Assess the scrotal area for any swelling when the neonate cries or ask the parents if they observe any swelling in the scrotal area when the neonate has a bowel movement.
- Assess for any congenital anomalies, such as hypospadias, epispadias, and cryptorchidism **(Figures 12-17** and **12-18)**.

Considerations for the Pediatric Patient
General
- UTIs usually do not occur until at least 2 to 6 years of age, unless caused by abnormal structure of the kidneys.
- Children younger than 2 years of age with UTIs have nonspecific complaints. They may have more gastrointestinal tract complaints than urinary complaints or just be irritable.
- If a previously toilet-trained child starts to wet in the day or night, this may be a sign of a UTI.
- An increased incidence of UTIs may be observed in adolescents who are sexually active.
- Determine whether an adolescent is sexually active.
- Determine if the adolescent has knowledge of reproductive function and determine the source of the information—for example, school or parents.

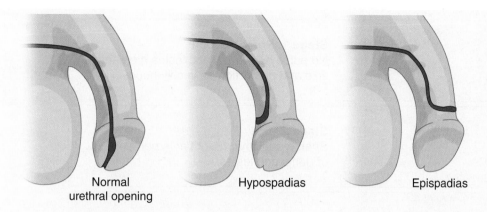

FIGURE 12-17 Positions of urethral opening.

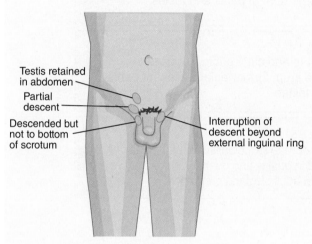

FIGURE 12-18 Varieties of cryptorchidism.

Inspection

- Inspect for any swelling, color changes, rashes, sores, or lesions on the penis and scrotum.
- Is there concern for sexual abuse—for example, findings of bruises, abnormal scarring on buttocks and around anus, or sores on penis?
- Inspect pubic hair and genital size for appropriate sexual development for age **(Figure 12-19)**.

Considerations for the Geriatric Patient

Note the following:

- There may be decreased bladder capacity in the older adult with frequent urination without the presence of disease.
- Certain medications that are prescribed for the older adult may cause urinary frequency and problems with starting urination.
- UTIs in the older adult are usually an incidental finding. Generally, the older adult presents to his healthcare provider or hospital with other complaints such as shortness of breath or chest pain.
- Determine whether there has been a change in the frequency of sexual activity or change in the desire for sexual activity, which may be related to the death of a spouse or sexual partner. Assess the patient for depression or a physical illness that is causing a change in sexual response. Determine whether there is a desire for sexual activity but inability to achieve an erection.

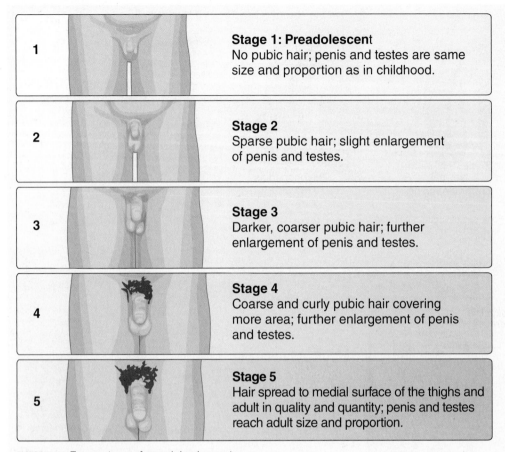

1		**Stage 1: Preadolescent** No pubic hair; penis and testes are same size and proportion as in childhood.
2		**Stage 2** Sparse pubic hair; slight enlargement of penis and testes.
3		**Stage 3** Darker, coarser pubic hair; further enlargement of penis and testes.
4		**Stage 4** Coarse and curly pubic hair covering more area; further enlargement of penis and testes.
5		**Stage 5** Hair spread to medial surface of the thighs and adult in quality and quantity; penis and testes reach adult size and proportion.

FIGURE 12-19 Tanner stages of sexual development.

- In the older male, it will take longer to achieve full erection and there is a longer time in between erections.
- Ejaculations are less forceful.
- The scrotum becomes pendulous.
- Pubic hair becomes thin and sparse.
- Sperm becomes less viable.

Case Study Review

Throughout this chapter, you have been introduced to Mr. J. This section of the chapter pulls together his history and demonstrates the documentation of his history and physical examination.

Chief Complaint

"It hurts when I urinate, and I go to the bathroom a lot."

Information Gathered During the Interview

PJ is a 78-year-old Caucasian male who presents with a 4-day history of pain with urination. Mr. J describes his urine as a little cloudy in appearance with a foul odor. He complains of going to the bathroom frequently and urinating only a small amount each time. He denies fever, chills, vomiting, or night sweats. He does complain of needing to urinate more during the night.

Mr. J had a urinary tract infection 4 weeks ago. He was treated with Bactrim. Mr. J is no longer sexually active. He has hypertension, which is treated with medication. He denies any history of past surgeries or trauma.

Mr. J reports that his father had hypertension and coronary artery disease and died of a heart attack at the age of 60. His mother died at the age of 84 of old age. Mr. J has one younger brother, age 70, who has hypertension. Mr. J has two adult children. His daughter is 48 and his son is 45. Both are alive and well.

Mr. J is married and lives with his wife on the second floor of a four-story apartment building. There is an elevator to his apartment. Mr. J worked as a carpenter for 35 years. He retired at the age of 60. Mr. J denies smoking, use of alcohol, and use of recreational drugs.

Clues	Important Points
A 4-day history with complaints of dysuria, urgency, and urinary frequency	May suggest problems with the prostate, but since complaints have been for the last 4 days, suggests a UTI.
Cloudy urine with a foul odor	Suggests UTI.
Nocturia	May suggest problems with the prostate.
Denies fever, chills, nausea, vomiting, and night sweats	Presence of symptoms would suggest pyelonephritis.
Previous UTI 4 weeks ago	The patient may have a persistent UTI or prostatitis.
Treated with Bactrim	The organism may be resistant to Bactrim. Appropriate antibiotic (ATB) therapy may not have been selected according to pharmacokinetics and spectrum of activity. The patient may not have completed the course of ATB therapy.
Pain in the costovertebral angles	Suggests UTI.

Name PJ	Date 5/15/15		Time 1500
	DOB 4/12/37		Sex M

HISTORY

CC

"It hurts when I urinate, and I go to the bathroom a lot."

HPI

78-year-old Caucasian male with a 4-day history of pain with urination. Describes his urine as a little cloudy in appearance with a foul odor; complains of going to the bathroom frequently and only urinating a small amount each time. Denies fever, chills, vomiting, or night sweats; needs to urinate more during the night.

Medications

Lisinopril 20 mg once a day

Allergies

NKDA

PMI

Illnesses

HTN; UTI 4 weeks ago (treated with Bactrim)

Hospitalizations/Surgeries

No history of hospitalizations/surgeries

FH

Father died of MI at 60; history of HTN and CAD.
Mother died at 84 of old age.
Brother alive at 70; history of HTN.

SH

Married; lives with his wife on the second floor of a four-story apartment building; worked as carpenter for 35 years, retired at age 60.
Has two adult children (ages 48 and 45).
Denies smoking, use of alcohol, or recreational drugs.

ROS

General	Cardiovascular
No fever or night sweats.	High blood pressure.
Skin	Respiratory
Denies changes.	No SOB or coughing.

Eyes	Gastrointestinal
Wears glasses.	Denies nausea and vomiting.
Ears	**Genitourinary/Gynecological**
Denies hearing loss.	UTI in the past, dysuria, frequency.
Nose/Mouth/Throat	**Musculoskeletal**
Wears dentures, denies problems.	Denies weakness.
Breast	**Neurological**
	Denies changes in mental status.

PHYSICAL EXAMINATION

Weight 160 lb	Temp 98.4	BP 120/72
Height 5'8"	Pulse 84	Resp 26

General Appearance
Well-developed, tired-looking male

Skin
Warm and dry to touch

HEENT
Normal cephalic; extraocular muscles intact; PERRL; hearing is intact to whisper in the right and left ears.
No nasal discharge, obstruction, or deviation.
Oropharynx is clear, with moist, pink, smooth mucous membranes; there is no tongue deviation.
Neck supple without adenopathy or thyromegaly.
Negative JVD.
Negative carotid bruits bilaterally.

Cardiovascular
Regular rate and rhythm; normal S_1, S_2; no S_3 or S_4; no murmurs, rubs, or clicks appreciated.

Respiratory
Clear throughout all lung fields.

Gastrointestinal
Normal bowel sounds.
Abdomen soft and tympany to percussion.
No bruits appreciated.
Rectum normal; no hemorrhoids noted.

Genitourinary
Positive costovertebral angle tenderness bilaterally.
Prostate gland palpated; smooth, no nodules palpated, about a grade 1.
Slight tenderness noted.

Musculoskeletal
Strengths 5/5.

Neurological
Cranial nerves II–XII intact, deep tendon reflexes 2+, Babinski absent.

Other

Lab Tests

Na 140 Hgb 13.5 Hct 42%	WBC 15.8	UA
K 4.0	75% Neutrophils	Nitrite (+)
Cl 99	15% Bands	Bacteria (+)
CO_2 22	13% Lymphs	Urine for C J S pending results
BUN 32	2% Monocytes	

Special Tests

Final Assessment Findings

1. Recurrent UTI

2. Possible prostatitis

Bibliography

Ferri, F. F. (1998). *Practical guide to the care of the medical patient.* St. Louis, MO: Mosby.

Foxman, B. (2003). Epidemiology of urinary tract infections: Incidence, morbidity, and economic costs. *Disease-a-Month, 49*(2), 53–70.

Frankel, S., Smith, G. D., Donovan, J., & Neal, D. (2003). Screening for prostate cancer. *Lancet, 361,* 1122–1128.

Grindel, C. G., Crowley, L. V., & Johnston, C. A. (1997). *Anatomy and physiology.* Philadelphia, PA: Lippincott-Raven.

Guyton, A. C., & Hall, J. E. (2011). *Textbook of medical physiology* (13th ed.). Philadelphia, PA: W. B. Saunders.

Holroyd-Leduc, J. M., Tannenbaum, C., Thorpe, K. E., & Straus, S. E. (2008). What type of urinary incontinence does this woman have? *Journal of the American Medical Association, 299*(12), 1366–1356.

Kiel, R. J., & Nashelsky, J. (2003). Does cranberry juice prevent or treat urinary tract infection? *Journal of Family Practice, 52*(2), 154–155.

Longo, D. L., Fauci, A. S., Kasper, D. L., Hauser, S. L., Jameson, J. L., & Loscalzo, J. (Eds.). (2012). *Harrison's principles of internal medicine* (18th ed.). New York, NY: McGraw-Hill.

Nicolle, L. E. (2003). Urinary tract infection: Traditional pharmacologic therapies. *Disease-a-Month, 49*(2), 111–128.

Ronald, A. (2003). The etiology of urinary tract infection: Traditional and emerging pathogens. *Disease-a-Month, 49*(2), 71–82.

Schaeffer, A. (2003). The expanding role of fluoroquinolones. *Disease-a-Month, 49*(2), 129–147.

Vaughn, G. (1999). *Understanding and evaluating common laboratory tests.* Stamford, CT: Appleton & Lange.

Zollo, A. J. (1995). *The portable internist.* St. Louis, MO: Mosby.

Chapter 13

Female Genitourinary and Breast Disorders

ADVANCED ASSESSMENT OF THE FEMALE GENITOURINARY SYSTEM

Anatomy and Physiology Review of the Female Genitourinary System

The primary functions of the female genitourinary system include the following:

- Removing and filtering waste products in the body
- Maintaining volume states and fluid composition in the body, accomplished through reabsorption and secretion of various substances in the kidneys
- Assisting in the regulation of acid–base balance of the body by secretion of hydrogen ions
- Regulating blood pressure (through the renin–angiotensin system)
- Serving as the site of reproduction

External Genitalia

The external genitalia, or vulva, is readily visible and can be identified by inspection, as depicted in **Figure 13-1.** The external structures extend from the mons pubis to the anus. The mons pubis is a fatty tissue covering the symphysis pubis. After puberty, the mons pubis is covered by a triangular pattern of pubic hair. The mons pubis protects the symphysis pubis during coitus. The labia majora are two skin folds that extend from the mons pubis to the perineum. The inner edges of the labia are

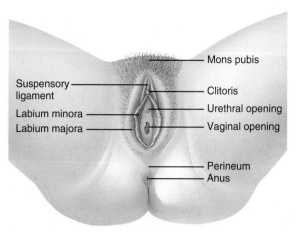

FIGURE 13-1 External genitalia.

hairless and smooth; pubic hair covers the outer edges. The labia minora are two smooth skin folds that lie within the labia majora. The labia minora extend from the clitoris toward the perineum and end at the fourchette, which is above the perineum. The upper portion of the labia minora divides into an upper and lower lamella. The upper lamellae of the labia minora join to form the prepuce of the clitoris, and the lower lamellae join below to form the frenulum of the clitoris.

The clitoris is a small organ composed of erectile tissue, analogous to the penis. It consists of the glans, the corpus, and the crura, although only the glans clostridia is visible. The corpus extends toward the pubis under the skin and divides into two crura, which are attached to the pubic bones.

The vestibule—a boat-shaped region between the labia minora—is visible when the labia minora are separated. Within the boundaries of the vestibule are the urethral and the vaginal orifices. The urethral or urinary meatus is located anterior to the vaginal orifice. The urethra opens externally at the meatus. On each side of the urethral meatus are two small depressions containing the Skene's glands, also called the paraurethral ducts, which are located below the outer part of the meatus; they usually are not visible but secrete mucus that keeps the vaginal area moist.

The vagina introitus (orifice) lies behind the urethra. The hymen is a membranous fold at the vaginal opening. When the hymen is imperforated, it is a continuous membrane; after perforation, fragments of hymen attach to the introit margins and are called hymen caruncles.

The Bartholin's glands, located on each side of the vaginal orifice deep within the perineal structures, secrete mucus, especially during coitus, for lubrication of the vaginal orifice and canal.

Internal Genitalia

The internal genitalia are composed of the vagina, cervix, uterus, ovaries, and fallopian tubes. **Figure 13-2** depicts the internal reproductive organs. The vagina is a pink, rugated, musculomembranous canal, approximately 9 to 10 cm in length, that connects the vulva with the uterus. It is highly elastic and extends upward and backward from the vulva. The rugae allow the vagina to expand during intercourse and during a vaginal delivery. The vagina is influenced by the hormone estrogen and has mucus-producing cells. The pH of the vagina is acidic; the acidic environment maintains the flora of the vagina, which prevent vaginal infections. The distal end of the vagina is cup-shaped, with the cervix located in the cup.

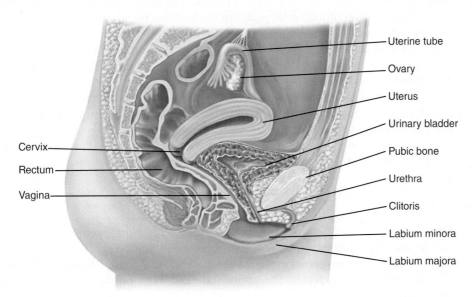

FIGURE 13-2 Lateral view of reproductive organs.

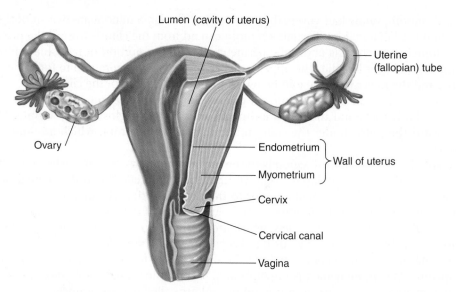

FIGURE 13-3 Ovaries, fallopian tubes, uterus, and vagina.

The uterus is a pear-shaped muscular organ, located in the pelvis between the bladder and rectum. It is composed of smooth muscles, muscle fibers, and connective tissue, all of which expand in all directions during pregnancy. The uterine wall comprises three layers: the endometrium, the myometrium, and the peritoneum (**Figure 13-3**). The endometrium is made up of epithelium, connective tissue, and blood vessels. Estrogen and progesterone influence the thickness of the endometrium. A portion of the endometrium is shed during menses and childbirth. When the endometrium grows outside the uterus, it causes endometriosis. The myometrium is composed of three layers of smooth muscles. The peritoneum, the outer layer, separates the uterus from the abdominal cavity.

The uterus has two main parts: the corpus and the cervix. The corpus forms the upper two-thirds of the uterus, while the cervix forms the lower portion. The cervix is a canal extending into the vagina. The opening into the vagina is called the external os. The upper end of the cervical canal ends at the internal os. Stratified squamous cells make up the mucous membrane cells of the cervix. The endocervix, or cervical canal, is lined with columnar epithelium cells. If the columnar epithelium cells come in contact with the lower pH of the vagina, a transformation called squamous metaplasia takes place. The columnar epithelium cells are replaced by squamous epithelium, and this area is now called the transformation zone.

The ovaries, two oval bodies, are considered the genital glands of the female. The ovaries are located in the pelvis, on either side of the uterus, and below the anterosuperior iliac spine. They produce and store ova and secrete estrogen and progesterone.

The fallopian tubes transfer the ovum from the ovaries to the uterus. The muscular tubes are 8 to 12 cm long. The tubes are composed of four parts: interstitial, the isthmus, the ampulla, and the fimbria.

The Menstrual Cycle

Hormones that affect fertility and childbearing also influence the female reproductive system. The hypothalamus, ovaries, and pituitary gland secrete hormones that affect the menstrual cycle, as depicted in **Figure 13-4**. The menstrual cycle ranges from 22 to 34 days (usually 28 days) and is regulated by fluctuating hormone levels. The menstrual flow starts on day 1 and usually lasts for approximately 5 days.

On day 1, the beginning of the menstrual or preovulatory phase, low estrogen and progesterone levels in the bloodstream stimulate the hypothalamus to secrete gonadotropin-releasing

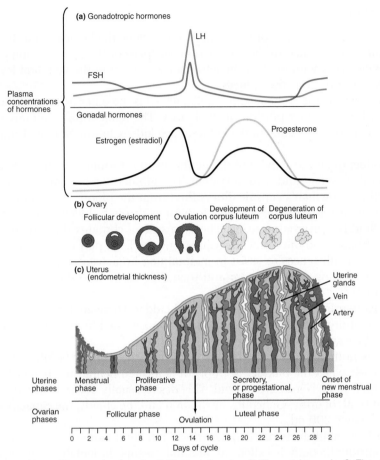

FIGURE 13-4 The menstrual cycle. **A.** Hormonal cycles. **B.** The ovarian cycle. **C.** The uterine cycle.

hormone (GnRH). GnRH stimulates the anterior pituitary to secrete follicle-stimulating hormone (FSH) and luteinizing hormone (LH). When the FSH level increases, the LH level increases.

The proliferative, or follicular, phase starts on day 6 and lasts until day 14. The LH and FSH act on the ovarian follicle, which contains the ovum, causing estrogen secretion. This in turn stimulates the endometrium to build up. At mid-cycle, estrogen levels peak, FSH secretion declines, and LH secretion increases. Late in the cycle, estrogen declines and the follicle matures, causing ovulation.

The luteal or secretory phase lasts from day 15 to day 28. In the luteal phase, FSH and LH levels decline and the estrogen and progesterone levels initially decline as the corpus luteum begins functioning. In this phase, the endometrium responds to the progesterone stimulation by becoming thick and secretory in preparation for implantation of the fertilized ovum. About 10 to 12 days after ovulation, the estrogen and progesterone levels reach a point too low to sustain the endometrium lining and the lining is shed (menses). The next cycle begins as the low estrogen and progesterone levels stimulate the hypothalamus.

During menopause, which usually occurs between the ages of 40 and 55, menses will cease. This cessation of menses is due to the lack of ovarian follicles and failure to respond to FSH and LH. Estrogen and progesterone hormone levels decrease, and testosterone hormone levels increase. Women still produce a weak estrogen form, called estrone; it is released by the peripheral tissue. This estrogen decrease stimulates changes in the vasomotor systems, causing hot flashes and urogenital tissue atrophy. Tissue atrophy promotes thinning and the loss of elasticity of the muscles of the vagina wall and the bladder, which can cause urine frequency.

The Urinary System

The female urinary system consists of the kidneys, the ureters, the bladder, and the urethra.

The two kidneys are located in the retroperitoneal space of the upper abdomen, with the right kidney usually lying slightly lower than the left. They extend from the vertebral level of T12 to L3. The peritoneal fat layer protects the kidneys.

Each kidney is composed of the renal medulla, which is the outer portion of the kidney, and the renal cortex, which is the inner portion of the kidney. The renal cortex contains nephrons, which are considered the functioning units of the kidney. Each kidney has more than 1 million functioning nephrons.

The end product of all the activity of the nephrons in the kidneys is urine. Each nephron consists of a glomerulus system and a tube system. The glomerulus system, which is enclosed in a membrane called the Bowman's capsule, filters fluid from the blood. Blood enters the glomerulus through the afferent arteriole and leaves the glomerulus through the efferent arteriole. In the tube system, filtered fluid is converted to urine. The tube system contains the proximal convoluted tubule, the loop of Henle, and the distal convoluted tubule. Each part of the tubule system absorbs and secretes different substances to assist in maintaining homeostasis in the body. Each nephron empties into the collecting tubule system and then fluid flows into the base of the pelvis of the kidney into the ureters.

The ureters carry urine from the kidneys to the bladder. There are two ureters. The left ureter is longer than the right ureter, because the left kidney is positioned higher in the body. Urine travels down the ureters by way of peristaltic action.

The bladder is normally located in the pelvis. When the bladder is full, it is displaced under the peritoneal cavity; when the bladder is empty, it is located behind the pelvic bone. The bladder holds the urine until there is a desire to void. This desire usually occurs when the bladder reaches approximately 500 mL of urine. Generally, in children and the elderly, the capacity of the bladder is less than approximately 200 mL.

The urethra is a small duct that carries urine from the bladder to the outside of the body. Its opening to outside the body is called the urethral meatus. In females, it is approximately 3 to 5 cm long and is located above the vagina introitus.

Health History

History of present illness (HPI), past medical illnesses/history (PMI), social history (SH), family history (FH), and the review of systems (ROS) are essential to diagnosis and to formulation of a treatment plan. A thorough health history helps detect such factors as a family history of gynecological cancer or unsafe sexual practices.

Chief Complaint and History of Present Illness

"I'm having pelvic pain."

> KC is a 24-year-old Caucasian woman who comes to the clinic with a chief complaint of pelvic pain. She has experienced pelvic pain for the last 6 months. Ms. C says the pain has progressively become worse. It started as an intermittent, dull pain, but now it is a constant, sharp pain. She says she is itchy and has minimal discharge, which she describes as grayish in color and without odor. She denies swelling, masses, lesions, odor, or nausea and vomiting. She says she has felt feverish, but has not taken her temperature. She denies vaginal bleeding and says her last menses was 2 weeks ago but was not normal. She says her menses was very heavy. She is experiencing dysuria. She has taken birth control pills for the last 3 years.

Common genitourinary chief complaints (CCs) include pelvic pain, vaginal bleeding, discharge, lesions, dysuria, hematuria, frequency or urgency, and incontinence. Pelvic pain, abnormal vaginal bleeding, discharge, and dysuria are discussed here.

Pelvic Pain

Pelvic pain is a common complaint in women. A localized or a generalized problem may cause this symptom. Pelvic pain is commonly associated with menstruation, infections, tumors, and pregnancy.

Onset	Was the pain sudden or gradual?
	An acute onset may be associated with pregnancy or urinary tract infection (UTI).
	An acute onset with a fever suggests infection.
Duration and pattern	How long has the patient had the pain?
	Is the pain recurring?
	Pain recurring every month suggests that it is related to the menstrual cycle.
Quality and severity	Where is the pain located? Does it radiate?
	Is the pain preventing the patient from activities of daily living (ADLs)?
	Appendicitis or pelvic inflammatory disease (PID) may cause severe pain that interrupts or prevents the patient from engaging in ADLs.
Associated symptoms	Is the patient experiencing pruritus, discharge, bleeding, urinary symptoms, or fever?
	PID often presents with pain, bleeding, and discharge.
	Pelvic pain with a burning sensation during urination suggests a urinary tract infection.
	Uterine cancer may present with pain and bleeding.
Alleviating and aggravating factors	What alleviates the pain? Did the patient try prescription or nonprescription drugs? How effective have the patient's efforts to treat the pain been?
	Do positional changes increase or decrease pain?
	A patient with gallstones may sit still to decrease pain.
Last menstrual period	When was the patient's last menstrual period? Was it normal? If not, describe how.
	Ask the patient if she could be pregnant.

Abnormal Vaginal Bleeding

Abnormal bleeding includes several types of bleeding. Metrorrhagia is bleeding at irregular intervals. Menorrhagia is excessive bleeding during the menstrual cycle; excessive bleeding could be increased flow or duration. Amenorrhea is a cessation of menstrual bleeding.

Onset	Was the onset sudden or gradual?
Pattern; quality	Is the bleeding acute or chronic?
	The patient's response may help in diagnosing the cause. For example, acute bleeding may be associated with uterine fibroids.
Associated symptoms	Ask about associated symptoms, including pain, discharge, weight loss or gain, or fatigue.

Uterine cancer may be associated with bleeding, pelvic pain, and weight loss.

Abnormal bleeding presenting with weight loss or gain may be thyroid dysfunction. Amenorrhea is often associated with anorexia.

Medications	Ask the patient what medications she is taking, including birth control.
	Some medications may affect menses.

Leukorrhea

Patients may complain of vaginal discharge, also called leukorrhea. Eliciting a thorough description of the discharge can greatly help narrow the diagnosis.

Onset	Was the onset sudden or gradual?
Quality	Ask the patient to describe the discharge, including color, amount, odor, and consistency.
	Bacterial vaginosis presents with a thin, foul-smelling, white or gray discharge.
	Candida vulvovaginitis presents with a thick, white discharge.
	Trichomoniasis often presents with grayish-green or yellow discharge.
Associated symptoms	Ask about associated symptoms, including pruritus, edema or erythema in the vaginal area, lesions, and bleeding.
	Vaginitis presents with discharge, erythema, and edema.
	Sexually transmitted diseases often present with lesions.
Precipitating factors	Ask about precipitating factors.
	Intercourse may cause an increase in the amount of discharge and bleeding in patients with PID.

Dysuria

Dysuria is difficulty or pain with urination and is a common complaint.

Onset	Was the onset sudden or gradual?
Quality; location	How severe is the pain with urination?
	Where do you feel the pain?
	The location of the pain may provide diagnostic clues. For example, with urinary tract infection (UTI), the pain is usually experienced in the suprapubic area, whereas interstitial cystitis may present with diffuse perineal, vaginal, suprapubic, or bladder pain that increases with urination.
Associated symptoms	Ask about associated symptoms, including frequency or urgency, vaginal discharge or pruritus, fever, chills, and nausea.
	Dysuria with vaginal discharge and pruritus suggests vulvovaginitis.
	Urethritis presents with vaginal discharge.
	Fever, chills, and nausea are often associated with UTI.

Past Medical History

Ms. C states that she has been in good health. She has had upper respiratory infections and a recent urinary tract infection, which she says was treated with an antibiotic (she cannot remember the name). She has no history of recent trauma. She denies any surgeries. Her last gynecological examination was 2 years ago, and she says that the Pap smear was normal. Ms. C has been pregnant once and has one child, delivered vaginally. She is married and monogamous. Prior to her marriage, she was diagnosed with chlamydia, which was treated.

The healthcare provider asks detailed questions about all past medical illness, trauma, surgeries, and pregnancy. This will provide information for a diagnosis and a treatment plan.

Menstrual history	When was the onset of menses? Ask the patient to describe her menstrual pattern. Is her menstrual cycle regular? Has she experienced any change in her menstrual pattern? Does she use tampons or pads?
Presence of recurring genitourinary problems	Has the patient experienced genitourinary problems in the past? If so, has the severity or pattern changed?
Sexual activity	Ask the patient to describe her sexual history, including the number of partners and use of contraceptives. *Sexual history can provide clues about diagnoses, such as sexually transmitted diseases.*
Pregnancies	Ask the patient about past pregnancies (gravida), including live births (para), miscarriages, and abortions. Were deliveries vaginal or cesarean sections?
Past health conditions or surgeries	Does the patient have any chronic diseases? *Some chronic diseases may manifest with genitourinary symptoms.* *Type 2 diabetes mellitus may cause polyuria or urinary tract disorders. Hyperthyroidism may cause amenorrhea.* Ask the patient about past surgeries. Ask about past trauma, especially to the abdominal and genital regions.
Last gynecological examination	Ask the patient about her last pelvic examination and Papanicolaou (Pap) smear. Were the results normal or abnormal?

Family History

Ms. C does not have a family history of gynecological or breast cancer. Ms. C's maternal grandparents are deceased. Her grandfather died of a heart attack, and she thinks her grandmother had some form of dementia. Her paternal grandmother is deceased; Ms. C thinks she died of complications from diabetes. Her paternal grandfather is alive and in good health. Ms. C's father has high blood pressure and is taking medications for it. Her mother is in good health. She has two brothers, ages 35 and 37, and one sister, age 30. Her oldest brother has type 2 diabetes mellitus. Her other brother is in good health. Ms. C's sister has been diagnosed with endometriosis.

Many disorders, particularly cancers, have familial patterns.

Age of living relatives	Include the relationship and health of parents, siblings, and children.
Deaths	Include the relationship of the deceased person to the patient and the cause of death (specifically disorders that affect the genitourinary system, such as uterine cancer).
Chronic diseases; genitourinary disorders	Ask about chronic diseases in the family; include the relationship of the patient to the family member with the disease. Focus on genitourinary disorders or disorders that have genitourinary manifestations. *Cancers and diseases, such as endometriosis, tend to run in families.*
Genetic defects	Is there a history of congenital birth defects?

Social History

Ms. C lives with her husband and 4-year-old daughter. She works at a grocery store as a cashier and occasionally stocks shelves. She likes to hike and go camping, but she has not done either recently. She uses low-dose birth control pills. She quit smoking 5 years ago, drinks alcohol only occasionally, and denies using recreational drugs. Before marriage, she had several sexual partners and was treated once for an STD, a *Chlamydia* infection. She denies any sexual problems with her husband.

A patient's social history often helps narrow the diagnosis.

Family	Ask the patient to describe the current family unit.
Occupation	Ask about the patient's occupation.
Stress and stress management	Ask about stress level and stress management techniques. *Stress may affect the menstrual cycle.*
Hobbies	Ask about hobbies and activities. *Long-distance runners and women with low percentages of body fat may experience amenorrhea.*
Personal hygiene	Ask the patient about personal hygiene. Has she recently used any new products or douches? *Douches, bubble baths, and other products may cause allergic vaginitis.*
Use of tobacco	Ask about tobacco use, including types, amounts, duration of use, and exposure to secondary smoke. *Nicotine is a vasoconstrictor and may contribute to urinary problems.*
Use of alcohol	Does the patient drink alcohol? If so, which type and how much does she drink? *Alcohol use may be associated with dysuria.*
Use of recreational drugs	Is the patient using recreational drugs? If so, which drugs and how much? *Many recreational drugs, such as heroin, affect menstruation.*

Review of Systems

Many genitourinary diseases and disorders have manifestations in systems other than the genitourinary system. A comprehensive review of systems should be performed whenever possible; however, due to time and other types of constraints, the provider may be able to perform only a focused review of systems. During a focused review of systems, the provider targets questioning at the systems in which genitourinary problems are most likely to have manifestations. Following is a summary of common manifestations of female genitourinary problems.

System	Symptom or Sign	Possible Associated Diseases/Disorders
General	Fever	Uterine cancer, nephrolithiasis, urolithiasis, pyelonephritis, acute renal failure
	Chills	Pyelonephritis, urolithiasis
Respiratory	Orthopnea, dyspnea	Poststreptococcal glomerulonephritis
Gastrointestinal	Nausea and vomiting	Urolithiasis, pyelonephritis
	Mild nausea	Bacterial cystitis
Neurologic	Altered mental status in elderly patient	Urinary tract infection

Physical Examination

Equipment Needed

- Sterile gloves
- Speculum (Graves or Pederson)
- Cytology liquid or slides with slide covers with fixative
- Spatula
- Brush
- Broom
- Water-soluble lubricant
- Light source
- Chlamydia and gonorrhea kit
- Test tube (optional)
- Vaginal pipette (optional)
- KOH (optional)
- Sodium chloride (optional)

Components of Urinary Examination

Percussion and Palpation

For this examination, it is helpful if the patient is wearing a gown so that the abdomen and back can be exposed as needed. Remember to provide appropriate draping.

Action	Rationale
1. Percuss the kidneys. Ask the patient to sit upright. Expose the patient's back; drape as needed. To use the indirect method, place the palmar surface of one hand against the costovertebral angle. Using the other hand, make a fist and use the ulnar surface to strike the first hand. To use the direct method, make a fist and use the ulnar surface to strike the costovertebral angle directly.	1. The patient should not experience any tenderness or pain. Pain and tenderness may indicate glomerulonephritis or glomerulonephrosis.

Action	Rationale

Whichever method you use, strike the costovertebral angle with enough force to cause the patient to receive a painless jolt. Observe the patient for any pain or discomfort in this area.

2. Palpate the kidneys. Ask the patient to lie in a supine position. Expose the patient's abdomen, draping as appropriate.

   a. To palpate the left kidney: Stand on the patient's right side. Reach across the patient with your left arm and place your hand behind the patient's left flank area. Then, lift the left flank area with your left hand and palpate deeply with the palmar surface of your right hand.

     a. This will displace the kidney anteriorly. Normally, the left kidney is not palpable.
     A tender, painful kidney indicates an infection.
     An enlarged kidney may indicate hydronephrosis or polycystic disease.

   b. To palpate the right kidney: Remain on the patient's right side and lift the right flank area with your left hand. Use your right hand to palpate deeply.

     b. The right kidney is more often palpable. The kidney should feel firm, smooth, and solid. Chronic renal disease may cause the kidney to feel soft.

3. Percuss for bladder volume.

   3. Percussion of the suprapubic area can detect the dullness of bladder volume. The volume in the bladder must be approximately 400 to 600 mL before dullness is noted. A distended bladder may also be detected during percussion.

4. Palpate the bladder.

   4. The bladder is not usually palpable unless it is distended.

Components of Gynecological Examination

A chaperone should be in the room with the provider to assist with the examination as well as to serve as a witness. The patient should not have had sexual intercourse or used a douche for at least 24 hours before the examination. Ask the patient to empty her bladder before examination.

The equipment should be assembled and ready to use before the patient is in the room. Ensure that the room is a comfortable temperature and that privacy can be maintained.

For the examination, the patient should be undressed, wearing a gown, and draped. Assist the patient into lithotomy position; her buttocks should be at the edge of the table (**Figure 13-5**). Have the patient place her feet in the stirrups. Cover the stirrups with oven mitts or have the patient leave her socks on to make the examination more comfortable.

Gloves must be worn during this examination. Some examiners prefer to wear two pairs of gloves in case one pair must be discarded. Then when the provider removes a glove, there is still a clean glove on the hand. This also protects the provider and patient from contamination if a glove has a hole in it.

Always explain the examination to the patient, informing her of what you are doing as the examination proceeds. The examiner can ask questions during the examination or ask the patient if she has any questions. This distracts the patient and allows for a more open communication.

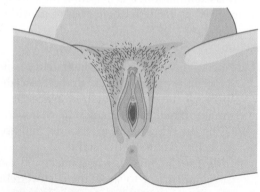
FIGURE 13-5 Lithotomy position.

External Genitalia: Inspection and Palpation

The patient should be positioned as described previously, and the examiner should sit at the foot of the examination table.

Action	Rationale

1. Assess the mons pubis for general hygiene, pubic hair distribution, and condition of the underlying skin.	1. Pubic hair should be coarse and cover the mons pubis, appearing as an inverse triangle. The texture of pubic hair may vary according to race. The underlying skin should be smooth and free of lesions. Some patients may have shaved pubic hair.
	
	    Small brown lice may be seen at the base of hair with pubic lice (pediculosis) infestation.
	
	    Hormonal problems may present with sparse hair.

2. Inspect the vulva for lesions, edema, color, or discharge.	2. Skin tone of the labia majora should be consistent with the rest of the patient's skin tone. The labia minora should appear pink. The vulva should be free of lesions and edema. Herpes simplex (**Figure 13-6**) presents with groups of vesicles on an erythematous base or crusted papules.

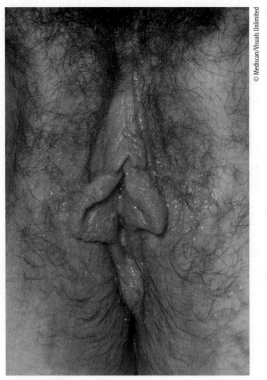

FIGURE 13-6 Herpes simplex.

© Mediscan/Visuals Unlimited

Action

Rationale

Genital warts, or condylomata acuminata, present as tiny pink or red painless swellings on the vulva and vaginal walls. In progressive disease, the warts may spread up the perineum and grow larger in size (**Figure 13-7**).

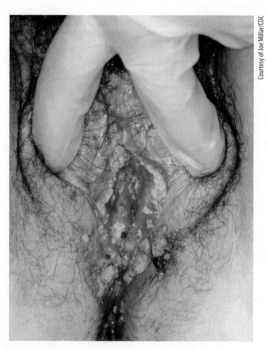

Courtesy of Joe Millar/CDC

FIGURE 13-7 Genital warts.

Syphilis usually presents with a single ulceration with a well-defined border.

Edema may occur with inflammatory infections.

3. Inspect the clitoris. Note the size.

3. The clitoris is usually about 2 cm in length and 0.5 cm in width.

An enlarged clitoris may suggest excess testosterone.

4. Examine the urethral orifice. Note the color and presence of discharge.

4. The urethral orifice should be pink and without discharge.

5. Inspect the vaginal introitus.

5. A small amount of clear or white discharge is normal.

Bulging of vaginal tissue through the orifice may be related to a cystocele.

Action	Rationale
6. Palpate the Bartholin's glands for masses, tenderness, or edema **(Figure 13-8)**.	6. The Bartholin's glands should be smooth. Tenderness and edema may indicate an abscess, and the patient should be referred to a specialist. A mass may indicate cancer; the patient should be referred to a specialist.

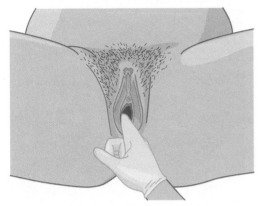

FIGURE 13-8 Palpating the Bartholin's glands.

Internal Genitalia: Inspection

Examination of the internal genitalia involves inspection and palpation. The examiner uses a speculum to inspect the internal structures. **Box 13-1** describes techniques for using a speculum. There are two types of speculum: the Graves and the Pederson (specula are depicted in **Figure 13-9**). The Graves speculum is plastic and comes in various sizes and lengths; most of these devices have an opening in which to insert a light source. The Pederson speculum is smaller and can be used on patients with a narrow introitus.

BOX 13-1   TECHNIQUES FOR USING A SPECULUM

The speculum helps the provider visualize internal structures. Use the following technique:

1. Explain the examination to the patient. Request that the patient relax her legs. Because this can be a traumatic experience, explain to the patient what you are going to do, show her the equipment, and explain how the equipment will be used.
2. Select an appropriately sized speculum—one that is comfortable for the patient and allows the examiner to clearly view the cervix.
3. Lubricate the tips of the speculum blades and gloves with warm water. Commercial lubricants may alter the results of Pap smears and cultures.
4. Spread the labia and open the introitus with your nondominant hand.
5. With your dominant hand, hold the speculum at a 45-degree angle with the blades pointed slightly down.
6. Gently insert the speculum into the vagina **(Figure A)**.
7. When the blades are in the vaginal vault, rotate the speculum to a horizontal position, so the blades are pointed downward **(Figure B)**. (If the patient is obese, the vagina walls may collapse. You may use a finger from a sterile glove or condom with the tip cut off to prevent the walls from collapsing and obstructing the view.)
8. Slowly open the blades **(Figure C)**.
9. The cervix should now be visible **(Figure D)**. Lock the speculum in place.

(continues)

BOX 13-1   TECHNIQUES FOR USING A SPECULUM *(continued)*

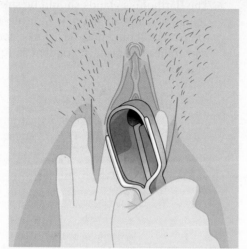

FIGURE A Inserting speculum into vagina.

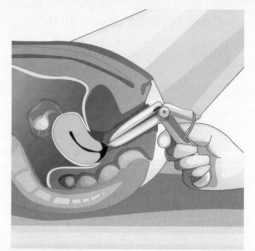

FIGURE B Speculum inserted in the vagina.

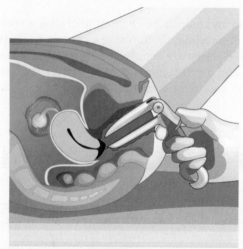

FIGURE C Examining the cervix.

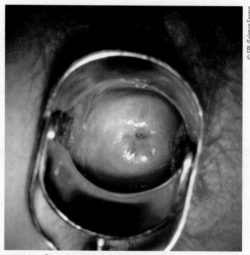

FIGURE D Opening the speculum.

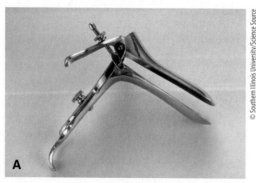

A

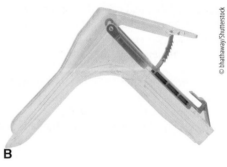

B

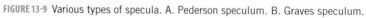

FIGURE 13-9 Various types of specula. A. Pederson speculum. B. Graves speculum.

Action	Rationale
1. Insert the speculum as described in Box 13-1. A large cotton swab may be used to mop up any excessive fluid.	1. This allows for clear visualization of internal structures.

2. Inspect the cervix.
   a. Note the color and texture.
	a. The cervix should be smooth, firm, pink, and protrude into the vagina. It should be symmetrical and round. There should not be any lesions, masses, ulcerations, strawberry spots, or discharge. The cervix may have a bluish hue in early pregnancy.
	   Table 13-1 depicts abnormal cervical findings.

Table 13-1   Abnormal Cervical Findings

Finding/Diagnosis	Description	Illustration
Nabothian cysts	Small, translucent, yellow nodules; appear as a result of chronic cervicitis or a cervical gland obstruction.	Nabothian cysts
Cervical eversion	Columnar epithelium from endocervix is everted; transformation zone is rough and deep red; tissue is friable.	Columnar epithelium / Squamous epithelium
Polyps	Bright red, soft protrusions from the external os; arise from cervical tissue.	Cervical polyps

(continues)

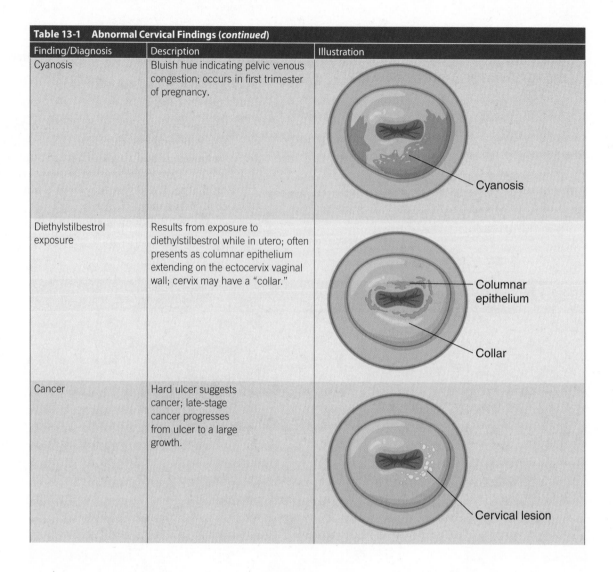

Table 13-1	Abnormal Cervical Findings (continued)	
Finding/Diagnosis	Description	Illustration
Cyanosis	Bluish hue indicating pelvic venous congestion; occurs in first trimester of pregnancy.	Cyanosis
Diethylstilbestrol exposure	Results from exposure to diethylstilbestrol while in utero; often presents as columnar epithelium extending on the ectocervix vaginal wall; cervix may have a "collar."	Columnar epithelium Collar
Cancer	Hard ulcer suggests cancer; late-stage cancer progresses from ulcer to a large growth.	Cervical lesion

Action	Rationale
b. Inspect the cervical os.	**b.** The os can be various shapes (**Figure 13-10**). In a nulliparous woman, the os is small and round. In a parous patient, it has a slit-like appearance.

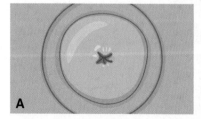
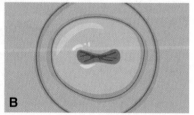

FIGURE 13-10 Shapes of the os. A. Nulliparous cervical os. B. Parous cervical os.

c. In the young adult, you will see the transformation zone. In the geriatric patient, the transformation zone will be in the os canal.	**c.** The transformation zone is an irregular, erythemic area that is friable.

Action	Rationale
3. As you withdraw the speculum, inspect the vagina. Check the vagina for color, discharge, rugae, lesions, and irritation.	**3.** The vagina is pink, moist, and free of lesions and irritation. There may be clear to white discharge. Any other color discharge is abnormal, as depicted in **Figure 13-11**.

At this point in the examination, the examiner may obtain smears and cultures as described in **Box 13-2**.

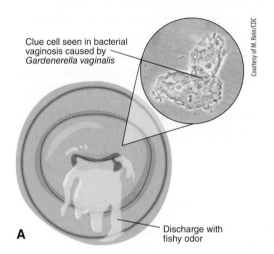

Clue cell seen in bacterial vaginosis caused by *Gardenerella vaginalis*

Discharge with fishy odor

Courtesy of M. Rein/CDC

A

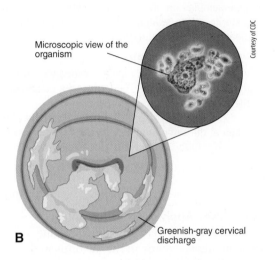

Microscopic view of the organism

Greenish-gray cervical discharge

Courtesy of CDC

B

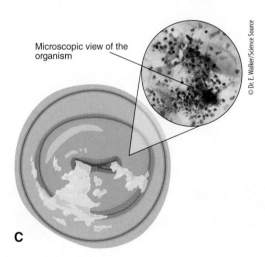

Microscopic view of the organism

© Dr. E. Walker/Science Source

C

FIGURE 13-11 Vaginitis. A. Bacterial vaginosis. B. Trichomonal vaginitis. C. Candidal vaginitis.

Bimanual Examination

Bimanual examination involves palpation of internal structures. As with all other aspects of this examination, explain what you are going to do to the patient.

BOX 13-2   CULTURES AND SMEARS

Cultures and smears all should be performed during the pelvic examination. Sterile gloves must be worn.

CULTURE SAMPLES FOR SEXUALLY TRANSMITTED DISEASES

Cultures for sexually transmitted diseases (STDs) should be performed before the Pap smear. The Centers for Disease Control and Prevention recommends testing any patient younger than the age of 25 years, any patient who is at high risk, or any patient who requests the testing.

To obtain a culture: Insert a sterile cotton swab into the os. Rotate it 360 degrees and leave it in the os for approximately 30 seconds. Remove the swab and place it in the vial.

CULTURES FOR INFECTION

Take samples for *Trichomonas* vaginitis, candidal vaginitis, and bacterial vaginosis after STD testing. Insert a sterile cotton swab into the os for approximately 20 seconds and swab in the vagina. Put the swab into a clean vial with sodium chloride.

PAPANICOLAOU SMEAR

Visualize the cervix. Scrape the exocervix with the wooden spatula; rotate the spatula 360 degrees. Spread the specimen on a glass slide. Insert a cytobrush 2 cm into the cervical canal and rotate it 180 degrees. Roll the brush onto the slide. Apply fixative.

If using the Thinprep, the plastic broom allows the samples from around the os and inside the os to be taken at the same time. Rotate the broom several times to take cells from all areas. Insert the broom into the fixative solution and swirl it around. Discard the broom.

Action	Rationale
1. Put on clean gloves. Apply the water-soluble jelly to the third and fourth fingers of your dominant hand. Insert the fingers gently in the introitus and with the other hand press on the lower abdomen, as depicted in **Figure 13-12**.	**1.** Clean gloves prevent cross-contamination. Water-soluble jelly decreases friction and is more comfortable for the patient.

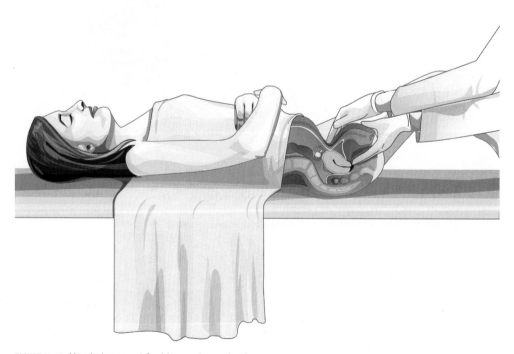

FIGURE 13-12 Hand placement for bimanual examination.

Action	Rationale
2. Palpate the vagina.	**2.** The vagina should be without masses or tenderness. A cystocele (protrusion of the bladder into the vagina) or rectocele (protrusion of the rectum into the vagina) may be palpated. A mass may indicate cancer of the vagina.
3. Palpate the cervix. Sweep the fingers around the protruding knob in the area of the fornices. Note the size, mobility, and firmness.	**3.** The cervix should be firm, soft, and mobile without tenderness. If the cervix is tender when moved, this suggests pelvic inflammatory disease. If the cervix extends into the vagina more than 3 cm, suspect a pelvic or ovarian mass. Endometriosis or a tumor may cause the cervix to be fixed. A cervix located low in the vagina may indicate vagina prolapse. Any masses or ulceration should be assessed and referred to a specialist.
4. Move your fingers slightly forward to palpate the uterus (**Figure 13-13**), including the fundus (the large upper end of the uterus). Push the uterus up toward the abdomen. With your other hand, gently press on the abdomen between the symphysis pubis and the umbilicus.	**4.** The uterus and fundus are located behind the cervix and within the pelvis.

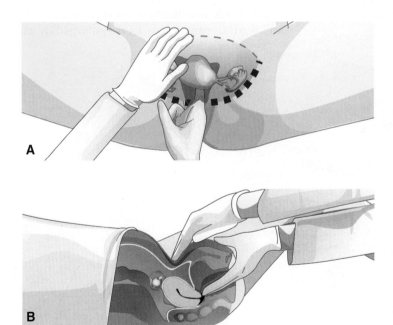

FIGURE 13-13 Palpating the uterus.

Action	Rationale

a. Note the position and mobility of the uterus. **Figure 13-14** depicts various positions of the uterus.

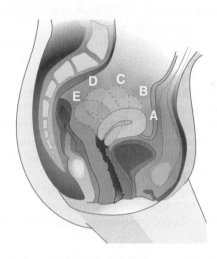

FIGURE 13-14 Positions of the uterus. A. Anteflexion. B. Anteversion (normal position). C. Midposition. D. Retroversion. E. Retroflexion.

b. Palpate for masses and tenderness.

5. Move your hand that is on the abdomen to the left. Press gently on the abdomen, pushing the hand slightly forward. Gently move the intravaginal hand to the left and palpate the ovary (**Figure 13-15**). Repeat on the other side.

5. The ovaries should be smooth, flat, mobile, and not tender.

You may not be able to palpate the ovaries in an obese or geriatric patient.

Polycystic ovarian syndrome, ovarian cysts, and ovarian cancer may cause enlarged ovaries.

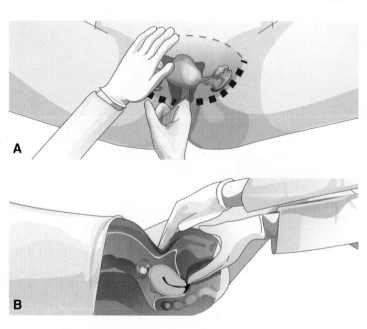

FIGURE 13-15 Palpating the ovaries.

Rectovaginal Examination

The rectovaginal examination is an important part of a pelvic examination, especially in postmenopausal women and women who complain of fullness or incontinence. As with all aspects of genitourinary examination, explain what you are going to do before you proceed.

Action	Rationale
1. Put on clean gloves. If wearing two pairs of gloves, pull off the first pair to reveal clean gloves. Apply water-soluble jelly to the second and third fingers.	1. Clean gloves will prevent cross-contamination of microorganisms from the vagina to the rectum.
2. Ask the patient to relax, and gently insert the second or index finger into the vagina and the third finger into the rectum. With your nondominant hand, press down on the abdomen (**Figure 13-16**).	2. These areas should be smooth, firm, movable, and not tender. Polyps, lesions, and hemorrhoids can be palpated in the sigmoid regions. Pain may indicate endometriosis. Palpate the internal vagina structures through the anterior rectum wall. Palpate the area behind the cervix, the cul-de-sac, and the rectovaginal septum. Finally, with a clean glove (lubricated with water-soluble jelly), slide the index finger into the anus and take a small stool sample for guaiac.

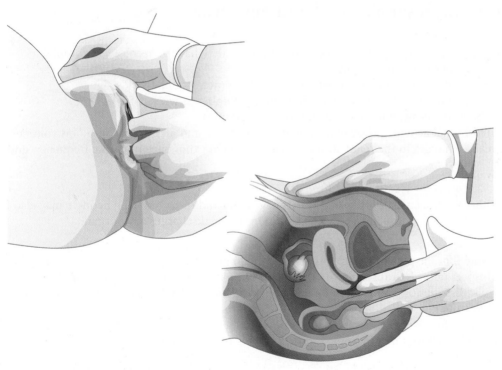

FIGURE 13-16 Performing rectovaginal examination.

Diagnostic Reasoning

Based on findings in the health history and physical examination, the clinician should formulate her or his assessment and plan. For example, a patient may report symptoms that suggest many possible diagnoses; however, findings in the past medical history and during the physical examination

Table 13-2   Differential Diagnosis of Pelvic Pain

Differential Diagnoses	Significant Findings in the Patient's History	Significant Findings in the Patient's Physical Examination	Diagnostic Tests
Ectopic pregnancy	Vaginal bleeding, pain that occurs on one side or that radiates to the middle, history of PID	Tenderness on palpation, cervical pain on movement of the cervix	β-hCG, ultrasound
Spontaneous abortion	Crampy pelvic pain, lower back pain, abnormal vaginal bleeding	Visualization of the cervix shows dilation or tissue passing through the cervical os	Ultrasound
Pyelonephritis	Flank pain, chills, fever, nausea	Costovertebral angle tenderness	Urinalysis, urine culture, IVP
Pelvic inflammatory disease	Pelvic pain, vaginal discharge, abnormal bleeding, dysuria	Abdominal tenderness, cervical discharge, cervical motion tenderness	CBC, ultrasound

Abbreviations: β-hCG, serum beta-human chorionic gonadotropin; CBC, complete blood chemistry; IVP, intravenous pyelography; PID, pelvic inflammatory disease.

might narrow the possible diagnoses down to one or two. Pelvic pain is a common chief complaint. **Table 13-2** illustrates the differential diagnosis of common disorders associated with pelvic pain.

Genitourinary Assessment of Special Populations

Considerations for the Pregnant Patient

Pregnant patients usually visit their obstetrician when they have gynecological complaints.
- Note physiological changes:
  - The cervix of a pregnant patient is bluish, known as Chadwick's sign.
  - The uterus will enlarge depending on the number of weeks of pregnancy.
- Use a cotton swab to take the endocervical samples.
- Hormonal activity, pressure from a growing uterus, and an increase in blood volume cause changes in the renal structure. Patients often experience nocturia, frequency, and urgency.

Considerations for the Neonatal Patient

The mother's estrogen causes the neonate to have a mucoid discharge. The neonate may also have some bloody spotting, called pseudomenstruation. These discharges are normal.

Considerations for the Pediatric Patient

- Note that the pediatric patient has soft labia majora.
- Inspect pubic hair distribution and breast budding to determine the Tanner stage. Pubic hair distribution and growth begin in puberty. **Figure 13-17** depicts stages of pubic hair growth.
- Inspect for discharge, ecchymosis, and bleeding; none should be apparent. Pediatric patients can have *Candida* infections for various reasons, especially prolonged wearing of wet garments.
- Inspect the hymen. A completely closed hymen will prevent discharge of blood during menses and should be referred to a specialist. (A torn hymen needs further investigation and should be referred to a specialist immediately, as this finding is an indication of possible sexual abuse.)
- Ask about sexual activity. A sexually active patient should have yearly pelvic and Pap examinations. If the patient is not sexually active, pelvic examinations should begin at age 21.

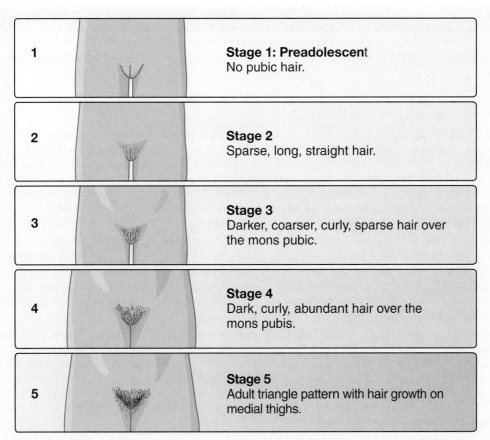

1 **Stage 1: Preadolescent**
No pubic hair.

2 **Stage 2**
Sparse, long, straight hair.

3 **Stage 3**
Darker, coarser, curly, sparse hair over
the mons pubic.

4 **Stage 4**
Dark, curly, abundant hair over the
mons pubis.

5 **Stage 5**
Adult triangle pattern with hair growth on
medial thighs.

FIGURE 13-17 Tanner stages of development.

- If sexual abuse is suspected, refer the patient to a specialist.
- The menstrual cycle is irregular during the first 2 years of onset because of physiological anovulation.
- Kidney function is comparable to that of an adult by age 2.

Considerations for the Geriatric Patient

Note that menopausal and postmenopausal patients show gynecological changes primarily due to decreased estrogen levels.

- The external genitalia and labia majora, are thin and atrophied. The pubic hair is sparse, gray, and thin.
- The vagina is pale, has decreased rugae and elasticity, and is dry; the cervix is pale.

Note physiological changes in the urinary system:

- In the elderly, muscles become weak; this is especially true of bladder muscles, which can lead to urine retention and incomplete emptying of the bladder. This leads to frequent urinary tract infection and nocturia. Weak pelvic floor muscles can lead to incontinence, such as stress incontinence.
- The pH of the vagina changes post menopause, leading to the demise of lactobacilli and increasing the incidence of vaginal infections, vaginal dryness, and UTIs in some older females.
- Renal failure will manifest as peripheral edema, periorbital edema, shortness of breath, change in blood pressure, and neurological changes.

Case Study Review

Throughout the first half of this chapter, you have been introduced to Ms. C. This section of the chapter pulls together her history and demonstrates the documentation of her history and physical examination.

Chief Complaint

"I'm having pelvic pain."

Information Gathered During the Interview

KC is a 24-year-old Caucasian woman who comes to the clinic with a chief complaint of pelvic pain. She has experienced pelvic pain for the last 6 months. Ms. C says the pain has progressively become worse. It started as an intermittent, dull pain, but now it is a constant, sharp pain. She says she is itchy and has minimal discharge, which she describes as grayish in color and without odor. She denies swelling, masses, lesions, odor, or nausea and vomiting. She says she has felt feverish, but has not taken her temperature. She denies vaginal bleeding and says her last menses was 2 weeks ago but was not normal. She says her menses was very heavy. She is experiencing dysuria. She has taken birth control pills for the last 3 years.

Ms. C states that she has been in good health. She has had upper respiratory infections and a recent urinary tract infection, which she says was treated with an antibiotic (she cannot remember the name). She has no history of recent trauma. She denies any surgeries. Her last gynecological examination was 2 years ago, and she says that the Pap smear was normal. Ms. C has been pregnant once and has one child, delivered vaginally. She is married and monogamous. Prior to her marriage, she was diagnosed with chlamydia, which was treated.

Ms. C does not have a family history of gynecological or breast cancer. Ms. C's maternal grandparents are deceased. Her grandfather died of a heart attack, and she thinks her grandmother had some form of dementia. Her paternal grandmother is deceased; Ms. C thinks she died of complications from diabetes. Her paternal grandfather is alive and in good health. Ms. C's father has high blood pressure and is taking medications for it. Her mother is in good health. She has two brothers, ages 35 and 37, and one sister, age 30. Her oldest brother has type 2 diabetes mellitus. Her other brother is in good health. Ms. C's sister has been diagnosed with endometriosis.

Ms. C lives with her husband and 4-year-old daughter. She works at a grocery store as a cashier and occasionally stocks shelves. She likes to hike and go camping, but she has not done either recently. She uses low-dose birth control pills. She quit smoking 5 years ago, drinks alcohol only occasionally, and denies using recreational drugs. Before marriage, she had several sexual partners and was treated once for an STD, a *Chlamydia* infection. She denies any sexual problems with her husband.

Clues	Important Points
Pelvic pain and vaginal discharge	These findings may suggest PID, STDs, *Candida* infection, or bacterial vaginosis.
History of urinary tract infections	Previous urinary tract infections are a risk factor for UTIs.
Fever	A fever suggests an infection.
Cervical motion tenderness and adnexal tenderness	These findings suggest PID.

Name KC	Date 8/2/15	Time 1000
	DOB 6/16/91	Sex F

HISTORY
CC "I have pelvic pain."
HPI 24-year-old female with a 6-month history of pelvic pain, which has become worse in the last 2 weeks. Started as intermittent and dull; has become constant and sharp. Reports pruritus in the genital region; scant, grayish discharge; and dysuria. Reports feeling feverish. Denies swelling, masses, lesions, odor, nausea, and vomiting. Denies vaginal bleeding. LMP = 2 weeks ago (7/20/15); was abnormally heavy.

Medications
1. Birth control pill (unknown name), 1 tablet PO daily
2. Ibuprofen, 200 mg, PO qid prn for pain

Allergies
NKA

PMI
Illnesses
Hx of chlamydia, URI, and a recent UTI. No hx of recent trauma. Last gyn exam was 2 years ago; she reports a normal Pap smear. Gravida 1, para 1.

Hospitalizations/Surgeries
Denies any surgeries.

FH
No FH of breast or gynecological cancer. Father has HTN and is taking medication. Mother is in good health. Maternal grandparents are deceased. Her grandfather died of a heart attack and her grandmother had some form of dementia. Paternal grandmother died of complications of type 2 diabetes; her grandfather is alive and well. Her oldest brother has diabetes and is taking medication for it; her other brother is in good health. Her sister was diagnosed with endometriosis. Her husband and daughter are in good health.

SH
Lives with husband and daughter. Works as a cashier at a grocery store. Occasionally hikes and goes camping. Quit smoking 5 years ago. Drinks alcohol only occasionally. Denies recreational drug use. Monogamous; prior to marriage had several sexual partners and was treated for a chlamydia infection.

ROS

General	Cardiovascular
Feels feverish.	Denies chest pain, edema.
Skin	Respiratory
Denies nonhealing sores.	Denies SOB.
Eyes	Gastrointestinal
Denies any problems or changes.	Denies nausea and vomiting.
Ears	Genitourinary/Gynecological
Denies any problems.	See HPI.
Nose/Mouth/Throat	Musculoskeletal
Denies any problems.	Denies any problems.
Breast	Neurological
Denies any lumps, tenderness, or discharge.	Denies any problems.

PHYSICAL EXAMINATION

Weight 140 lb	Temp 100.5	BP 148/86
Height 5'8"	Pulse 98	Resp 20

General Appearance
24-year-old Caucasian female in acute distress, slightly bent and holding her pelvic area. Tall, slender, well groomed, and pleasant. States she is in pain; on a scale of 1–10 her pain level is 7.

Skin
Warm and dry to touch; no ecchymosis or lesions; few freckles on the nose.

HEENT
Normal hair distribution. No ear pain or drainage; tympanic membrane pearly gray, cerumen. Scleras are white; no excessive tearing; PERRL; EOMs intact. No caries or bleeding gums. Neck is supple; no lymphadenopathy.

Cardiovascular
Regular rhythm, no murmur; radial pulse +3; femoral pulse +3.

Respiratory
Lungs clear to auscultation.

Gastrointestinal
Abdomen soft and flat; bowel sounds normal; no masses.

Genitourinary

Vulva: Shaved pubic hair; no lesions or erythema.

Vagina: Slight odor and grayish discharge present. Vagina is red; no lesion.

Cervix: Firm, transformation zone visible, small Nabothian cyst at 1100, friable, os open to Q-tip; cervical motion tenderness present.

Uterus: Firm, oval shaped; no masses palpated.

Adnexa: Motion tenderness present; no masses palpated.

Rectovaginal: No masses palpated, but tender to palpation.

Musculoskeletal

Full range of motion without pain; no edema; strength 4/5.

Neurological

Alert and oriented × 3; no tremors; CNS II–XII intact.

Other

Lab Tests

Sodium: 142 mmol/L

Potassium: 4.2 mmol/L WBC 11.5 × 103

Chloride: 105 mmol/L RBC 4.1 × 106

CO^2: 28 mmol/L Hgb 13.5 g/dL

Anion gap: 8 Hct 39.0%

BUN: 18 mg/dL MCV 88 fl

Creatinine 0.9 mg/dL MCHC 32.2 g/dL

Glucose: 100 mg/dL RDW 12.0%

Calcium: 8.9 mg/dL PLT 311 × 103

Total protein: 5.9 g/dL

Bilirubin: total 0.3 mg/dL, urinalysis

Alk phos: 82 U/L, color: brown

AST (SGOT): 13 U/L, turbidity: cloudy

ALT (SGPT): 12 U/L, sp. gr. >1.030

Urinalysis

Fasting: No

Color: brown

Turbidity: cloudy

Sp gr: > 1.03

pH 7.4

Glucose: negative

Urobilinogen: present

Nitrite: present

Leukocytes: present

Blood: present

Special Tests

Pelvic ultrasound found a tubo-ovarian abscess on the left side.

Chlamydia and gonorrhea tests were negative.

Wet mount for bacterial vaginosis, *Candida*, and *Trichomonas* was negative.

Final Assessment Findings

1. PID
2. UTI

ADVANCED ASSESSMENT OF THE BREASTS

Anatomy and Physiology Review of the Breast and Lymph Nodes

The Breast

The breasts are mammary glands, secondary reproductive glands, and modified sebaceous glands. Their main function is to provide nutrition in the form of milk to newborns. They have a secondary function as a sexual attraction and a sexual stimulation. Females start to develop breasts late in pre-adolescence; the breasts continue to develop until the female reaches maturity. The male has breasts but they are not functional and do not develop after puberty due to hormone changes. The hormones estrogen and progestin from the ovaries control the growth and development of the breasts. Occasionally the male breast will enlarge (referred to as gynecomastia), which is due to hormones or body mass.

The female breasts (**Figure 13-18**) are located over the pectoralis major and serratus anterior muscles of the anterior chest wall. They extend from the second rib to the sixth rib and from the sternal edge to the axillary line. A triangle of breast tissue extends into the axilla (called the tail of Spence).

Each breast has a nipple and areola, which are darker in color than the patient's surrounding skin. The nipple is centrally located in the breasts and has tiny openings that allow milk to pass from the lactiferous ducts. The areola that surrounds the nipple contains sebaceous glands, also called Montgomery glands. These glands are irregular, elevated, small, round papules. They secrete a lipid, which lubricates the area during lactation to prevent fissures and dryness. The periphery of the areola also has hair follicles embedded in it and smooth erectile muscle. The smooth muscles cause the nipple to become erect during sexual stimulation or by the stimulation of a feeding infant. During embryonic development, the fetus may develop supernumerary nipples along the milk lines.

The breasts are composed of three tissue types: glandular, fibrous, and adipose. Breast size depends on the amount of the three tissues. The amount of the tissue depends on body size, hormone cycle, age, nutritional status, and genetics.

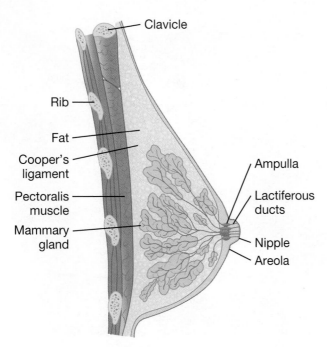

FIGURE 13-18 Anatomy of the breast.

The glandular tissue consists of 15 to 20 lobes arranged in a circle. The lobes are made of lobules and the secreting alveolar, or acini cells, which are arranged in clusters. The alveoli produce milk. The milk flows through mammary ducts, which merge to form a single lactiferous duct. The lactiferous duct delivers milk to the nipple. If the female is breastfeeding, milk is stored in the lactiferous sinus.

Breasts are supported by the fibrous tissue, known as Cooper's ligaments. These ligaments start at the skin and extend through the breasts and attach to the deep muscle fascia of the anterior chest wall.

The glandular tissue is embedded in the adipose (fatty) tissue. The fatty tissue, as well as the subcutaneous and retromammary fat, gives the breasts size and shape.

Lymph Nodes

The breasts of females and males have a lymphatic system that drains impurities and lymph to the blood (**Figure 13-19**). This network consists of superficial and deep parenchymatous nodes.

The pectoral (anterior) lymph nodes are located at the lower border of the pectoralis major inside the anterior axillary fold; they drain most of the breast and the anterior chest wall. The brachial or lateral nodes are located in the upper humerus and drain most of the arm. The subscapular or posterior nodes are located in the lateral scapular border and deep in the posterior axillary fold; they drain the rest of the arm and the posterior chest wall. The pectoralis, brachial, and subscapular nodes drain into the midaxillary nodes. The parenchymatous nodes are not palpable; located deep within the breast, they drain the lobules.

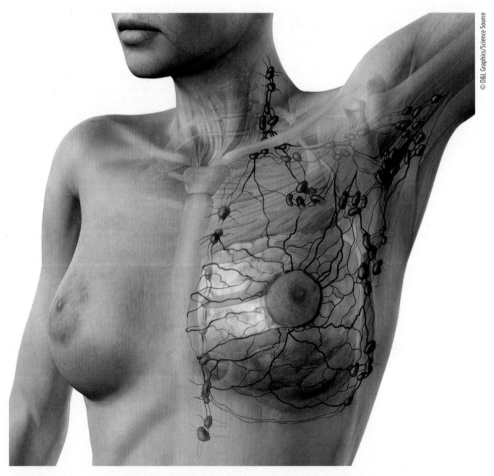

FIGURE 13-19 Lymphatic system of the breast and axilla.

Health History

A thorough health history helps diagnose and detect breast disorders and diseases, especially breast cancer. A family history of breast cancer is a risk factor for breast cancer.

Chief Complaint and History of Present Illness

"I found a lump in my right breast."

JM is a 56-year-old African American woman who comes to the clinic with a chief complaint of a lump in her right breast. She reports a clear discharge from the right nipple. Ms. M says she felt the lump about 3 months ago and it seems to be getting larger. She denies pain and says the lump does not seem movable.

Breast Lump (Mass)

A breast mass or lump can be benign or malignant and can be caused by various medical problems, such as fibroadenoma, fibrocystic disease, fat necrosis, abscess, or cancer. Benign breast conditions and tumors are depicted in **Figure 13-20**.

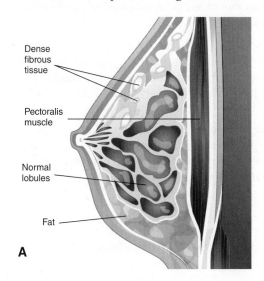

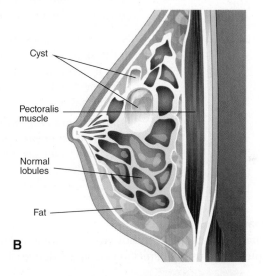

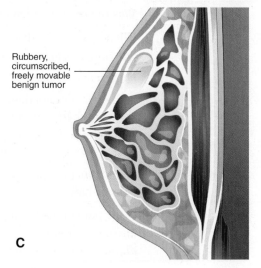

FIGURE 13-20 Benign breast conditions. A. Fibrocystic changes. B. Cysts. C. Fibroadenoma.

Fibroadenomas are either round, lobular, or ovoid. They are firm, well-defined, singular, mobile, and usually not tender. They usually occur between puberty and menopause. Fibrocystic disease or benign breast disease is the presence of well-defined, round, elastic, mobile, tender cysts. They usually occur between 30 years of age and the onset of menopause, after which they become less noticeable or disappear. Fat necrosis is a rare finding but can cause skin or nipple retraction. The fat necrosis mass is round, usually tender, and there is ecchymosis. A breast abscess is also rare in women who are not lactating but can occur around the areola. The mass is ecchymotic and tender, and it can drain purulent discharge. Malignant breast mass is usually nontender, firm, irregularly shaped, and fixed to the underlying tissue.

Onset	Was the onset acute or gradual? Is the lump related to the menstrual cycle?
	Before the menstrual cycle, the breast may be "lumpy" and tender.
Quality	Is the lump tender or mobile?
	Has the lump changed in size or shape?
	A malignant breast mass is usually nontender, firm, and irregular in shape. Tenderness may be due to mastitis, interductal papilloma, cystic mastitis, or cystic adenosis.
Associated symptoms	Is there any redness or dimpling of the breast? Are there any changes in the skin color or texture? Is the patient experiencing any pain, and does it occur at specific times? Is the patient experiencing discharge from the nipple? If so, ask her to describe the color and consistency of the discharge.
	Inflammation may indicate an infection. Dimpling and a texture similar to an orange peel (peau d'orange) suggest cancer. Pain before and during menses may be a side effect of some oral contraceptives. Pain is also a sign of late-stage cancer. Purulent discharge may indicate an abscess.

Discharge

Discharge is another common chief complaint. The nature of the discharge, along with associated symptoms, helps the clinician determine diagnosis.

Onset	Was the onset sudden or gradual?
Quality	What color is the discharge? Is it bloody or blood-tinged?
	A bloody discharge suggests cancer.
	Duct ectasia produces a green or brown discharge.
Location	Is the patient experiencing discharge bilaterally or from one breast? Is the discharge from one or multiple ducts?
	Discharge emanating from one duct suggests cancer, whereas multiple duct involvement suggests infection.
Associated symptoms	Is the patient experiencing associated symptoms, such as tenderness or pain or lumps?
Medication taken	Is the patient taking any medications?
	Medications such as oral contraceptives, steroids, phenothiazines, digitalis, and diuretics cause a clear discharge.

Past Medical History

Ms. M states she had gallbladder surgery 2 years ago, an appendectomy when she was 16, and a tonsillectomy as a child. She had pertussis, measles, and mumps as a child. She has high blood pressure and is taking medication for it. Her last physician told her she is borderline diabetic. Ms. M denies any trauma to her chest.

She says she started her menses at the age of 12. She took birth control pills from age 20 to 23. Ms. M has five children; all were vaginal deliveries. She reports that onset of perimenopause occurred when she was 48 years old and lasted 5 years. Although she did not have a lot of hot flashes or night sweats, her provider prescribed hormone replacement therapy "to prevent heart disease, strokes, and bone loss."

Her last breast examination and mammogram were 3 years ago, but she does breast self-examinations monthly. She says that her mammogram showed some calcifications but was otherwise normal.

Past health conditions or surgeries	Ask the patient about past or chronic health conditions. Has the patient had any breast disorders?
	A history of breast cancer increases the patient's risk for cancer.
	Does the patient have history of breast surgeries or biopsies? Does the patient have, or has the patient ever had, breast implants?
	Implants, especially silicone implants, can cause breast problems. Surgery may change the shape and appearance of breasts.
Trauma	Has the patient ever experienced any trauma to the chest?
Onset of menses and/or menopause	Ask the patient about the onset of menses. If the patient is menopausal or postmenopausal, ask her about the onset of menopause.
	Patients who began menses before the age of 13 or who began menopause after the age of 52 have a higher risk of breast cancer.
Last menses	Ask the patient the date of her last menstruation.
	Hormone-related tenderness, swelling, and lumpiness are decreased after menstruation.
Number of pregnancies	How many times has the patient been pregnant?
	Women who have never given birth or who have given birth after the age of 30 have a higher risk of cancer.
Last clinical breast examination or mammogram	When were the patient's last breast examination and mammogram, and what were the results?
	A lump may have been found previously.

Family History

Ms. M reports that her paternal grandfather died of a heart attack and her paternal grandmother died of a stroke. Her maternal grandfather died of heart failure, and her maternal grandmother died of breast cancer. Her father died in a car accident when she was an infant and her mother remarried. Her stepfather and mother are alive. Her mother has arthritis and high blood pressure and is taking medications. Ms. M has two half-brothers, 54 and 51 years old, and one half-sister, 52 years old. The older half-brother was diagnosed with colon cancer 2 years ago. He had surgery and chemotherapy, and his cancer is in remission. Her other half-brother has a heart murmur and takes a lot of medications. Her half-sister was diagnosed with breast cancer 1 year ago. She had a left mastectomy with 21 lymph nodes removed, radiation therapy, and chemotherapy, and is now doing well. Ms. M has five children: three sons and two daughters. Her daughters, ages 32 and 28, are well. Her oldest and youngest sons, ages 30 and 22, have type 2 diabetes mellitus. The 30-year-old takes insulin; the youngest son takes an oral medication. Both of the diabetic sons also have high blood pressure and are on blood pressure medications. Her middle son, age 26, is well.

Age of living relatives	Include the relationship and health of parents, siblings, and children.
Deaths	Include the relationship of the deceased person to the patient and the cause of death (specifically, disorders that affect the breast, such as breast cancer).
Chronic diseases; genitourinary disorders	Ask about chronic diseases in the family; include the relationship of the patient to the family member with the disease. Focus on breast disorders, specifically breast cancer, or disorders that have genitourinary manifestations. *A family history of breast cancer increases a patient's risk for the disease.*

Social History

Ms. M works as a certified nursing assistant for a home health agency. She is divorced and lives alone. Ms. M is not sexually active. Her children all live in the area and visit her frequently. She has many friends and enjoys visiting museums. She is a smoker; she says she smokes about eight cigarettes per day. She denies alcohol or recreational drug use.

Family	Ask the patient to describe the current family unit.
Occupation	Ask about the patient's occupation. Is the patient exposed to chemicals? *Chemicals increase the risk of cancer.*
Use of tobacco	Ask about tobacco use, including types, amounts, duration of use, and exposure to secondary smoke.
Use of alcohol	Does the patient drink alcohol? If so, which type and how much does she drink?
Use of recreational drugs	Is the patient using recreational drugs? If so, which drugs and how much?
Medications taken	Is the patient taking hormones, contraceptives, or antipsychotic drugs? *Hormones and some antipsychotic drugs may cause breast engorgement. Oral contraceptives may increase the risk of cancer. Haloperidol may cause galactorrhea.*

Review of Systems

Unlike most disorders, breast diseases and disorders usually do not have manifestations in other systems. A comprehensive review of systems should still be performed whenever possible. Due to time and other types of constraints, the provider may be able to perform only a focused review of systems. During a focused review of systems, the provider targets questioning at the systems in which breast problems are most likely to have manifestations. Infections, such as mastitis or mammary abscess, may present with fever or chills. On rare occasions, late-stage breast cancer may present with bone pain.

Physical Examination

Equipment Needed

- Draping
- Gown
- Gloves
- Equipment for culture (optional)

Components of the Physical Examination

The breast examination involves inspection and palpation. The patient should be wearing a gown, and the clinician should use drapes to provide privacy.

Inspection

Action	Rationale
1. Ask the patient to sit at the edge of the examination table and to remove (fold down) the top of the gown. Have the patient let her arms rest at her sides (**Figure 13-21**). Inspect the breasts for size and symmetry.	1. The breasts should be symmetrical and approximately equal in size. It is normal for one breast to be slightly larger than the other. In the male, the breasts lie flat against the chest wall with a protruding nipple.

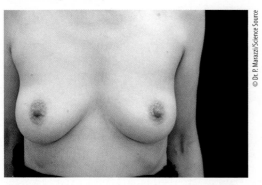

FIGURE 13-21 Initial position for inspecting the breasts.

Action	Rationale
2. Inspect the skin for texture and color. Inspect the venous system.	2. The skin should be smooth and soft. Nevi, seborrheic keratosis, striae, or supernumerary nipples are normal findings. A unilateral predominant venous system indicates engorged veins from a disease and is associated with malignant tumors.
3. Inspect the nipples and areola.	3. The color is darker than the surrounding skin. The nipples should be the same size and shape bilaterally. Occasionally, one or both nipples will be inverted. A recently developed, unilateral inverted nipple suggests fibrosis and malignancy.

Montgomery tubercles are visible on the areola in females and males.

A crusty, red, scaly nipple may indicate Paget's disease (**Figure 13-22***).

Except during pregnancy or lactation, discharge without palpation is always abnormal.

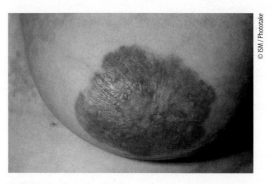

FIGURE 13-22 Paget's disease.

Action	Rationale
4. Inspect the breasts for masses, retraction, dimpling, or ecchymosis. To inspect further for dimpling, have the patient put her hands on her hips. Then have her raise her arms over her head. Inspect the axillae. Next have her stand, place her hands on her hips, and lean forward slightly. **Figure 13-23** depicts the additional positions for inspection.	4. These positions allow the provider to check for dimpling and free movement of the breasts. There should be no retraction, dimpling, or ecchymosis. Dimpling indicates a tumor, which has caused shortening of the fibrotic areas or the Cooper's ligaments. Ecchymosis indicates infection or inflammation. Females often shave the axillae. In men, there will be hair. Skin tags are a normal finding.

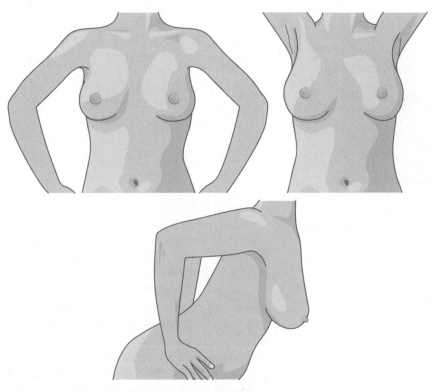

FIGURE 13-23 Additional positions for inspecting the breasts.

Palpation

Action	Rationale
1. Assist the patient into a supine position with her arms above her head (**Figure 13-24**). Place a small pillow or rolled-up towel under the back. The breasts can be divided into four quadrants plus the tail of Spence to identify any abnormalities (**Figure 13-25**).	1. The pillow or rolled-up towel helps spread the breast.

Action   **Rationale**

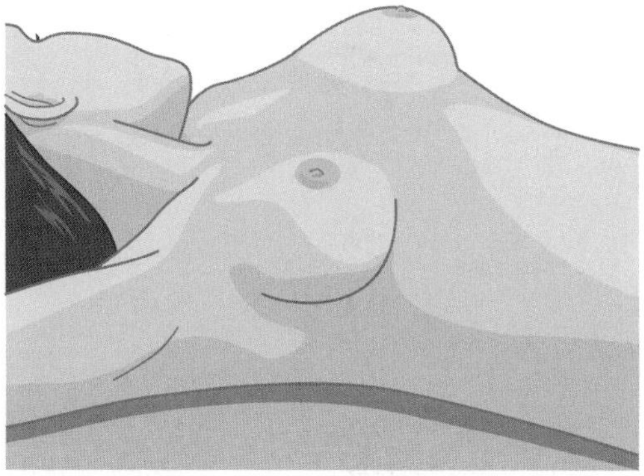

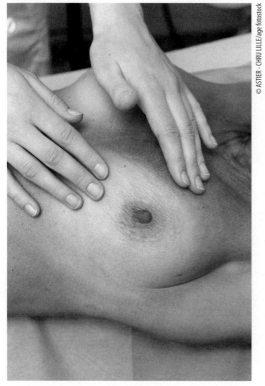

FIGURE 13-24 Position for palpating the breasts.

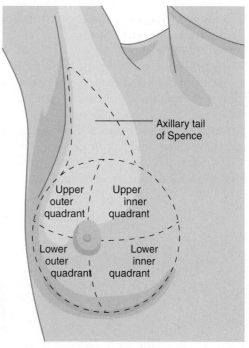

© ASTIER - CHRU LILLE/age fotostock

FIGURE 13-25 Quadrants of the breast, used to describe findings.

FIGURE 13-26 Palpating the breast.

2. Palpate the breast (**Figure 13-26**). You may use the circular, wedged, or vertical strip technique to palpate the breast. The vertical strip technique is the preferred method for palpation; it is the most effective in detecting abnormalities.

2. In young women, the breast may be lobular. Premenstrually, palpation may reveal cysts, which are well defined, freely mobile, and tender. A malignant tumor usually presents as a single mass in one breast. The lump is usually nontender, firm, irregularly shaped, and fixed to the surrounding tissue.

Action   **Rationale**

Circular: Use the three middle-finger pads of your dominant hand and palpate gently in a circle, starting either at the tail of Spence or from the center near the areola.

Wedged: Use the three middle-finger pads of your dominant hand and palpate gently toward the nipple or from the nipple to the edge of the breast tissue.

Vertical strip: Use the three middle-finger pads of your dominant hand and palpate gently up and down the breast, starting at the outer edge of the breast.

Figure 13-27 depicts these techniques.

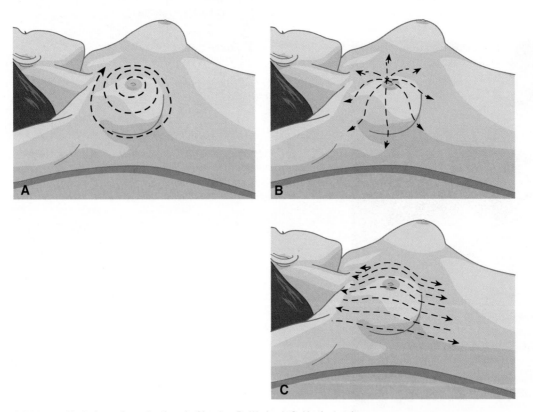

FIGURE 13-27 Techniques for palpation. A. Circular. B. Wedged. C. Vertical strip.

3. Palpate the nipple (**Figure 13-28**). Using the index finger, gently compress the nipple.

3. There should be no masses or tenderness. Assess any discharge for color and consistency. Bloody discharge suggests intraductal papilloma. Bilateral, clear, or milky discharge that increases during menses suggests benign breast disease. Greenish nipple discharge suggests duct ectasia.

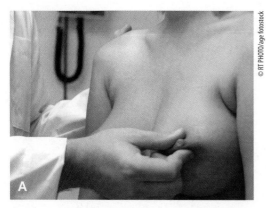
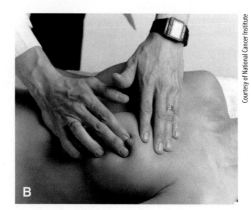

FIGURE 13-28 Palpating the nipple. A. For masses. B. For discharge.

Action	Rationale
4. Ask the patient to sit up and move to the edge of the examination table. Support the patient's arm with your nondominant hand. With the dominant hand, gently palpate from the center of the axilla downward toward the ribs. Then, palpate the lymph nodes along the upper arm by pressing your fingers into the inner arm.	4. The axilla should be smooth. Any lymph nodes should be small, movable, and nontender. You should not feel any masses or enlarged or tender lymph nodes.

Encourage the patient to perform breast self-examination. **Box 13-3** describes the recommended technique.

BOX 13-3   BREAST SELF-EXAMINATION

STEP 1

- Stand before a mirror.
- Check both breasts for anything unusual.
- Look for discharge from the nipple and puckering, dimpling, or scaling of the skin.

The next two steps check for any changes in the contour of your breasts. As you do them, you should be able to feel your muscles tighten.

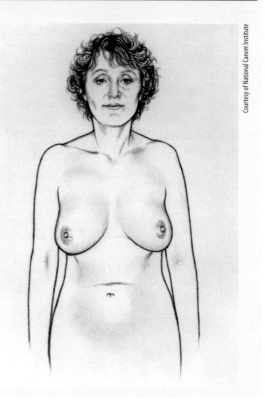

(continues)

BOX 13-3   BREAST SELF-EXAMINATION *(continued)*

STEP 2

- Watch closely in the mirror as you clasp your hands behind your head and press your hands forward.
- Note any change in the contour of your breasts.

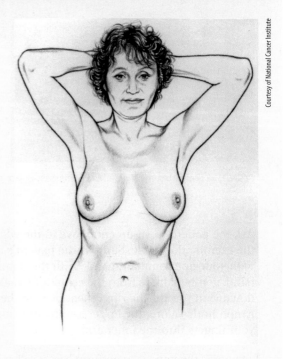

Courtesy of National Cancer Institute

STEP 3

- Press your hands firmly on your hips and bow slightly toward the mirror as you pull your shoulders and elbows forward.
- Note any change in the contour of your breasts.

Some women perform the next part of the examination in the shower. Your fingers will glide easily over soapy skin, so you can concentrate on feeling for changes inside the breast.

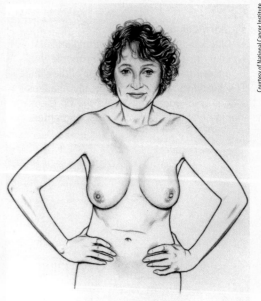

Courtesy of National Cancer Institute

BOX 13-3 BREAST SELF-EXAMINATION *(continued)*

STEP 4

- Raise your left arm.
- Use three or four fingers of your right hand to feel your left breast firmly, carefully, and thoroughly.
- Beginning at the outer edge, press the flat part of your fingers in small circles, moving the circles slowly around the breast.
- Gradually work toward the nipple.
- Be sure to cover the whole breast.
- Pay special attention to the area between the breast and the underarm, including the underarm itself.
- Feel for any unusual lumps or masses under the skin.
- If you have any spontaneous discharge during the month—whether or not it is during your BSE—see your doctor.
- Repeat the examination on your right breast.

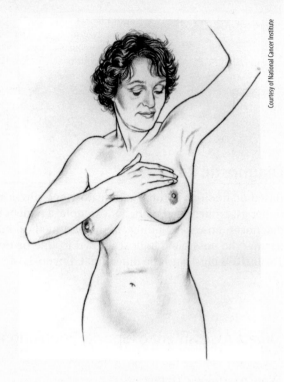

Courtesy of National Cancer Institute

STEP 5

- Lie flat on your back with your left arm over your head and a pillow or folded towel under your left shoulder. (This position flattens your breast and makes it easier to check.)
- Repeat the actions of Step 4 in this position for each breast.

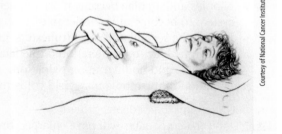

Courtesy of National Cancer Institute

Text reproduced from Smeltzer, S. C., & Bare, B. (2004). *Brunner and Suddarth's textbook of medical–surgical nursing* (10th ed.). Philadelphia, PA: Lippincott Williams & Wilkins. Modified from U.S. Department of Health and Human Services, & Public Health Service. (2003). *What you need to know about breast cancer*. Bethesda, MD: National Institutes of Health.

Table 13-3 Differential Diagnosis of Breast Lumps			
Differential Diagnoses	Significant Findings in the Patient's History	Significant Findings in the Patient's Physical Examination	Diagnostic Tests
Breast cancer	New nontender lump, family history of breast cancer, older age, late menopause, early menarche, nulliparity	Single, firm, irregularly shaped, nontender, fixed lump; dimpling; retraction; bloody nipple discharge; asymmetry of breasts	Mammogram, biopsy, or aspiration
Fibroadenoma	Mobile lump, younger age	Mobile, well-defined lump	Mammogram, biopsy
Fat necrosis	Single lump, history of trauma to the chest, may have pain	Single, fixed, irregular lump	Biopsy

Diagnostic Reasoning

Based on findings in the health history and physical examination, the clinician should formulate his or her assessment and plan. For example, a patient may report symptoms that suggest many possible diagnoses; however, findings in the past medical history and during the physical examination might narrow the possible diagnoses down to one or two. A breast lump is a common chief complaint. **Table 13-3** illustrates the differential diagnosis of common disorders associated with a breast lump.

Breast Assessment of Special Populations

Considerations for the Pregnant Patient
Note physiologic changes:
- Increased levels of estrogen and progesterone cause fullness and sensitivity early in pregnancy.
- Nipples and areolae become more pigmented. Richer blood supply causes the venous system to become more noticeable.
- During the second and third trimesters, growth of the mammary glands causes the breasts to enlarge. Due to proliferation of the lactiferous ducts and lobularalveolar tissue, breasts feel coarse and nodular upon palpation.
- Palpation of the nipple may yield colostrum (a premilk fluid).

Considerations for the Neonatal Patient
Female and male neonates will have enlarged breasts caused by the mother's estrogen; the breast will assume normal size within 2 weeks to 3 months. The nipples may secrete a white fluid, known as witch's milk. This is normal.

Considerations for the Pediatric Patient
Breast development usually begins around the age of 10. **Figure 13-29** depicts stages of development. During inspection, it is normal to note asymmetry during the growth period.

Considerations for the Geriatric Patient
- Inspection reveals a more pendulous or flatter breast.
- Upon palpation, the breasts feel more granular. The breast tissue is not firm and elastic. The inframammary ridge is often palpable.
- Reinforce the importance of regular breast self-examination and mammograms.

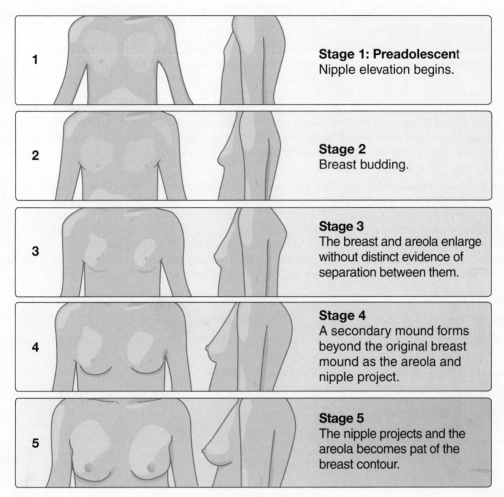

1
Stage 1: Preadolescent
Nipple elevation begins.

2
Stage 2
Breast budding.

3
Stage 3
The breast and areola enlarge without distinct evidence of separation between them.

4
Stage 4
A secondary mound forms beyond the original breast mound as the areola and nipple project.

5
Stage 5
The nipple projects and the areola becomes pat of the breast contour.

FIGURE 13-29 Tanner stages of breast development.

Case Study Review

Throughout the second half of this chapter, you have been introduced to Ms. M. This section of the chapter pulls together her history and demonstrates the documentation of her history and physical examination.

Chief Complaint

"I have a lump."

Information Gathered During the Interview

JM is a 56-year-old African American woman who comes to the clinic with a chief complaint of a lump in her right breast. She reports a clear discharge from the right nipple. Ms. M says she felt the lump about 3 months ago and it seems to be getting larger. She denies pain and says the lump does not seem movable.

Ms. M states she had gallbladder surgery 2 years ago, an appendectomy when she was 16, and a tonsillectomy as a child. She had pertussis, measles, and mumps as a child. She has high blood pressure and is taking medication for it. Her last physician told her she is borderline diabetic. Ms. M denies any trauma to her chest.

She says she started her menses at the age of 12. She took birth control pills from age 20 to 23. Ms. M has 5 children; all were vaginal deliveries. She reports that onset of perimenopause occurred when she was 48 years old and lasted 5 years. Although she did not have a lot of hot flashes or night sweats, her provider prescribed hormone replacement therapy "to prevent heart disease, stroke, and bone loss."

Her last breast examination and mammogram was 3 years ago, but she does breast self-examinations monthly. She says that her mammogram showed some calcifications but was otherwise normal.

Ms. M reports that her paternal grandfather died of a heart attack and her paternal grandmother died of a stroke. Her maternal grandfather died of heart failure, and her maternal grandmother died of breast cancer. Her father died in a car accident when she was an infant and her mother remarried. Her stepfather and mother are alive. Her mother has arthritis and high blood pressure and is taking medications. She has two half-brothers, 54 and 51 years old, and one half-sister 52 years old. The older half-brother was diagnosed with colon cancer 2 years ago. He had surgery and chemotherapy and his cancer is in remission. Her other half-brother has a heart murmur and takes a lot of medications. Her half-sister was diagnosed with breast cancer 1 year ago. Ms. M had a left mastectomy with 21 lymph nodes removed, radiation therapy, and chemotherapy, and is now doing well.

Ms. M has five children: three sons and two daughters. Her daughters, ages 32 and 28, are well. Her oldest and youngest sons, ages 30 and 22, have type 2 diabetes mellitus. The 30-year-old takes insulin; the youngest son takes an oral medication. Both of the diabetic sons also have high blood pressure and are on blood pressure medications. Her middle son, age 26, is well. Ms. M works as a certified nursing assistant for a home health agency. She is divorced and lives alone. Ms. M is not sexually active. Her children all live in the area and visit her frequently. She has many friends and enjoys visiting museums. She is a smoker; she says she smokes about 8 cigarettes per day. She denies alcohol or recreational drug use.

Clues	Important Points
Nontender, irregular and fixed, hard lump	Characteristics suggest breast cancer.
Nipple discharge	One nipple has discharged spontaneously, which suggests cancer or infection.
Older than 50 years of age	Age is the highest risk factor for breast cancer.
Early menses	Menarche before the age of 13 is a risk factor for breast cancer.
Family history of breast cancer	Breast cancer has a tendency to run in families.
Smoker	Nicotine is a carcinogen.

Name JM	Date 8/4/15	Time 1100
	DOB 7/11/59	Sex F

HISTORY

CC
"I have a lump in my right breast."

HPI
56-year-old African American female with a 3-month history of a right breast lump, which is growing in size; right nipple expresses clear discharge; lump is immobile and painless.

Medications
Unknown medication for HTN

Allergies
PCN, codeine

PMI
Illnesses
Childhood diseases include pertussis, measles, and mumps. Diagnosed with high blood pressure. Reports that doctor told her she is a borderline diabetic. Menarche at 12. Birth control from age 20–23. Gravida 5, para 5 (vaginal deliveries). Perimenopause at 48 years of age; took HRT; lasted 5 years. Last breast exam 3 years ago; reports mammogram showed calcifications but otherwise normal.

Hospitalizations/Surgeries
Gallbladder surgery, appendectomy, tonsillectomy. Denies recent trauma.

FH
Paternal grandparents deceased (MI and CVA). Maternal grandparents deceased (HF and breast cancer). Mother has arthritis and high blood pressure. Her half-sister (52) has breast cancer, which is in remission; half-brother (54) has colon cancer, which is in remission; half-brother (51) has a heart murmur. She has five children. Her two daughters are well. Two sons have diabetes mellitus; her other son is well.

SH
Divorced; works as a CNA. Lives alone, but children visit often. Not sexually active. Smokes 8 cigarettes per day; denies alcohol or drug use.

ROS	
General Denies fever, chills, and malaise.	Cardiovascular Denies chest pain.
Skin Denies changes in color or texture.	Respiratory Denies SOB or cough.
Eyes Wears glasses.	Gastrointestinal Denies any problems.
Ears Denies any problems.	Genitourinary/Gynecological Denies any problems.
Nose/Mouth/Throat Wears dentures.	Musculoskeletal A little stiff in the mornings.
Breast See HPI.	Neurological Denies any problems.

PHYSICAL EXAMINATION		
Weight 228	Temp 98.6	BP 158/98
Height 5'4"	Pulse 80	Resp 20

General Appearance
56-year-old obese, African American in no distress; well groomed.

Skin
Warm and dry to touch; no discoloration or lesions.

HEENT
Normal hair distribution. No ear pain or drainage; tympanic membrane pearly gray, cerumen. Scleras are white; no excessive tearing; PERRL; EOMs intact. No caries or bleeding gums. Neck is supple; no lymphadenopathy.

Cardiovascular
Regular rhythm, no murmur; radial pulse 3; femoral pulse 3.

Respiratory
Lungs clear to auscultation.

Gastrointestinal
Abdomen soft, large; BS hyperactive; no masses palpated.

Genitourinary
Not examined.

Musculoskeletal
Strengths 5/5 and symmetrical, full range of motion with pain, no edema.

Neurological
No tremors; CN I–XII intact.

Other
Breasts: Large, no dimpling, retraction, ecchymosis, lesions, or scars; venous system is slightly prominent.
Right breast: Not firm, granular. Irregular-shaped mass, approximately 3 × 1 cm, palpated in upper quadrants at 12:00. Palpated inframammary ridge. Left breast: No masses palpated, granular, not firm.
Nipples: No retraction. Discharge from the right nipple (guaiac positive for blood). No discharge from left nipple.
Lymph nodes: No tenderness or enlargement.

Lab Tests

Special Tests
Mammogram: The breast parenchyma is heterogeneously dense and nodular in configuration. There is extensive benign-appearing calcification formation in both breasts. There is a 2- to 2.5-cm area of architectural distortion in the upper midportion of the right breast in the general location of the palpable concern. The area of architectural distortion contains radiating strands of density and relative central lucency. This is a category 4 mammogram (suspicious abnormality—biopsy should be considered).
Fine-needle biopsy (FNB): Sections show multiple needle cores of breast tissue; many have multiple ducts involved by low- to intermediate-grade DCIS. Some of the ducts have associated microcalcifications.

Final Assessment Findings
Breast cancer—DCIS

Bibliography

Anderson, M. R., Klink, K., & Cohrssen, A. (2004). Evaluation of vaginal complaints. *Journal of the American Medical Association, 291*(11), 1368–1379.

Apgar, B., Brotzman, G., & Spitzer, M. (2008). *Colposcopy principles and practices* (2nd ed.). Philadelphia, PA: W. B. Saunders.

Bastian, L., Smith, C. M., & Nanda, K. (2003). Is this patient perimenopausal? *Journal of the American Medical Association, 289*(7), 895–902.

Bent, S., Nallamothu, B. K., Simel, D. L., Fihn, S. D., & Saint, S. (2002). Does this woman have an acute uncomplicated urinary tract infection? *Journal of the American Medical Association, 287*(20), 2701–2710.

Bereks, J. S. (2011). *Berek and Novak's textbook of gynecology* (15th ed.). Baltimore, MD: Lippincott Williams & Wilkins.

Carlson, K. J., Eisenstat, S. A., Frigoletto, F. D., & Schiff, I. (2002). *Primary care of women* (2nd ed.). St. Louis, MO: Mosby.

DeCherney, A. H., & Nathan, L. (2007). *Current obstetric and gynecology diagnosis and treatment* (10th ed.). New York, NY: Lange Medical Books/McGraw-Hill.

Habermann, T. M., & Steensma, D. P. (2000). Lymphadenopathy. *Mayo Clinic Proceedings, 75,* 723–732.

Physical assessment of the well woman. University of Manitoba. Archived from the original on September 28, 2006. Retrieved October 31, 2012.

Smeltzer, S. C., & Bare, B. (2004). *Brunner and Suddarth's textbook of medical–surgical nursing* (10th ed.). Philadelphia, PA: Lippincott Williams & Wilkins.

Smith, R. P. (2002). *Netter's obstetrics, gynecology and women's health.* Teterboro, NJ: Icon Learning Systems.

U.S. Department of Health and Human Services, & Public Health Service. (2003). *What you need to know about breast cancer.* Bethesda, MD: National Institutes of Health.

Chapter 14

Endocrine Disorders

The endocrine system regulates metabolic processes of the body. Generally speaking, the primary functions of the endocrine glands include the following:

- Regulating reproduction
- Regulating metabolism
- Controlling extracellular fluid and electrolytes (sodium, potassium, calcium, and phosphates)
- Maintaining an optimal internal environment such as regulation of blood glucose levels
- Stimulating growth and development during childhood and adolescence

Performing assessment of a patient's endocrine system is challenging because the locations of the majority of these glands (with the exceptions of the thyroid gland and testes) make it impossible to inspect, palpate, percuss, or auscultate. It is also difficult to assess this system because of the different effects the hormones have on various systems throughout the body. Assessment of endocrine function depends on clustering data and recognizing the underlying pattern of an endocrine disorder.

Anatomy and Physiology Review of the Endocrine System

The endocrine system is the body's control mechanism. It comprises a complex network of glands that are distributed throughout the body (see **Figure 14-1**):

- Hypothalamus
- Pituitary gland
- Thyroid and parathyroid glands
- Pancreas
- Adrenal glands
- Gonads

These glands secrete hormones directly into the bloodstream. Hormones are chemical messengers that are secreted into the circulation and then carried to various tissues, where they signal and affect target cells that have appropriate receptors. They then act on these cells to cause a specific cell function. Most hormones are regulated by a negative feedback mechanism. Increased levels of a particular hormone will inhibit secretion, and decreased levels of a particular hormone will stimulate secretion. **Table 14-1** provides a summary of the source and major action of selected hormones.

Hypothalamus

The hypothalamus secretes thyrotropin-releasing hormone (TRH), which stimulates secretion of thyroid-stimulating hormone (TSH); corticotropin-releasing hormone (CRH), which causes release of adrenocorticotropic hormone (ACTH); growth hormone-releasing hormone (GHRH), which causes release of growth hormone (GH); somatostatin, also known as growth hormone inhibitory hormone (GHIH), which inhibits release of growth hormone; and prolactin-inhibiting factor (PIF), which inhibits release of prolactin.

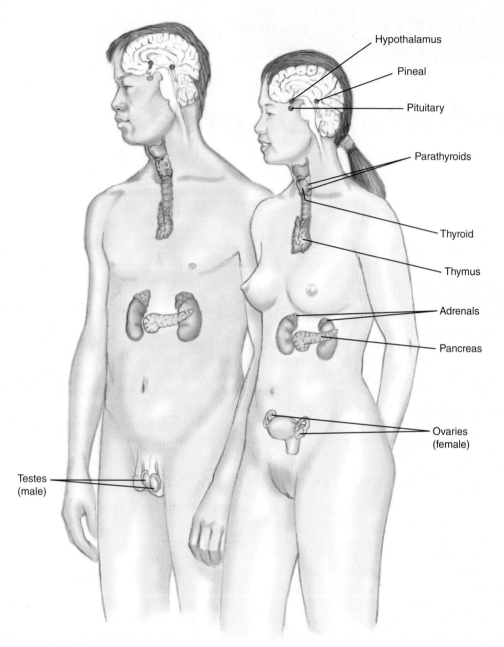

FIGURE 14-1 Endocrine system.

Pituitary Gland

The pituitary gland (also known as the hypophysis) consists of the anterior and posterior components.

Anterior Pituitary Gland

Glandular tissue in the anterior pituitary lobe synthesizes and secretes six hormones. These hormones include GH, which stimulates protein synthesis and overall growth of most cells and tissues; TSH, which stimulates synthesis and secretion of thyroid hormones; ACTH, which stimulates synthesis and secretion of adrenal cortical hormones; prolactin (PRL), which promotes development of the female breasts and secretion of milk; follicle-stimulating hormone (FSH), which causes growth of follicles of the ovaries and sperm maturation in cells of the testes; and luteinizing hormone (LH), which stimulates the testicular testosterone production, ovulation, and ovarian estrogen and progesterone production.

Table 14-1   Major Action and Source of Selected Hormones

Source	Hormone	Major Action
Hypothalamus	Releasing and inhibiting hormones	Control the release of pituitary hormones.
	Corticotropin-releasing hormone (CRH)	
	Thyrotropin-releasing hormone (TRH)	
	Growth hormone-releasing hormone (GHRH)	
	Gonadotropin-releasing hormone (GnRH)	
	Somatostatin	Inhibits CH and TSH.
Anterior pituitary	Growth hormone (GH)	Stimulates growth of bone and muscle, promotes protein synthesis and fat metabolism, decreases carbohydrate metabolism.
	Adrenocorticotropic hormone (ACTH)	Stimulates synthesis and secretion of adrenal cortical hormones.
	Thyroid-stimulating hormone (TSH)	Stimulates synthesis and secretion of thyroid hormone.
	Follicle-stimulating hormone (FSH)	Female: stimulates growth of ovarian follicle, ovulation.
		Male: stimulates sperm production.
	Luteinizing hormone (LH)	Female: stimulates development of corpus luteum, release of oocyte, production of estrogen and progesterone.
		Male: stimulates secretion of testosterone, development of the interstitial tissue of the testes.
	Prolactin	Prepares the female breast for breastfeeding.
Posterior pituitary	Antidiuretic hormone (ADH)	Increases water reabsorption by the kidney.
	Oxytocin	Stimulates contraction of pregnant uterus, milk ejection from breasts after childbirth.
Adrenal cortex	Mineralocorticosteroids, mainly aldosterone	Increase sodium absorption, potassium loss by kidney.
	Glucocorticoids, mainly cortisol	Affect metabolism of all nutrients; regulates blood glucose levels, affects growth, has anti-inflammatory action, and decreases effects of stress.
	Adrenal androgens, mainly dehydroepiandrosterone (DHEA) and androstenedione	Have minimal intrinsic androgenic activity; they are converted to testosterone and dihydrotestosterone in the periphery.
Adrenal medulla	Epinephrine Norepinephrine	Serve as neurotransmitters for the sympathetic nervous system.
Thyroid (follicular cells)	Thyroid hormones: triiodothyronine (T_3), thyroxine (T_4)	Increase the metabolic rate; increase protein and bone turnover; increase responsiveness to catecholamines; necessary for fetal and infant growth and development.
Thyroid C cells	Calcitonin	Lowers blood calcium and phosphate levels.
Parathyroid glands	Parathyroid hormone (PTH)	Regulates serum calcium.
Pancreatic islet cells	Insulin	Lowers blood glucose by facilitating glucose transport across cell membranes of muscle, liver, and adipose tissue.
	Glucagon	Increases blood glucose concentration by stimulation of glycogenolysis and glyconeogenesis.
	Somatostatin	Delays intestinal absorption of glucose.
Kidney	1, 25-dihydroxyvitamin D	Stimulates calcium absorption from the intestine.
Ovaries	Estrogen	Affects development of the female sex organs and secondary sex characteristics.
	Progesterone	Influences the menstrual cycle; stimulates growth of the uterine wall; maintains pregnancy.
Testes	Androgens, mainly testosterone	Affect development of male sex organs and secondary sex characteristics; aid in sperm production.

Posterior Pituitary Gland

The posterior pituitary stores two hormones: antidiuretic hormone (ADH) and oxytocin. ADH increases water reabsorption by the kidneys and causes vasoconstriction and increased blood pressure. Oxytocin stimulates milk ejection from the breasts and causes uterine contraction.

Thyroid and Parathyroid Glands

The thyroid gland secretes two distinct amino acid hormones that compose thyroid hormone: thyroxine (T_4) and triiodothyronine (T_3). Iodine molecules are bound to the amino acid structure of these hormones; T_4 has four iodine atoms and T_3 has three. The thyroid gland requires iodine to synthesize its hormones. Thyroid hormone is produced and stored within the cells of the thyroid gland until needed for release into the bloodstream. The secretion of T_3 and T_4 by the thyroid gland is controlled by TSH, which is secreted by the anterior pituitary gland.

The function of the thyroid hormones, T_4 and T_3, is to increase the rate of chemical reactions in most of the cells of the body, thereby increasing the metabolic rate. T_4 is the weaker hormone and functions to maintain a steady body metabolism. T_3 is five times stronger than T_4 and exhibits a more rapid metabolic action.

Another hormone produced by the thyroid gland is calcitonin, which promotes deposition of calcium in the bones and decreases extracellular fluid calcium ion concentration.

The parathyroid glands secrete parathyroid hormone (PTH), which regulates serum calcium by increasing absorption by the intestines and kidneys and releasing calcium from the bones.

Pancreas

The endocrine component of the pancreas contains the islets of Langerhans. These islets consist of A, B, and D cells. A cells secrete glucagon, which increases the synthesis and release of glucose from the liver into the serum. B cells secrete preproinsulin, which is ultimately converted to insulin, which in turn promotes glucose entry in many cells. D cells secrete somatostatin, which extends the period of time over which food nutrients are assimilated into the blood and acts on insulin and glucagon secretion, decreasing the utilization of the absorbed nutrients by the tissues. Insulin is a hormone that regulates blood glucose concentrations and the metabolism of fat, protein, and carbohydrates.

Adrenal Glands

The adrenal glands are a pair of endocrine glands located on the kidneys. Each of the adrenal glands consists of an adrenal medulla and a cortex. The adrenal medulla secretes catecholamines, including epinephrine and norepinephrine. These hormones cause a range of metabolic effects and are liberated in the "flight or fight" response. The adrenal cortex secretes steroid hormones, including glucocorticoids, mineralocorticoids, and androgens and estrogens. The most potent glucocorticoid is cortisol, which has anti-inflammatory effects and performs multiple metabolic functions in controlling metabolism of proteins, carbohydrates, and fats. The major mineralocorticoid is aldosterone, which affects potassium and hydrogen ion secretion and reabsorption of sodium.

Gonads

The testes produce testosterone, which promotes development of the male reproductive system and male secondary sexual characteristics. The ovaries produce estrogens, which promote growth and development of the female reproductive system and produce female secondary sexual characteristics. The ovaries also release progesterone, which causes secondary female sexual characteristics.

Other Sources of Hormones

The kidney produces renin, 1,25-dihydroxycholecalciferol, and erythropoietin. Renin catalyzes conversion of angiotensinogen to angiotensin 1; 1,25-dihydroxycholecalciferol increases intestinal absorption of calcium and bone mineralization; and erythropoietin increases erythrocyte production.

The heart produces atrial natriuretic peptide (ANP), which increases sodium excretion by the kidney, thereby reducing blood pressure. The stomach produces gastrin, which stimulates hydrochloric acid (HCl) secretion by the parietal cells of the stomach. The small intestines produce secretin and cholecystokinin (CCK). Secretin stimulates pancreatic cells to release bicarbonate and water, and CCK stimulates gallbladder contraction and release of pancreatic enzymes.

Health History

In assessing endocrine disorders, the practitioner needs to obtain an accurate history. Collect data relevant to the reason for the clinic appointment (chief complaint [CC]). A determination should be made regarding the onset, location, duration, quality, and severity of the signs and symptoms (history of present illness [HPI]). While interviewing the patient, assess mental status. With many endocrine disorders and altered metabolic functioning, the patient may experience restlessness, agitation, and a short attention span.

Chief Complaint and History of Present Illness

"I can't sleep very well even though I am always tired, and I can feel my heart racing and pounding all of the time."

> JK is a 54-year-old woman who presents with a 2-month history of fatigue, insomnia, palpitations, and increased perspiration. Ms. K also complains of changes in the appearance of her eyes, a red rash, and bruising of her arms and legs.

Common chief complaints associated with endocrine disorders include fatigue, insomnia, palpitations, weight changes, integumentary changes, changes to facial features, and temperature intolerance.

Fatigue, insomnia, palpitations, weight changes, and integumentary changes are described in detail here. Many endocrine disorders manifest with changes to facial features. Eyelid retraction and ptosis occur with hyperstimulation (thyrotoxicosis) or understimulation (hypothyroidism or Wilson's syndrome). This is due to nervous stimulation of eyelid muscles via cranial nerve III, which is either understimulated or overstimulated by the general tone of the reticular activating system (RAS). Cushing's syndrome may cause "moon face," a rounding of the face.

Heat or cold intolerance is also common because metabolic rate influences body temperature. Patients with hypothyroidism may present with cold intolerance, whereas patients with hyperthyroidism often experience heat intolerance.

Fatigue

Fatigue is a common complaint of people with endocrine disorders. When the endocrine system is not functioning optimally, fatigue or exhaustion can occur. It is often chronic in nature and commonly is associated with hyperthyroidism, hypothyroidism, hyperparathyroidism, Addison's disease, Cushing's syndrome, diabetes mellitus, diabetes insipidus, and deficient levels of TSH or ACTH.

Onset	Was the onset sudden or gradual?
	Sudden onset of fatigue is associated with hypoglycemia of diabetes mellitus. A more gradual onset of fatigue is associated with hyperthyroidism, hypothyroidism, hyperparathyroidism, hypopituitarism, Addison's disease, and Cushing's syndrome.
Duration and pattern	How long has the patient had fatigue? Is the fatigue a daily occurrence or does it come and go? Is the fatigue associated with any activity? Does the patient have insomnia? Does the patient have sleep apnea?
	Patients with thyrotoxicosis and Graves' disease often have fatigue that is constant. Patients with diabetes often experience fatigue due to the body's inability to utilize glucose.
	Does the patient have any mental health issues that might prevent adequate rest?

Quality and severity	Does the fatigue interfere with activities of daily living?
	Patients with thyrotoxicosis or hyperthyroidism (Graves' disease) often report fatigue that interferes with normal activities of daily living.
	Has the fatigue caused personality changes such as anger, irritability, or inability to handle stress?
Associated symptoms	Ask about associated symptoms, including weight loss or gain, excessive perspirations, anorexia, nausea, vomiting, depression, irritability, intolerance to heat or cold, and palpitations.
Alleviating factors	Is the patient taking any prescription or nonprescription drugs? Does the patient self-treat with increased resting/sleeping periods, herbal remedies, meditation, yoga, and so on? How effective are the treatments in reducing fatigue levels?

Palpitations

Palpitations are irregular or rapid heartbeats sensed by the patient. They are commonly described as intermittent sensations of beating, flip-flopping, or pounding in the substernal region or neck and can be a common symptom even with a normal heart rhythm. Palpitations can occur for many reasons and may be caused by disorders associated with various systems. Endocrine disorders such as hypertension, congestive heart failure, myocardial infarction, thyroid disease, and metabolic syndrome can all produce palpitations.

Onset	Was the onset of the palpitations sudden or gradual?
Duration	How long has the patient noticed the palpitations? When the palpitations occurred, how long did they last? Did the patient do anything that stopped them?
	Each time the palpitations occurred, did they last the same amount of time?
Frequency of occurrence; regularity	How many times a week does the patient experience the palpitations? At which time of day do they occur most frequently? Are there any preceding symptoms that warn the patient of impending palpitations? Are the palpitations recurring more often?
	The palpitations associated with endocrine abnormalities occur frequently. Disorders such as Addison's disease, Cushing's syndrome, pheochromocytoma, thyroid disease, and diabetes are most often associated with changes in the cardiovascular system.
Associated symptoms	Do the palpitations occur in association with any other signs and symptoms? During the palpitations, did the patient experience any shortness of breath (SOB), dizziness, syncope, or pain?
	Palpitations clustered with exophthalmos, insomnia, increased perspiration, and elevations in blood pressure, pulse, and respirations may be indicative of thyrotoxicosis.
	Increased stroke volume and increased heart rate (tachycardia) together with palpitations are indicative of thyrotoxicosis. If tachycardia is caused by thyrotoxicosis, the resting pulse rate is usually 90 or greater.

Congestive heart failure may occur along with palpitations in the patient with thyrotoxicosis because of increased metabolism and increased adrenergic-like sensitivity of the heart to catecholamines, resulting in decreased reserve.

Episodes of fainting and severe headache, together with palpitations, are indicative of pheochromocytomas (adrenal tumors).

Precipitating factors	What precipitated them? Did the patient experience any stressful event before the palpitations occurred? Did you consume unusual amounts of caffeine before the event?
Medications	Is the patient taking any medications, including prescription or nonprescription drugs and social substances, that might cause or affect palpitations?

Insomnia

Onset	Was the onset of insomnia sudden or gradual? Is this a new onset?
Duration and pattern	Has the patient had a long history of sleeping disorders? Is the insomnia recurring? *Diseases such as diabetes, hypertension, and pheochromocytoma all produce disturbances in sleep patterns. Hyperanxiety states or extreme exhaustion may significantly affect the patient's activities of daily living, and they play an important role in how the patient responds to subsequent treatment.*
Associated symptoms	Is the patient experiencing restlessness, fatigue, emotional lability, and/or short attention span? *Along with insomnia, the patient can have serious anxiety stages— highs and lows—that affect every area of the patient's life. If sleep is disturbed, the body is unable to replenish itself or regroup to respond to the next day's activities. A constant state of wakefulness, as seen in patients with diabetes, adrenal disease, or thyroid disease, greatly alters the body's immune system response to disease.*
Efforts to treat and effectiveness of treatment	Is the patient taking any prescription or nonprescription medications; using any herbal remedies or natural techniques; or using lifestyle changes (e.g., decreasing caffeine/stimulant use) to self-treat the insomnia? How effective were the substances in treating the insomnia?

Weight Changes

Weight gain or loss is common with endocrine disorders. A careful history will help narrow diagnosis.

Onset	Was the onset sudden or gradual?
Quality	Has the patient lost or gained weight? How much? *Hypothyroidism and Cushing's syndrome often present with weight gain. Thyrotoxicosis, Addison's disease, hyperthyroidism, adrenocortical insufficiency, diabetes insipidus, and diabetes mellitus often present with weight loss.*

Associated symptoms	Ask about associated symptoms, including fatigue, anxiety, muscle weakness, temperature changes, gastrointestinal problems, and changes to facial appearance.
	Hypothyroidism may cause inability to tolerate cold, fatigue, lethargy, and constipation.
	Hyperthyroidism may present with nervousness/anxiety, rapid pulse, heat intolerance, and muscle weakness.
	Cushing's syndrome may cause a heavy trunk, "buffalo hump," and moon face.
	Adrenocortical insufficiency often presents with muscular weakness, fatigue, gastrointestinal problems, and mood alterations.

Integumentary Changes

Patients with endocrine disease may experience skin dryness, petechiae, hair loss, or excessive hair growth. Remember to consider unusual body odor and changes in skin pigmentation when questioning the patient about his symptoms.

Onset	Was the onset of symptoms sudden or gradual?
Quality	Describe the changes.
	Patients with thyrotoxicosis often have petechiae and bruising, probably because an excessive amount of thyroid hormones causes degradation of protein to exceed the synthesis. Protein within the blood vessels may be reduced, resulting in increased fragility.
	Hypothyroidism may cause thick, puffy skin and hair loss.
	Hyperthyroidism often presents with profuse perspiration and moist, warm skin.
	Patients with Cushing's syndrome may have thin, fragile skin; striae; and ecchymoses.
Duration	How long has the patient noticed the changes in skin, hair, or nails? Have the changes occurred suddenly or over the past few years?
	Any changes in hair, nails, and skin need to be carefully reviewed to differentiate normal from abnormal variations.
Associated symptoms	Ask about associated symptoms, including weight changes, temperature intolerance, fatigue, vocal changes, and mood alterations.
Efforts to treat	Is the patient taking any prescription or nonprescription drugs, particularly aspirin-containing products, to try to alleviate the symptoms—for example, special shampoos or creams?

Past Medical History

Ms. K reports that she has had "eye burning" for some time. She has experienced lack of energy and difficulty in sleeping on and off for the last 6 years. She denies a history of diabetes, cancer, coronary artery disease, or mental health problems. She denies a history of trauma or hospitalizations.

Ask detailed questions focusing on all past medical illnesses/history (PMI). This information may be critical in formulating an appropriate plan of care.

Past health conditions or surgeries	Inquire about past health conditions or surgeries.
	Treatment sequelae or resulting disabilities are critical data to obtain.
	Ask if the patient has been diagnosed with any arrhythmias, renal disorders, gastrointestinal disturbances, or neurovascular complaints.
	Remember that the endocrine system controls basic metabolic functions, which in turn affect every body system.
Recent hospitalization or clinic visits	Ask about hospitalizations or office visits for any endocrine or other conditions.
	Frequently, patients with endocrine disorders are hospitalized for other conditions, particularly cardiac conditions.
	Approximately 40% of older patients with thyrotoxicosis will have atrial fibrillation and may be hospitalized or have a clinic appointment not because of a thyroid problem, but because of the arrhythmia.
Medications	Ask about all medications, both prescription and over-the-counter products.

Family History

Ms. K has never been married and has no children. Her mother is 82 and has a significant history of cardiac disease. Recently, her mother was diagnosed with hypothyroidism. Ms. K's father died at age 78 of idiopathic pulmonary fibrosis. Ms. K has no brothers or sisters. She has two aunts and three uncles, all of whom are alive. Two uncles have coronary artery disease (CAD) and one aunt has diabetes. Grandparents on both sides died of "old age."

Family history (FH)—information about the medical status of family members—helps the healthcare provider determine possible genetic and heredity factors that may play a role in the patient's disease.

Age of living relatives	Include the relationship and health of parents, brothers, sisters, and children.
Deaths	Include the relationship, age, and cause of death.
Chronic diseases	Ask about chronic diseases in the family. Include the relationship to the family member with disease and how the long family member has had disease.
	Many diseases and disorders are familial/genetic, and careful screening and prevention or health promotion activities can assist the patient in leading as normal a lifestyle as possible. Patients often have a family history of endocrine disorders or family history of benign or malignant thyroid disease.
Genetic defects	Include any family genetic disorders and congenital birth defects.
	History of familial genetic or congenital birth defects can assist in screening and health promotion activities.

Social History

> Ms. K has a very quiet social life. She states she has always had a hard time making friends. Ms. K has always been overweight, and her hair is thin and chronically hard to manage. She denies smoking, drinking alcohol, and taking drugs. She is active in church activities. She works as a secretary in a large toy factory and has been there for 20 years. She has no hobbies but loves to read and go online.

Hobbies, lifestyle, health habits, and the local environment (social history [SH]) can all affect a person's endocrine system. Many endocrine disorders affect a person's appearance or emotional or mental state.

Family	Ask the patient to describe the current family unit.
Occupation	Ask about past positions, volunteer activity, and community activities.
	If the patient is retired, ask how long she or he has been retired and how she or he is adjusting.
	Has the patient had exposure to toxic substances?
Hobbies	Ask about hobbies.
	With significant changes in metabolic function, energy levels are often impaired, resulting in lack of interest or energy to participate in hobbies. Patients with endocrine disease may have inattention, may have difficulty with "staying on task," and may not participate in hobbies.
Stress and stress management	Ask the patient about how she or he deals with stress.
	With impaired metabolic functions, the body's ability to deal with stress is grossly impaired. Stress may affect the endocrine system and regulation of hormone levels within the body.
Use of tobacco	Include the type of tobacco used, duration, and amount (pack-years = number of years of smoking × number of packs smoked per day).
	Because of the nervousness associated with many endocrine disorders, patients may have difficulty quitting smoking and may increase their tobacco use.
Use of alcohol	Does the patient drink alcohol? How much? Which type (wine, beer, liquor)? At which time of day? How long?
	Patients with endocrine disorders may drink to "calm their nerves" or improve their mood.
Use of recreational drugs	Does the patient use recreational drugs? How much? Which type? At which time of day? Does the patient need to use drugs to reduce nervousness or increase energy levels?
Environment	Ask the patient about exposure to radiation, living in an iodine-deficient area, or ingestion of goitrogenic drugs.

Review of Systems

Many endocrine disorders have manifestations in systems other than the endocrine system. A comprehensive review of systems (ROS) should be performed whenever possible; however, due to time and other types of constraints, you may be able to perform only a focused review of systems. During a focused review of systems, questioning is targeted at the systems in which endocrine problems are most likely to have manifestations. Following is a summary of common manifestations of endocrine problems.

System	Symptom or Sign	Possible Associated Diseases/Disorders
General/constitutional	Weight loss	Thyrotoxicosis, diabetus mellitus, diabetes insipidus, and Addison's disease
	Weight gain	Hypothyroidism and Cushing's syndrome
	Fatigue	Thyrotoxicosis and hypothyroidism
	Altered emotional state (nervous, easily irritated, energetic)	Hyperthyroidism
	Altered emotional state (lethargic, complacent, disinterested)	Hypothyroidism
Head and face	Exophthalmos	Thyrotoxicosis
	Strabismus and/or diplopia	Thyrotoxicosis
	Sunken eyes and lack of tearing	Dehydration associated with diabetes insipidus, diabetic ketoacidosis, or hyperglycemic hyperosmolar nonketosis (HHNK)
	Periortibal edema or generalized facial edema	Hypothyroidism or syndrome of inappropriate antidiuretic hormone (SIADH)
	Coarse features, enlarged jaw, and increased distance between the upper and lower lips	Acromegaly
	Changes in pigmentation	Hyperthyroidism and Addison's disease
Neck	Deviation of the trachea	Thyroid cancer and goiters
	Enlarged thyroid	Goiters because of limitation of iodine in the diet or because of Hashimoto's disese, an autoimmune disorder; benign conditions and cancer can also cause enlargement or nodules within the thyroid
	Neck vein distention	May indicate congestive heart failure, a common sequela of thyrotoxicosis
	Hoarseness	Hypothyroidism
Skin	Clammy skin	Thyrotoxicosis and hypoglycemia
	Reddish color to the skin	Thyrotoxicosis
	Cool, pale skin	Hypothyroidism or hypoglycemia
	Brittle, thin hair	Thyrotoxicosis and hypothyroidism
	Excessive facial hair and male pattern baldness in the female	Cushing's sydnrome
	Lack of body hair and bronzing	Addison's disease
	Sparse, short head hair with split ends	Thyrotoxicosis and hypothyroidism
	Separation of the layers of the nails (onycholysis)	Thyrotoxicosis and hypothyroidism
	Dry skin with poor turgor	HHNK or ketoacidosis
Cardiovascular	Elevated blood pressure	Thyrotoxicosis and arteriosclerosis from diabetes mellitus; severe hypertension may reflect a pheochromocytoma
	Tachycardia	Diabetes insipidus and hypoglycemia
	Bradycardia	Addison's disease and hypothyroidism
	Orthostatic hypotension	Addison's disease
	Lowered blood pressure	Addison's disease, hypothyroidism, and diabetes insipidus
	Congestive heart failure (CHF)	Thyrotoxicosis and volume overload in patients with SIADH and Cushing's syndrome
	Arrhythmias	Thyrotoxicosis and ketoacidosis (due to factors such as electrolyte distrubances)
Respiratory	Adventitious breath sounds (crackles)	Thyrotoxicosis
	Increased respiratory rate with dyspnea	Thyrotoxicosis

(continues)

System	Symptom or Sign	Possible Associated Diseases/Disorders
	Lung muscle degeneration; reduced vital capacity; pleural effusions; hypoventilation	Hypothyroidism
Gastrointestinal	Increased frequency of bowel movements	Hyperthyroidism
	Constipation	Hypothyroidism
Female genitourinary	Amenorrhea, scant flow	Hyperthyroidism
	Menorrhagia	Hypothyroidism
Musculoskeletal	Increasing weakness (especially proximal muscles)	Hyperthyroidism
	Lethargic, but good muscle strength	Hypothyroidism

Physical Examination

Equipment Needed

- Stethoscope
- Small cup of water
- Gown

Components of the Physical Examination

The patient should change into a gown. Use draping as appropriate.

Inspection

Action

1. Weigh the patient. Note any significant change in weight (loss or gain).

2. Have the patient sit. Inspect facial features.

3. Inspect the eyes for position, alignment, and extraocular movements. Note irritation, strabismus, exophthalmos, periorbital edema, lid lag, globe lag, or poor convergence.

Rationale

1. Ask the patient if there has been a change in weight. With endocrine disease, there is a disruption in metabolism, resulting in weight loss or weight gain.

2. Many endocrine disorders manifest with changes to facial features/characteristics (**Box 14-1**).

3. Eyes should be in alignment with each other and should not protrude. The lid should overlap the iris slightly during up-to-down midline movement. Converging eyes will follow an object to within 5 to 8 cm of the nose.

   Patients with thyrotoxicosis often have a bright-eyed "stare." With this stare, the upper eyelid is retracted (**Figure 14-2**), which is evidenced by the presence of a rim of sclera between the lid and limbus. A lid lag, in which the upper lid lags behind the globe of the eye when the patient is asked to look downward, is also present (**Figure 14-3**).

   A globe lag, in which the globe lags behind the upper lid when the patient gazes slowly upward, is present. The movements of the lids are jerky, and a fine tremor of the closed lids may be present. These manifestations may be related to increased adrenergic activity.

BOX 14-1 FACIAL MANIFESTATIONS OF ENDOCRINE DISORDERS

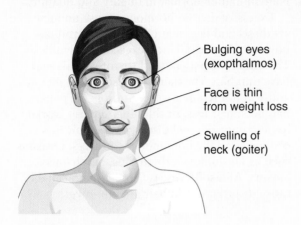

Bulging eyes (exopthalmos)

Face is thin from weight loss

Swelling of neck (goiter)

Hyperthyroidism (thyrotoxicosis) facies

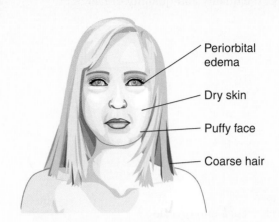

Periorbital edema

Dry skin

Puffy face

Coarse hair

Hypothyroidism (myxedema) facies

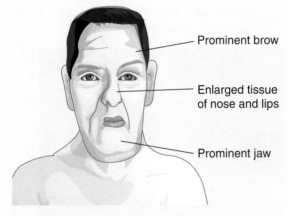

Prominent brow

Enlarged tissue of nose and lips

Prominent jaw

Acromegaly facies

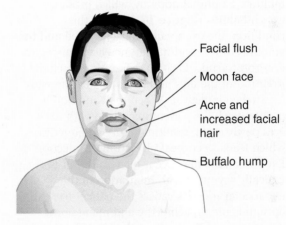

Facial flush

Moon face

Acne and increased facial hair

Buffalo hump

Cushing's syndrome facies

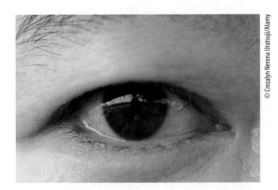

© Crezalyn Nerona Uratsuji/Alamy

FIGURE 14-2 Retracted eyelid.

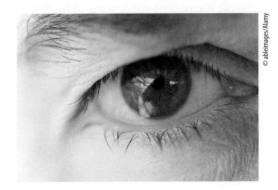

© ableimages/Alamy

FIGURE 14-3 Lid lag.

Action	Rationale
4. Inspect the quality and quantity of hair.	**4.** Hair should be normal in quality and quantity. Excessive thyroid hormones cause an increased synthesis and degradation of protein and fat; however, the degradation exceeds the synthesis. Therefore, the patient with thyrotoxicosis may have thin hair. The hair may also have split ends and will not retain a wave. Androgenic pattern baldness, hair loss, or thinning requires workup to determine adrenal disease. Most hair loss is connected to the immunologic process. Diseases such as Hashimoto's thyroiditis, pernicious anemia, Addison's disease, and vitiligo can all cause disturbances in hair growth integrity.

5. Inspect trachea and thyroid.
a. Note the position of the trachea, symmetry of the neck muscles, and the size of the thyroid.
   A major manifestation of Graves' disease is infiltrative ophthalmopathy, which produces exophthalmos (**Figure 14-4**). With this condition, the extraocular muscles swell and the amounts of retro-orbital fat increase, causing the eyes to protrude. Early manifestations include irritation of the eyes and excessive tearing with injected conjunctivae. When the condition is pronounced, the patient may sleep with the eyes partly open, resulting in dry conjunctiva, which leads to corneal ulceration or infection. Exophthalmos may occur bilaterally, but is typically asymmetrical. Infiltration of the extraocular muscles causes the patient to have difficulty in achieving and maintaining convergence. Hence, the patient may have difficulty in focusing and may have diplopia.
	a. The trachea should be midline and the space should be symmetrical on both sides. The neck muscles should be symmetrical, and there should be no visible enlargement of the thyroid.
	   An enlarged thyroid or a tumor may cause deviation of the trachea.
	
	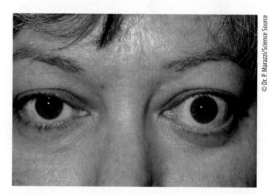
	FIGURE 14-4 Exophthalmos.

b. Observe the patient swallowing to inspect the upward movement, size, and symmetry of the throat. Ask the patient to take a drink of water. While the patient swallows, observe the thyroid tissue.	**b.** Normally, the thyroid tissue, thyroid cartilage, and cricoid cartilage move upward symmetrically when the patient swallows (**Figure 14-5**). No swelling, enlargement, or lumps are normally seen in the thyroid tissue.
	   Note diffuse enlargement or nodular lump(s), which will rise on swallowing. Most thyroid swellings are accurately discernible by observing the patient swallow (**Figure 14-6**).
	   Failure to observe before palpating the thyroid gland may lead to missing a large retrosternal goiter arising from beneath the sternum and clavicles.

Action   **Rationale**

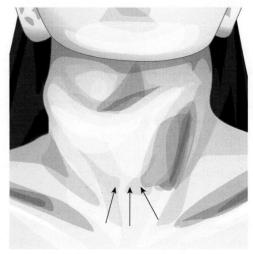

FIGURE 14-5 Normal thyroid seen upon swallowing.   FIGURE 14-6 Swollen thyroid seen upon swallowing.

6. Inspect the skin. Note its color, moisture, and texture.

6. The patient with endocrine disease may exhibit significant skin changes, including dryness or excessive oiliness; petechiae; excessive bruising; flushed, red appearance; warmth; excessive moisture; increased perspiration; palmar erythema; thin skin; patchy vitiligo; or increased pigmentation.

In some patients with endocrine disorders, increased bilirubin levels may cause jaundice and itching. In Cushing's syndrome, the patient will have hirsutism and purple striae over the abdomen. Addison's disease will cause significant skin pigmentation.

7. Inspect the fingers and fingernails.

7. Fingers and fingernails should be uniform in size, shape, and coloring.

A patient with endocrine disease may have soft and friable nails that separate. This is a characteristic finding in patients with thyroid disease and is known as Plummer's nails. It refers to a separation of the distal margin of the nail from the nail bed with irregular recession of the junction. Dirt may accumulate between the nails, giving the appearance of dirty nails. Clubbing is rare but could possibly occur with long-standing hypoxia. The color between the nails should be the same color as the patient's hand.

There should be no splinter hemorrhages. Nail texture should be the same on all nails with no grooves, pits, lines, or spooning.

8. Inspect the strength and tone of the extremities. Note if wasting has occurred.

8. Strength and tone of extremities should be within the normal range for the patient's age.

Hyperthyroidism, Cushing's syndrome, and adrenocortical insufficiency may cause muscle wasting and weakness.

Action	Rationale
9. Measure the respiratory rate.	**9.** The normal respiratory rate should be between 14 and 20 breaths per minute. Thyrotoxicosis may present with increased respiratory rate with dyspnea. Hypothyroidism may cause hypoventilation.
10. Observe for tremors. Ask the patient to extend the hands. Observe for movement. To facilitate this observation of potential nervous system effects, ask the patient to keep the hand extended and to abduct the fingers. Lay a piece of paper on the hand.	**10.** No tremors should be noted. In thyroid disease, the patient's hands move if fine tremors are present.
11. Assess reflexes (biceps, triceps, brachioradialis, patellar, and Achilles tendon reflexes).	**11.** In most endocrine diseases, especially the thyroid disorders, patients may exhibit exaggerated deep tendon reflexes.
12. Ask the patient to lay supine. Inspect the abdomen. Look for bruises, evidence of recent trauma, or scars from surgery or trauma. Inspect for asymmetry, looking down on the abdomen and across the abdomen.	**12.** Pink-purple striae are often seen with Cushing's syndrome. Spider angiomas indicate increased intra-abdominal pressure, often seen with liver failure.

Palpation

Action	Rationale
1. Palpate the lymph nodes. Palpate the cervical chain as well as the posterior triangle of lymph nodes. Palpate for the presence of a delphian node just above the thyroid isthmus and cricoid cartilage.	**1.** Normally no enlarged lymph nodes are felt on palpation. Palpation of enlarged jugular nodes immediately adjacent to a thyroid nodule may indicate papillary thyroid cancer.
2. Determine the position of the trachea. Place the thumbs on each side of the trachea in the suprasternal notch and move the trachea from side to side along the upper edges of each clavicle and in the spaces above to the inner borders of the sternocleidomastoid muscle (**Figure 14-7**).	**2.** A slight deviation to the right is considered normal. A large deviation may indicate thyroid disease. 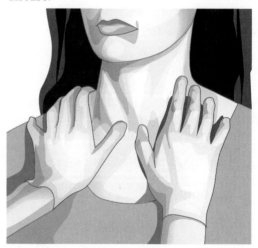 FIGURE 14-7 Palpating the trachea.
3. Palpate the isthmus, main body, and lateral lobes of the thyroid gland. Note the following during palpation: size, shape, configuration, consistency, tenderness, and nodules. Ask the patient to flex the neck slightly forward, to relax the sternomastoid muscles, and to move the neck laterally toward the side being examined.	**3.** When palpable, the thyroid lobes should be small (4 cm at the broadest point), smooth (free of small or large lumps), and rubbery. When the patient swallows, the isthmus should rise freely.

Action

When palpating the thyroid, it is important to do so gently. Lightly pass your fingers over the gland to identify the presence of nodules or altered positions of the thyroid. There are two approaches to palpating the thyroid—posterior and anterior.

Posterior Approach

Place the fingers of both of your hands on the patient's neck so that your index fingers are just below the cricoid cartilage (**Figure 14-8**). Ask the patient to sip water; as the patient swallows, you should feel the thyroid isthmus rise up under your fingers. Sometimes it is not palpable. Displace the trachea to the right with the fingers of your left hand. With the fingers of your right hand, palpate the right lobe of the thyroid between the trachea and the sternomastoid muscle. Examine the left lobe of the thyroid in the same manner.

Anterior Approach

Stand facing the patient. Use the fingers of your right hand to displace the trachea to the person's right (**Figure 14-9**). Place the fingers of your left hand around the sternomastoid muscle and palpate for lobe enlargement as the patient swallows. Examine the right lobe of the thyroid in the same manner.

Rationale

If an enlarged thyroid is palpated, note whether the enlargement is diffuse, whether it is multinodular, or whether a single nodule is present (**Figure 14-10**). Diffuse enlargement of the thyroid indicates Graves' disease, Hashimoto's thyroiditis, or endemic goiter. Multiple nodules indicate a metabolic process (commonly) or malignancy (rarely). Palpation of a single nodule may indicate a benign tumor, a cyst, or a cancerous tumor. The thyroid will feel soft in Graves' disease and firm in Hashimoto's thyroiditis or malignancy.

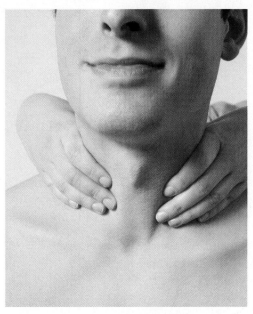

FIGURE 14-8 Palpating the thyroid (posterior technique).

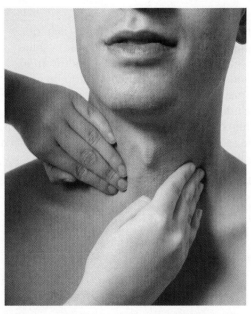

FIGURE 14-9 Palpating the thyroid (anterior technique).

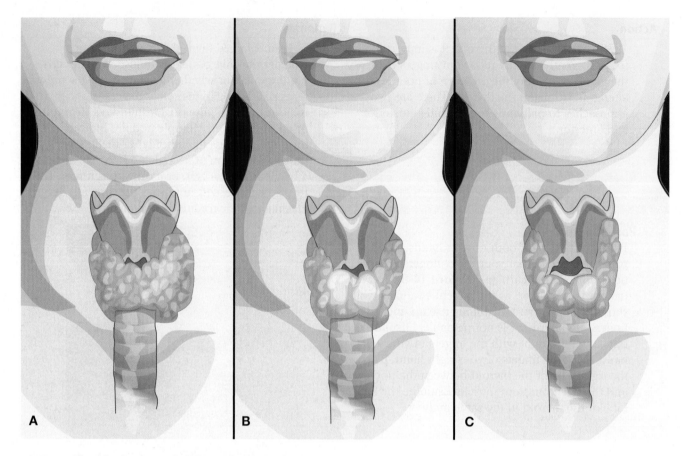

FIGURE 14-10 Thyroid enlargement. A. Diffuse enlargement. B. Multinodular. C. Single nodule.

Auscultation

Action	Rationale
1. Auscultate the thyroid. Auscultate each lobe of the thyroid when enlargement or nodules are suspected. To distinguish a bruit from a venous hum, ask the patient to stop breathing momentarily to reduce breath sounds that may occlude auditory perception of the practitioner. While compressing the jugular vein on the same side as the lobe being auscultated, listen with a stethoscope.	1. Compression of the jugular will remove a venous hum but not a bruit. A soft, rushing sound or bruit may indicate thyrotoxicosis.
2. Auscultate the lungs.	2. Assess for adventitious breath sounds. No adventitious breath sounds should be heard on auscultation. Crackles may indicate congestive heart failure (CHF), which is frequently found in thyrotoxicosis.

Action	Rationale
3. Have the patient lay supine, and auscultate the abdomen. Follow path defined in Gastrointestinal Disorders chapter. *After auscultating*, palpate the abdomen.	3. Use an organized method for auscultation, and determine the presence of bowel sounds, vascular sounds such as bruits, venous hums, and friction rubs. Any muscle guarding, facial grimacing, pulsation, mobility, and movement with respiration provide clues as to presence of fluid and should be duly noted.

The physical examination of a patient with a suspected endocrine disorder is very limited. The practitioner must rely heavily on the health history and laboratory and diagnostic test results in conjunction with the physical examination to determine the patient's diagnosis. **Box 14-2** provides a list of common laboratory and diagnostic tests for the endocrine system.

BOX 14-2 LABORATORY AND DIAGNOSTIC TESTS USED IN ASSESSMENT OF THE ENDOCRINE SYSTEM

THYROID PROFILE TESTS

Thyroid-Stimulating Hormone (TSH)
Many clinicians believe that circulating level of TSH is the single most sensitive test of thyroid function.
- Normal blood levels of thyrotropin (TSH) are between 0.4 and 4 mIU/mL.
- Decreased levels of TSH are found in Graves' disease and toxic nodular goiter.
- Increased levels of TSH are found in primary hypothyroidism, Hashimoto's thyroiditis, and thyrotoxicosis due to pituitary tumor.
- Low T_4 levels indicate thyroid destruction (e.g., end-stage Hashimoto's thyroiditis).

Total Thyroxine and Serum-Free Thyroxine
The total thyroxine (TT_4) is commonly obtained to rule out hypothyroidism and hyperthyroidism. Free thyroxine (FT_4) estimates are not performed as a routine screening tool in thyroid disease. Use of this test is confined to cases of early hyperthyroidism in which TT_4 levels may be normal but FT_4 levels are raised.
- Reference values are TT_4 55–150 nmol/L and FT_4 10–26 pmol/L.
- Increased TT_4 levels are found in hyperthyroidism (Graves' disease, goiter) and acute thyroiditis; decreased TT_4 levels are found in hypothyroidism.

Total Triiodothyronine and Free Triiodothyronine
Levels of total triiodothyronine (TT_3) and free triiodothyronine (FT_3) are not used in the routine investigation of thyroid function.
- Reference values are TT_3 1.5–3.5 nmol/L and FT_3 3–9 pmol/L.
- FT_3 is most useful in confirming the diagnosis of early hyperthyroidism, in which levels of FT_4 and FT_3 rise before TT_4 and TT_3.

T_3 Resin Uptake
A blood sample is taken and radioactive iodine is added in the laboratory. The advantage is that the patient does not have to ingest iodine. Results are as follows:
- More than 19% iodine uptake by RBCs = hyperthyroidism
- Less than 11% iodine uptake by RBCs = hypothyroidism

Radioactive Iodine Uptake
Radioactive iodine is given orally (PO); 24 hours later, the iodine level in the thyroid is checked.
- A high percentage of iodine indicates an overactive gland.
- A low percentage of iodine indicates an underactive gland.

Note: Do not use iodine products before administering the test; check for allergy to iodine or shellfish before administering the test.

(continues)

BOX 14-2 LABORATORY AND DIAGNOSTIC TESTS USED IN ASSESSMENT OF THE ENDOCRINE SYSTEM *(continued)*

Thyroid Ultrasound or Computed Tomography (CT) Scan/Magnetic Resonance Imaging (MRI)
These tests are used to rule out tumor/goiter.

Fine-Needle Aspiration Cytology
This simple and low-risk technique involves inserting a 23-gauge needle into the thyroid swelling; several passes are made while aspirating the syringe. These slides are stained by Papanicolaou or Wright's stains and observed under the microscope. Skilled cytopathologists can accurately diagnose the majority of thyroid diseases using this technique, with a high degree of specificity. This test is less accurate in patients with thyroid nodules and a history of familial nonmedullary thyroid cancer and in patients with a previous history of exposure to low-dose therapeutic radiation. Benign and malignant thyroid tumors are common in such patients, and the tumors usually are multifocal.

BLOOD CHEMISTRIES

Hormone Level Tests
Serum levels of hormones of target organs (e.g., thyroid, adrenal, pituitary, and so on) assist in diagnosis if other information is inconclusive.

Glucose Tests
These tests aid in diagnosing types 1 and 2 diabetes.

URINE TESTS

24-Hour Urine (Hormone Levels)
A 24-hour urine collection is used to assess adrenal gland disorders (e.g., Addison's disease, pheochromocytoma).

Fluid Deprivation Test
This test is done to detect diabetes insipidus. Fluids are withheld for 8–12 hours, or until 3% to 5% of body weight is lost. Plasma and urine osmolality tests are performed at the beginning and end of the test. The inability to increase specific gravity and osmolality of the urine is characteristic of diabetes insipidus.

DIAGNOSTIC TESTS

CT Scans and MRI
These imaging studies are used in diagnosis of tumors of various endocrine glands.

Diagnostic Reasoning

Based on findings in the health history and physical examination, the examiner should formulate the assessment and plan. For example, a patient may report symptoms that suggest many possible diagnoses; however, findings in the past medical history and during the physical examination might narrow the possible diagnoses down to one or two. Fatigue is a common chief complaint with endocrine disorders. **Table 14-2** illustrates the differential diagnosis of common endocrine disorders associated with fatigue.

Table 14-2 Differential Diagnosis of Fatigue			
Differential Diagnosis	Significant Findings in the Patient's History	Significant Findings in the Patient's Physical Examination	Diagnostic Tests
Hyperthyroidism	Gradual onset of constant fatigue, heat intolerance, nervousness, palpitations, skin thinning, goiter, weight loss	Exophthalmos, rapid pulse, thyroid gland may be palpable	TSH, T_3, T_4 blood tests (thyroid profile), MRI, or thyroid scan
Hypothyroidism	Fatigue and lethargy, weight gain, cold intolerance	Thick, puffy skin; periorbital edema; reduced attention span; thinning of hair	TSH, T_3, T_4 blood tests (thyroid profile)
Adrenocortical insufficiency	Fatigue, weight loss, dehydration, gastrointestinal problems	Muscle weakness, irritability or anxiety, hyperpigmentation	CBC, 24-hour urine studies
Diabetes mellitus	Fatigue, weight loss, polyuria	Blurred vision	Fasting blood glucose

Abbreviations: CBC, complete blood count; MRI, magnetic resonance imaging; T_3, triiodothyronine; T_4, thyroxine; TSH, thyroid-stimulating hormone.

Endocrine Assessment of Special Populations

Considerations for the Pregnant Woman

- The clinician needs to be aware of and screen for thyroid disorders (e.g., undiagnosed Graves' disease, acute thyroiditis).
- The signs and symptoms of abnormal thyroid function can mimic the signs and symptoms of typical pregnancy.
- Hyperthyroidism can occur in the pregnant client from increased secretion of human chorionic gonadotropin with a molar pregnancy. Women with hyperthyroidism are at an increased risk of complications from preeclampsia and thyroid storm. Hypothyroidism in pregnancy is a possibility.
- Inspect and palpate the thyroid gland. Symmetrical enlargement is expected. Marked or asymmetrical enlargement is not characteristic of pregnancy.

Considerations for the Neonatal Patient

- Newborn screening (which tests for various disorders, including phenylketonuria [PKU], congenital adrenal hyperplasia, hypothyroidism, sickle cell anemia), performed after 24 hours of age, is required by many (if not all) states.
- Thyroid hormone is essential for embryonic growth, particularly the tissues of the brain. The infant will be mentally retarded if no T_4 is available during fetal life. This effect can be partially reversed with the administration of T_4 at birth.
- Thyrotoxicosis is virtually nonexistent in the newborn.
- Congenital hypothyroidism may occur with clinical manifestations not evident until about 4 months of age because most cases of intrauterine thyroid failure do not occur until the third trimester. Hypothermia, delayed meconium passage, enlarged posterior fontanelle, signs of respiratory distress in the term newborn, and prolonged neonatal jaundice are suggestive signs of hypothyroidism. Clinical manifestations of hypothyroidism include feeding difficulties, hoarse cry, and protruding tongue. In addition, there may be hypotonic muscles of the abdomen, constipation, abdominal protrusion, and umbilical hernia; subnormal temperature; lethargy; excessive sleeping; bradycardia; delayed dentition; and cold, mottled skin (**Figure 14-11**). The skeletal growth is stunted. If not treated, congenital hypothyroidism can become fatal.

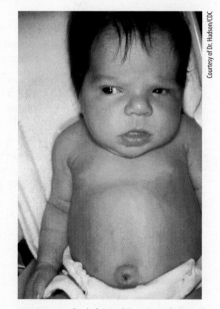
Courtesy of Dr. Hudson/CDC

- There is an increased risk of congenital hypothyroidism in children with Down syndrome. Therefore, children with Down syndrome should be screened for hypothyroidism at birth, at 6 months of age, and at each birthday.

Considerations for the Pediatric Patient

- Thyrotoxicosis occurs in approximately 2 per 1000 children younger than 10 years of age. Affected children may have hypermetabolism and accelerated linear growth, staring eyes (not true exophthalmos, which is very rare in children), and an enlarged thyroid gland.
- The majority of the cases of acquired juvenile hypothyroidism are caused by Hashimoto's thyroiditis. Signs and symptoms are similar to those manifested by adults but also include decreased growth (less than 4 cm per year), delayed puberty, and delayed tooth eruption.

FIGURE 14-11 An infant with congenital hypothyroidism.

Considerations for the Geriatric Patient

- As people age, it is not uncommon for them to experience changes in the endocrine system. Take time to do a careful health history, including both past and present medical information.
- Most older adults take numerous medications for various chronic conditions. These medications can often produce or disrupt metabolic balance.
- Pay special attention to questions related to depression, weight loss or gain, heart rate changes, increased thirst, and excessive thirst or appetite.
- Thyroid disease presents differently in older adults, with fewer signs of hyperactivity but pronounced changes in mental status reflected by apathy, depression, and emaciation. Atrial fibrillation is common in thyroid disease.
- Hypothyroidism is the most frequent thyroid disorder and is easy to misdiagnose because hair, eye, and nail changes are often associated with the normal aging process.
- The incidence of diabetes increases with age.
- Individuals older than the age of 60 may have clinical manifestations of thyrotoxicosis that are more subtle or dramatically different than those noted in younger patients. Thyrotoxicosis may be manifested as apathetic hyperthyroidism, in which the older adult is not motivated to eat, move, or interact with others. Many of these individuals are mistakenly diagnosed as having a major depression.
- In the older adult, the thyroid may become fibrotic, feeling more nodular or irregular upon palpation.

Case Study Review

Throughout this chapter, you have been introduced to Ms. K. This section of the chapter pulls together her history and demonstrates the documentation of her history and physical examination.

Chief Complaint

"I can't sleep very well even though I am always tired, and I can feel my heart racing and pounding all of the time."

Information Gathered During the Interview

JK is a 54-year-old woman who presents with a 2-month history of fatigue, insomnia, palpitations, and increased perspiration. Ms. K also complains of changes in the appearance of her eyes, a red rash, and bruising of her arms and legs.

Ms. K reports that she has had "eye burning" for some time. She has experienced lack of energy and difficulty in sleeping on and off for the last 6 years. She denies a history of diabetes, cancer, coronary artery disease, or mental health problems. She denies a history of trauma or hospitalizations.

Ms. K has never been married and has no children. Her mother is 82 and has a significant history of cardiac disease. Recently, her mother was diagnosed with hypothyroidism. Ms. K's father died at age 78 of idiopathic pulmonary fibrosis. She has no brothers or sisters. Ms. K has two aunts and three uncles, all of whom are alive. Two uncles have CAD and one aunt has diabetes. Grandparents on both sides died of "old age."

Ms. K has a very quiet social life. She states she has always had a hard time making friends. Ms. K has always been overweight, and her hair is thin and chronically hard to manage. She denies smoking, drinking alcohol, and taking drugs. She is active in church activities. She works as a secretary in a large toy factory and has been there for 20 years. She has no hobbies but loves to read and go online.

Clues	Important Points
Two-month history of palpitations	Patients with hyperthyroidism (thyrotoxicosis) frequently have palpitations.
Pulse 94; BP 140/90; respirations 20	Increased thyroid hormones cause an adrenergic-like activity, causing an increase in pulse and blood pressure. Because of an increase in metabolism, respirations are often increased to increase oxygen intake and to expel carbon dioxide.

Irregular pulse	A rapid and irregular pulse is a common finding in hyperthyroidism. An irregular pulse may indicate atrial fibrillation.
Exophthalmos	A classic manifestation of hyperthyroidism is exophthalmos.
Petechiae and bruising	Because protein degradation exceeds synthesis of protein, blood vessels may become fragile, resulting in petechiae and bruising.
Fatigue and insomnia	Because of the adrenergic-like effects of the excessive thyroid hormones, the patient may have difficulty sleeping.

Name JK	Date 10/12/15		Time 14:40
	DOB 8/11/61		Sex F

HISTORY

CC

"I can't sleep very well even though I am always tired, and I can feel my heart racing and pounding all of the time."

HPI

2-month history of palpitations, insomnia, fatigue, and increased perspiration. Petechiae and bruising on arms and legs.

Medications

Denies use of any medications except ASA (2) about once a week for headache.

Allergies

No known allergies.

PMI

"Eye burning," lack of energy, difficulty in sleeping on and off for the last 6 years. Denies diabetes, cancer, CAD, or mental health disorders.

Hospitalizations/Surgeries

None.

FH

Mother (age 82), cardiac condition; diagnosed with hypothyroidism 10 years ago. Father died (at age 78) of idiopathic pulmonary fibrosis. Aunt with diabetes. Uncle with CAD.

SH

Denies tobacco, alcohol, or drug use. Employed as secretary. Unmarried, no children. Quiet social life.

ROS

General	Cardiovascular
Weakness, insomnia almost every night, weight loss.	"Fluttering feelings," racing heart.
Skin, Hair, Nails	Respiratory
Changes in texture of hair and skin color; increased intolerance to hot and cold.	Occasional SOB.
Eyes	Gastrointestinal
Eye irritation, double vision, lid lag bilaterally.	No complaints or significant history.
Ears	Genitourinary/Gynecological
No complaints or significant history.	No complaints or significant history.
Nose/Mouth/Throat	Musculoskeletal
Choking sensation and tightness in neck.	Weakness.
Breast	Neurological
No complaints or significant history.	Shaky feelings with tremors.

PHYSICAL EXAMINATION

Weight 180 lb	Temp 98.8		BP 140/90
Height 5'5"	Pulse 94, irregular		Resp 20, regular

General Appearance

Well-developed Hispanic female who appears nervous.

Skin

Warm, moist, and erythematous. Petechiae and bruising noted on arms and legs bilaterally, no specific pattern.

HEENT
Normal cephalic, extraocular muscles intact in six cardinal fields of gaze; pupil response, visual fields, corneal reflexes intact. Bilateral exophthalmos. Hearing intact to whisper on both sides. Tonsils present; bilaterally equal in size. Oropharynx is erythematous but clear; no obvious mucosal lesion; no deviation or fasciculation of the tongue.
Neck/Lymphatic
No JVD; no difficulty swallowing noted; cervical nodes nonpalpable; trachea midline and mobile; thyroid nonpalpable, nontender.
Cardiovascular
HR, 109; irregular rate and rhythm; no S3 or S4 or murmurs noted. Pulses present at all pulse sites 2+.
Respiratory
Clear to auscultation; no adventitious sounds noted. Tactile and vocal fremitus equal in all areas. Sounds symmetrical, respiratory excursion, A&P diameter, WNL.
Gastrointestinal
Hyperactive bowel sounds with tympany. Obese, soft, nontender abdomen. No masses, organomegaly, or rebound tenderness noted. No pulses, bruits.
Genitourinary
Not examined.
Musculoskeletal
Strength 4–5/5 throughout and symmetrical. No clubbing, cyanosis; no discrete masses, scars. No cutaneous temperature differences bilaterally.
Neurological
Fine motor tremors bilaterally, disappearing at rest. Gait and posture normal, ROM all muscle/extremity; cranial nerves intact. Deep tendon reflexes; hyperactive sensory impulses present and appropriate to pain, temperature, and touch/vibration.
Laboratory Tests
Serum TSH: 1 U/mL T_3: 38 mg/dL T_4: 22
Final Assessment Findings
Hyperthyroidism

Bibliography

American Diabetes Association. (n.d.). *Position statement: Screening for diabetes.* Retrieved from http://www.diabetes.org/clinicalrecommendations/Supplement101/S21.htm.

Hinkle J. L., & Cheever K. (2014). *Brunner & Suddarth's textbook of medical-surgical nursing* (13th ed.). Philadelphia, PA: Lippincott Williams & Wilkins.

Kim, K., Kim, S., Sung, K., Wook, Y., Seok, K., & Park, W. (2012). Management of type 2 diabetes mellitus in older adults. *Diabetes and Metabolism Journal, 36*(5), 336–344. doi: 10.4093/dmj.2012.36.5.336

Porth, C. M. (2005). *Pathophysiology: Concepts of altered health states* (7th ed.). Philadelphia, PA: Lippincott Williams & Williams.

Porth, C. M. (2010). *Pathophysiology: Concepts of altered health states* (8th ed.). Philadelphia, PA: Lippincott Williams & Wilkins.

Samuels, M. H. (1998). Subclinical thyroid disease in the elderly. *Thyroid, 8,* 803–813.

Toft, A. D. (2001). Subclinical hyperthyroidism. *New England Journal of Medicine, 345,* 512–516.

Tuomilehto, J., Lindström, J., Eriksson, J. G., Valle, T. T., Hämäläinen, H., Ilanne-Parikka, P., . . . Uusitupa, M., for the Finnish Diabetes Prevention Study Group. (2001). Prevention of type 2 diabetes mellitus by changes in lifestyle among subjects with impaired glucose tolerance. *New England Journal of Medicine, 344,* 1343–1350.

Chapter 15

Musculoskeletal Disorders

The major functions of the musculoskeletal system are as follows:

- Providing a framework that supports the body
- Allowing movement of the body
- Protecting internal organs
- Serving as storage sites for minerals and producing red blood cells
- Generating body heat

Assessment of the musculoskeletal system (see **Figure 15-1**) can be difficult. Many musculoskeletal injuries and complaints can have a variety of causes that may be difficult to identify, especially when trying to pinpoint the mechanism of the complaint. Being able to perform an evidence-based assessment will increase the likelihood of making the differential diagnosis that leads you to develop a treatment plan and a positive outcome for your patient. Understanding anatomy and physiology of the problem area helps guide assessment and development of an accurate differential diagnosis.

Anatomy and Physiology Review of the Musculoskeletal System

Bones provide a system of levers (rigid rods that can be moved about a fixed point) on which a group of specialized tissues (muscles) act to produce motion. The human skeleton is made up of a total of 206 bones.

Bones are a solid network of moist living cells (osteocytes), living tissue, and fibers (collagen) that are supported by a matrix of calcium salts. Calcium salts aid in strength and protection. Osteocytes regulate the amount of calcium salts that are deposited in, or removed from, the bone matrix. They are responsible for bone growth and changes in the shape of bones. Each bone is surrounded by a tough membrane called the periosteum, which is a fibrous connective tissue membrane whose collagen fibers merge with the tendons and ligaments that are attached to the bones. The periosteum contains a network of blood vessels, which supply oxygen and nutrients to the bone. The jointed surfaces of bones are covered with articular cartilage, which provides a smooth surface for movement.

Beneath the periosteum is a thick layer of bone tissue, known as compact bone. Compact bone is very dense, similar in texture to ivory,

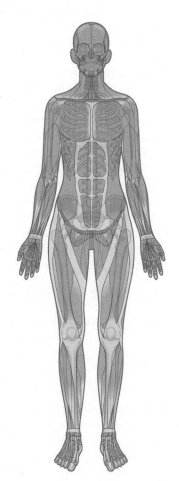

FIGURE 15-1 Musculoskeletal system.

357

but it is not solid. This thick layer of compact bone enables the shaft of long bones (called the diaphysis) to endure the large amount of stress it receives upon impact with a solid object. Compact bone also contains nerves and blood vessels carrying nourishment to the cells of the living bone tissue.

The second type of bone tissue is spongy bone, which is the inside layer of compact bone. Spongy bone is not actually soft and spongy; it is quite strong. Near the ends of any bone (called the epiphysis) where force is applied, spongy bone is organized into structures that resemble the supporting girders of a bridge. It is arranged along points of pressure or stress, making bones both light and strong. The structure of spongy bone helps add strength to bone without increasing its mass. Growth occurs in the epiphyseal disc or plate (growth plates) at the junction of the diaphysis with each epiphysis.

The cavities of bones contain a soft tissue, called bone marrow. Bone marrow produces red blood cells and special white blood cells (lymphocytes) and other elements of blood (platelets). The actual "bony" system is divided into the axial and the appendicular skeleton. The axial skeleton is composed of the skull (which consists of more than two dozen bones), the facial bones, the 12 pairs of ribs (which are attached to the vertebrae dorsally and serve as a scaffolding for the upper body torso), and the vertebral column (which extends from the base of the skull to the hip bones and contains 24 separate vertebrae plus a sacrum and a coccyx). The appendicular skeleton houses the pectoral girdle and upper limbs as well as the pelvic girdle and lower limbs.

Joints are where two bones come together; they allow movement of the bones without damaging each other. The joints can be described by the amount of movement that they have. They can be either synovial (the most common type), cartilaginous, or fibrous. Synovial joints are oily and allow the bones to move freely; they are stabilized by ligaments (e.g., the ball-and-socket joints of the hips or the hinge-like joints of the knee). Cartilaginous joints have no gap, are held together by cartilage, and move only a little (e.g., those between the vertebrae). Fibrous joints have no gap between the bones and hardly move (e.g., the flat cranial bones).

The outer layer of the joint capsule produces synovial fluid, which forms a thin lubricating film over the surface of a joint and protects the ends of bones from friction. This lubricating film enables the cartilage found on the ends of the bones to slip past each other more smoothly as the joint moves. In some freely movable joints, small pockets of synovial fluid called bursae form. Bursae reduce the friction between the bones and joints and act as tiny shock absorbers.

Ligaments and tendons are soft collagenous tissues. Ligaments connect bone to bone, and tendons connect muscles to bone. Tendons carry tensile forces from muscle to bone. When wrapped around bone like a pulley, they carry compressive forces. A sprain is a type of joint injury characterized by tearing of the ligaments and capsule. Injury to tendons or the muscles themselves is called a strain. Muscles provide movement of body parts and resist movement of body parts (postural stability). Skeletal muscles consist of muscle fibers. Connective tissue (perimysium) binds the muscle fibers into a fascicle. The epimysium binds the fasciculi together. Most muscles are attached to bones.

The Upper Extremities

The upper extremities include the shoulder, elbow, forearm, wrist, and hand. The upper extremities are prone to both acute and overuse complaints due to exposure and the nature of their use.

The Shoulder
The bones and muscles that make up the shoulder are an extremely complex region of the body.

Bones and Ligaments
The function of the shoulder involves the thorax and three bones—the humerus, the scapula, and the clavicle—and nearly 30 muscles (**Figure 15-2 A–C**). The capsule that surrounds the shoulder joint is a very strong ligament that helps to keep the ball and socket normally aligned. In the shoulder, the joint capsule is formed by a group of ligaments that connect the humerus to the glenoid. These ligaments are the main source of stability for the shoulder. They help hold the shoulder in place and keep it from dislocating.

Another ligament links the coracoid to the acromion; this ligament can thicken and cause impingement syndrome. Ligaments attach the clavicle to the acromion in the acromioclavicular (AC)

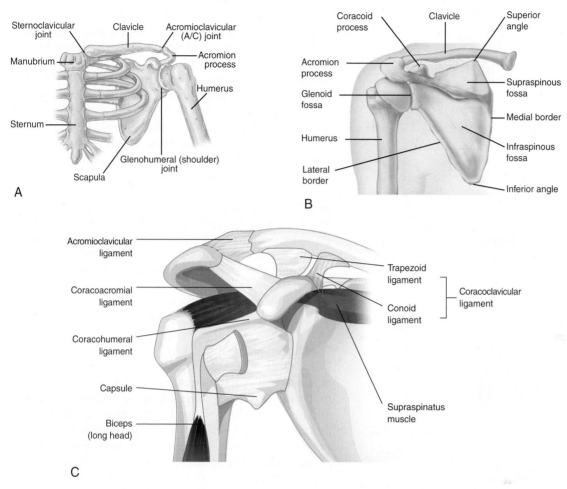

FIGURE 15-2 The shoulder. A. Anterior shoulder. B. Posterior shoulder. C. Ligaments of the anterior shoulder.

joint. Two ligaments connect the clavicle to the scapula by attaching to the coracoid process, a bony ridge on the scapula. The rotator cuff tendons are a group of four tendons that connect the deepest layer of muscles to the humerus. They are the tendons of the rotator cuff muscles.

In addition, four areas of articulation (i.e., acromioclavicular, sternoclavicular, glenohumeral, and scapulothoracic) must move normally for the shoulder to function correctly. Several bursae are located in the shoulder joint, with the subacromial bursa being the most important. This bursa is located between the acromial arch and the synovial capsule and is reinforced by the supraspinous tendon.

Muscles

The muscles of the shoulder act as reinforcement to the joint itself by offering stability to this weak, bony, and ligamentous area. The superficial muscles arise from the thorax and attach to the humeral shaft, while the deeper muscles originate from the scapula. They attach at the humeral head. These deeper muscles, consisting of the supraspinous, infraspinous, subscapular, and teres minor and major, make up the "rotator cuff" area. The supraspinatus arises from the suprascapular fossa and inserts at the humeral head. It abducts the humeral head and acts as a humeral head depressor. The infraspinous arises from the infraspinous fossa and comes together with the teres minor posteriorly. It is responsible for externally rotating and horizontally extending the humerus. The subscapularis arises from the front of the scapula and is supplied by two nerves of the brachial plexus. It is responsible for internally rotating the humerus. The teres minor externally rotates and extends the humerus.

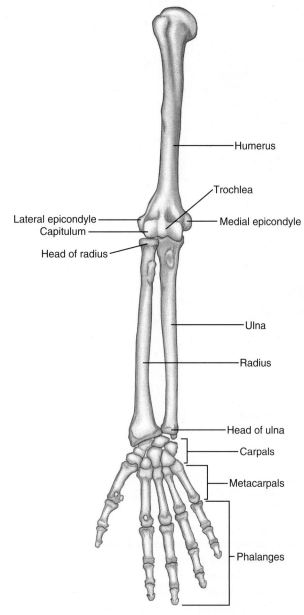

FIGURE 15-3 Anterior view of the bones of the elbow.

Labels on figure:
Humerus
Trochlea
Lateral epicondyle
Capitulum
Medial epicondyle
Head of radius
Ulna
Radius
Head of ulna
Carpals
Metacarpals
Phalanges

Shoulder Joint

The glenohumeral joint, considered a true joint, exists between the humerus and the scapula. The glenoid fossa, which acts as a receptacle for the humeral head, is located on the anterior, superior lateral margin of the scapula. The fossa is a shallow void. The area contains no cartilage, but primarily fibrous tissue, and becomes a redundant fold of the anterior capsule. Only a small portion of the humeral head is in contact with the fossa at any given time. This leads to more of a gliding movement as opposed to the ball-and-socket type joint seen in the hip.

Blood and Nerve Supply

In addition to the bones, ligaments, and muscles of the shoulder complex, there are important nerve and blood supplies that innervate this area. The subclavian artery lies distal to the sternoclavicular joint, moving downward posteriorly over the clavicle and in front of the first rib. The brachial plexus is a complex nerve network that supplies the shoulder, arms, and the hands.

The Elbow

When assessing the elbow, consider the relationship of the elbow as part of a kinetic chain that extends from the neck to the fingers. The elbow is made up of the humerus, radius, and ulna, with the lower end of the humerus forming two articulating areas known as condyles. The medial epicondyle lies on the medial aspect (the ulna side) of the humerus (**Figure 15-3**). The lateral epicondyle is the tendon on the outside (radial aspect) of the arm or elbow.

The design of the elbow permits flexion and extension at these articulating areas. The pronation and supination of the forearm are made possible because of the freedom of movement of the head of the radius.

The biceps brachii protects the capsule of the elbow anteriorly, with the triceps brachii protecting it posteriorly. The biceps act in flexion and supination, with extension under the control of the triceps. The brachial and medial arteries lie deep within the antecubital fossa and supply blood to the elbow. While assessing injury, it is important to consider the high likelihood of neurovascular problems. These nerves arise from the cervical area of C5–C8 and the thoracic region and control all of the movement of the elbow. They then branch into the antecubital fossa, and further branch into the medial radial and ulnar nerves.

The Forearm

The bones of the forearm consist of the radius and ulna. The ulna is the long, straight bone that is thicker proximally to the elbow. The radius is thicker distal to the elbow (see Figure 15-3). These bones have three articulations: the superior, middle, and distal radioulnar joints. The muscles of the forearm can be put into two categories: the flexors and the pronators on the anterior aspect, and the extensors and the supinators lying on the posterior surface.

The major blood supply to the forearm originates with the brachial artery, which divides in the forearm into the radial and ulnar arteries. The radial nerve supplies the extensor muscles, while the median nerve supplies most of the flexor muscles (with the exception of the flexor carpi ulnaris and part of the flexor digitorum profundus).

The Hand

Assessment of the hand depends on a thorough knowledge of the anatomy of this complex structure. It is important that the hand and wrist have all the structures and sensation intact, along with pain-free active movement. The wrist and hand bones (**Figure 15-4**) include the carpals (bones of the wrist); the metacarpals (bones of the hand); and the proximal, middle, and distant phalanges (bones of the fingers).

Carpals

The wrist is an articulating joint that is formed by the distal ulna, the radius, and three of the eight carpal bones. The carpal bones articulate with one another and are stabilized by numerous ligaments. Being able to identify the bones of the wrist is especially important to the clinician when assessing for any injury. An easy way to remember the bones of the wrist is to use the mnemonic "Stop Letting Those People Touch The Cadaver's Hand" to help recall the first letter of each bone name:

Scaphoid
Lunate
Triquetral
Pisiform
Trapezium
Trapezoid
Capitate
Hamate

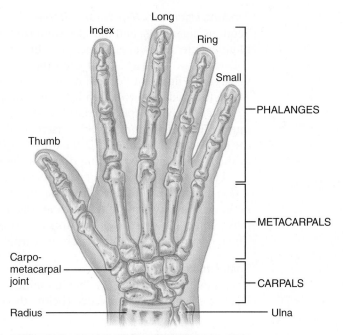

FIGURE 15-4 Bones of the wrist and hand.

With this mnemonic in mind, the proximal row (with which the radius and ulna align on the thumb side) is the scaphoid (also called the navicular). The scaphoid is probably one of the most significant bones of the hand as well as the most frequently injured carpal bone. The scaphoid lacks a good blood supply, which can lead to problems such as non-union and arthrosis if an injury is not identified promptly. Next to the scaphoid are the lunate (which articulates with the radius), the triquetral (which does not articulate with the radius but with a disc that separates the radioulnar joint from the wrist), and the pisiform (a pea-shaped bone on top of the triquetral bone) bones.

The next row of bones that begin closest to the thumb starts with the trapezium, the trapezoid, the capitate (the largest of the carpal bones), and the hamate (touches the fourth metacarpal).

The proximal row of carpal bones is smooth and perfectly articulate with the concave distal ends of the radius and ulna. These bones also articulate among themselves as gliding joints and glide along with the movement of the radiocarpal joint (which permits flexion, extension, abduction, and circumduction) and the carpometacarpal joints. Remember, these joints do not articulate with the ulna.

Metacarpals and Phalanges

The metacarpal bones are the five bones that join the carpals and the phalanges to each other and have ligaments that reinforce them. There are 14 phalanges of the hand: three for each finger and two for the thumb. They are described as being either the distal, middle, or proximal phalanges (working from the fingertip to the base of the hand).

The interphalangeal articulations are similar to hinges that only flex and extend. They also have major tendons (deep flexors and superficial flexors) that stabilize these bones.

Tendons, Ligaments, Muscles, and Nerves

Tendons, ligaments, and muscles stabilize the bones of the wrist. The three major ligaments are the ulnar collateral ligament (which attaches the styloid process of the ulna to the pisiform), the radial collateral ligament (which connects the styloid process of the radius to the navicular), and the transverse carpal ligament (located on the volar aspect of the wrist, it forms the roof of the carpal tunnel where the median nerve often becomes compressed).

There are two types of muscles—extrinsic and intrinsic. The extrinsic muscle originates in the muscle belly of the forearm and inserts in the hand. The extrinsic flexors are on the volar aspect of the hand, with the extensor on the dorsal aspect. Intrinsic muscles are small and are entirely confined to the region distal to the long bones of the forearm.

The three major nerves of the hand are the ulnar, radial, and median nerves, which provide sensation and motor control to the wrist, fingers, and hand. **Table 15-1** describes the nerves. The ulnar nerve passes between the pisiform and hamate and intervenes at the front of the hand. The radial nerve enters the wrist from the dorsal area of the forearm and terminates in the back of the hand. The median nerve travels through the carpal tunnel to the palm of the hand (**Figure 15-5**).

Volar Landmarks

Volar landmarks include the thenar eminence (the muscles are below the thumb on the palmar surface), the hypothenar eminence (below the fifth digit), and numerous creases. The dominant hand

Table 15-1	**Nerves and Motor Function of the Hand**	
Nerve	Sensations (Areas Controlled by Nerve)	Motor Control
Median	Palmar surface of the thumb, index, long, and radial half of the fourth digit (ring)	Controls opposition of the thumb and fifth digit.
	Dorsal surface of the index and long digits with radial half of the (fourth) ring digit from the DIP to the tip	Allows for control of fine pincer grip. Innervates the thenar muscle.
		Tests opposition of the thumb to each finger.
Radial	Dorsal surface of the thumb, index, and long digit, and half of the fourth (ring) digit from MCP to the DIP	Controls flexing and extension of the wrist and deviation of the wrist radially.
		Innervates the extrinsic wrist and finger extensors.
		Tests wrist and hand extension against resistance.
Ulnar	Fifth digit and ulnar aspect of half of the fourth (ring) digit, both palmar and dorsal aspects	Controls abduction of the fingers and allows the ability to cross the fingers. Allows for power grip.
		Tests finger abduction against resistance.

Abbreviations: DIP, distal phalanges; MCP, metacarpal phalanges.

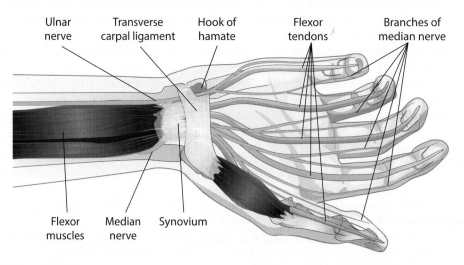

Ulnar nerve   Transverse carpal ligament   Hook of hamate   Flexor tendons   Branches of median nerve

Flexor muscles   Median nerve   Synovium

FIGURE 15-5 Carpal tunnel.

has deeper palmar creases. On the dorsal aspect, the landmarks are the ulnar and radial styloids and the anatomical snuffbox (the area just distal to the radial styloid over the navicular). The snuffbox is the depression formed by the tendons and the navicular carpal bone. Visualization of the extensor pollicis longus on the ulnar side and the abductor pollicis longus on the radial side can be done easily by having the patient extend her or his thumb.

The Lower Extremities

Hip, Pelvis, and Thigh

The ischium is the "V"-shaped bone that forms the posteroinferior part of the pelvis. It is one of the three bones—the ilium, ischium, and pubis—that form the os coxae. The ischial tuberosity is the roughened projection that protrudes posteroinferiorly from the body of the ischium.

The bony ring formed by the sacrum and the coccyx is referred to as the pelvis, with its major function being to support the spine and transfer weight and any forces from the spine and upper extremities to the lower extremities. The pelvis also provides protection to the pelvic organs, along with serving as an area of attachment for the trunk and thigh muscles. Also found in this region is the area in which the hip articulates with the femur in the deep socket, which forms a vacuum known as the acetabulum.

Of the many strong ligaments that reinforce the hip, the strongest is the iliofemoral ligament. This ligament prevents hyperextension, controls external rotation, and limits the pelvis from rotating the femur backward with weight bearing.

The gluteus maximus forms the buttock region of the hip and allows the body to rise from a sitting position to a standing position. It also assists with flexion of the knee. Nerves from the fourth and fifth lumbar, along with the first through third sacral areas, form the sacral plexus, which in turn merges with other nerves to form the sciatic nerve, which innervates the thigh. This anatomy can be important when assessing individuals with back pain.

The thigh is considered the area between the hip and knee. The femur—the long bone of the thigh—is the longest and strongest bone of the body. The head of the femur is round and smooth and articulates with the acetabulum of the pelvis. The femoral neck is the constricted area distal to the head of the femur. Most of the blood supply to the head of the femur courses along the surface of the neck. Fractures of the neck of the femur may result in avascular necrosis of the head. The greater trochanter is a large process that projects superiorly from the junction of the neck and shaft of the femur. The greater trochanter is the insertion site of the gluteus medius muscle, gluteus minimus, and obturator internus. The gluteal tuberosity, a roughened area located on the posterior surface of the femur, is one of the insertion sites of the gluteus maximus.

On the posterior surface, you can find the hamstrings, which act as extensors of the hip and flexors of the knee. The gluteus maximus muscles also act as extensors of the hip.

The adductors work at the hip to adduct the thigh. The largest adductor is the adductor magnus, which is located in the median aspect of the thigh. It originates from the tibial tuberosity and attaches to the femur with innervation of the sciatic nerve distally. The muscles of the thigh consist of the quadriceps femoris, the hamstrings, the adductors (sartorius, gracilis, and adductor longus and brevis), and the tensor fascia lata.

The quadriceps is the strongest muscle of the thigh. This muscle group's major function is the extension of the lower leg. The only flexor found in this group is the rectus femoris, which attaches at the pelvis. The femoral nerve innervates this muscle group.

The Knee

The knee is another of the complex joints of the body. It must withstand extreme stressors that are put on it in all our activities of daily living (ADLs) and recreational activities. The knee is a modified hinged joint (ginglymus) that permits the two actions of flexion and extension while working to absorb or transmit shock.

The femur articulates with the tibia (not the fibula) at the knee. The distal end of the femur forms the medial and lateral condyles, which enable it to articulate with the tibia and patella. The patella lies within the tendon of the quadriceps, and its major function is to protect the knee joint and increase leverage during extension.

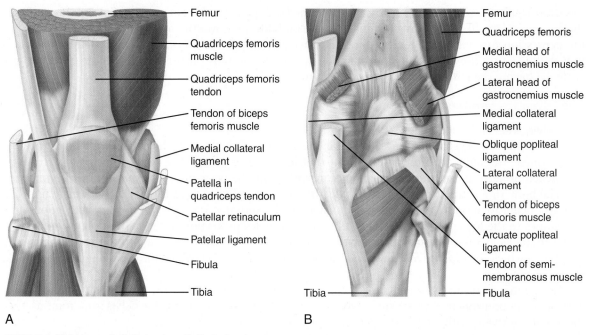

FIGURE 15-6 Right knee. A. Anterior view. B. Posterior view.

The menisci are two oval-shaped cartilages that articulate with the tibia and decrease stress to the knee itself. The medial meniscus is "C"-shaped and the lateral meniscus is more "O"-shaped. Generally, the meniscus has a poor blood supply, but the inner two-thirds are bathed in synovial fluid.

The stabilizing ligaments of the knee are made up of the cruciate, capsular, and collateral ligaments, with the major stabilizers being the cruciates. The anterior cruciate ligament (ACL) attaches just below and in front of the tibia and then proceeds to the back of the knee and attaches to the lateral condyle. The posterior cruciate ligament (PCL) is the stronger of the two ligaments and comes across the back of the tibia (up, forward, and medial) and attaches to the anterior portion of the medial condyle of the femur (**Figure 15-6**). The ACL prevents posterior movement of the femur during weight bearing and prevents the tibia from any abnormal rotation. It is tight in extension and loosened in flexion. The PCL prevents hyperextension with a gliding motion during weight bearing. The capsular and collateral stabilizing ligaments ensure that the femur, knee, and tibia move in the correct way without rotation.

The knee has approximately 11 bursa sites, which are situated in areas where the probability of friction is high. The prepatellar bursa (located over the patella) is often injured with a contusion to the patella. The infrapatellar bursa is located superior to the tibial tubercle; when inflamed, it appears as an area of swelling inferior to the patella (i.e., bursitis).

The Foot and Ankle

The foot consists of 26 bones whose major functions are strength, flexibility, and coordinated movement. The largest tarsal bone is the calcaneus, which supports the irregularly shaped talus (the major weight-bearing bone) and makes up the shape of the heel (**Figure 15-7**). Its major function is to convey weight from the body to the ground and act as a lever with the calf muscle. The calcaneus is also the area in which the plantar fascia originates before ending at the proximal heads of the metatarsals. The plantar fascia is a thick fibrous band that supports the foot against downward forces.

The ankle is a hinge joint formed by the articulation of the tibia/fibula and talus in an area called the mortise. Because of the bony and fortified ligamentous arrangement that exists in the ankle, this joint is quite strong, with the medial aspect being stronger than the lateral.

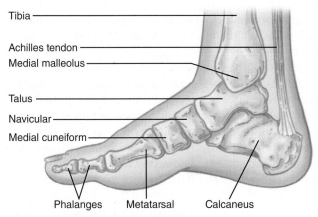

FIGURE 15-7 Medial view of the right foot.

The Spine

The spine is composed of 33 vertebrae (7 cervical, 12 thoracic, 5 lumbar, 5 sacral, and the coccyx), with 24 being movable (with the remaining 9 immovable). The spine's design (four sagittal curves) provides strength, flexibility, and balance. The five lumbar vertebrae are the strongest and most massive of the vertebrae, with most of the flexion occurring at L5–S1 (**Figure 15-8**).

An important joint in this area, the sacroiliac (SI) joint, is the point where the sacrum and the ilium are joined. This joint transmits a lot of the body's weight when standing and sitting occur. Several ligaments connect the vertebrae and muscles along the spine allow for movement.

Health History

The history is one of the most essential components in the management of any patient with musculoskeletal problems. An accurate patient history will serve as a guide to the etiology of the problem. Carefully listening to the patient's concerns often provides important clues (i.e., chief complaint [CC] and history of present illness [HPI]). As with complaints in any other body system, the history must include a detailed past medical history (PMI), family history (FH), social history (SH), and review of systems (ROS).

Chief Complaint and History of Present Illness

"My right hip and hand hurt."

PD is a 25-year-old female who presents with pain to her right hip and hand after falling off a mountain bike. Ms. D explains that while she was testing a new mountain bike, she tried to jump a curb and was thrown over the handlebars and landed on her right side. She was wearing a helmet and there was no loss of consciousness. After the incident, she was able to stand up and limp back to the store with the bike as a crutch, and then to her car. Ms. D took some acetaminophen (Tylenol) last night, but when she awoke this morning, she was unable to move her right wrist and shoulder or bear weight on her right leg. She has a large abrasion and ecchymotic area on her right thigh with no swelling. She states that she had a difficult time putting her bra on and brushing her teeth this morning. She prefers to lie supine because sitting makes her right hip hurt.

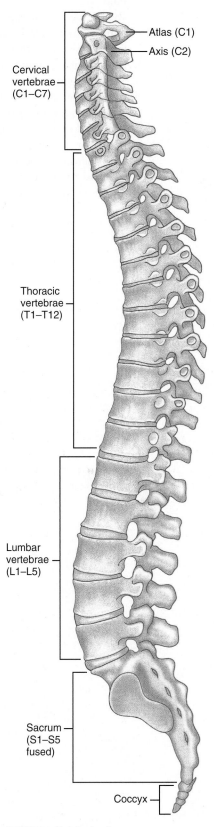

FIGURE 15-8 Vertebral column.

Pain

Pain is a common complaint seen when assessing musculoskeletal problems and may be exacerbated with normal activities or work-related activities. It is usually the body's protective response to possible injury. This protective mechanism not only has physiologic characteristics (as seen with the pain with movement and numbness), but it can also have emotional (perception of the degree of pain) elements. This emotional component many times makes it difficult to adequately assess the problem. Knowing the type of pain and location, along with the mechanism of injury, is a good indicator of injury probability.

Inflammation is one of the most common causes of pain and can be identified by redness, edema, heat, and even a decrease in function of the affected area. When inflammation occurs, potent chemical mediators stimulate nociceptors to begin a "chemical chain reaction" that, if not intercepted, can lead to numerous pathophysiologic consequences. Careful and accurate assessment of an individual's pain will assist you in ensuring an effective plan of care along with an effective outcome for your patient.

Onset	Was the pain sudden, acute, gradual, insidious, or a combination of these? (Let the patient describe in his or her own words.)
	Keep in mind that the mechanism of injury can be an excellent indicator of the injury probability.
	Acute onset suggests a fracture or a large tear. Gradual onset suggests inflammation.
Duration	How long has the pain been going on?
	If it has been constant and unremitting, consider malignancy. Be sure to elicit a history that will allow you to look for signs and symptoms of systemic illness.
	If the pain is constant, consider an acute condition, such as a sprain or bursitis. If the pain is felt only after repeating the mechanism of injury, consider a localized lesion. If the pain is reproduced only in certain directions, consider a muscle or ligament injury. If the pain occurs only after repeated movement, consider an overuse injury.
Location; radiation	Where on the body is the pain located? Think about the anatomy of the area in question and what may be lying under that area.
	For example, if the pain is in the lateral shoulder, consider glenohumeral arthritis, supraspinous tendinitis, or subacromial bursitis. If the patient has posterior shoulder pain, consider infraspinatus tendinitis. If the patient has radicular pain, consider a disc problem associated with back pain. Ask the patient to point to the area where she or he is having pain. Local pain tends to be more superficial and the patient is able to easily point to the painful area.
	Keep in mind that the pain may be referred. For example, abdominal pain may refer pain to the shoulder. Referred pain tends to come from deep structures and nerves.
Quality; severity	Does this pain keep the patient from doing ordinary activities or does she or he become fatigued much more easily? Use a pain scale (e.g., scale of 1–10 or face scale) to allow the patient to rate the pain objectively so that you can measure outcomes. Is it sharp, dull, burning (think nerves), or aching (deep tissue)? Any numbness or tingling?
	Sharp pain is seen frequently with injuries to the skin, tendon, superficial muscles or ligaments, and bursae. Aching pain is seen with deep tissue problems. Burning pain is seen with skin injuries such as blisters, fungal foot infections, or nerve injury. It is also seen when a muscle is being overworked/stressed, as in exercise.

Disability	Was there immediate disability or did the symptoms occur later (e.g., the next morning)? Did the patient continue with the activity that he or she was participating in when the pain started? Could the patient bear weight or use the area in question? Is there any locking of the joint or other area?
Associated symptoms	Ask about associated symptoms, including noises, swelling, or discoloration.
	Did the patient hear a "pop," crunch, clicking, or a snap before the onset of pain or when he or she experiences pain now?
	If so, this may suggest that the pain may be caused by a severe tear or break. Common sites for loose bodies are in the joints, which will have a clicking, locking, or popping sound.
	Did the swelling occur immediately or develop overnight while sleeping?
	If the swelling was immediate, consider severe tear or fracture. If the swelling occurred more gradually, consider inflammation. Typically, the more immediate the swelling, the more likely blood is causing the inflammation. This may be an unreliable sign, and the swelling may increase the perceived pain due to inflammation and irritation.
Precipitating factors	Does the time of day make a difference in when the pain occurs?
	If the patient reports morning pain, consider inflammation; disc problems may get better at night.
	Do you have pain with specific activities?
	For example, sneezing and coughing will affect disc problems. If there is pain medial to the scapular over the trapezius, consider myofascial pain syndrome.
	Has the patient experienced any pain flare-ups? If so, what does the patient think may have caused them?
Alleviating factors	Is the pain relieved by certain activities or rest?
	Ongoing back pain unrelieved by activity or rest suggests pancreatitis, abdominal aortic aneurysm, or a malignancy, and excludes musculoskeletal or disc disease.

Change in Motor Function

It is necessary to assess and evaluate the nature and degree of motor and functional deficits. Being able to consistently and objectively assess and evaluate the nature and degree of motor and functional deficits is key.

Onset	Was the onset acute or gradual?
	Acute onset suggests a rupture of a muscle (e.g., supraspinatus or AC separation). Gradual onset suggests inflammation or swelling of the muscle, tendon, or ligaments.
Location	In what part of the range of motion (ROM) does this change in motor function occur?
	Specific parts of the ROM help to pinpoint what type of injury the patient may have. Arthritis or any type of inflammation affects the entire ROM. Pain with overhead motion and a decrease in the entire ROM of the shoulder suggests impingement.

Quality	Do you feel any snaps or catches with the ROM? Are there any restrictions to the ROM (e.g., trauma, swelling, noxious stimuli)?
	Restrictions to the ROM can be caused by swelling or tearing of a muscle or a tendon (e.g., rotator cuff or biceps tendon rupture).
Associated symptoms	Is there any obvious swelling of the joints (acute or gradual)? Are there any problems with other systems? Have you noticed any changes in strength associated with the change in motor function? If so, were they acute or gradual?
	Other symptoms may limit the time that these motor functions can revert to their normal limits or prevent them from reverting to normal at all.
Mechanism of injury	How was the injury sustained? In which position was the affected region when injured (i.e., flexion, extension, supination, pronation)?
	Knowing the mechanism of injury and underlying anatomy can give cues for a differential diagnosis (e.g., a fall on an outstretched wrist should make you think of a radius or scaphoid fracture). Falling onto a flexed wrist increases the risk of rupture to the radiocarpal ligaments. A history of lifting, twisting, or a sudden change of load may lead to low back strain.

Alteration in Sensation

Assessing the changes in sensation can almost always be related to the cellular level of function (e.g., if the tissue is receiving the correct amount of perfusion).

Onset	Was the onset acute or gradual?
Quality	Have you experienced changes in proprioception (e.g., tingling, numbness, and warmth)?
	Nerve impingement can often change sensation owing to swelling or injury to the nerve.
Associated symptoms	Have you noticed any changes in skin color?
	Redness indicates infection or inflammation. Pale/chalky skin indicates circulatory compromise. Note: During the physical examination, be sure to check pulses above and below the site of injury.
	Have you experienced any change in body temperature?
	An increased body temperature indicates inflammation or infection.
	A decreased body temperature indicates circulatory compromise.

Past Medical History

Ms. D has no past history of previous injury to her shoulder, hand, or leg. She denies any surgeries. Her only medications are NSAIDs for pain. Ms. D denies any chronic conditions.

The past medical history often provides substantial clues to diagnosis. Be sure to note any history of musculoskeletal trauma.

Past trauma or surgery	Ask about recent trauma and past surgeries.
	This information will enable you to again distinguish between acute and chronic problems. If this is a chronic problem, determine what may have exacerbated this problem. If this is a recurring problem with similar intensity/location, it may be the result of overuse of the affected area.
	Direct trauma may result in disruption to neurological pathways, so be sure to evaluate for any secondary injuries. If the patient experienced recent trauma, start considering soft-tissue injury versus bony injury. If the patient has a history of a recent surgery, the cause could be an infectious process or residual problems.
Presence of impaired senses	Ask about impaired senses (sight or hearing), impaired gait, dizziness/vertigo, and slow tissue healing.
	Any impairment in these areas may cause a delay or influence the recovery of the patient.
Past health conditions	Ask about past or ongoing health conditions.
	The presence of chronic illnesses (e.g., osteoporosis, diabetes mellitus, cancer, renal or neurological problems) may increase the risk of injury, decrease the rate of healing, and decrease muscle mass.
Skeletal deformities/ congenital anomalies	Ask about congenital abnormalities and deformities.
Medications	Ask about use of medications.
	Some medications may lead to change in gait and predispose a patient to injury.

Family History

> Ms. D has a maternal grandmother who suffers from arthritis. Ms. D's mother is alive and well. Her father has coronary artery disease, and her paternal grandfather died at the age of 67 from coronary artery disease. Ms. D's paternal grandmother and aunt are on medication for osteoporosis. There is no family history of lung disease, diabetes, or cancer.

Information obtained in this section can determine any genetic or hereditary factors that may be playing a role in the patient's chief complaint. This may assist the provider in determining which diagnostic and screening procedures should be included in the patient's plan of care.

Age of living relatives	Include the relationship and health of parents, siblings, and children.
Deaths	Include the relationship of the deceased person to the patient and the cause of death (specifically, disorders that affect the musculoskeletal system).
Chronic diseases	Do any members of the family have chronic diseases? Identify the relationship of the patient to the affected family member, the age of the affected family member, and at which age this family member developed the disease. Identify any risk factors for osteoporosis; arthritis (rheumatoid, osteoarthritis, or gout); scoliosis/back problems; ankylosing spondylitis; or genetic disorders (dwarfism, osteogenesis imperfecta).
Prenatal health	Inquire whether the patient's mother was healthy during her pregnancy with the patient. Inquire about any congenital abnormalities of the patient (especially feet or hip).

Social History

Ms. D is a graduate student in town. She denies use of tobacco and drugs. She reports a social drinking history of about two glasses of wine a month. She denies ever receiving a blood transfusion. She is an avid outdoors person and loves to mountain bike.

Family	Ask the patient to describe the current family unit.
Occupation	Ask the patient to describe the nature of her work, in regard to physical and emotional effort and stress (overuse injury). Does the job carry a potential for injury? Does the patient use any safety precautions, such as spinal support belt, splints, or an ergonomically correct workstation? Is there a presence of environmental hazards at the workplace (e.g., working too long at a computer may cause carpal tunnel syndrome or back pain; carpet layers indicate an increased risk of knee problems; swimmers [especially those doing the butterfly stroke] will have an increased risk for rotator cuff problems)? Work-related musculoskeletal disorders can be associated with the following work postures and movements: repetitive movements and pace of work, force of movements, vibrations, and temperature.
Hobbies or leisure activities	Ask the patient to list all leisure activities and hobbies. Has the patient experienced any decrease in the ability to participate in usual activities? At which level of intensity does she or he complete this activity? Are any of these activities placing undue stress on the joints? Which type of physical conditioning is she or he involved in? Does the patient adhere to a warm-up/cool-down period with each activity? Does the patient play any contact sports? What is the level of competition? Be sure to note the technique and equipment (e.g., shoes and athletic gear) used. Is the patient in a period of rapid growth (e.g., childhood, adolescence)?
	All of these questions are important when assessing overuse injuries. The patient may also be involved in activities that are exacerbating the musculoskeletal problem.
	Is there any increase in the amount of time spent watching TV?
	An increase in passive activities often decreases the amount of regular exercise and increases the risk for injury when the patient participates in sporadic exercise (i.e., "weekend warrior").
Nutritional status, weight changes	Ask about nutrition and dietary intake (specifically, calcium, protein, and vitamin D).
	During adolescence, young women should be taking in approximately 1500 mg of calcium/day (adolescents may be at an increased risk for ACL injury when menstruating). Anorexia/bulimia increases the risk of fractures.
	Poor nutrition leads to a decrease in muscle mass that leads to a decrease in protection to connective tissue and bones.
	Has the patient experienced any recent weight gain or loss?
	Obesity will increase the risk for osteoarthritis, back pain, and joint problems.

Use of tobacco	Ask about tobacco use, including types, amounts, duration of use, and exposure to secondary smoke.
	Tobacco use may delay healing.
Use of alcohol	Does the patient drink alcohol? If so, which type and how much does the patient drink?
	Alcohol use may delay healing or may even increase/worsen any injury.
Use of recreational drugs	Is the patient using recreational drugs? If so, which drugs and how much?
	Use of recreational drugs increases the risk of injury due to impaired thought processes.

Review of Systems

Many musculoskeletal diseases and disorders have manifestations in systems other than the musculoskeletal system. A comprehensive review of systems should be performed whenever possible; however, due to time and other types of constraints, the provider may be able to perform only a focused review of systems. During a focused review of systems, the provider targets questioning at the systems in which musculoskeletal problems are most likely to have manifestations. Most musculoskeletal disorders have manifestations limited to the musculoskeletal system; however, following is a summary of other systemic manifestations of musculoskeletal problems.

System	Symptom or Sign	Possible Associated Diseases/Disorders
General	Fever, chills	Osteomyelitis, septic arthritis, metastatic bone disease, JRA, gout
	Weight loss	Metastatic bone disease, JRA, osteomalacia
	Fatigue	RA
Respiratory	Dyspnea	JRA
Cardiovascular	Chest pain	JRA
	Changes in pulses and sensation, warmth	Fracture, dislocation, Raynaud's syndrome
Genitourinary	Bowel/bladder dysfunction	Cauda equina syndrome

Abbreviations: JRA, juvenile rheumatoid arthritis; RA, rheumatoid arthritis.

Physical Examination

Equipment Needed

- Tape measure
- Reflex hammer

Components of the Physical Examination

When examining the musculoskeletal system, always consider the high likelihood that a musculoskeletal problem may have a neurovascular problem in conjunction. Consider the entire skeletal system as part of a kinetic chain. If cues are missed, these problems can become long-term disabilities.

While performing a musculoskeletal examination, think of the "five P's":

Pain
Paralysis
Paresthesia
Pallor
Pulselessness

BOX 15-1   GENERAL STRATEGIES FOR MUSCULOSKELETAL EXAMINATION

Place the patient in a comfortable position. Make sure the room is warm. These actions make the examination easier and less painful. Be sure the patient removes all rings, earrings, and bracelets that may compromise circulation if the area becomes edematous.

INSPECTION

Note the gait when the patient enters the room. Also, note how the patient sits, takes off clothing, and even stands up from a sitting position. This will enable you to assess the patient without her or him knowing that you are watching her or him. While taking the history, note any use of the affected area when the patient is talking with you and describing the injury or complaint. You can determine a lot about range of motion when the patient is not aware of what she or he may be doing (e.g., you can rule out a c-spine injury if the individual turns the head from side to side while speaking). Pay close attention to the patient's posture and positioning of any injured area.

Inspect the joints carefully (anterior and posterior) for contour, unusual skin markings, ecchymosis, redness, swelling (local or diffuse), atrophy/hypertrophy, changes in the integrity of the skin (e.g., lacerations and abrasions), guarding, deformity, or discoloration. Note any pallor, cyanosis, or bleeding. Compare the joints anteriorly and posteriorly, as well as bilaterally. Ruptures cause an "unusual shape" or dislocation.

PALPATION

Encourage the patient to relax. Putting her or him at ease will allow you to passively move the injured area. Patient anxiety, edema, and extreme pain may make it difficult to examine the joint thoroughly for ligamentous stability.

Palpate the joints. Note any tenderness, masses, crepitus, bony deformities, or lesions. Assess capillary refill, temperature of the area, and pulse.

RANGE OF MOTION

Test range of motion (ROM) both passively and actively. (Remember that passive ROM is what the patient can do on his or her own; active ROM requires your assistance in completing the movement.) Passive and active ROM should be the same. Any discrepancies may indicate that there is true muscle weakness or a problem in the joint. Note any crepitus or tenderness with movement.

MUSCLE STRENGTH

Evaluate the strength of each muscle group. Ask the patient to flex and hold it while you apply an opposing force. The patient should not move the joint with this test. Perform this test bilaterally and then grade the muscle strength on a scale from 0 to 5:

> 5 Normal
> 4 Good
> 3 Fair
> 2 Poor
> 1 Trace

Using the five P's will assist you in performing a more concise examination in any musculoskeletal problem.

Musculoskeletal examination involves inspection, palpation, testing ROM, and testing muscle strength. General strategies for these parts of the exam are described in **Box 15-1**.

Examining the Shoulder

The shoulder is a complex structure. Being aware of the structures that make up the shoulder will aid in your assessment. **Table 15-2** summarizes common shoulder problems.

Table 15-2 Common Shoulder Problems	
Problem/Diagnosis	Assessment Findings
Myofascial pain	■ Asymmetrical "trigger points" that are medial to the scapula and over the trapezius. ■ Stress and/or previous neck injuries.
Subacromial bursitis	■ Tenderness that can be palpated over the head of the humerus many times on the dominant extremity; it is due to inflammation of the bursae, and pain will be elicited with internal and external rotation at 90 degrees and abduction greater than 30 degrees. ■ Pain at night. ■ Abrupt onset, but without any known trauma. ■ Overuse pattern (identified when you question the patient further about her or his occupation).
Acromioclavicular (AC) joint separation	■ History of a direct fall or blow to the "point" of the shoulder (x-rays [with weights] will confirm).
Shoulder dislocation	■ Any trauma to the shoulder with a mechanism of injury involving external rotation with abduction. ■ Loss of the normal contour of the shoulder (x-rays will confirm). ■ Marked instability: when moving anteriorly, the shoulder moves too far forward; when moved posteriorly, it moves too far back. *Note: Be sure that you palpate pulses distally to be sure that they are present.*
Frozen shoulder (adhesive capsulitis)	■ Total restriction of normal range of motion with an insidious onset of pain. ■ Cause thought to be an inflammatory process, holding it dependent, or prolonged immobilization. ■ Common in women, after age 50, and in diabetics.
Clavicle fractures	■ Direct trauma to the clavicle. ■ Obvious deformity to the mid-shaft. ■ Pain on palpation to the region.

Inspection

Action	Rationale
1. Assess both the anterior and posterior shoulder. Inspect the contour of the clavicles, scapula, and shoulders. Look for any wasting of the deltoid or swelling of the joint.	1. These structures should be symmetrical in contour. Any asymmetry or a hollow rounded area in the contour suggests a shoulder dislocation. The patient may even be guarding the area (not allowing you to move the area or not using the area him or her self).
2. Inspect for "winging" of the scapula. (Winging is when the scapula is very pronounced, an outward prominence of the scapula.) Test the function of the serratus anterior by asking the patient to push against a wall.	2. Winging is an abnormal finding that may be caused by a weakness or paralysis of the serratus anterior, which may be secondary to a brachial plexus injury. If there is "winging" of the scapula, suspect a disruption of the nerves or muscles in this area.
3. Inspect for discoloration of the skin (e.g., bruising, or redness).	3. The color of bruising helps indicate whether the injury is acute or old (blue versus yellow-green). Redness suggests infection or inflammatory process.

Palpation

Action	Rationale
1. Ask the patient to place the arms at her or his sides. Palpate the sternoclavicular joint, acromioclavicular (AC) joint (**Figure 15-9**), acromion process, clavicles, spine of the scapula, and greater trochanter of the humerus. Palpate shoulders separately to obtain the best assessment; assess the noninjured side first.	1. No discomfort should occur when you are palpating an area. Any tenderness to these areas may be suggestive of a rupture to the ligaments or muscles. Palpation of the AC joint may reveal discomfort, pain, and hollowing. Hollowing indicates a shoulder dislocation. Pain over the supraspinatus suggests rotator cuff tendinitis.

Action

Rationale

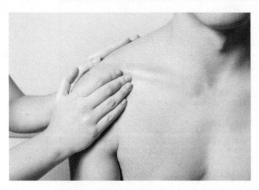

FIGURE 15-9 Palpating the acromioclavicular joint.

2. Palpate the groove of the biceps and triceps. Have the patient flex her or his arm to contract the biceps muscles. Then, have the patient abduct and hold the arm midway between flexion and extension.

2. Abnormal findings include pain, tenderness, and muscle spasm.

Range of Motion and Special Tests
A quick test for range of motion is "arms above the head and arms behind the back"; however, you should test for mobility in a systematic way (as described in step 1). This mobility testing should be done both actively (patient's own strength) and passively (done by you).

Action

Rationale

1. Test range of motion.
   a. Have the patient reach straight forward with arms horizontal to the ground.

   b. Assess abduction and adduction (**Figure 15-10**). Ask the patient to reach overhead and past the ear as far as he or she can (abduction). Remember that 0 degrees is with the hand by his or her side and 180 degrees is with the hand fully extended over the head. Then, ask the patient to reach down and across his or her chest as far as he or she can.

   c. Assess external and internal rotation (**Figure 15-11**). To test external rotation, have the patient flex the elbow 90 degrees. Hold the patient's elbow against his or her side, and have him or her externally rotate the arm to the point that begins to bring on discomfort. Assess internal rotation by having the patient move the shoulder as if he or she were going to "scratch his or her back." With the elbows at the patient's side, have him or her raise the thumb up the spine as far as he or she can.

   a. The patient should be able to raise the arms without difficulty. If sharp pains occur with this motion, consider rotator cuff impingement.
   b. With a complete rotator cuff tear, the patient will not be able to adduct the shoulder. When attempting this maneuver, he or she will instead have a look of "shrugging" of the shoulder.

   c. During internal rotation, reaching T7 is normal.

Action   **Rationale**

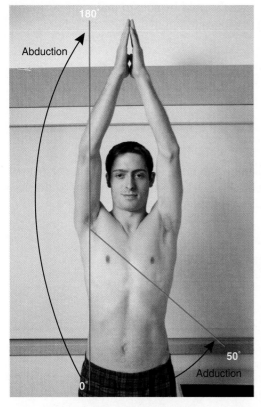

FIGURE 15-10 Testing shoulder abduction and adduction.

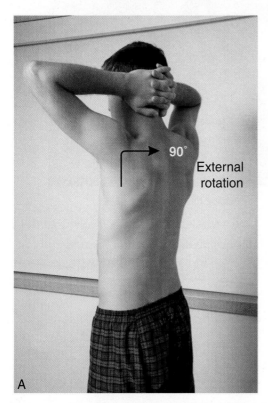

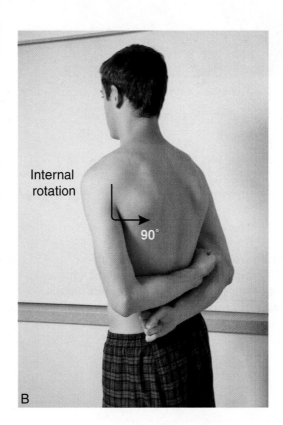

FIGURE 15-11 Assessing external (A) and internal (B) rotation.

Action	Rationale

2. Test the rotator cuff strength both externally and internally.

   a. To test external strength, have the patient sit with arms at his or her sides and elbows bent at 90 degrees. Apply internal resistance while the patient maintains the elbow positioning.

   b. Internal resistance can be tested as described previously, but have the patient attempt to rotate internally while you apply external resistance.

3. Test biceps and triceps function.

   a. To test the biceps, ask the patient to flex the elbow against resistance (**Figure 15-12**).

   b. To test the triceps, have the patient push against your hands (**Figure 15-13**).

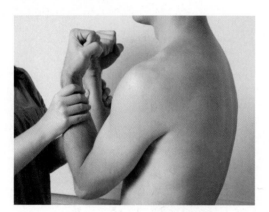

FIGURE 15-12 Testing biceps strength.

4. Perform the cross-arm horizontal adduction test. Ask the patient to place his or her hand on the opposite shoulder, while you exert force horizontally (**Figure 15-14**).

2. The patient should be able to maintain position when resistance is applied.

3. The patient should be able to perform these tasks without pain. Decreased strength may be due to a tear or an inflammation.

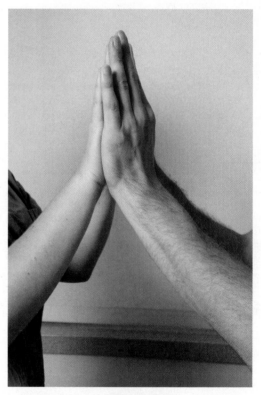

FIGURE 15-13 Testing triceps strength.

4. Pain indicates possible pathology. Cross-arm test is for acromioclavicular joint disorder.

Action   **Rationale**

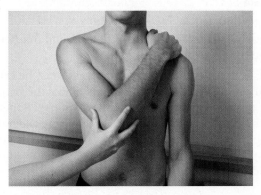

FIGURE 15-14 Assessing cross-arm adduction.

5. Test for impingement. Use the following two techniques.
   a. Hold the scapula down and pronate and flex the forearm (Neer's sign).

   b. Perform the Hawkin's test. Have the patient stand with the shoulder abducted 90 degrees while you internally rotate the forearm.

    a. Pain indicates a positive Neer's sign; consider rotator cuff tendinitis in patients with a history of dull, achy pain of gradual onset.
    b. Pain is caused by overstretching of the ligaments, causing the greater tuberosity to impinge against the acromion. This test is to determine subacromial impingement or rotator cuff tendinitis.

6. Perform the drop arm test. Have the patient hold the arm up to the side (fully abduct the arm). Then, ask the patient to slowly lower it to the side *or* lightly tap the patient's wrist and see if it falls to the side.

6. The drop arm test is designed to find tears of the rotator cuff. An abnormal finding is when the patient is unable to hold the affected arm at 90 degrees. Consider a rotator cuff tear in patients with a positive history of night pain and an inability to initiate abduction.

7. Perform the apprehension test, which tests for anterior instability. Have the patient's arm abducted to 90 degrees while you externally rotate the arm and apply anterior pressure to the humerus.

7. Normally the patient will allow you to perform the entire ROM. Positive findings indicate shoulder instability (dislocation).

8. Perform the laxity test. With the patient supine, stabilize the scapula and slide the humeral head anteriorly and posteriorly within the glenoid fossa to evaluate stability of the joint. Note the axial load being applied to the elbow.

8. This test assists in the diagnosis of glenohumeral laxity. Normally the patient will be able to perform the entire ROM without pain or loss of strength.

Examining the Elbow

Remember that all the joints of the elbow are very stable due to the bony structure of the elbow. The joints of the elbow aid in prevention of hyperextension and lateral deviation. The joint capsule limits flexion. While assessing the elbow, keep in mind that any injury to the elbow has a high likelihood of neurovascular problems.

Inspection

Action	Rationale
1. Ask the patient to flex and extend the elbow while you observe the contour of the elbow. Watch how she or he carries the elbow.	1. If the elbow is hyperextended, it may make individuals more prone to irritation and injury to the biceps tendon.
2. Inspect for swelling, deformities, and nodules.	2. Swelling over the olecranon process must be cared for immediately; chronic bursitis places the patient at risk for tendon rupture with trauma. A "Popeye" arm with localized bulging of the biceps when the elbow is flexed and an inability of the patient to supinate with the examiner's fingers on the elbow indicates a biceps tendon at risk for rupture.

Palpation

Action	Rationale
1. Palpate for tenderness over the extensor surface of the ulna and the medial and lateral epicondyles. Position the patient with the elbow flexed and the shoulder hyperextended.	1. Any swelling, bogginess, fluctuant swelling, point tenderness, or increased pain with supination and pronation suggests tendinitis or epicondylitis.
2. Palpate the ulnar nerve (funny bone). Consider this nerve involvement with any injury to the elbow. Flex elbow and test the ulnar nerve for sensation and motor function.	2. Normally, there should not be tenderness or decreased sensation. Impingement shows decreased sensation and motor function of hand and fingers. Chronic damage may lead to the patient not being able to make a fist.
3. Palpate the olecranon process (**Figure 15-15**). With the patient's elbow flexed, palpate the proximal end of the ulna and also the groove of the humerus.	3. Abnormal findings include tenderness and redness. Limited movement suggests infection or bursitis. If nodules are noted, consider rheumatoid arthritis.
4. Palpate the radial head. With the patient's shoulder abducted and elbow flexed, palpate the epicondyle; the radial head is approximately 1 to 1½ cm distal to the lateral epicondyle.	4. Pain indicates inflammation due to infection, fracture, or tendinitis.

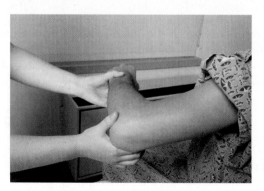

FIGURE 15-15 Palpating the olecranon process.

Range of Motion and Special Tests

Action	**Rationale**
1. Examine extension, flexion, supination, and pronation (**Figure 15-16**). Bend and straighten the elbow and observe the full ROM. With the patient's elbow flexed at 90 degrees, rotate the hand (or supinate and pronate).	1. Flexion should be approximately 150–160 degrees; extension should be approximately 180 degrees. The normal hand rotation movement is approximately 90 degrees. Inflammation, swelling, infection of the bursae, and arthritis limit ROM.

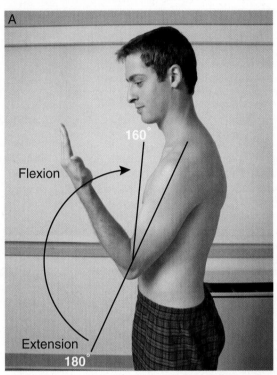
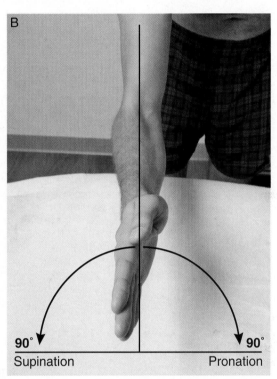

FIGURE 15-16 Assessing the range of motion of the elbow. A. Flexion and extension. B. Supination and pronation.

Action	**Rationale**
2. Test for lateral epicondylitis (tennis elbow). With the patient's elbow almost fully extended, push on her or his wrist.	2. With lateral epicondylitis, the opposing force will cause pain at the lateral epicondyle due to tendon inflammation at the insertion on the lateral epicondyle.
3. Test for medial epicondylitis (golfer's elbow or Little League elbow). Assess wrist flexion against resistance.	3. Medial epicondylitis will cause pain medially when resistance is applied.

Examining the Wrist, Hand, and Fingers

Remember that the hands and wrist are in constant motion and are involved in many activities. When these areas are extended beyond their normal ROM, the underlying tissue and ligaments will become injured. The amount of injury depends on the mechanism of injury and the amount of force expended on the area, along with the amount of time that the force was applied. Being able to diagnose injuries to this area correctly can minimize disability later. The most commonly missed injuries that are noted to the wrist are fractures to the carpals (especially the navicular). If you are unable to diagnose the exact injury, immobilize the wrist (using a thumb spica splint) and reevaluate the patient in 7 to 10 days. **Table 15-3** describes common wrist, hand, and finger problems.

Table 15-3 Common Wrist, Hand, and Finger Problems	
Problem/Diagnosis	Assessment Findings
Colles' fracture	■ History of a fall on an outstretched hand (FOSH). ■ Pain, edema, and limited range of motion (ROM) with an obvious deformity ("dinner fork") of the wrist.
Navicular fracture	■ History of FOSH injury with the impact on the fingers or distal palm. ■ Tenderness over the anatomical snuffbox, which increases with the movement of the wrist. ■ Possible swelling. *Note: If you are unsure of a fracture, you should immobilize the wrist and reevaluate it in 2 weeks because a missed fracture can result in avascular necrosis or nonunion.*
Carpal tunnel syndrome	■ Pain that increases at night. ■ Clumsiness, with distribution of numbness located in the median nerve distribution (in the thumb, index, and long fingers and radial aspect of the ring finger). ■ Possible wasting of the thenar eminence. ■ Tinel's sign (percussion over the median nerve reproduces the pain and tingling). ■ History of performing repetitive movements. *Note: Carpal tunnel syndrome is often seen in pregnant women (due to edema), alcoholics, and patients with arthritis and hypothyroidism.*
De Quervain's tenosynovitis	■ Pain in the radial aspect of the wrist that is aggravated with ulnar deviation of the hand with the thumb flexed (such as when turning a doorknob). ■ A thickening sheath or nodule in the area of tenderness upon palpation. ■ Positive Finkelstein test (having the patient flex the thumb into his or her palm and then cover with the other fingers, and passively ulnar—deviating the wrist elicits pain in the affected area).
Ganglion cyst	■ A nodule on the dorsum aspect of the wrist (this nodule is really a synovial cyst from a herniated tendon lining). ■ Painless to a dull ache if the nodule is really large.
Gamekeeper's thumb/ skier's thumb (ulnar collateral ligament tear)	■ History of a sudden, forceful abduction of the thumb. ■ Pain on the ulnar side of the thumb with swelling of the metacarpal phalanges. ■ Stress testing reveals laxity (Stress testing is performed by stabilizing the metacarpophalangeal joint in flexion and radially deviating the thumb. More than 30 degrees deviation or more than 20 degrees deviation compared with the opposite side suggests significant damage to the ulnar collateral ligament.)

Inspection

Action	Rationale
1. Have the patient place the hand on a pillow or table. Inspect the palm and dorsum. Observe the thenar and hypothenar eminences. Note the color of the fingernails and tips. Inspect for any swelling, nodules, edema, and abnormal positioning. Inspect the joints of the wrist for swelling or redness.	1. Atrophy of the hand decreases the palmar depression (thenar atrophy is due to the compression of the median nerve as in carpal tunnel, whereas ulnar nerve problems cause hypothenar atrophy). Nodules indicate arthritis (rheumatoid arthritis often involves the metacarpophalangeal proximal joints). Swelling indicates an inflammatory process.

Palpation

Action	Rationale

1. Palpate for tenderness.
  a. Palpate the entire wrist for the point of maximum tenderness, which will help you locate a specific area of injury.
  b. To assess the palmar aspect of the wrist, apply pressure over the radial styloid and carpal bones.
	a. Any tenderness should alert you to an injury or inflammation.
	
	b. Normally, the area should be smooth and without pain. Pain at the hypothenar eminence suggests a fracture of the hamate.

Action	**Rationale**
c. Palpate the "snuffbox" (**Figure 15-17**), which is located just beyond the radial styloid, between the tendons of the extensors pollicis brevis and pollicis longus. This area contains the navicular (scaphoid), the radial artery, and the radial collateral ligament.	**c.** Any tenderness of the navicular bone in the snuffbox suggests a navicular fracture. Tenderness with "clicking" in this area suggests a ligamentous injury.

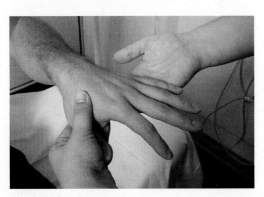

FIGURE 15-17 Palpating the snuffbox.

Action	**Rationale**
d. Palpate the joints of the wrist and fingers. Use both of your thumbs to palpate the metacarpal joints, and your thumb and index finger to palpate the interphalangeal joints. Palpate the dorsal aspect of the wrist with your thumbs and the palmar aspect with your fingers.	**d.** Normally, you would feel depressions between the joints. With inflammation or degenerative joint diseases, the depressions will disappear. Joint surfaces should be smooth. A firm mass at the dorsal aspect of the wrist may be a ganglion cyst.
2. Assess vascular status.	
a. Palpate the radial and ulnar pulses; note the warmth and color of the fingers, and the capillary refill of the nailbeds.	**a.** Normally, the hand and wrist should be pink, warm to touch, and have equal pulses bilaterally. Normal capillary refill should be less than 2 seconds.
b. Perform Allen's test. Occlude the radial artery with one hand and the ulnar artery with the other and have the patient rapidly flex his or her fingers until the palm blanches. Then, alternately release pressure from one artery to the other. Be sure you complete an ongoing serial evaluation of this area to note any subtle changes.	**b.** If the hand is filled in 5 seconds, then the collateral circulation is good. Slow filling time indicates an inadequate collateral circulation.
3. Assess sensory status. Carefully assess sensation over the dorsal and palmar surfaces, the radial and ulnar surfaces of the wrist, and the palmar and dorsal aspects of the hand and fingers. Light touch and two-point discrimination is helpful to reveal the more subtle abnormalities. Be sure a serial evaluation is done.	**3.** Note any isolated areas of decreased sensation (see **Table 15-1**), noting the innervation of the median, ulnar, and radial nerves.

Range of Motion and Special Tests

Action	Rationale

1. Assess range of motion of the wrist.
   a. Test flexion and extension of the wrist (**Figure 15-18**). To test flexion, stabilize the patient's arm and have him or her bend the wrist downward as far as he or she can. To check extension, stabilize the patient's arm and have him or her bend his wrist upward as far as he or she can.

    a. The patient should have a flexion of 90 degrees and extension of 70 degrees.

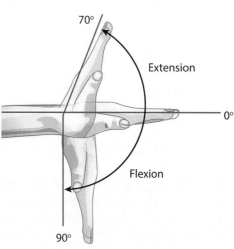

FIGURE 15-18 Extending and flexing the wrist.

   b. Test radial and ulnar deviation. Place one hand on the patient's elbow. With your other hand, hold the patient's hand and deviate the wrist both ulnar and radially.
   c. Test pronation and supination. Holding the patient's hands in yours, supinate (turn them palm side up) and then pronate (turn them palm side down).

    b. Ulnar deviation should be about 55 degrees; radial deviation should be about 20 degrees. Limited ROM indicates some type of inflammation or dislocation.
    c. Limited ROM indicates inflammation.

2. Perform Phalen's test (**Figure 15-19**). Have the patient flex the wrist facing downward and apply resistance between the wrists for 1 minute.

    2. A positive test will involve the reproduction of the symptoms (e.g., pain) and suggests carpal tunnel syndrome.

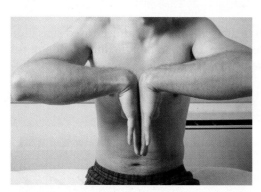

FIGURE 15-19 Performing Phalen's test.

Action	Rationale
3. Test thumb extension, abduction, adduction, and opposition. To test extension, have the patient "hitchhike." To test adduction, have her or him reach the thumb to the index finger. To test opposition, have the patient reach the thumb across to the fifth digit.	3. The patient should be able to perform all of these activities without pain.
4. Observe movements of fingers from extension to flexion. Test both active and passive ROM.	4. Any limitations in ROM are indicative of inflammation or disruption of the tendon.
5. Test flexor digitorum profundus function. Hold the patient's proximal interphalangeal joint extended and ask the patient to flex the finger.	5. Successful finger flexion indicates the tendon is intact. Pain, decreased movement, or instability may indicate rupture or partial rupture of the flexor tendons (flexor digitorum superficialis or flexor digitorum profundus).
6. Test flexor digitorum superficialis function. Hold the other fingers extended while you ask the patient to flex the finger being tested.	6. Successful flexion indicates the tendon is intact. Pain or decreased movement indicates that the tendon is not intact.
7. Assess metacarpal joint hyperextension. Have the patient bend the fingers back as far as she or he can.	7. Normally, fingers should bend back approximately 10–20 degrees past full extension.
8. Assess ulnar nerve/interosseus muscle function. Ask the patient to abduct his or her fingers while slowly pushing the hands together until the weaker one collapses.	8. Normally, the patient should demonstrate good strength.
9. Assess median nerve function.	9. Normally, the thumb can pronate with the nail of the ring finger at or around 180 degrees. If it cannot, then there is an injury to the median nerve.
10. Assess the function of the hand with the fine pinch grip. Have the patient grip a paperclip.	10. Normally, the patient can hold a paperclip between fingers with good strength.

Examining the Hip and Pelvis

When assessing the hip and pelvis, you must always evaluate the patient's gait and examine the back and lower extremities. With the hip and pelvis being part of the kinetic chain, any forces or impact to the spine can cause problems to the hip and pelvis. The main function of the hip and pelvis is to transfer the weight and any forces from the upper extremities and spine to the lower extremities. Therefore, the hip and pelvis must be very stable structures and joints. The muscles that are involved in this area balance themselves, adding to the stability of this region. **Table 15-4** describes common hip problems.

Table 15-4 Common Hip Problems	
Problem/Diagnosis	**Assessment Findings**
Slipped capital femoral epiphysis	*Note: Findings are subtle in this common hip problem.* ■ Child with a history of hip, knee, groin, and/or thigh pain and a limp. ■ Decreased range of motion during internal rotation of the femur. ■ Possible pain with hip abduction and flexion. ■ Hip is externally rotated with the foot facing to the side when the patient walks. ■ Flexion of the hip causes external rotation. *Note: This problem is seen more frequently in boys during a growth spurt.*

(continues)

Table 15-4 Common Hip Problems *(continued)*	
Problem/Diagnosis	Assessment Findings
Legg-Calvé-Perthes disease	*Note: The assessment findings vary depending on the age of the child and the stage of the disease.* ■ Child displays a limp, which is often painless and intermittent. ■ Possible pain noted in the anterior groin, inner thigh, or knee; also atrophy of the thigh and buttocks. ■ Limitation and pain are noted with internal rotation. ■ Limitation of abduction, particularly in flexion. ■ Positive Catterall's sign (passive hip flexion causes external rotation).
Stress fracture	■ Pain on palpation at the iliac crest, due to poor running technique (running with arms swinging from side to side, causing the abdominal muscles to pull on the iliac crest).
Avulsion fracture	■ Pain on palpation at the greater trochanter or at the anterior superior iliac spine (ASIS). ■ Possible crepitus or bony fragments felt during palpation. ■ Pain with active movement and passive stretching of the involved muscle. ■ May have some "popping" with the acute pain. ■ History of running (runners may pull this tendon with some type of forceful muscle contraction).
Ischial bursitis	■ Pain radiating to the hamstrings when the patient lies on her or his side with the hip flexed. ■ History of long-distance running.
Hip fracture	■ Pain with pressure/palpation to the iliac crest. ■ Patient's inability to lift the leg while on his or her back. ■ The foot on the injured side is usually turned outward (laterally rotated). ■ History of feeling of pressure on the bladder and feeling like he or she has to void. ■ History of trauma.

Inspection

Action	Rationale
1. Inspect the hips anteriorly and posteriorly. Note any asymmetry of the iliac crests and the size of the buttocks.	1. Landmarks should be symmetrical. If landmarks are asymmetrical, it may be due to scoliosis or unequal leg length. Be sure to consider the patient's posture. Weak abdominal muscles and lordosis can cause an anterior pelvic rotation. A flat back will usually be seen with a posterior pelvic tilt. Watch for motion that may cause discomfort. Do the hips look even? If not, consider a leg-length discrepancy and/or abnormal muscle contraction on one side of the hip.
2. Inspect the sacrum.	2. There should be no redness, swelling, or atrophy. If the patient has a red, painful swollen area at the sacrum that descends into the gluteal crease, consider a pilonidal cyst.
3. Observe the patient's gait and posture.	3. Gait should be coordinated and symmetrical.

Palpation

Action	Rationale
1. Palpate the bony areas anteriorly. 　a. Start by palpating the anterior superior iliac spine (ASIS). The ASIS is an important landmark because it is the origin of the sartorius and is a common site for avulsion fractures. Also, it is the last epiphysis to close.	a. There should be no pain, tenderness, or crepitus.

Action	Rationale
b. Progress inferiorly to the iliac crest; palpate the posterior edge of the greater trochanter of the femur. It is covered by the gluteus medius.	**b.** There may be areas of tenderness at the iliac crest of the pelvis or greater trochanter (hip pointer). Make sure to consider internal organ injury (e.g., spleen) when you evaluate hip pointers. If there is pain to the iliac crest with trauma, consider a pelvic fracture.
2. Palpate the bony areas posteriorly. 　**a.** The posterior superior iliac spines (PSIS) are the dimpling (indentations) above the buttocks. From these points you can palpate the posterior portion of the iliac crests.	**a.** Normally there should be no pain. Any pain in this area should make you suspicious of sacroiliac disease. Pain can also be seen here with avulsion fractures in adolescents who do extreme splits.
b. In the middle of each buttock is the ischial tuberosity, which can be palpated when the hip is flexed. This area is where the sciatic nerve comes through and is where the hamstring originates.	**b.** Pain or tenderness suggests inflammation and compression on the nerve.
c. Palpate the sacrum, the large broad bone at the end of the spinal column.	**c.** Pain or swelling indicates a fracture.
3. Palpate the soft tissue. 　**a.** Palpate the groin. Note lymph node enlargement in the groin or bulge between the pubic tubercle and the ASIS.	**a.** Enlargement or bulges indicate an inflammatory process.
b. Palpate the gluteus maximus for tone, size, and shape.	**b.** The gluteus maximus may be tender with lumbar and hamstring strains.
4. Palpate for pain.	**4.** Localized pain indicates something superficial, such as a tendon, muscle, or bursa injury. Diffuse pain may mimic pain from other systems. Pain in the groin, medial thigh, hip, or knee may indicate inguinal/femoral hernia (groin), inflammation of underlying visceral organs, tumors, enlarged lymph nodes, circulatory problems, pubic ramus stress fracture, or pubic symphysis instability. Pain in the posterior buttock/thigh may indicate lumbar spine nerve root irritation, posterior thigh compartment syndrome, piriformis syndrome, hamstring strain, ischiogluteal bursitis, and sciatic nerve contusion. Anterior pain may indicate rectus femoris strain/tendinitis, iliopsoas strain/tendinitis, symphysis pubis, iliofemoral tendinitis, lymphatic edema, and pubic fracture. Lateral pain may indicate trochanteric bursitis, gluteus medius strain, iliac crest contusion, and hip joint dysfunction.

Range of Motion and Special Tests

Action	Rationale
1. Test ROM. 　**a.** Have the patient lie supine. Ask her or him to raise each leg with knee extended and then with the knee flexed.	**a.** Flexion with knee extended should be 90 degrees; flexion with knee flexed should be 130–150 degrees.

Action	Rationale
b. Have the patient flex the knee and hip. Hold the patient's thigh with one hand and her or his ankle with the other hand. Rotate both internally and externally.	b. Internal rotation should be 35–40 degrees; external rotation should be 40–50 degrees. Any restriction noted with rotation indicates hip disease. Any shortening of external rotation suggests a hip fracture.
c. Test abduction and adduction. Ask the patient to extend the leg. Hold the patient's thigh with one hand and the ankle with the other hand. Abduct and adduct the leg.	c. Abduction should be 45 degrees; adduction should be 20–30 degrees.
2. Test strength.	2. Restriction is indicative of disease or inflammation.
3. Perform the Thomas test. With the patient supine, have him or her draw his or her knee to chest, while you observe the opposite hip.	3. If the hip rises, suspect tight hip flexor that may be masked by lordosis. The leg may abduct with a tight iliotibial (IT) band. If there is pain, consider a lesion in the iliopsoas or an inflamed iliopectineal bursa.
4. Ask the patient to sit up. Test iliopsoas function by asking the patient to lift his or her thigh off the seat while you apply resistance.	4. Groin pain occurs with iliopsoas tendinitis. The motion of hip flexion will also be weak and may cause pain even without resistance in severe cases. Tenderness may be present along the course of the tendon and at the insertion.
5. Perform the Trendelenburg test. Have the patient stand on one leg with the knee flexed enough to allow the foot to be clear of the ground. Support the patient by holding the arm on the stance side.	5. This tests the gluteus medius strength and also hip dislocation. Once the patient is balanced, note any asymmetry.

Examining the Knee

The knee is a complex structure that must withstand extreme stressors during ADLs and recreational activities. An imbalance in the major muscle groups (quadriceps and hamstrings) causes problems with the knees. **Table 15-5** describes common knee and leg problems.

Table 15-5 Common Knee and Leg Problems	
Problem/Diagnosis	Assessment Findings
Quadriceps tear	<ul><li>Tear is visible upon inspection.</li><li>Patient will not be able to lift her or his leg.</li></ul>
Trochanteric bursitis	<ul><li>Pain over the greater trochanter at the widest protrusion of the hip, which may radiate to the knee.</li><li>Complaint of pain when lying on the affected side.</li></ul>
Patellofemoral syndrome (chondromalacia)	<ul><li>History of chronic aching type of pain that may be described as "knife-like" along the anterior-medial aspect of the knee; pain on the front of the patella that radiates to the inner and outer aspects of the knee.</li><li>Pain occurs after sitting for long periods of time with legs flexed, going up and down stairs/hills, or squatting.</li><li>No swelling is noted, but at times the patient may have some "puffiness".</li><li>Patient may even feel like the knee is going to "give out".</li><li>Crepitus and a positive inhibition test (have patient straighten the leg and push the patella into the femur).</li></ul>
Iliotibial band syndrome	<ul><li>History of running or cycling.</li><li>Pain over the lateral femoral condyle with "grinding" or "snapping" felt over the knee.</li><li>Tenderness 2–3 cm proximal to the lateral joint line.</li><li>Positive Ober's test. (Ober's test consists of positioning the patient on the side with the symptomatic leg up and the lower hip flexed. Stand behind the patient and have him or her flex the knee and hip 90 degrees, abduct the hip and extend it neutrally, and then allow it to adduct by gravity.)</li></ul>

Table 15-5   Common Knee and Leg Problems *(continued)*

Problem/Diagnosis	Assessment Findings
Anterior cruciate ligament (ACL) tear	■ History of doing a cutting or pivoting activity with the leg planted. ■ History of sudden "pop" or "snap" heard and feeling like the knee is coming apart. ■ Quick onset of swelling with a large effusion. ■ Patient walks on tiptoes and cannot straighten the leg. ■ Positive Lachman's or draw test.
Meniscal tear	■ History of some type of crushing force between the femoral condyles and the tibia. ■ Pain on the joint line. ■ Swelling with intra-articular effusion. ■ Locking of the knee with a positive McMurray test or Steinmann sign (flex knee and forcibly rotate the tibia). *Note: Women commonly will have lateral tears and men medial tears.*
Medial collateral ligament (MCL) tear	■ History of knee injury with a force to the lateral knee. ■ Knee caves in to the medial side, but rarely swells. ■ Pain noted over the MCL. *Note: Injury is seen often in breaststrokers due to the whip kick that they use to swim this stroke.*
Posterior cruciate ligament tear (PCL)	■ History of injury with hyperextension, such as falling on a flexed knee, which will force the tibia posteriorly on the femur. ■ Positive posterior draw test.
Hamstring strain	■ History of injury with activities that require sudden bursts of speed. ■ Patient reports sudden onset of pain and swelling diffusely over the hamstring.
Shin splints	■ History of a dull intermittent pain over the distal third of the tibia that often developed slowly and became aggravated over a period of time.
Osgood-Schlatter disease	■ Onset of pain is gradual, and begins as a mild ache in the morning when the patient gets out of bed; pain worsens over a 2-week period of time. ■ Pain over the tibial tubercle that is exacerbated by activities of repeated extension and flexion (squatting, climbing stairs) and direct impact on site (jumping, running); knee extension causes pain. ■ Tenderness and swelling. ■ Many patients have tight hamstrings and look as if they have two knees because of a bump just below the patella on the tibia tubercle. *Note: Injury is seen in girls older than age 11 and boys older than age 13.*
Baker's cyst	■ Inspection reveals swelling behind the medial knee. ■ Pain or pressure with full flexion. ■ Palpation reveals a firm palpable mass behind the knee on the medial side, which is most easily seen with the patient standing. ■ In a ruptured cyst, the calf will usually be enlarged, but is usually not as taut or as painful as a deep vein thrombosis. ■ With very large cysts, venous return from the lower extremity may be impaired, resulting in edema of the extremity.
Septic arthritis	■ History of fever, chills, and malaise. ■ Intense pain in the joint, with the area around the knee frequently being hot and erythematous. ■ Septic arthritis is seen most commonly in the knee but can involve the hip, shoulder, wrist, ankle, and elbow. ■ Usually seen in the patients with rheumatoid arthritis, immunocompromised patients, and IV drug abusers.

Inspection

Action	Rationale
1. With the patient in a supine or sitting position with legs dangling: a. Inspect the knee for coloring and swelling. Note any deformity and the muscle tone.	a. If you note localized swelling, consider a bursa rupture. With generalized swelling, consider some type of intra-articular problem. Redness indicates inflammation. Bruising suggests trauma. Bulging indicates fluid in the knee joint.

b. Inspect the contour of the knee and alignment of the patellae. Compare bilaterally.

b. When comparing the patellae and knees, note that women commonly have genu valgum (knock-knees). Genu valgum creates a serious problem of the joints. The excessive angling of the "Q angle" (where the femur and lower leg meet) causes the patient to bear weight on the inside of the knee. A Q angle of greater than 10 degrees in men and 15 degrees in women predisposes them to knee problems. Genu varus (bowlegs) places undue stress on the patella and IT band.

Palpation

Action	Rationale
1. Palpate the bones.	
a. With the patient supine or sitting, palpate the femur, starting from the proximal portion and moving to the distal end.	a. The area should be smooth with no masses or atrophy. If palpation reveals masses on the femur caused by trauma, consider bleeding secondary to a fracture.
b. Palpate the tibia. Landmarks for the tibia are the tibial plateau (which runs medial to lateral and is where the medial and lateral meniscus are found) and the tibial tubercle (where the quadriceps inserts).	b. The tibia will be flat until a child is weight bearing and then slowly begins to move to a horizontal position. The area should be smooth with no masses or swelling.
c. Palpate the patella (**Figure 15-20**). The patella or "kneecap" sits within a tendon and is attached to the tibia and has a ridge that runs up and down. Check its movement medially and laterally.	c. The patella is a large sesamoid bone. The joint should feel smooth but firm without any tenderness or crepitus. Crepitus and tenderness indicate inflammation.

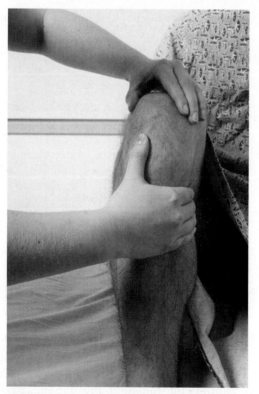

FIGURE 15-20 Palpating the bones of the knee.

Action	**Rationale**
d. Palpate the fibula. The fibula is difficult to palpate on the proximal end but can be palpated distally; it is more laterally located than the tibia. The lateral femoral epicondyle lays lateral to the lateral femoral condyle (which is covered by the patella).	d. The lateral femoral condyle is a common region for patellofemoral pain, and the lateral femoral epicondyle is a common area for IT band syndrome.
2. Palpate the soft tissue. Note its temperature.	2. Warmth may indicate blood in the joint (blood is usually warmer than synovial fluid).
a. Palpate the popliteal space for any tenderness, swelling, or masses. b. Palpate the IT band (a thick band of connective tissue that begins at the pelvis, crosses the hip, and inserts below the knee joint at the outer edge). It can be palpated when the knee is slightly bent.	a, b. Any pain or tenderness of this area would indicate inflammation.

Range of Motion and Special Tests

Be sure to test both active and passive ROM.

Action	**Rationale**
1. Test ROM. Examine the patient for flexion, extension, and hyperextension.	1. Normal flexion is approximately 135 degrees. Normal extension should be 180 degrees.
2. Test strength. Have the patient keep the knee flexed and extended while you apply an opposing force against it. It is graded as any other muscle/joint.	2. You should note stability of this joint. No give should be noted.
3. Perform Apley's distraction test. Have the patient lie prone with the knee flexed at 90 degrees. Stabilize the thigh by placing your hand on the posterior thigh while you pull the ankle upward, internally and externally rotating the tibia.	3. If there is pain, consider collateral ligament injury. Pain is typically caused by meniscal injury as the injured meniscus is pinched between the femur and the tibia.
4. Perform Lachman's test. With the patient lying supine, grasp the femur with your left hand and grasp the proximal tibia with your right hand. Flex the knee to 30 degrees and pull anteriorly and posteriorly. Note: If your hands are not large enough to do this, you can anchor the foot distally with your lower body or you can use your forearm instead of your hands.	4. Excessive motion in either direction may mean disruption of the respective ligament. Look for a firm endpoint. Compare to the nonaffected side and make sure the patient's quadriceps are relaxed.
5. Perform McMurray's test. Have the patient sit or lie down with the knee flexed. Externally rotate the tibia at the ankle and then extend the knee **(Figure 15-21)**.	5. A palpable click in the initial degrees of flexion suggests a posterior tear of the medial meniscus; a palpable click with the knee almost extended suggests a tear more anteriorly.

Action   **Rationale**

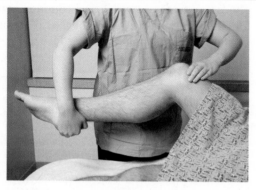

FIGURE 15-21 Performing McMurray's test.

6. Test anterior draw. Have the patient lie supine with the knee flexed to 90 degrees and the hip and ankle flexed at 45 degrees. Cup your hands around the knee with your fingers at the insertion of the lateral and medial hamstrings and thumbs on the joint line. Draw forward on the tibia and watch for any movement of the tibia (**Figure 15-22**).

6. This tests the integrity of the ACL.

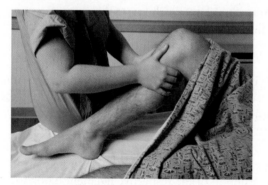

FIGURE 15-22 Positioning for anterior draw.

7. Test posterior draw. Have patient sit with the knee flexed over the side of table. Move the proximal tibia posteriorly and rotate externally to test posterior cruciate ligaments.

7. The ligaments should be strong and stable. Instability is indicative of posterior cruciate ligament injury.

8. Perform a valgus stress test.
   Test the PCL. Have the patient lie supine with the knee flexed at 90 degrees. Place the patient's foot between your legs and use the palms of your hands to push the tibia posteriorly. Inspect for stability from the lateral view of the knee. Evaluate posterior displacement by using your thumb to palpate the area.

8. Laxity is graded on a 1–4 scale. The ligament should be strong with not a lot of movement (or laxity).

Action	Rationale

Test the MCL. With the patient supine, support the thigh and flex the knee 20–30 degrees. Stabilize the femur and palpate the medial joint line with one hand. Place the other hand on the distal tibia. Place the joint surface in the starting position and abduct the tibia on the femur, restricting axial rotation. Estimate the medial joint space and evaluate the stiffness of motion.

9. Perform a varus stress test. Place the patient in the supine position, with the knee flexed 20–30 degrees and the thigh supported. Stabilize the femur and palpate the lateral joint line with one hand. Place the other hand on the distal tibia. Begin with the joint in the standing position and adduct the tibia on the femur, restricting axial rotation.

9. This test reveals the laxity of the medial stabilizing complexes, especially the collateral ligaments of the knee.

Examining the Foot and Ankle

When examining the foot and ankle, you will find that the majority of the acute problems tend to be clear (especially when using the Ottawa criteria for ankles; see **Box 15-2**). In contrast, chronic problems tend not to be so cut and dried and require a more comprehensive history and evaluation. Consider other problems with the lower extremity, and think of the ankle and foot as being one link on a chain that works together to make the whole (the lower extremity) work correctly. The foot and ankle can affect the back, the knee, and even the hip if the patient's biomechanics are off. If the knee is out of alignment, it can cause problems with the ankle and increase the incidence of injury. If possible, examine the patient's foot and ankle while the patient is sitting, standing, and walking. **Table 15-6** lists common problems of the foot and ankle, and **Box 15-3** discusses injury mechanisms to the ankle.

BOX 15-2   THE OTTAWA ANKLE RULES

An ankle radiographic series is required only if there is any malleolar pain and any of the following findings:
- Bone tenderness at the posterior edge or tip of either malleolus
- Tenderness at the navicular or base of the fifth metatarsal
- Instability to bear weight both immediately and/or ambulate only four steps

---

BOX 15-3   INJURY MECHANISMS TO THE ANKLE

- Inversion injury: The most common mechanism of injury to the ankle is due to overstretch. With this injury, the anterior talofibular ligament is usually injured with some rolling of the tibia. It causes lateral ankle sprain.
- Eversion injury: Eversion injury is not as common as inversion injury because the natural tendency of the ankle is to invert. It injures the deltoid ligament, and because of the strength of this ligament, a subsequent avulsion fracture of the distal tibia may occur.
- Plantar flexion injury: These types of injuries are uncommon but may be seen in combination with either of the previously mentioned movements.
- Overuse: Overuse injury is seen with improper training techniques, improper footwear, muscle imbalances, and poor body mechanics.

Table 15-6   Common Foot and Ankle Problems

Problem/Diagnosis	Assessment Findings
Shin splints (medial tibial stress syndrome)	▪ Pain due to the periosteum separating from the bone; onset of pain is gradual after exercise. ▪ History of doing a lot of jumping, "cutting sport activities," running, or not stretching well before or after exercise.
Stress fractures	▪ History of pain with exercise; patient describes the pain as unbearable. ▪ Obesity. ▪ History of jobs that require the patient to stand for prolonged periods of time on a hard surface.
Achilles tendinitis	*Note: Stress fractures may be confused with shin splints, but are due to repetitive activities that cause stress to a particular bone or tissue.* ▪ Pain at the insertion or at areas 2–6 cm proximal to the insertions of the tendon at the posterior aspect of the heel. ▪ Crepitus may be noted with chronic problems. ▪ Patient may be wearing poor-fitting shoes or high heels. ▪ History of long-distance running or not stretching before/after exercising.
Achilles tendon rupture	▪ Seen in the "weekend athlete" who is playing basketball or any other activity that may require a directional change. ▪ Patient reports hearing a "pop" at the back of the heel and is not able to bear weight on the area. ▪ Positive Thompson's test.
Plantar fasciitis	▪ Heel pain with weight bearing; pain is usually at its maximum after long periods of non-weight bearing or first thing in the morning. ▪ Increased pain with dorsiflexion of the toe. ▪ There is usually no edema or redness noted in the area; no numbness or tingling. ▪ Palpable diminution in the tension of the plantar fascia. ▪ Individuals with flat feet or very high arches are more prone to this.
Calcaneal apophysitis (Sever's disease)	▪ Pediatric patient (9 to 12 years old) who is active. ▪ Child will limp and complain of heel pain that is worsened by jumping or running. ▪ Palpation at the posterior-plantar junction reveals pain. ▪ Increased pain with stretching of the heel cord. ▪ There may or may not be any edema, but the area is never warm or red.
Jones fracture	▪ Pain at the base of the fifth metatarsal after an inversion type of injury. ▪ Possible swelling of the area.
Talar dome fractures	▪ History of an inversion and eversion ankle injury. *Note: The initial x-ray at the time of the injury may not reveal a fracture, but the patient will experience persistent stiffness, intermittent joint pain, or instability 2–3 weeks after an "ankle sprain."*

Inspection

Action	Rationale
1. Inspect the area for edema, ecchymosis, or deformity. Be sure to inspect bilaterally. Be sure to look at the toes to see if they are proportional and in good position.	1. When evaluating for swelling, note the amount and if the swelling is pitting. (This type of swelling would alert you to dependent fluid that may indicate heart problems or peripheral vascular disease [PVD]). A longer second toe is referred to as a Morton's toe, which can become irritated if shoes are too small. A subungual hematoma can cause an aching pain due to the pressure of the blood under the nail itself. This can be due to direct trauma (an object falling on the toe). It can be relieved by drilling a hole through the nail to allow the blood collected under the toe to escape. A *bunion*, usually found on the inside of the great toe (first metatarsophalangeal joint), is a bursa that becomes irritated due to severe pronation caused by incorrect footwear (too small shoes). *Hammertoes* are noted as a hyperextension of the metatarsophalangeal joint and flexion only at the distal phalangeal joint. *Corns* are pressure points on the foot due to irritation from contact.

Action	Rationale
	With a swollen, warm great toe, suspect *gout*. Inspect the arch and consider if the patient has *pes cavus* (high arches) or *pes planus* (flat feet).
2. Inspect the patient's gait.	2. A limp may indicate a fracture, inflammation, or a degenerative disease.

Palpation

Action	Rationale
1. Palpate the ankle. a. Palpate the talus.	a. The talus is easily palpated with pes planus. Note tenderness of any structure and note the stability of the Achilles tendon.
b. Palpate the medial malleolus and lateral malleolus. (The medial malleolus is the distal end of the tibia and is found on the medial aspect of the ankle. The lateral malleolus is the distal end of the fibula and is found on the lateral aspect of the ankle. It is longer than the medial.)	b. Masses or abnormal indentations are abnormal findings.
c. Palpate the heel or calcaneus and the proximal tibia/fibula.	c. Normally, there should not be any pain on palpation. If the patient experienced an eversion type of injury, there will be tenderness on the proximal tibia/fibula.
d. With your thumb, palpate the anterior aspect of the ankle joint.	d. It should be smooth and without pain.
e. Palpate the Achilles tendon. Note any nodules or tenderness.	e. The tendon should insert at the heel. If there is an indented area, consider an Achilles tendon rupture.
2. Palpate the foot.	2. The foot should be warm to the touch, with strong pulses. If not, consider disruption of the nerves or vascular system (PVD, dislocation, fracture).
a. Palpate pedal pulses and assess the temperature of the foot and ankle. b. Note any areas of tenderness along the tarsals, metatarsals, and joints.	

Range of Motion and Special Tests

Action	Rationale
1. Test ROM of the foot and ankle. a. Test dorsiflexion and plantar flexion of the foot at the ankle (or the tibiotalar joint).	a. Dorsiflexion should be 20 degrees. Plantar flexion should be 45 degrees. If there is limited ROM, consider a degenerative disease, dislocation, or inflammation.
b. Stabilize the ankle (at the distal tibia/fibula) with one hand, grasp the heel with the other hand, and invert and evert the talus (**Figure 15-23**).	b. Increased laxity indicates injury to the ligaments.

Action

Rationale

c. Test ROM of the transverse joint by stabilizing the heel and inverting and everting the forefoot (**Figure 15-24**).

c. Increased laxity indicates a ligamentous injury.

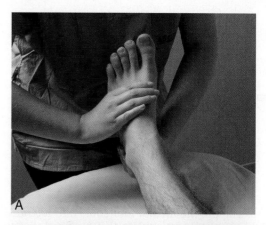

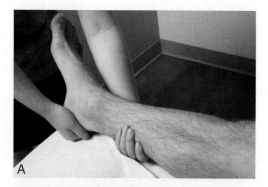

FIGURE 15-23 Inversion (A) and eversion (B) of the talus.

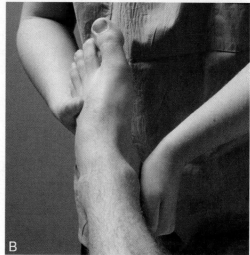

FIGURE 15-24 Inversion (A) and eversion (B) of the forefoot.

d. Flex the toes at the metatarsophalangeal joint.

d. Diminished ROM may be due to inflammation or degenerative disease (arthritis).

2. Test sensation distally. Test for proprioception. Ask the patient to close her or his eyes. Hold the patient's great toe with your thumb and index finger, pull it away from the other toes, and actively move it up and down. Then ask the patient if she or he can determine the direction in which the toe is being moved.

2. The patient should be able to sense position. Inability to do so suggests neurological (nerve) impairment.

3. Test anterior draw. Have the patient sit on the side of the examining table with the foot hanging in a neutral position. Position one hand on the patient's anterior tibia just above the joint line to stabilize the tibia and fibula. Use the other hand to cup the calcaneus and displace it anteriorly (this stresses the anterior talofibular ligament).

3. Normal movement is only about 3 mm. If there is more movement, suspect a ligament tear.

Action	Rationale
4. Perform a side-to-side test. Have the patient sit on the side of the examining table with the leg hanging and the ankle in a neutral position. With one hand just above the joint line, stabilize the tibia and fibula. Put the other hand around the heel and apply a lateral and medial force to see how much the mortise opens.	4. A positive test will elicit pain and even a "thud." This also tests for talofibular ligament stability.
5. Perform Thompson's test. Have the patient lie prone with the knee flexed at 90 degrees. Squeeze the middle third of the calf to produce plantar flexion of the foot.	5. No plantar flexion indicates a complete tear of the Achilles tendon.

Examining the Spine

Back pain is one of the most common complaints that you will encounter. It might seem like a relatively straightforward problem, but many times it becomes very complicated. Taking a thorough and accurate history about the precipitating events helps narrow the diagnosis. Keep in mind that back pain is frequently a cumulative process that includes a repetitive deconditioning component (i.e., poor posture, poor body mechanics, and poor "maintenance" of the muscles in the back). When assessing for spinal injuries, you should perform a neurological examination. Also, remember that some abdominal disorders may present with back pain. Be sure to assess the abdomen. **Table 15-7** lists common causes of lower back pain.

Table 15-7 Common Back Problems

Problem/Diagnosis	Assessment Findings
Compression fracture/back pain	▪ Point tenderness to any bony area of the geriatric patient after a minor trauma. ▪ Weakness. ▪ Pain. ▪ Reflexes and proprioception need to be assessed to determine if there is any nerve involvement.
Low back strain	▪ Limited range of motion. ▪ Slow gait. ▪ Pain to low back (paravertebral muscular area, not bony). ▪ Reflexes intact; proprioception intact. ▪ Abdomen without bruits or masses.
Malignancy or tumor	▪ Back pain that lasts longer than 2–4 weeks. ▪ Point tenderness. ▪ Weight changes. ▪ Diminished reflexes. ▪ Pain at night when supine.
Ankylosing spondylitis	▪ Back pain that improves with activity. ▪ Decreased chest expansion. ▪ Decrease in spinal flexion.
Cauda equina syndrome	▪ Back pain. ▪ Urinary or fecal incontinence. ▪ "Saddle" anesthesia (numbness or decreased sensation of the perianal area involving the nerve roots of S2–S4). ▪ Sphincter laxity. ▪ Recent chiropractic manipulation, infection, or a tumor.
Herniated disc	▪ Pain that is exacerbated by Valsalva maneuver or coughing. ▪ Pain radiating below the knee.

Inspection

Action	Rationale
1. Observe the patient's gait as she or he enters the room. Ask the patient to walk heel to toe (placing one foot in front of the other) to test the gastrocnemius.	1. If the patient is unable to ambulate, then this will not be possible. If the patient has short strides and leans to the side that is painful, consider a hip problem.
2. Assess posture (**Figure 15-25**).	2. If inspection reveals an accentuation of lordosis, consider a muscle spasm or maybe an inflamed disc. Note any other changes in posture, such as lordosis, scoliosis, kyphosis, or a pelvic tilt (**Figure 15-26**).

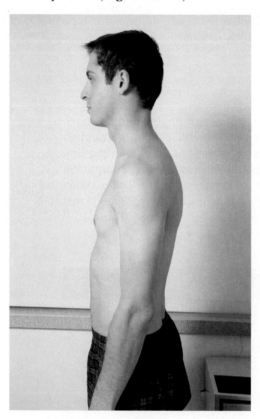

FIGURE 15-25 Assessing posture.

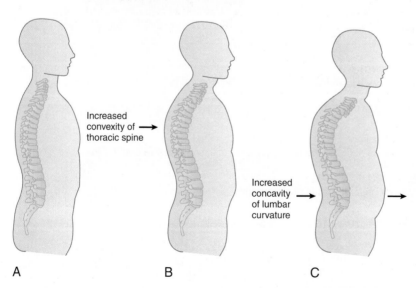

Increased convexity of thoracic spine →

Increased concavity of lumbar curvature →

A   B   C

FIGURE 15-26 Abnormal curvatures of the spinal cord. A. Normal. B. Kyphosis. C. Lordosis. D. Scoliosis.

Action	Rationale

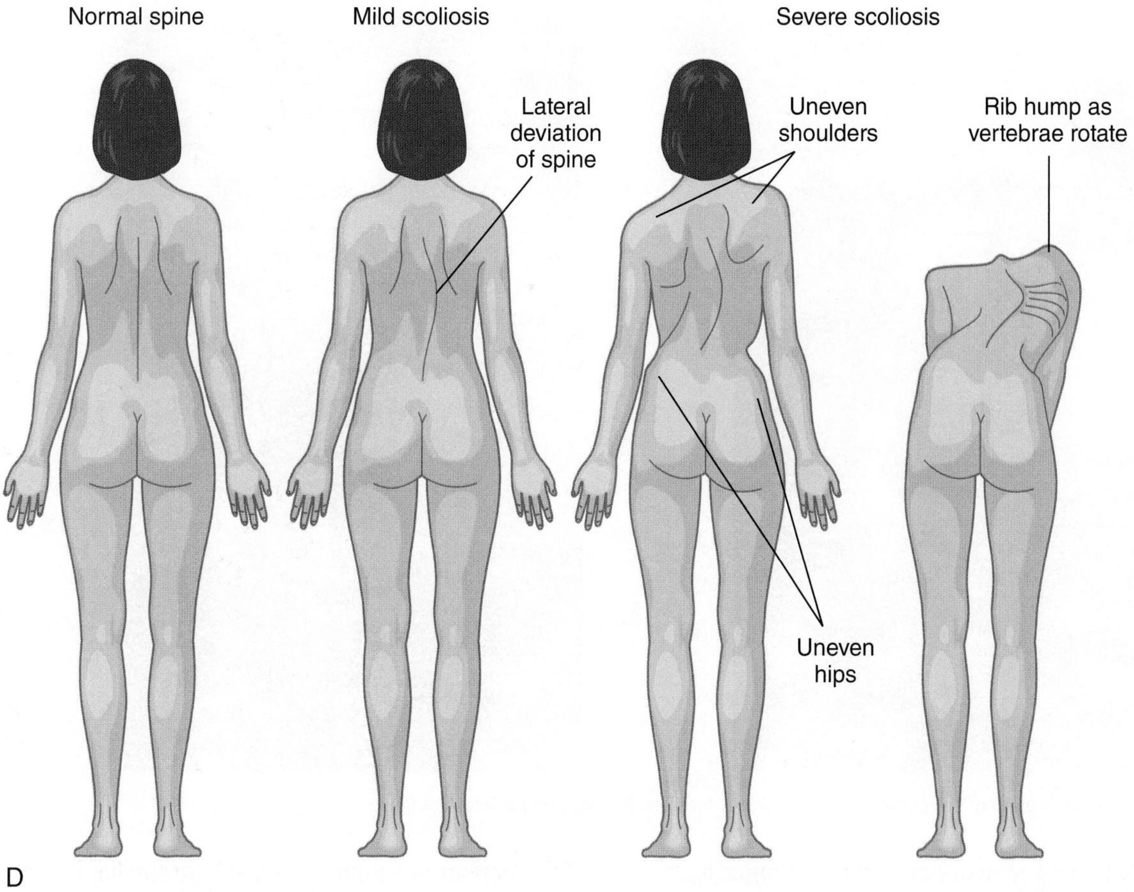

FIGURE 15-26 Abnormal curvatures of the spinal cord. A. Normal. B. Kyphosis. C. Lordosis. D. Scoliosis. (*continued*)

Palpation

Action	Rationale
1. Palpate the back, including the spinal column and paravertebral muscles.	1. Note any vertebral tenderness, paraspinal tenderness, or spasm. Masses may indicate a tumor.
2. Palpate for warmth and distal pulses.	2. Warmth would indicate inflammation and perfusion. Make sure to note change in strength of pulses distally.

Range of Motion and Special Tests

Action	Rationale
1. Observe ROM. Have the patient flex as if she or he were trying to touch her or his toes, extend, and move side to side (**Figure 15-27**).	1. Flexion should be 90 degrees; extension should be 30 degrees. Reduction of flexion suggests a problem with a disc. Right and left lateral flexion should be 35 degrees.
2. With the patient seated, test the foot strength on dorsiflexion.	2. Toe raising or foot dorsiflexion provides information about L5 and S1. If the patient is unable to do these movements, investigate a lesion of this area.

Action   **Rationale**

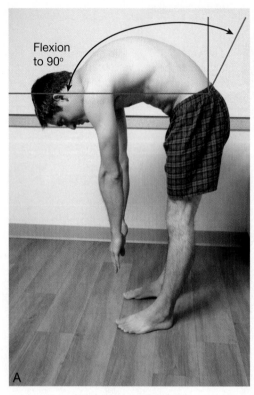

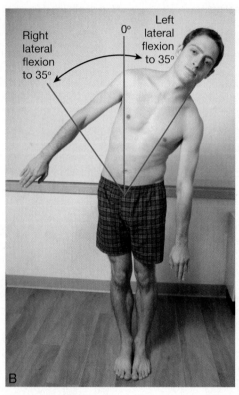

FIGURE 15-27 Range of motion of the spine. A. Flexion and extension. B. Right and left lateral flexion.

3. With the patient seated, perform the straight leg raise.

3. If the patient has pain on the side of the leg being raised, consider a disc problem. A more specific test for possible disc problems is raising the opposite leg with resulting pain on the affected side. To guard against pain, the patient will normally lean backward when you raise the leg.

4. Test the sacroiliac (SI) joint. With the patient on her or his side, have her or him pull the lower leg into a fetal position and extend the upper leg.

4. SI pain will be reproduced with this movement. A positive test may indicate a disc problem or ulcerative colitis.

Diagnostic Reasoning

Based on findings in the health history and physical examination, the clinician should formulate the assessment and plan. For example, a patient may report symptoms that suggest many possible diagnoses; however, findings in the past medical history and during the physical examination might narrow the possible diagnoses down to one or two. Hip pain is a common chief complaint. **Table 15-8** illustrates differential diagnosis of common disorders associated with hip pain.

Table 15-8 Differential Diagnosis of Hip Pain			
Differential Diagnosis	Significant Findings in the Patient's History	Significant Findings in the Patient's Physical Examination	Diagnostic Tests
Hip fracture	Recent trauma, osteoporosis	Pain on palpation, shortening of leg with external rotation, unable to bear weight, bruising	X-ray of the pelvis
Sciatica	Recent trauma to the hip or pelvis, sitting for long periods of time, tingling, burning down leg	Numbness, decreased/abnormal sensations to the thigh and lower extremity; weakness of the leg and foot; difficulty walking	MRI to rule out any other problems (fracture/tumor)
Bursitis	History of trauma or overuse of the area	Joint pain and tenderness, warmth over the affected area, swelling, crepitus	CBC
Osteoarthritis	Obesity, age older than 50, slowly developing pain	Pain in the front part of the thigh, pain with movement, decreased ROM	X-ray of the hip/femur

Abbreviations: CBC, complete blood count; MRI, magnetic resonance imaging; ROM, range of motion.

Musculoskeletal Assessment of Special Populations

Considerations for the Pregnant Patient

General Considerations

Remember the following:

- Falls and tripping are common during pregnancy due to the laxity of the ligaments in the pelvic region, fatigue, and unstable gait. The weight of the uterus shifts the center of gravity forward during the third trimester, making the pregnant woman's stature that of lordosis. This lordosis is an effort to shift the center of gravity back over her lower extremities but not without her throwing back her head and shoulders. Remember that heels will increase lordosis, so remind pregnant women to wear flat shoes with arch support.
- Pregnancy is a hypervolemic and hyperdynamic state.
- Pregnancy is characterized by a relaxation of the sacroiliac joint and a softening of the pelvic cartilages. The pelvis widens (almost doubles in width) by the third trimester. Because of this widening and relaxation of the SI joint, the pelvis is less susceptible to fractures.
- During the second trimester, the pregnant woman may experience painful muscle cramps at night, especially in the thigh, gastrocnemius, or the gluteal muscles.

Targeted Health History Questions

Remember to elicit the following information:

- What is the estimated date of conception?
- Has there been any increase in laxity of any joints (hips especially)?
- Which type of exercise does the patient perform?
- Does she experience any muscle cramps, back pain, or any other musculoskeletal problems?
- Which type of shoes does the patient wear?

Considerations for the Neonatal Patient

Inspection

To inspect the hip, place the infant frog-legged; the groin crease should not be below the anus. If it is, consider a dislocation.

Special Tests

- Perform the Barlow–Ortolani test (maneuver). This test is performed on infants during their first year to detect hip dislocation. Place your hands on the inner thigh with your thumbs at the knees and fingertips on the hip. Adduct the hip so that the thumbs touch. Apply downward pressure and then slowly abduct the thighs while applying pressure. The Ortolani sign consists of a palpable click when the dislocated hip is reduced by abduction.

- Test for Allis's sign. Position the infant lying supine on the bed with both knees flexed and the femurs aligned. If one knee is lower than the other, this test is "positive" for a hip dislocation.

Considerations for the Pediatric Patient
General Considerations

Remember the following:

- Fractures are more difficult to diagnosis in children. Be sure to obtain comparison views.
- Bones in this population are pliable, secondary to the periosteum being thicker and stronger. This leads to the pediatric fracture often being undisplaced and incomplete.
- Fracture of the growth plate (the area located between the epiphysis and the metaphysis at both the proximal and distal ends of long bones) is of greatest concern.
- Younger children are more likely to have a "buckle" fracture than older children due to the porous nature of bones at this age.
- Bones heal faster in children due to the capability of the periosteal covering to produce great amounts of bone.
- The toddler's and child's center of gravity is higher (T11 to T12) compared with the adult's center of gravity (L4 to L5). This factor, along with underdeveloped muscles, makes it difficult for a toddler to keep her or his balance.
- The child has a large head in proportion to his or her body until he or she is approximately 6 to 8 years old.
- Children are easily distracted and have little concept of danger.
- Children who just wear lap belts in vehicles have an increased risk of midlumbar/vertebral fractures (particularly L2–L4).
- The cervical spine is less protected.
- Subluxations are common secondary to a sudden forceful, longitudinal pull on the extremity. The most common subluxation is the "nursemaid's elbow."
- Children have difficulty understanding various terms used by medical professionals. Be sure to consider their developmental stage and use appropriate descriptors, such as "funny," "different," or "asleep" to assist them in verbalizing how it feels to them.
- Rapid growth during adolescence results in a decrease in strength in the epiphyses and even less flexibility, leading to increased potential for injury. (Remember that bone growth is completed by approximately age 20.)

Targeted Health History Questions

Remember to include the following elements:

- Birth history: Did the child experience any perinatal trauma? Did the mother have prenatal care? Was the delivery normal?
- Motor and speech development: Is the child's fine and gross motor development in line with her or his age?
- Possible ingestions: Did the child ingest any medications or alcohol (either accidentally or recreationally)?
- Nonaccidental trauma: Did the child experience any physical abuse or neglect (poor nutrition, failure to thrive)?
- Immunization status: Is the child up to date with immunizations?
- Participation in sports: Does the child participate in sports (specify type)? How often does he or she train for the sport? Does the child perform other cross-training or physical conditioning?
- Medications: Which medications does the child take (e.g., NSAIDs, aspirin, acetaminophen, muscle relaxants, over-the-counter drugs, herbs, weight reduction medications, calcium)?

Considerations for the Geriatric Patient

General Considerations

Remember the following points when assessing this population:

- Geriatric patients have decreased ability to perceive hazards due to the brain's diminished ability to rapidly process, coordinate, and react to stimuli.
- Older adults often have decreased visual acuity and attention.
- They may have limited neck rotation due to degenerative disease or arthritis.
- Atherosclerotic changes may cause limited ability to respond to stress.
- Osteoporosis may cause a brittle skeleton, which increases older adults' risk for fractures.
- Bony prominences become more apparent with age because of the changes in muscle mass.
- Tendons are less elastic in older adults.
- Arthritic changes may cause limited mobility.
- Older adults will have an increase in minor injuries from falls or tripping due to gait problems and vision, but may not want you to know because this will decrease their independence.
- Pain restriction to range of motion is different from mechanical restrictions.
- Always assess flexion, extension, supination, and pronation and associated pain that is caused by a decrease in range of motion and a change in sensation.
- Degenerative changes to the joints of this population may make it difficult to identify fractures on x-ray.
- Geriatric patients have an increased incidence of falls:
  - One out of three elderly individuals fall each year, with 84% happening at home.
  - Thirteen percent of the falls are preceded by an acute "medical condition" (e.g., dizziness, paralysis, myocardial infarction).
  - Environmental problems/objects (furniture, rugs, electrical cords, uneven pavements) are associated with falls in this population.
  - Intrinsic factors such as gait and balance problems are also associated with falls and the subsequent musculoskeletal problems. These factors may be exacerbated with alcohol consumption.

Targeted Health History Questions

- Does the patient experience other medical problems, such as peripheral vascular disease or previous fracture? Ask about weakness (is it sudden or gradual?).
- Which medications does the patient take? Ask about NSAIDs, aspirin, muscle relaxants, over-the-counter drugs, calcium, glucosamine, antirheumatics, and corticosteroids. What has the patient done to relieve pain (e.g., medications, ice, splints, home remedies)?
- Is the patient on multiple medications? Consider multiple interactions and side effects from multiple medication use.
- Is the patient ingesting an adequate diet? Inadequate nutrition and fluid intake can alter the body's capacity to respond to stress. Inadequate nutrition may be due to economic problems, living alone, or an inability to prepare food due to changes in strength and motor function.
- Is the older adult being treated well? Older adults can be subjected to maltreatment; those who have preexisting illnesses are at higher risk for maltreatment. Maltreatment may be difficult to identify because of the individual's fear of rejection or isolation.
- Does the patient have pain with vague signs and symptoms? Older individuals have a higher incidence of developing painful conditions with vague signs and symptoms.

Case Study Review

Throughout this chapter, you have been introduced to Ms. D. This section of the chapter pulls together her history and demonstrates the documentation of her history and physical examination.

Chief Complaint

"My right hip and hand hurt."

Information Gathered During the Interview

PD is a 25-year-old female who presents with pain to her right hip and hand after falling off a mountain bike. Ms. D explains that while she was testing a new mountain bike, she tried to jump a curb and was thrown over the handlebars and landed on her right side. She was wearing a helmet and there was no loss of consciousness. After the incident, she was able to stand up and limp back to the store with the bike as a crutch, and then to her car. She took some acetaminophen (Tylenol) last night, but when she awoke this morning, she was unable to move her right wrist and shoulder or bear weight on her right leg. Ms. D has a large abrasion and ecchymotic area on her right thigh with no swelling. She states that she had a difficult time putting her bra on and brushing her teeth this morning. She prefers to lie supine because sitting makes her right hip hurt.

Ms. D has no past history of previous injury to shoulder, hand, or leg. She denies any surgeries. Her only medications are NSAIDs for pain. Ms. D denies any chronic conditions.

Ms. D has a maternal grandmother who suffers from arthritis. Ms. D's mother is alive and well. Her father has coronary artery disease, and her paternal grandfather died at the age of 67 from coronary artery disease. Ms. D's paternal grandmother and aunt are on medication for osteoporosis. There is no family history of lung disease, diabetes, or cancer.

Ms. D is a graduate student in town. She denies use of tobacco and drugs. She reports a social drinking history of about two glasses of wine a month. She denies ever receiving a blood transfusion. She is an avid outdoors person and loves to mountain bike.

Clues	Important Points
Fall from bike	The mechanism of injury suggests blunt trauma to her right side.
Unable to move the shoulder	Associated with blunt trauma and suggests either a contusion or a strain.
Large abrasion and ecchymotic area on right thigh	Ecchymosis is consistent with bleeding under the skin and trauma to underlying tissue and may involve bony areas.
Walked with a limp last night and now unable to bear weight on the leg	A limp suggests contusion; not being able to bear weight may indicate a fracture or increased swelling of the area that would increase pain and compromise mobility.
Trouble putting her bra on and brushing teeth	Supports contusion/strain of the shoulder.
Unable to move wrist	Is this due to swelling/pain or fracture?
Preferred position of comfort is supine and not sitting upright	Supports the fracture diagnosis.

Name PD		Date 8/1/15	Time 10:30
		DOB 6/10/90	Sex F
HISTORY			
CC "My right hand and hip hurt."			
HPI Fell off mountain bike yesterday while trying to "jump curb." Wearing helmet. Used acetaminophen. This AM unable to move her right wrist and shoulder and unable to bear weight on right leg. Large abrasion and ecchymotic area on right thigh. No swelling. Difficulty putting on bra and brushing teeth. Prefers to lie supine; sitting up causes hip pain.			

Medications
Acetaminophen

Allergies
NKDA

PMI
Illnesses
Denies past trauma or chronic illness.
Hospitalizations/Surgeries
Denies surgeries or hospitalizations.
FH
Maternal grandmother with arthritis; father, CAD; paternal grandfather, died age 67 from CAD; paternal grandmother and aunt, osteoporosis.
SH
Graduate student. Denies tobacco or drug use. Drinks 2 glasses of wine/month. Avid outdoors person.

ROS	
General	Cardiovascular
Denies weight change; mild headache; no loss of consciousness.	No chest pain or palpitations.
Skin	Respiratory
Abrasions and ecchymosis to thigh.	No SOB or respiratory difficulties.
Eyes	Gastrointestinal
No change in vision or double vision.	No abdominal pain, nausea, or vomiting.
Ears	Genitourinary/Gynecological
No changes in hearing or vertigo.	LMP 2 weeks prior; grav 0 para 0; no blood noted in urine.
Nose/Mouth/Throat	Musculoskeletal
No changes.	Limited ROM of right wrist, shoulder; unable to bear weight on right leg; able to walk right after incident.
Breast	Neurological
No changes.	No numbness or tingling, no blackouts; weakness of lower extremity on the right due to pain.

PHYSICAL EXAMINATION		
Weight 112 lb	Temp 98.1	BP 100/56
Height 5'4"	Pulse 100	Resp 16

General Appearance
Healthy-appearing, thin, white female. Does not appear uncomfortable.
Neck
Supple with no lymphadenopathy. No bony deformity or tenderness.
Skin
Abrasion and ecchymotic area on right thigh and knee. Skin is warm and dry.
HEENT
Normal cephalic, no signs of trauma. PERLA with EOMs intact, conjunctiva clear. Ears, TMs pearly and mobile. Nose, clear without discharge, deviation, or obstruction. Oropharynx, clear with no obvious lesions, uvula is midline, and tonsils are symmetrical.
Cardiovascular
Rate is slightly tachycardic but regular with no murmurs or abnormal heart sound noted.
Respiratory
Lungs clear bilaterally. Chest intact with no signs of trauma.
Gastrointestinal
No signs of trauma; soft, nontender, with bowel sounds in all 4 quadrants; no rebound tenderness or masses noted.
Genitourinary
Not examined.

Musculoskeletal

Ecchymotic area on right thigh with difficulty bearing weight on the right leg. Shoulder pain on the right with limited ROM, strong; tenderness over the AC joint with no obvious deformity; able to raise arm overhead after it is actively raised to 30 degrees. Is able to abduct and adduct slowly due to pain; no swelling noted. Wrist tenderness over the snuffbox with limited ROM due to pain; good sensation distally. Color pink, warm to touch, capillary refill < 2 sec. CMS intact. Lower extremity: Right thigh shows a swollen, ecchymotic area approximately 3 cm in diameter with an abrasion just distal to it measuring 2.5 cm in diameter. Pain is noted on palpation to the posterior hip and groin. No tenderness over the proximal or distal femur. Strong inguinal, popliteal, and pedal pulses noted, with good sensation distally. Color pink, warm to touch, capillary refill < 2 sec. Able to wiggle toes bilaterally. Strength of the right leg is 3/5. Reflexes brisk and intact.

Neurological

No numbness or tingling. CN II–XII grossly intact; A&O × 3; unable to ambulate due to right hip pain and weakness. Deep tendon reflexes intact 2; negative Babinski.

Other

Lab Tests

CBC
Hgb: 14 g/dL
Hct: 40%
WBC: 10.1×10^3/mm^3
Neutrophils: 75%
Bands: 9%
Lymphs: 13%
Monocytes: 3%
Urinalysis: Clear yellow urine; specific gravity, 1.005; pH, 5.0; negative WBCs and RBCs; no ketones, bilirubin, or protein; no bacteria

Special Tests

X-rays
Right shoulder: Mild AC separation with no fractures noted.
Right hip: Nondisplaced hip fracture, pelvic ring intact. Degenerative changes noted to all the bony areas.
Right wrist: Scaphoid (navicular) fracture, nondisplaced.

Final Assessment Findings

Fracture of the right hip: Non-weight bearing; use of crutches
Right wrist fracture: Thumb spica splint applied
Right AC separation: Sling applied
Possible early osteoporosis

Bibliography

Adkins, S., & Figler, R. (2000). Hip pain in athletes. *American Family Physician, 61,* 2109–2120.

American Society for Surgery of the Hand (2003). *The hand: Primary care of common problems* (3rd ed.). New York, NY: Churchill Livingstone.

Biewen, P. C. (1999). A structured approach to low back pain. *Postgraduate Medicine Online, 106*(6), 102–107, 111–114.

Braunwalk, E., & Fauci, A. (2001). *Harrison's principles of internal medicine* (15th ed., pp. 111–163, 2369–2441). San Francisco, CA: McGraw-Hill.

Burkhart, S. (2000). A 26-year-old woman with shoulder pain. *Journal of the American Medical Association, 284,* 1559–1567.

Cardone, D., & Tallia, A. (2002). Diagnostic and therapeutic injection of the elbow region. *American Family Physician, 66,* 2097–2100.

Carragee, E. (2005). Persistent low back pain. *New England Journal of Medicine, 352,* 1891–1898.

Chapman, M. W. (2001). *Chapman's orthopaedic surgery* (3rd ed., pp. 2247–2265). Philadelphia, PA: Lippincott Williams & Wilkins.

Chumbley, E., O'Connor, F., & Nirschl, R. (2000). Evaluation of overuse elbow injuries. *American Family Physician, 61,* 691–702.

Daniels, J., Zook, E., & Lynch, J. (2004). Hand and wrist injuries: Part I. Non-emergent evaluation. *American Family Physician, 69*, 1941–1948.

Daniels, J., Zook, E., & Lynch, J. (2004). Hand and wrist injuries: Part II. Emergent evaluation. *American Family Physician, 69*, 1949–1956.

D'Arcy, C., & McGee, S. (2000). The rational clinical examination: Does this patient have carpal tunnel syndrome? *Journal of the American Medical Association, 283*, 3110–3117.

Deyo, R., & Weinstein, J. (2005). Low back pain. *New England Journal of Medicine, 344*, 363–370.

El-Gabalawy, H. S., Duray, P., & Goldbach-Mansky, R. (2000). Evaluating patients with arthritis of recent onset. *Journal of the American Medical Association, 284*, 2368–2373.

Emergency Nurses Association (Ed.) (2003). Pediatric trauma. In *ENPC provider manual* (3rd ed., pp. 9–10). Park Ridge, IL: Emergency Nurses Association.

Felson, D. (2006). Osteoarthritis of the knee. *New England Journal of Medicine, 354*, 841–848.

Griffin, L. (2015). *Essentials of musculoskeletal care* (15th ed.). Rosewood, IL: American Academy of Orthopedic Surgeons.

Hoppenfeld, S., & Hutton, R. (1976). *Physical examination of the spine and extremities.* New York, NY: Prentice-Hall.

Jackson, J. L., O'Malley, P. G., & Kroenke, K. (2003). Evaluation of acute knee pain in primary care. *Annals of the Institute of Medicine, 139*, 575–599.

Levine, J. D., & Reichling, D. B. (1999). Peripheral mechanisms of inflammatory pain. In P. D. Wall & R. Melzack (Eds.), *Textbook of pain* (4th ed., pp. 59–84). Philadelphia, PA: W. B. Saunders.

Lonner, J. H. (2003). A 57-year-old man with osteoarthritis of the knee. *Journal of the American Medical Association, 289*, 1016–1025.

Luime, J. J., Verhagen, A. P., & Miedema, H. S. (2004). Does this patient have an instability of the shoulder or a labrum lesion? *Journal of the American Medical Association, 292*, 1989–1999.

Magee, D. J. (2002). *Orthopedic physical assessment* (4th ed.). Philadelphia, PA: W. B. Saunders.

McCaffery, M., & Pasero, C. (1999). *Pain: Clinical manual* (2nd ed.). St. Louis, MO: Mosby.

Smith, C. C. (2004). Evaluating the painful knee: A hands-on approach to acute ligamentous and meniscal injuries. *Advanced Studies in Medicine, 4*, 362–369.

Solomon, D. H., Simel, D. L., & Bates, D. W. (2001). Does this patient have a torn meniscus or ligament of the knee? *Journal of the American Medical Association, 286*, 1610–1620.

Woodward, T. W., & Best, T. M. (2000). The painful shoulder—Part I. *American Family Physician, 61*(10), 3079–3088.

Chapter 16

Neurological Disorders

Anatomy and Physiology Review of the Nervous System

The neurological, or nervous, system is a highly organized system that directs all body functions through both voluntary and autonomic responses. Anatomically, the nervous system is divided into two parts: the central nervous system (CNS) and the peripheral nervous system (PNS) (**Figure 16-1**). The central division of the nervous system includes the brain and the spinal cord, which direct coordinated signals to other systems throughout the body. The PNS consists of 12 symmetrically arranged pairs of cranial nerves and 31 symmetrically arranged pairs of spinal nerves. Each nerve contains a sensory (dorsal) root and a motor (ventral) root, which are used to relay information to and from the CNS. The autonomic nervous system (ANS), which is considered part of the efferent division of the PNS, regulates body systems through the control mechanisms of the sympathetic and parasympathetic systems. These systems are designed to manage internal processes by carrying impulses to effector organs, thereby creating needed change for adaptation and survival. A basic understanding of the microstructure and macrostructure of the neurological system is essential for gaining insight into certain disease processes.

Nervous Tissue Cells

The cells of the nervous system can be divided into two types: neurons and supporting cells. The supporting cells serve to protect the neurons and provide them with metabolic support. Neurons are often referred to as the functional units of the nervous system. They transmit information to other neurons, muscle cells, or gland cells. Each neuron is composed of three basic components: a cell body, dendrites, and an axon (**Figure 16-2**). The cell body is responsible for the metabolic properties of the cell. It contains the nucleus and cytoplasmic organelles that are responsible for storing of proteins, support, and scavenging. Dendrites are branching fibers that extend

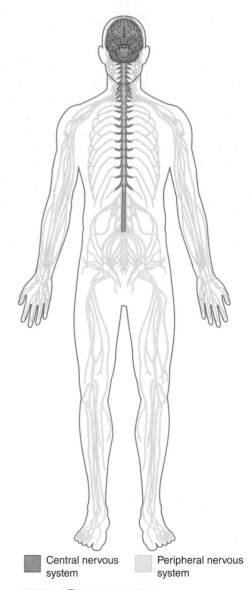

Central nervous system

Peripheral nervous system

FIGURE 16-1 The nervous system.

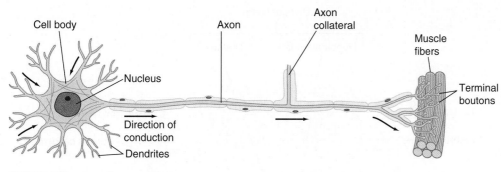

FIGURE 16-2 Structure of a neuron.

only a short distance from each cell body and conduct impulses toward the cell body. Each neuron contains only one axon; however, an axon may have multiple branches. An axon conducts impulses away from the cell body.

As their name implies, supporting cells mainly serve to support neurons. The layered myelin wrapping of supporting cells results in myelin sheaths; groups of axons (from various neurons) are bundled in myelin sheaths, which act as insulation for the conduction of nerve impulses (action potentials). The white matter of the CNS is composed of myelinated fiber tracts. Loss of myelin sheath integrity, as in multiple sclerosis (MS), disrupts nerve impulse transmission. Nerve tracts are not continuous, but have gaps called nodes of Ranvier. These periodic constrictions are present where the axon is exposed.

Nerve cells communicate by synapses, where the terminal branches of an axon from one neuron and the dendrites of another neuron lie close to each other but do not make direct contact. There are two types of synapses: electrical and chemical. Electrical synapses allow currents to travel in either direction. The more common type of synapse is chemical synapses. Synaptic transmission is a chemical process involving the release of neurotransmitters. This process allows unidirectional conduction of an impulse from the presynaptic terminal at the end of the axon across the postsynaptic cleft. Neurotransmitters can be categorized as excitatory or inhibitory.

Excitatory neurotransmitters promote conduction, whereas inhibitory neurotransmitters cause an increased resistance to depolarization, slowing the impulse. The main endogenous neurotransmitters are acetylcholine, norepinephrine, dopamine, gamma-amino butyric acid (GABA), and serotonin.

Nervous System

The CNS consists of the brain and the spinal cord. The CNS is surrounded by several structures designed to provide protection from manipulation, invasion of foreign fragments, or blunt trauma. These structures are the skull, meninges, cerebrospinal fluid, and the vertebrae. The skull, or cranium, forms the bony container that surrounds the brain. The skull opens at the base, where the brain stem protrudes (foramen magnum). It is covered by both fibrous and fatty vascular tissue layers (scalp). The brain is also protected by the meninges. The meninges are connective sheaths that suspend and protect the brain inside the skull (and the spinal cord inside the vertebral column). Cerebrospinal fluid (formed in the ventricles of the brain) is a protective, supportive fluid in which the brain and the spinal cord float.

Brain

Structures of the Brain

The brain is composed of the cerebrum, cerebellum, and the brain stem. **Figure 16-3** depicts the structures of the brain.

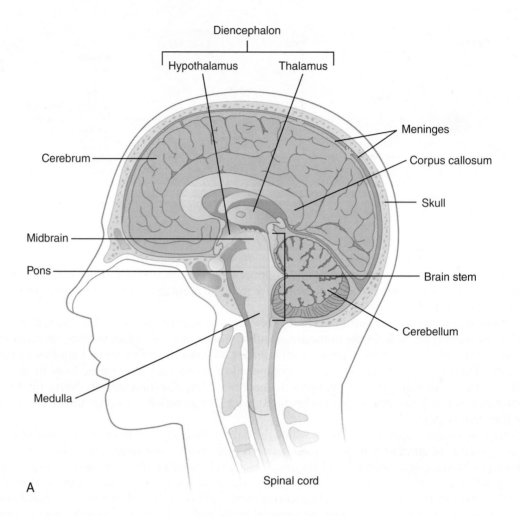

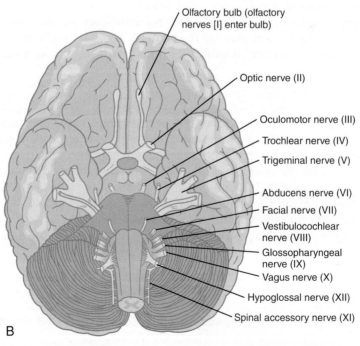

FIGURE 16-3 Structures of the brain. A. The major regions of the central nervous system. B. The cranial nerves.

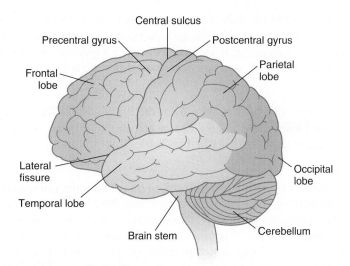

FIGURE 16-4 Lobes of the brain.

Cerebrum

Two cerebral hemispheres form the cerebrum. The right hemisphere controls the left side of the body, while the left hemisphere controls the right side.

Each hemisphere is divided into four lobes (**Figure 16-4**). The *frontal lobe* contains the motor cortex associated with voluntary skeletal movement and fine repetitive motor movements. It is responsible for higher mental functions such as judgment, foresight, affect, and personality. The *parietal lobe* is responsible for sensory function. It assists with interpretation of tactile sensations such as temperature, pressure, and pain, as well as visual, gustatory, olfactory, and auditory sensations. Higher-level processing, such as proprioception, depends on the parietal lobe. The *occipital lobe* contains the primary vision center and provides interpretation of visual stimuli. The *temporal lobe* perceives and interprets sounds, and determines their source. It is also involved in the integration of taste, smell, and balance, as well as behavior and emotion.

The cerebral cortex—the thin outer layer—houses the higher mental functions and is responsible for visceral functions, perceptions, and behavior. The complex network of fibers connected throughout each hemisphere, called commissural fibers, forms a communication pathway between both motor and sensory function.

The basal ganglia, composed of several subcortical nuclei located deep within white matter of the cerebral hemispheres, provide a pathway and assist in processing information associated with motor function. They influence postural reflexes and can suppress muscle tone. The basal ganglia's function is driven through extrapyramidal motor pathways.

The diencephalon is the central core of the cerebrum and includes the thalamus, hypothalamus, and epithalamus. The thalamus is divided into several nuclei. It receives specific sensory input for interpretation and transmission and plays a role in motor function. The hypothalamus regulates temperature, food and water intake, aggressive behavior, and autonomic responses.

The limbic system—the medial aspect of the cerebrum organized in bands of cortex—is responsible for patterns of behavior such as mating, aggression, fear, and affection. Disturbances of the limbic system result in altered behavioral states and memory deficits.

Cerebellum

The cerebellum is located posterior and inferior to the cerebrum. It aids the motor cortex of the cerebrum in influencing muscle tone and coordinating muscle action. Integrated with the vestibular system, the cerebellum also utilizes the sensory data for reflexive control of equilibrium and posture.

Brain Stem

The brain stem lies between the cerebral cortex and the spinal cord, controlling many involuntary functions. Its structures include the medulla oblongata, pons, and midbrain. The reticular activating system (RAS) formation of the brain stem communicates with the thalamus, cortex, spinal cord, and cerebellum. The ascending RAS is essential for arousal from sleep, alert wakefulness, attention, and perceptual association. The descending RAS inhibits activity of motor neurons controlling skeletal musculature. Respiratory, circulatory, and vasomotor activities are coordinated in the brain stem.

Cranial Nerves

Cranial nerves are peripheral nerves that arise from the brain stem. They provide both motor and sensory interpretation and responses. Cranial nerves are numbered with Roman numerals, starting with the most anterior nerve, and are described in **Table 16-1**.

Cerebral Blood Supply

Cerebral circulation requires approximately 750 mL of blood flow per minute. This system lacks the ability to create a reserve of oxygen or glucose and, therefore, functionally deteriorates with alterations in adequate supply. The internal carotids, vertebral arteries, and basilar artery are responsible for delivering blood to the brain. The two separate circulations are connected at the base of the brain by vessels referred to as the circle of Willis, which permits collateral circulation should occlusion of one of the arteries occur. Anteriorly, at the level of the cricothyroid junction, the common carotid splits to form the external and internal carotid arteries.

These arteries deliver blood to such structures as the face, scalp, skull, optic nerve, eyes, brain stem, and cerebellum. Cerebral blood flow (CBF) varies with changes in cerebral perfusion pressure and the diameter of the cerebrovascular bed. Cerebral perfusion pressure (CPP) is the difference between mean arterial pressure (MAP) and intracranial pressure (ICP): CPP = MAP − ICP.

Changes in the diameter of the vascular bed are influenced by auto-regulation of arterioles by means of vasoconstriction or vasodilation. Increases in $PaCO_2$ cause vasodilation and decreases in $PaCO_2$ cause vasoconstriction, leading to increases or decreases in CBF, respectively. Hypoxemia leads to vasodilation of cerebral arteries, albeit to a lesser extent than $PaCO_2$ changes. Venous drainage is accomplished by both the external and internal venous systems, which empty into venous sinuses of the dura. Capillary flow moves to venules and then to cerebral veins, which empty into the sinuses located throughout the cranium. Blood from the sinuses travels to the superior vena cava and then back to the right atrium.

Table 16-1	Cranial Nerves and Their Functions		
Number	Name	Type	Function
I	Olfactory	Sensory	Smell
II	Optic	Sensory	Vision
III	Oculomotor	Motor	Extraocular movement, pupil constriction, and upper eyelid elevation
IV	Trochlear	Motor	Extraocular eye movement
V	Trigeminal	Motor	Mastication and lateral jaw movements
		Sensory	Transmission of stimuli from face and head, corneal reflex
VI	Abducens	Motor	Extraocular eye movement
VII	Facial	Sensory	Taste (receptors on anterior two-thirds of the tongue)
		Motor	Facial muscle movement, including muscles of expression
VIII	Vestibulocochlear	Sensory	Hearing, balance
IX	Glossopharyngeal	Sensory	Sensations from throat, taste (receptors on posterior one-third of the tongue)
		Motor	Swallowing movements
X	Vagus	Motor	Movement of palate, larynx, and swallowing; gag reflex; activity of the thoracic and abdominal viscera
		Sensory	Sensations from throat, larynx, and thoracic and abdominal viscera
XI	Spinal accessory	Motor	Shoulder movement, head rotation
XII	Hypoglossal	Motor	Tongue movement

Data from The Anatomical Chart Company. (2001). *Atlas of human anatomy.* Springhouse, PA: Springhouse.

Blood–Brain Barrier

The blood–brain barrier maintains the delicate balance of the brain's internal environment. It is responsible for the transport of water, waste, nutrients, and ions such as oxygen, carbon dioxide, and glucose through selective permeability. The passage of substances across the blood–brain barrier depends on that substance's size, lipid solubility, and protein binding. Any change in the composition of the barrier poses an increased risk for exposure to toxins, resulting in damage to cerebral tissue.

Spinal Cord

The spinal cord begins at the foramen magnum and is a continuation of the medulla oblongata, terminating at L1 or L2 of the vertebral column. It is a ropelike structure composed of white and gray matter.

White and Gray Matter

The white matter contains the ascending and descending tracts. The ascending tracts convey impulses, via the dorsal root of the spinal nerves, to various muscle groups controlling tone and posture. Descending motor tracts transmit impulses from the brain to motor neurons of the spinal cord and exit via the ventral root of the spinal nerves. The gray matter is arranged in a butterfly shape with anterior and posterior horns and a lateral column. The anterior gray column contains cell bodies of efferent or motor fibers, whereas the posterior horn contains cell bodies of afferent or sensory fibers. The lateral column contains preganglionic fibers of the autonomic nervous system.

The descending pathways from the brain to the spinal cord are composed of upper motor neurons. They serve to influence and modify spinal reflex arcs and circuits. The lower motor neurons are spinal and cranial motor neurons that directly innervate muscles.

Spinal Nerves

Segments of the spinal cord communicate with corresponding body parts via spinal nerves. Thirty-one symmetrical pairs of nerves arise from the spinal cord (**Figure 16-5**).

These nerves divide into branches. Intermixing branches form plexuses (nerve networks). Nerves arise from the plexus and then form smaller branches that communicate with skin and muscles.

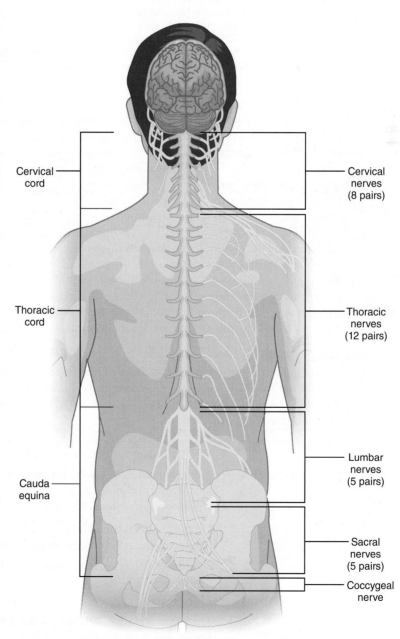

FIGURE 16-5 Spinal nerves and spinal cord in relation to the vertebral column.

Health History

Neurological system impairments include changes in consciousness, altered mobility (tremors, weakness, incoordination), altered sensation (numbness, tingling), dysphagia, dysphasia, and pain. Conducting a thorough examination upon initial presentation assists the practitioner in providing optimal care for the patient. When taking the health history, note general appearance, affect, voice, speech content, memory, logic, judgment, and speech patterns.

Chief Complaint and History of Present Illness

"I have frequent headaches, keep losing my balance, and sometimes have difficulty speaking."

KW is a 48-year-old woman who presents to the clinic accompanied by her husband. Mrs. W reports that over the last 2 weeks she has experienced frequent headaches and periods of dizziness that resolved spontaneously. Mr. W states that early this morning he found his wife unresponsive. Shortly thereafter, she regained consciousness but had no recollection of the morning's events. She is currently having difficulty speaking and is unable to ambulate due to left-sided weakness and numbness. She denies a history of seizures and dysphagia.

Common chief complaints (CCs) associated with neurological disorders include headaches, vertigo, loss of equilibrium, changes in level of consciousness, altered mobility, seizures, altered sensation, dysphagia, and dysphasia. Specific questions (regarding the history of present illness [HPI]) for vertigo, loss of equilibrium, changes in level of consciousness, headaches, and altered mobility are given here.

Seizures may be due to withdrawal from anticonvulsant or sedative medications, ethyl alcohol withdrawal, CNS infections, metabolic disorders, trauma, or cerebrovascular disease. A careful history will help the practitioner to determine the cause.

Altered sensation often relates to some types of CNS disorders, such as MS or cerebrovascular accident (CVA), or PNS disorders. Altered sensations include tingling, numbness, and loss of sensation. Determining the quality, location, pattern, and associated symptoms helps narrow the diagnosis.

Dysphagia, or difficulty swallowing, is often related to neurological disorders, such as CVA, brain tumors, spinal cord injuries, Parkinson's disease, and MS.

Dysphasia is an alteration in language comprehension, a complete or partial loss of the ability to understand, speak, read, and write. Dysphasia is a hallmark sign associated with dysfunction of the temporal lobe by cerebral tumor, CVA, or trauma.

Headaches

Careful assessment of the descriptive qualities of headaches may indicate various forms of intracranial/extracranial pathologies. For example, vascular headaches are characterized by their intermittence and throbbing pain. Further testing may be necessary to determine possible obstruction, intracranial hypertension, bleeding, or infection.

Onset	Was the onset sudden or gradual?
	Causes of sudden headaches include spontaneous subarachnoid hemorrhage, rupture of an intracranial aneurysm or arteriovenous malformation, and subdural hematoma.
Duration, frequency, and pattern	How long does the headache last? Are the headaches frequent? Do they progressively increase in frequency?
	Migraines are recurring headaches; the frequency of their occurrence varies.
	Cluster headaches occur in clustered cycles.
	Transient ischemic attacks (TIAs) usually present with a history of headaches with a duration of days.

	Trigeminal neuralgia causes sudden, severe, brief episodes of unilateral facial pain.
	Intracranial tumors present with a constant, progressing pain.
Quality; location	Describe the headache. Is it burning, aching, deep, superficial, or throbbing? What is the intensity? Is the headache continuous or intermittent? Where is it located? Does it radiate?
	Tension headaches are often described as mild or moderate in severity, causing "tightness," and with a gradual onset.
	Migraines without aura often present with a unilateral, severe, throbbing pain that may become bilateral.
	Cluster headaches present with increasing sharp, unilateral pain, often located in the ocular area.
	Brain abscesses often present with a poorly localized, dull pain.
Associated symptoms	Ask about associated symptoms, including neurological deficits, fever, photophobia, nausea, vomiting, excessive tearing or redness of the eye, sweating, and nuchal rigidity.
	Migraines often present with photophobia, nausea or vomiting, and phonophobia.
	Cluster headaches are often accompanied by excessive tearing or redness of the eyes and sweating.
	TIAs often present with intermittent neurological deficit, vertigo, weakness, and numbness.
	CVA may present with altered sensation and motor ability and dysphagia.
	Rupture of an intracranial aneurysm or arteriovenous malformation (AVM) may present with altered consciousness, vertigo, visual disturbances, and nausea.
	Meningitis often presents with fever, altered mental status, and nuchal rigidity.
	Encephalitis may present with altered level of consciousness, fever, seizures, or altered mood.
Precipitating factors	Does anything specific precipitate the onset of the headaches? Ask about medications, coughing, straining or physical exertion, emotional tension, and menses. Has the patient recently experienced any trauma?
	Benign exertional headaches are related to coughing, sneezing, and physical exertion.
	Cluster headaches may be precipitated by stress, exertion, or alcohol intake.
	Tension, menses, and excessive noise or light may precipitate migraines.
	Stress and fatigue may precipitate tension headaches.
Alleviating and aggravating factors	What relieves the pain (medications, sleep)? What makes the pain worse?

Vertigo or Loss of Equilibrium

Vertigo can be the result of a neurological dysfunction or caused by the lack of cerebral blood flow. A proper clinical and diagnostic evaluation helps differentiate between problems associated with benign positional vertigo and cerebral abscesses, infection, or sclerosis.

Onset	Is the onset sudden or gradual?
	Acute or sudden onset may indicate stroke.
Quality	Is there loss of balance upon ambulation? Are there fainting spells or a feeling of the room spinning?
	Acoustic neuroma often presents with increasing loss of equilibrium.
Pattern	When does this happen? How often does it occur?
Associated symptoms	Is there recent hearing loss, tinnitus, fatigue, weakness, impaired speech, dysphagia, or headache?
	Ménière's disease often presents with tinnitus and hearing loss.
	Vestibular neuronitis does not present with hearing loss. Acoustic neuroma may present with tinnitus and unilateral hearing loss.
	Multiple sclerosis presents with various neurological symptoms, including fatigue, weakness, vision disturbances, sensory disturbances, dysphasia, and dysphagia.
	Transient ischemic attacks may present with weakness and a history of headaches.
Alleviating factors	What relieves the problem (positional changes, medications)? How effective is it?

Changes in Level of Consciousness

Altered level of consciousness often indicates neurological dysfunction. Altered level of consciousness has varying degrees and ranges from confusion (or inability to understand and respond) to coma.

Quality; severity	Ask the patient to describe the change and to describe the events before and after the change in level of consciousness. What is the patient's mental/physical state after the event?
	Rupture of an intracranial aneurysm or AVM may present with loss of consciousness. Meningitis may present with confusion.
Frequency, duration, and pattern	Is there a history of fainting, blackouts? How often are these changes occurring? What are they brought on by? How long do these episodes last? How long after the event until the patient's level of consciousness returns to normal?
Associated symptoms	Ask about associated symptoms, including headache, numbness, dysphagia, nausea, vomiting, and fever.
	TIA presents with headaches and numbness.
	CVA presents with sudden, severe headache; numbness, weakness, or loss of motor function on one side of the body; visual difficulties; and dysphagia.

Altered Mobility

A change in level of mobility may indicate a neurological disorder. The practitioner should differentiate between changes that indicate Parkinson's disease (tremors at rest) and tics that point to multiple neurological pathology requiring further testing.

Quality	Which kind of change is the patient experiencing: tremors, shaking, twitches, jerks, weakness, problems with coordination, balance, frequent falling or tripping, or a tendency to favor one side or fall toward one side? Is there a change in walking pattern?
	CVA may present with loss of motor ability on one side of the body.
	Bradykinesia (slowness of movement), loss of spontaneous movement, and resting tremors suggest Parkinson's disease.
	Weakness, tremor, and incoordination may suggest MS. Decreased circulation to the brain, such as with a CVA, causes symptoms of weakness, loss of coordination, and difficulty in moving parts of the body.
Precipitating factors	What precipitates the event? Does a particular activity trigger the change?

Past Medical History

Mrs. W denies a history of trauma. She states that she was diagnosed with hypertension 10 years ago but has been noncompliant with antihypertensive medications because of their adverse effects. Mrs. W also has a history of hyperlipidemia; she has been noncompliant with medication regimen because of the cost. Mrs. W had a right carotid endarterectomy 2 years ago.

The healthcare provider should ask detailed questions focusing on any/all past medical illnesses/history (PMI), traumatic events, and surgeries, including elective surgeries. This critical information will aid in the formulation of a detailed plan of care.

Past health conditions or surgeries	Ask about past or ongoing health conditions.
	Some conditions, such as cardiovascular (coronary artery disease, hypertension, hyperlipidemia, aneurysm) or metabolic conditions (thyroid disease, diabetes mellitus, leukemia, cancer, lipid storage diseases), may contribute to neurological problems.
	Question the patient about a history of neurological disorders, such as CVA, cerebral aneurysm, chronic subdural hematoma, AVMs, seizures, or neuropathies. Has the patient been treated by a neurologist or neurosurgeon?
	Inquire about exposure to communicable diseases, such as meningitis, encephalitis, poliomyelitis, AIDS, botulism, syphilis, cat scratch disease, rickettsial infections, toxoplasmosis, and malaria, all of which may have neurological manifestations.
	Inquire about a history of psychological disorders. Ask about past surgeries, including craniotomy, laminectomy, carotid endarterectomy, transsphenoidal hypophysectomy, cordotomy, aneurysmectomy or repair, and cardiac surgery.
Trauma	Ask about past trauma, such as head trauma, CNS insult, birth trauma, spinal cord injury, and peripheral nerve damage. If the patient has a history of trauma, how and when did it happen? Was she or he treated? If so, how?
	Head trauma may result in intracranial bleeding, or soft tissue or other neurological damage.

| Medications | Does the patient take any medications, such as anticonvulsants, sedatives, anticoagulants, aspirin, antidysrhythmics, or antihypertensives? For which conditions? How long has the patient been taking the medication? |

Family History

> Mrs. W denies any history of coronary artery disease, diabetes, neurological disease, or cancer. She is an only child. Her father, age 78, has hypertension. Her mother, age 75, is alive and well. She does not have any children.

The family history (FH)—information about the medical status of family members—helps the health-care provider determine possible genetic factors that may play a role in the patient's chief complaint.

Age of living relatives	Include the relationship and health of parents, siblings, and children.
Deaths	Ask about the relationship of the deceased person to the patient and the cause of death; specifically explore disorders that may have neurological implications, such as hypertension and CVA.
Chronic diseases; neurological disorders	Ask about chronic diseases. Is there a history of neurological disease in the family? If so, what is the relationship of family member with the neurological disease? How long has the family member had the disease? *Specifically, explore the patient's family history of brain tumors, degenerative disease, and dementia, as these tend to run in families.*
Genetic defects	Is there a history of familial genetic or congenital birth defects?

Social History

> Mrs. W lives with her husband in a one-bedroom apartment and has worked as a receptionist for the past 20 years. Recently, she has had trouble completing tasks at work. She reports that she smokes one pack of cigarettes a day and has been smoking since she was 18 years old. Other than an occasional glass of wine with dinner, she does not drink. Mrs. W denies recreational drug use. She does not have a regular exercise regimen.

In taking the social history (SH), try to determine the patient's ability to interact with others in healthy ways. Also, clues such as inability to perform activities of daily living (ADLs) provide insight into the severity of the patient's diagnosis.

Family	Ask the patient to describe the current family unit.
Occupation	What does the patient do for a living? Has the patient had any recent trouble functioning at work? *A change in ability to focus and complete work may indicate impaired cognitive status or altered level of consciousness.*
Stress	Ask about physical and emotional stress. Is the patient exposed to any toxic chemicals (e.g., lead, carbon dioxide, arsenic, insecticides, organic solvents)?

Hobbies	Ask about use of leisure time. Does the patient have difficulty concentrating on activities (reading or watching television) that once were enjoyable? Does the patient participate in contact sports or high-risk activities (e.g., football, soccer, hockey, boxing, race car driving, motorcycling)?
	Such activities may put the patient at risk for trauma, especially if the patient does not wear protective equipment.
Activity/exercise intolerance	Ask about diminished ability to carry on ADLs, immobilization or marked sedentary habits, and alteration in living habits or activities as a result of neurological symptoms.
	Neurological disorders, such as CVA, Parkinson's disease, MS, amyotrophic lateral sclerosis, Guillain–Barré syndrome, myasthenia gravis, and brain tumors, often manifest as diminished ability to perform ADLs.
Use of tobacco	Ask about tobacco use, including types, amounts, duration of use, and exposure to secondary smoke.
Use of alcohol	Does the patient drink alcohol? If so, which type and how much does he or she drink?
Use of recreational drugs	Is the patient using recreational drugs? If so, which drugs and how much?
	Recreational drugs affect the neurological system.
Sexual practices	Ask the patient about his or her sexual history.
	Sexually transmitted diseases may affect the neurological system (e.g., syphilis and AIDS).

Review of Systems

Many neurological diseases and disorders have manifestations in systems other than the neurological system. A comprehensive review of systems (ROS) should be performed whenever possible; however, due to time and other types of constraints, the provider may be able to perform only a focused review of systems. During a focused review of systems, the provider targets questioning at the systems in which neurological problems are most likely to have manifestations. Following is a summary of common manifestations of neurological problems.

System	Symptom or Sign	Possible Associated Diseases/Disorders
General	Fever, chills	Meningitis, encephalitis
	Sleeplessness	Parkinson's disease
	Fatigue	Multiple sclerosis, myasthenia gravis
	Dizziness	Ménière's disease
Skin	Petechial or purpuric rash	Meningitis
Eye	Visual disturbances/difficulty	CVS, rupture of intracranial aneurysm or AVM, encephalitis, multiple sclerosis, brain tumor, migraine
	Tearing or redness of eye	Cluster headaches
Respiratory	Respiratory irregularities	Guillain–Barré syndrome
Cardiovascular	Bruits, thrills	CVA
Gastrointestinal	Nausea, vomiting	Brain and spinal abscesses, rupture of intracranial aneurysm or AVM, brain tumor, migraine

(continues)

System	Symptom or Sign	Possible Associated Diseases/Disorders
Genitourinary	Urinary dysfunction (frequency, hesitancy, urgency, incontinence)	Multiple sclerosis, brain tumor
Musculoskeletal	Backache	Spinal abscess
	Nuchal rigidity	Meningitis
	Weakness	CVA
Mental Health	Depression	Parkinson's disease, multiple sclerosis

Abbreviations: AVM, arteriovenous malformation; CVA, cerebrovascular accident (stroke).

Physical Examination

Equipment Needed

- Penlight
- Tongue blade
- Tuning forks, 200 to 400 Hz and 500 to 1000 Hz
- Familiar small objects (such as coins, keys, and paper clips)
- Sterile needles
- Cotton wisp
- Reflex hammer
- Vials of aromatic substances (coffee, orange, peppermint extract, oil of cloves)
- Vials of solutions for tasting (glucose, salt, lemon or vinegar, and quinine)
- Vials containing hot and cold water for testing temperature sensation
- Snellen and Rosenbaum charts
- Denver Developmental Screening Test (for infants and children)

Components of the Physical Examination

A complete neurological assessment includes an assessment of mental status, sensation, cranial nerves, motor function, cerebellar function, and reflexes. To facilitate examination, make sure the room is a comfortable temperature, well lit, and quiet. When the patient enters the room, observe as she or he approaches. Note gait, posture, dress, grooming, hygiene, involuntary movements, and general appearance. Ask the patient to replace all street clothes with the examination gown provided.

Assessing Mental Status

A significant part of the neurological assessment is performed during the entrance and history. When taking the health history, the practitioner should note the patient's general appearance, affect, voice, speech content, memory, logic, judgment, and speech patterns. In most cases, the information obtained during the health history is sufficient to assess mental status. Use the Mini-Mental Status Examination to test cognitive function.

A more specific mental assessment should be performed if the following are noted: known or suspected brain lesion, memory deficits, confusion, vague behavioral complaints, aphasia, and irritability. (See the Mental Health Disorders chapter for more information.)

Testing Cranial Nerves

Alterations in cranial nerve (CN) function cause motor and/or sensory impairments. Table 16-1 (located in the "Anatomy and Physiology Review of the Nervous System" section) describes the function of each CN.

Action	Rationale
1. Assess CN I (olfactory nerve) function. Test the patient's recognition of familiar, nonirritating odors (cloves, coffee, perfume). Test each nostril independently.	**1.** Patients should be able to identify each odor. Unilateral anosmia (the loss of sense of smell) may result from compression of the olfactory tract or bulb by an intracranial neoplasm, such as meningioma of the sphenoid ridge. It may also be caused by sinusitis or trauma to the cribriform plate.
2. Test CN II (optic nerve). Evaluate visual acuity and visual fields.	**2.** Uncorrected strabismus from early childhood or from certain medical conditions, such as alcoholism, uremia, and diabetes mellitus, may result in the permanent loss of visual acuity. Pathology affecting the optic nerve—as seen in MS, tumors or abscesses in the nerve itself, optic atrophy, papilledema from increased ICP, optic neuritis, or neovascularization of the optic nerve with resultant hemorrhage—may result in visual deficits. It may also result from tumors or strokes or other neurological diseases.
3. Assess CNs III (oculomotor nerve), IV (trochlear nerve), and VI (abducens nerve). **a.** Test extraocular movements through the six cardinal fields of gaze. Assess for convergence.	**a.** Identify any nystagmus and the direction of gaze in which it occurs. Traumatic paralysis of one or more of the optic muscles may cause injury to the extraocular muscles or CNs II, III, IV, and VI by an orbital fracture near the foramen magnum. Extraocular muscle palsy from CN VI involvement may be caused by basilar skull fractures that involve the cavernous sinus. Infections such as herpes zoster, syphilis, scarlet fever, whooping cough, and botulism may affect CNs III, IV, and VI, contributing to extraocular muscle palsy. Increased ICP may cause compression of CN VI. Invasion of the wall of the cavernous sinus by parasellar meningiomas or tumors in the sphenoid sinus may affect CNs III, IV, and VI. Vertical gaze deviation may result from damage at the area of the midbrain–diencephalic junction, or tumors that compress the brain stem. Destruction of the motor region of the cerebral cortex leads to the inability of both eyes to look to the contralateral side, thereby causing deviation toward the side of the lesion. Demyelinization resulting from multiple sclerosis may create internuclear ophthalmoplegia, where the eyes converge but are unable to look medially. Skew deviation—where one eye deviates down and the other eye deviates up—may result from cerebellar disease or a lesion in the pons on the same side as the eye that is deviated down. Nystagmus can result from a lesion in the brain stem, cerebellum, vestibular system, or along the visual pathways in the cerebral hemispheres.

Action	**Rationale**
b. Examine the shape and size of the pupils. Assess the direct and consensual light reflex. Assess the accommodation reflex.	b. Certain medications (such as sympathomimetics or parasympathomimetics) or CN III paralysis, due to a carotid artery aneurysm or trauma, may cause abnormal papillary size. Optic nerve injury in the optic chiasm from trauma leads to damage of optic afferent pathways, which is tested by the papillary light reflex. In the presence of a midbrain lesion, stimulation of the pupil with light results in the hippus phenomenon, where the pupil initially constricts, then appears to rhythmically fluctuate in size while leaving accommodation intact.
c. Assess eyelid elevation. Observe the blinking of the eyes. Observe the patient's eyelids for drooping. Ask the patient to elevate the eyelids.	c. Excessive blinking can be the result of involuntary tonic spasms of the orbicularis oculi muscle involving CN VII lesions. Ptosis may be related to myasthenia gravis, paralysis of the levator muscle from injury, or disruption of neural pathways. The inability to bring about complete lid closure may be associated with Bell's palsy or stroke.
d. Assess for "doll's eyes." Briskly move the patient's head from side to side.	d. The "doll's eyes" test will demonstrate the integrity of the vestibular and oculomotor pathways. Eyes should move in the opposite direction of head movement. An abnormal doll's eyes phenomenon (fixed eyes when the head is moved) may result from lower brain stem lesions.
4. Assess CN V (trigeminal nerve).	
a. Evaluate sensation awareness of the forehead, cheeks, and jaw on each side of the face. Use a wisp of cotton for a light touch, a pin for superficial pain, and test tubes of hot and cold water for temperature.	a. Compression of the trigeminal nerve from lesions may lead to impaired sensory perception and/or facial pain. An abnormal, brief, paroxysmal unilateral facial pain that follows the distribution of the trigeminal nerve without motor weakness and is stimulated by touch or movement of the face is known as trigeminal neuralgia. Postherpetic neuralgia involves a constant, burning, aching pain with intermittent stabbing pains that may occur spontaneously or may be caused by touch.
b. For unconscious patients, stroke the cornea of each eye with a wisp of cotton. Observe for reflex blinking.	b. A diminished corneal reflex indicates either an acute lesion of the opposite hemisphere or an ipsilateral lesion in the brain stem. The absence of a corneal response results from a lesion involving the afferent limb of CN V and the efferent limb of CN VII of the reflex arc.
c. Palpate the masseter and temporal muscles with the patient's teeth clenched (**Figure 16-6**). Assess the strength of masseter muscles by pushing down on the mandible against the patient's resistance. Assess the patient's ability to chew.	c. Masseter muscle spasm occurs due to motor root involvement of the trigeminal nerve. Head trauma may result in facial anesthesia and paralysis of the muscles of mastication.

Action   **Rationale**

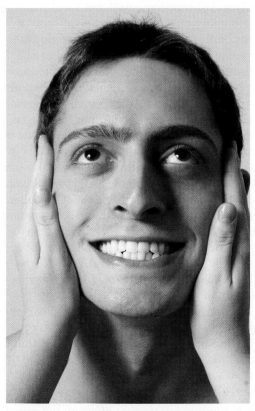

FIGURE 16-6 Palpating the masseter and temporal muscles.

5. Assess CN VII (facial nerve).
   a. Ask the patient to raise his or her eyebrows, frown, smile, and open eyes against resistance. Note the strength and symmetry of facial muscles.

   a. An upper motor neuron lesion of the facial nerve may result in supranuclear facial palsy evidenced by paralysis in the lower one-third to two-thirds of the face. Bell's palsy, characterized by total flaccid paralysis of facial muscles, results from injury to the facial nerve on the ipsilateral side.

   b. Evaluate the patient's recognition of sweet and salty taste on the anterior two-thirds of the tongue.

   b. Alterations in the gustatory sense may be due to lesions of the medulla oblongata and/or parietal lobe.

6. Assess CN VIII (vestibulocochlear nerve).
   a. Assess hearing acuity (see the Ear Disorders chapter for techniques).

   a. Sensorineural loss due to a disorder in the inner ear or to the nerve in the involved ear results in lateralization to the unaffected ear.

   b. Evaluate the vestibular division by assessing for vertigo, nausea, and anxiety. Note any evidence of equilibrium disturbances.

   b. Vertigo results from disruption of the labyrinth or the vestibular nerve.

Action

Rationale

---

7. Assess CNs IX (glossopharyngeal nerve) and X (vagus nerve).

8. Assess CN XI (spinal accessory nerve). Inspect the sternocleidomastoid and trapezius muscles for size and symmetry. Ask the patient to turn her or his head to one side and instruct the patient to resist your attempt to forcibly turn the head back to midline. Palpate opposite the sternocleidomastoid muscle. Evaluate each side independently. Ask the patient to push her or his head forward against your hand.

9. Assess CN XII (hypoglossal nerve).
  a. Assess the tongue for atrophy. Have the patient protrude the tongue and push it to the right and left. Check alignment of the tongue when it is protruded. Have the patient press his or her tongue against the inside of the cheek while you assess its strength bilaterally.

  b. Ask the patient to repeat lingual sounds such as "la."

7. Unilateral glossopharyngeal and vagal paralysis due to injury or skull fractures at the base of the skull may result in unilateral lowering and flattening of the palatine arch, weakness of the soft palate, deviation of the uvula to the unaffected side, mild dysphagia, regurgitation of fluids, nasal quality of voice, absence of gustatory sense in the posterior one-third of the tongue, and hemianesthesia of the palate. Bilateral vagus nerve paralysis will cause significant nasal quality of the voice, difficulty with guttural and palatal sounds, severe dysphagia with liquids, and inability of the palate to elevate on phonation. Cerebellar dysfunction can interfere with the coordination of the muscles innervated by these cranial nerves.

Ask the patient to say, "Ah." Observe for a symmetric rise of the palatal arch. Stroke the palatal arch with a tongue blade to observe for the presence of the gag reflex.

Evaluate speech for nasal quality, hoarseness, and articulation. If a deficit is noted, ask the patient to produce guttural and palatal sounds such as "k," "q," "ch," "b," and "d." Evaluate the patient's ability to swallow a small amount of water. Observe for control of oral secretions.

8. Injury, tumors, or infection affecting the spinal accessory nerve may cause unilateral paralysis of the sternocleidomastoid muscle and result in a flat, flaccid muscle and the inability to rotate the head toward the paralyzed side. In addition, there may be unilateral paralysis of the trapezius, causing asymmetrical shoulder and scapula height, a depressed outline of the neck, and the inability of the patient to lift that shoulder.

Assess the strength of the sternocleidomastoid muscles. Ask the patient to shrug the shoulders upward against resistance of your downward pressure on the shoulders. Observe for strength, atrophy, and fasciculation.

  a. Lesions of the hypoglossal nucleus or trauma to the nerve fiber may cause symptoms consisting of tongue deviation as a result of unilateral paralysis because the muscles on the paralyzed side are unable to oppose the strong muscles of the unaffected side. Inability of the patient to protrude the tongue results from bilateral paralysis of the tongue muscles.

  b. Lesions of the hypoglossal nerve may also impede pronunciation of lingual sounds.

Assessing Motor Function: Inspection and Palpation

Action	Rationale
Muscles	
1. Observe the size and contour of muscles. Note atrophy, hypertrophy, asymmetry, and joint malalignments.	1. Size and contour should fall within normal limits, and muscles should appear symmetrical bilaterally. Wasting of the arms, legs, and trunk suggests ALS or Guillain–Barré syndrome. Atrophy of a particular muscle group may indicate a peripheral nerve injury (PNI). For example, femoral nerve injury often presents with atrophy of the quadriceps.
2. Note involuntary movements.	2. Abnormal involuntary movements include fasciculations, fibrillation, spasms, tetany, chorea, tremors, tics, ballismus, athetosis, dystonia, myoclonus, and asterixis. These may result from various neurological pathologies. Parkinson's disease often presents with resting tremors.
3. If tenderness or spasm is suggested by the history or if muscles seem atrophic or hypertrophic, palpate muscles. Assess muscle strength and tone and note whether rigidity, spasticity, or hypotonia is elicited by passive motion.	3. Limbs involved in hemiparesis, paraplegia, or quadriplegia typically exhibit local atrophy. Neurological diseases of the lower motor neurons may manifest as flaccidity in the affected muscles. Spasticity may denote upper motor neuron dysfunction and is commonly seen with paralysis and cerebral palsy. **Table 16-2** describes findings associated with upper and lower neuron lesions. Unilateral weakness or paralysis may be related to a stroke, tumor, or trauma, whereas generalized diminution in muscle strength is associated with diffuse atrophy and deteriorating neuromuscular disorders such as ALS, muscular dystrophy, MS, myasthenia gravis, and Guillain–Barré syndrome.

Table 16-2 Common Findings with Upper and Lower Motor Lesions	
UMN Lesions	**LMN Lesions**
Muscle spasticity	Muscle flaccidity
Diminished strength without atrophy	Loss of strength and tone with atrophy
Hyper deep tendon/abdominal reflexes	Weak or absent reflexes
No fasciculations	Fasciculations
Damage above the level of the brain stem will affect the opposite side of the body	Ipsilateral changes noted
Possible paralysis of the lower side of the face	Palsy possible; coordination unimpaired
Positive Babinski reflex	Absent Babinski reflex
Clonus	No clonus

Abbreviations: LMN, lower motor neuron; UMN, upper motor neuron.

Action	Rationale

Cerebellar Function

1. Assess balance and gait.
   a. Instruct the patient to walk normally across the room. Observe the patient during transfer between the sitting and standing positions. Ask the patient to walk on tiptoes, then on heels. Ask the patient to walk in a straight line touching heel to toe. Instruct the patient to walk forward, then backward. Ask the patient to side-step to the left, then to the right.
   b. Instruct the patient to walk forward a few steps with the eyes closed. Note the patient's ability to maintain balance. Ask the patient to hop in place first on one foot and then on the other.

   c. Perform Romberg's test: Observe for swaying when the patient stands with the feet together, first with eyes open, then with eyes closed.

   d. Test for pronator drift. Ask the patient to stand and extend the arms with his or her palms up (**Figure 16-7**).

a. Movements should be smooth. Cerebellar disease, muscle weakness, paralysis, lack of coordination or balance, stiffness, fatigue, and pain may all result in abnormal gait.

Parkinson's disease may present with rigid and slow movement. Weakness and ataxia may suggest MS. A tumor in the cerebellar area may present with gait and balance disturbances.

b. The inability of the patient to remain balanced with the eyes opened and closed may be the result of cerebellar disease. An increase in the instability with eye closure may indicate posterior column disease with proprioceptive loss.

c. The patient should be able to maintain the position. A positive Romberg's test is when the patient cannot maintain balance with the eyes closed. MS often presents with a positive Romberg's test.

d. Downward drifting of an arm may indicate hemiparesis, which is evidence of a stroke.

Have the patient hold the position; observe for downward drifting of the patient's arm.

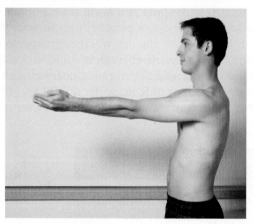

FIGURE 16-7 Testing pronator drift.

2. Assess coordination.

2. Cerebellar disease may be characterized by uncoordinated action of the muscle groups where the patient's movements appear jerky, irregular; impaired judgment of distance, range, speed, and force of movement where the patient overshoots; or the inability to perform rapid alternating movements.

Action	**Rationale**
a. Test for arm dystaxia using the finger-to-nose test. Ask the patient to sit on the examination table. Instruct him or her to close his or her eyes and to touch the tip of the nose with the index finger. Have the patient repeat this action using alternating hands.	**a.** Movements should be smooth and accurate.
b. Test rapid alternating movements (RAM). Ask the patient to slap his or her thigh first with the palm and then with the back of his or her hand in quick alternating movements.	**b.** The patient should be able to perform this task quickly and rhythmically.
c. Observe for leg dystaxia using the heel-to-shin test. Ask the patient to assume a supine position. Instruct the patient to run her or his heel from the opposite knee down the shin. Observe rate, rhythm, smoothness, and accuracy of the movements.	**c.** The patient should be able to quickly run her or his heel down the leg in a straight line.

Assessing Sensory Function

Action	**Rationale**
1. Assess exteroceptive sensation. All tests should be completed with the patient's eyes closed. **a.** Test light touch sensation. Apply a light stroking stimulus using a wisp of cotton (**Figure 16-8**), beginning with distal areas of the patient's limbs and moving proximally following the dermatomal distribution. 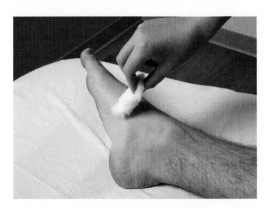 FIGURE 16-8 Assessing "light touch" sensation.	1. **(a, b, c)** The patient should be able to feel and discriminate between all sensations. Peripheral nerve lesions may cause anesthesia (absent touch sensation), hypesthesia (diminished touch sensation), or hyperesthesia (increased sensitivity to touch sensation) in the sensory distribution of the nerve involved. Lesions in the brain stem or spinal cord may cause anesthesia, paresthesia (abnormal sensation, such as burning, pricking, or tingling), or dysesthesia (abnormal sensation, such as loss of sensation just short of anesthesia, or abnormal sensations in the absence of stimuli). Lesions of the thalamus and peripheral nerves and nerve roots may cause analgesia (abnormal sensation where painful stimuli, although perceived, are not perceived as painful), hypalgesia (decreased sensation of pain), and hyperalgesia (extreme sensitivity to painful stimuli). An extensive lesion of the thalamus or a lesion laterally situated in the upper brain stem may manifest as complete unilateral loss of all exteroceptive sensation and gross disability. A "saddle" pattern of sensation deficit with a loss of leg reflexes and sphincter control may be due to a lesion of the cauda equina. Absent touch sensation in the hands and lower legs is common in polyneuritis of any cause.

Action	**Rationale**

b. Assess the patient's ability to sense superficial pain. Use a sharp object such as a sterile pin or edge of a broken tongue depressor (**Figure 16-9**). Randomly apply the dull and sharp edge of the object.

   Establish that the patient can accurately distinguish sharp and dull sensations by alternating stimuli.

c. Test temperature sensation. Apply vials containing warm water (40–45°C) and cold water (5–10°C) to the patient's skin to test temperature perception. (Temperatures greater or lower than these ranges will stimulate pain receptors.)

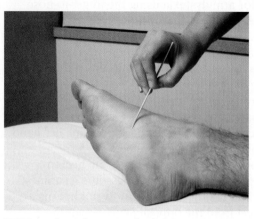

FIGURE 16-9 Assessing sense of pain.

2. Assess proprioceptive sensation.

a. Test motion and position sense. Grasp the patient's index finger or toe at the sides. Move the finger or toe up or down and ask the patient to report whether the finger or toe is being moved up or down (**Figure 16-10**). If there appears to be a deficit in motion sense, proceed to the proximal joints such as wrists or ankles, and repeat the test.

a. Position awareness may be affected by peripheral neuropathies, lesions of the thalamus, or lesions of the sensory cortex. An ipsilateral loss of position sense or vibratory sense deficit may indicate polyneuropathies or spinal cord lesions of the posterior column.

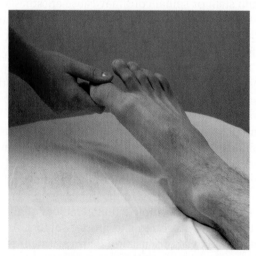

FIGURE 16-10 Assessing positional sense.

b. Test vibratory sense. Apply a vibrating tuning fork to the bony prominences and soft tissue, and ask the patient to report when vibration is being felt. Apply a fork to a toe or a finger, and place your finger under the digit (**Figure 16-11**). Note the length of time the patient feels the vibration. If a deficit

b. Loss of vibratory sense suggests peripheral neuropathies.

Action   **Rationale**

in vibratory sense in the peripheral bony
prominences is detected, progress toward the
trunk by testing ankles, knees, wrists, elbows,
anterior superior iliac crests, ribs, sternum, and
spinous processes of the vertebrae.

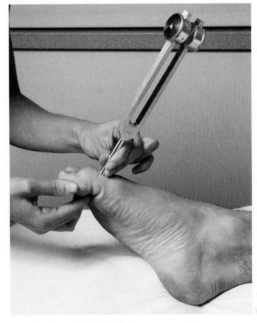

FIGURE 16-11 Testing vibratory sense.

3. Assess cortical sensation. All tests should be
   completed with the patient's eyes closed.
   a. Test stereognosis. Place a familiar object, such
      as a coin, in the hand (**Figure 16-12**). Ask the
      patient to identify the object.
   b. Assess graphesthesia. Have the patient close her
      or his eyes; ask her or him to identify letters or
      numbers as you trace them on the skin of the
      palms (**Figure 16-13**).

3. (**a, b, c, d**) The patient should be able to correctly
   discriminate each sensation. In the presence of
   intact tactile peripheral sensation, a dysfunction
   or lesion in the sensory cortex of the parietal lobe
   may result in impaired identification of objects
   via touch manipulation, impaired recognition of a
   number or letter drawn, and impaired two-point
   discrimination and extinction awareness.

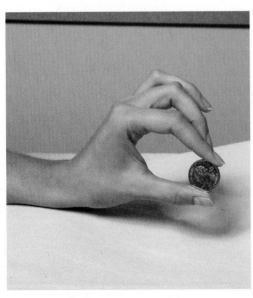

FIGURE 16-12 Assessing stereognosis.

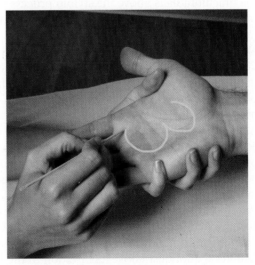

FIGURE 16-13 Assessing graphesthesia.

Action	Rationale

c. Test two-point discrimination. With two sterile pins or an unraveled paper clip, simultaneously touch the tip of the patient's fingers, hand, or foot with the objects apart. Continue to move the two pins closer together until the patient is unable to distinguish two points, noting the minimum distance between the points at which the patient reports feeling the objects separately.

d. Assess extinction. Simultaneously touch the patient on both sides of the body at the same location, such as the wrists. Ask the patient if one or two points are felt and where they are felt. Remove the stimulus from one side while maintaining the stimulus on the opposite side. Ask the patient if one or two points are felt and where.

Testing the Reflexes

Action	Rationale
1. Assess deep tendon reflexes (DTRs) (**Figure 16-14**). When testing DTRs, be sure to compare them bilaterally (**Table 16-3**). a. Biceps: Ask the patient to relax the arm. Flex the arm between 45 and 90 degrees and support it. Place your thumb over the tendon, just above the crease of the antecubital fossa. Strike your thumb with the reflex hammer. Observe for contraction of the biceps muscle and contraction of the elbow. b. Brachioradialis: With the patient's arm supported and flexed to 45 degrees, stimulate the tendon of the brachioradialis above the styloid process of the radius. Observe for flexion and supination of the forearm. c. Triceps: With the patient's arm supported and flexed to between 45 and 90 degrees, stimulate the triceps tendon just above its insertion above the olecranon process. Observe for contraction of the triceps muscle and extension of the arm. d. Assess the patellar reflex. Assist the patient to the edge of the examination table, so the legs hang over the sides. Stimulate the patellar region just below the patella with the reflex hammer. Observe for contraction of the quadriceps muscle and extension of the leg. e. Test the Achilles reflex. With the patient's feet dangling and slightly dorsiflexed, stimulate the Achilles tendon just above its insertion in the heel. Observe for contraction of the gastrocnemius, soleus, and plantaris muscles and plantar flexion of the foot.	1. A disruption in the reflex arc may manifest as decreased DTRs, whereas a complete severance of the reflex arc may demonstrate a total loss of DTRs. Diminished or absent DTRs may also be evident in deep coma, narcosis, deep sedation, increased ICP, or spinal shock. With a lack of inhibition of the higher centers in the cortex and reticular formation or lesions of the pyramidal system, DTRs may exhibit a hyperactive quality.

Action

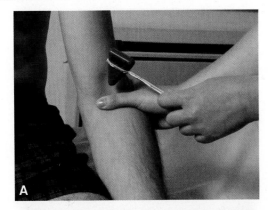

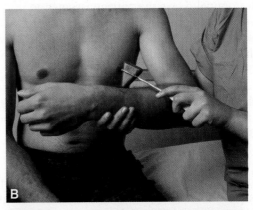

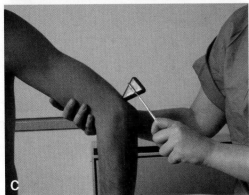

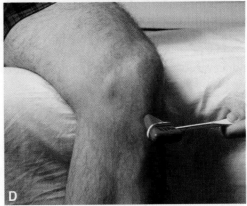

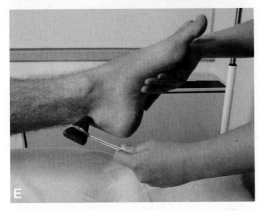

Rationale

Table 16-3	Deep Tendon Reflexes Grading System
Grade	Response
5+	Clonus
4+	Hyperactive
3+	More brisk than normal
2+	Normal
1+	Diminished
0	Absent

FIGURE 16-14 Assessing deep tendon reflexes: A. Biceps. B. Brachioradialis. C. Triceps. D. Patellar. E. Achilles.

2. Assess superficial reflexes.

2. Superficial reflexes involve the parietal areas and the motor centers of the premotor area and the pyramidal system. Lesions in the pyramidal tracts, dysfunction of the reflex arc, and deep sleep and coma may manifest as diminished or absent superficial reflexes. A positive bulbocavernosus reflex in a paraplegic patient following acute spinal cord injury implies that the initial phase of spinal shock has passed.

Action **Rationale**

  a. Abdominal: Have the patient assume the recumbent position. Use a sharp object to diagonally stroke the skin of the upper and lower abdominal quadrants. Observe for contraction of the upper and lower abdominal muscles with a deviation of the umbilicus toward the stimulus.
  b. Plantar: Stroke the outer aspect of the sole of the foot from the heel across the ball of the foot. Observe for plantar flexion of the toes.

For male patients:

  c. Cremasteric: In a downward direction, stroke the skin of the inner aspect of the thigh near the groin. Observe contraction of the cremasteric muscle with corresponding elevation of the ipsilateral testicle.
  d. Bulbocavernosus: Pinch the skin of the foreskin or the glans penis. Observe for a contraction of the bulbocavernosus muscle in the perineum at the base of the penis.

  3. Assess for pathological reflexes (**Table 16-4**).

  3. These primitive reflexes are normal in early development; however, later in life, they suggest dementia.

Table 16-4	Common Pathological Reflexes
Reflex	Description
Palmar grasp	Palmar stimulation results in grasp response.
Snout	Stimulation of oral region results in puckering response.
Sucking	Stimulation of lips, tongue, or palate results in sucking movement of the lips.
Rooting	Stimulation of the lips results in deviation of the head toward the stimulus.
Glabellar	Stimulation of glabellar region between eyes results in blinking each time.

Additional Tests

Action **Rationale**

  1. If you have any reason to suspect a vascular anomaly of the brain, auscultate over the skull for bruits.

  1. Auscultation of the skull is not routinely performed. In individuals who have developed diplopia, a bruit or blowing sound over the orbit may be rarely heard and may indicate an expanding cerebral aneurysm responsible for the diplopia.

  2. Auscultate over the carotid (**Figure 16-15**) and temporal (**Figure 16-16**) arteries, over the eyes, and below the occiput.

  2. A bruit over any of these areas indicates a vascular anomaly such as obstruction and decreased blood flow.

Action   **Rationale**

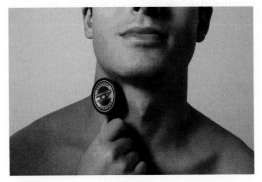

FIGURE 16-15 Auscultating over the carotid artery.

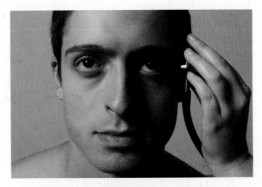

FIGURE 16-16 Auscultating over the temporal artery.

3. Palpate the skull for lumps, depressions, and tenderness.

3. Tumors or hydrocephalus may manifest as lumps and bulging on the skull surface. Depressions on the skull surface may indicate dehydration in the neonate. Tenderness may suggest tumor or infection.

4. Palpate carotid and temporal arteries.

4. Presence of pulsations over these areas signifies adequate blood flow to the brain.

5. Assess for meningeal irritation.

5. Meningeal irritation as a result of meningitis, subarachnoid hemorrhage, or stretching of irritated nerve roots and meninges may be exhibited as nuchal rigidity, Kernig's sign, or Brudzinski's sign.
  a. Nuchal rigidity is stiffness in the neck.

a. Assess for nuchal rigidity. With the patient in a supine position, flex the patient's neck. Note stiffness or resistance to flexing of the neck.

b. Test for Kernig's sign: With the patient in a recumbent position, lift the patient's leg and flex the knee at a right angle. Attempt to extend the patient's knee by pushing down on it (**Figure 16-17**). Note pain in the lower back and resistance to straightening the leg at the knee.

b. A positive Kernig's sign is when severe stiffness of the hamstrings causes an inability to straighten the leg when the hip is flexed to 90 degrees.

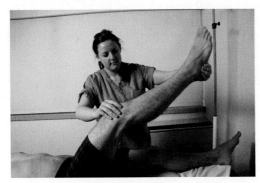

FIGURE 16-17 Assessing for Kernig's sign.

Action	Rationale
c. Assess for Brudzinski's sign. Ask the patient to assume the supine position. Place one hand under the patient's neck and the other hand on top of the patient's chest to prevent elevation of the body (**Figure 16-18**). Flex the patient's neck with a deliberate motion.	**c.** A positive Brudzinski's sign is involuntary flexion of the hips and knees upon flexing the neck.

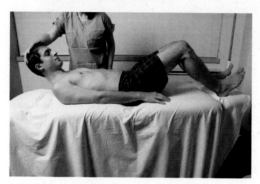

FIGURE 16-18 Assessing for Brudzinski's sign.

Patients who present to the practitioner in an altered state of consciousness should receive an immediate, thorough neurological evaluation. **Box 16-1** describes assessment procedure.

BOX 16-1   ASSESSMENT OF THE PATIENT WITH AN ALTERED STATE OF CONSCIOUSNESS

A complete neurological examination is performed when all major components are evaluated, including level of consciousness using the Glasgow Coma Scale (GCS), motor ability, cranial nerves, and vital signs.

LEVEL OF CONSCIOUSNESS

Determining a patient's level of consciousness entails evaluation of arousal or alertness, and subsequent behavioral responses to various forms of stimuli. Assessment of the stimuli necessary to arouse the patient reflects the capabilities of the reticular activating system. Arousal must be intact for awareness to become apparent. The patient's ability to give appropriate motor and verbal responses is noted and documented. The GCS is a standardized tool used to document such findings. Patient's responses are graded, and scores are summed. Scores range from 3 to 15, with a score of 15 being normal.

Scoring of eye opening:

4 Opens eyes spontaneously.
3 Opens eyes in response to speech.
2 Opens eyes in response to pain.
1 Does not open eyes in response to pain.

BOX 16-1 ASSESSMENT OF THE PATIENT WITH AN ALTERED STATE OF CONSCIOUSNESS (*continued*)

Scoring of verbal response:

5 Oriented to place, time, and person.
4 Converses, but is confused.
3 Speaks in inappropriate words (makes little sense).
2 Responds with incomprehensible words/sounds.
1 Does not respond verbally.

Scoring of motor response:

6 Obeys commands.
5 Localizes to pain.
4 Withdraws from pain.
3 Has abnormal flexion.
2 Extends upper and lower.
1 None.

If the patient can follow verbal commands, a proper evaluation of motor strength and tone can be performed. If he or she is unable to follow verbal commands, observing for spontaneous movement of extremities or movement with noxious stimuli is vital. Abnormal motor responses may indicate varying pathology, including metabolic disturbances, lesions, shock, or increased intracranial pressure (ICP).

Assessment of eye movement and pupillary function is an important component of the neurological examination of the unconscious patient. Pupillary reaction reflects the ability of the parasympathetic or sympathetic nervous system to innervate CN III, the oculomotor nerve. Adequately assessing for equal size, shape, and degree of reactivity to light is essential for determining possible changes in ICP on the oculomotor nerve. Difference in pupil size may indicate impending danger of herniation.

In the unconscious patient, assessing innervation of the medial longitudinal fasciculus pathway, which elicits a "doll's eye" reflex, demonstrates brain stem injury. Holding the eyes open, the practitioner briskly turns the patient's head to one side while observing eye movements, then briskly turns the head to the other side and observes. Absence of an oculocephalic reflex, in which the eyes remain midline and move with the head, indicates significant brain stem injury. Another test reflecting brain stem function is the cold caloric test, where 20 to 50 mL of ice water is injected into the external auditory canal. Dysconjugate eye movement is an abnormal result indicating a brain stem lesion.

Hemiparesis or hemiplegia may be detected by lifting both of the patient's arms off the bed and releasing them simultaneously. The hemiparetic side will fall more quickly and more limply than the other side. Resistance to passive movement, termed paratonia, accompanies forebrain dysfunction. It can also signal frontal lobe lesions and increased ICP when findings favor one side.

Decorticate posturing consists of flexion and adduction of the upper extremity, with internal rotation and plantar flexion in the lower extremity. It indicates possible cerebral or brain stem lesions. Decerebrate posturing is characterized by extension, adduction, and hyperpronation of the upper extremities and flexion of the lower extremities, which may demonstrate pontomesencephalic level lesions. Hyperreflexia and a positive Babinski reflex are also signs of reflecting obstructive lesions of the CNS.

Various changes in vital signs accompany CNS disturbances. Hyperthermia or hypothermia, respiratory dysrhythmias such as Cheyne–Stokes and Biot's breathing, and hemodynamic changes reflect advanced increases in ICP.

Diagnostic Reasoning

Based on findings in the health history and physical examination, the clinician should formulate the assessment and plan. For example, a patient may report symptoms that suggest many possible diagnoses; however, findings in the past medical history and during the physical examination might narrow the possible diagnoses down to one or two. Headache is a common chief complaint. **Table 16-5** illustrates differential diagnosis of common disorders associated with headache.

Table 16-5   Differential Diagnosis of Headache

Differential Diagnosis	Significant Findings in the Patient's History	Significant Findings in the Patient's Physical Examination	Diagnostic Tests
Cerebrovascular accident	Sudden severe headache; numbness, weakness, or impaired motor ability on one side of the body; dysphagia; dysphasia; visual difficulties; altered cognitive abilities	Loss of half of visual field, unilateral ptosis, unilateral hemiparesis, dysphasia	Carotid ultrasound, CT scan, cerebral angiography
Transient ischemic attacks	History of headaches with a duration of days. Carotid system involvement: dysphasia. Vertebrobasilar system involvement: vertigo, dysphagia	Carotid bruit. Carotid system involvement: unilateral weakness and/or numbness. Vertebrobasilar system involvement: bilateral weakness	Cerebral angiography; carotid angiography, CT scan (to rule out lesion or hemorrhage)
Rupture of an intracranial aneurysm or arteriovenous malformation	Sudden severe headache, nausea, vomiting, loss of consciousness, visual disturbances	Nuchal rigidity, no neurological deficit	CT scan, lumbar puncture, cerebral angiogram
Tumor	Headache, numbness, weakness, visual difficulties, cognitive difficulties	Visual deficits, impaired motor ability	CT scan, MRI
Meningitis	Headache, fever, rash, photophobia	Nuchal rigidity, positive Brudzinski's and Kernig's signs	CBC, lumbar puncture
Migraines	Gradual onset of severe, unilateral, throbbing headaches; nausea; vomiting; photophobia	N/A	Skull films and CT/MRI to rule out lesions or hemorrhage
Cluster headaches	Sudden, sharp, unilateral pain; occurs in clusters of 2 to 8 weeks; unilateral excessive tearing or redness of the eye	N/A	Skull films and CT/MRI to rule out lesions or hemorrhage

Abbreviations: CBC, complete blood count; CT, computed tomography; MRI, magnetic resonance imaging.

Neurological Assessment of Special Populations

Considerations for the Pregnant Patient
- While eliciting the history, note the following:
  - Estimated date of conception (EDC) and weeks of gestation
  - Seizures: history of, onset, frequency, duration, character of movement; pregnancy-induced hypertension or preeclampsia
  - Headache: onset, character, frequency, related to hypertension
  - Nutritional status: dietary supplements, herbal medications, prenatal vitamins, calcium, folic acid, sodium depletion
  - Exercise regimen and level of activity
- The pregnant patient may experience light-headedness or fainting from vasodilation, hypoglycemia, hypotension, or the fetus's pressure on the vena cava.
- The most frequently experienced neurological changes of pregnancy consist of headaches, numbness, and tingling. Other neuropathies include foot drop, facial palsy, fatigue, and inability to sleep at night.
- The pregnant patient normally has a side-waddling gait with broad-based support as a result of softening of the pelvic joints and instability. The pregnant patient may appear clumsy and tend to lose balance because of the shift in the center of gravity.
- Abnormal findings are a new onset of seizures or increased seizures from a preexisting condition; convulsions without prior history may signify the development of eclampsia. Additional abnormal findings include signs of multiple dystrophy or myasthenia gravis,

carpal tunnel syndrome, or hand numbness as a result of brachial plexus traction. Status returns to the prepregnant condition after delivery.

■ Establish a baseline evaluation of deep tendon reflexes during the initial assessment. Inpatient assessment should include laboratory values.

Considerations for the Neonatal Patient

■ If you are assessing a neonate, question the parent or caregiver regarding the following:
  • Prenatal history: maternal health/illness/injury; medications; radiation exposure; exposure to toxoplasmosis, syphilis, tuberculosis, rubella, cytomegalovirus, herpes; infections/toxemia; bleeding; history of trauma/stress/surgery; unremitting vomiting; pregnancy-induced hypertension; history of smoking/drug/alcohol use; mental disposition
  • Birth history: gestational age, birth weight, Apgar score, medications/instruments used during the birthing process, prolonged labor, fetal distress/trauma
  • Respiratory status at birth: spontaneous respirations, oxygen/ventilator requirements, prolonged apnea, cyanosis, resuscitative efforts
  • Neonatal health: infections, seizures, irritability, sucking and swallowing status, poor coordination, positive phenylketonuria, jaundice
  • Congenital anomalies/handicapping conditions

■ Significant brain growth and myelinization of the nervous system take place during the initial years of development. Primary reflexes in the newborn include yawning, sneezing, hiccupping, blinking at both bright lights and loud noises, constricting pupils in response to light, and withdrawing from painful stimuli. As brain development progresses, advanced cortical functions and voluntary control will take over, diminishing or inhibiting some of the more primitive reflexes.

■ Although cranial nerves are not directly evaluated in the newborn, several observations during the physical examination allow indirect evaluation.

■ Cerebellar function is demonstrated by coordinated sucking and swallowing.

■ At birth, the patellar tendon reflexes are present. The Achilles and brachioradial tendon reflexes appear at 6 months of age. A finger, rather than a reflex hammer, should be used to tap the tendon when deep tendon reflexes are being evaluated. Contraction of the muscle attached to the corresponding tendon should contract with each test. Findings should be interpreted as for adults. One to two beats of ankle clonus is typically observed.

■ Motor control advances in a cephalocaudal direction, starting at the head and neck and moving to the trunk and then to the extremities. Although variation may exist from one newborn to the next, functions generally progress in an orderly sequence.

■ It is essential to assess muscle strength and tone in the newborn; the neuromuscular development at the time of birth should be evaluated with the Dubowitz clinical assessment for gestational age.

■ Sensory integrity is evidenced by a withdrawal of all limbs from a painful stimulus.

■ Assess neonatal reflexes (**Table 16-6**).

■ The posture and movement of the developing infant are routinely assessed via primitive reflexes, which appear and disappear in a sequence corresponding with central nervous system development. The infant's spontaneous activity should be observed for symmetry and smoothness of movement. Rhythmic twitching of the facial, extremity, and trunk musculature, as well as any sustained asymmetric posturing, may indicate seizure activity.

■ At approximately 2 months of age, purposeful movement, such as reaching and grasping for objects, begins. A progression to taking objects with one hand at 6 months, transferring an object to the hand at 7 months, and purposefully releasing objects by 10 months of age should occur. This should take place without tremors or overshooting of movements.

■ The plantar reflex parallels the adult examination. Until the infant is 16 to 24 months of age, a positive Babinski sign, consisting of fanning of the toes and dorsiflexion of the great toe, is present.

Table 16-6	Neonatal Reflexes
Reflex	**Description**
Palmar grasp	Palmar stimulation results in grasp response.
Plantar grasp	Plantar stimulation results in a grasp response from the toes.
Babinski	Plantar stimulation results in dorsiflexion of the great toe and fanning of the toes.
Sucking	Stimulation of the lips, tongue, or palate results in a sucking movement of the lips.
Rooting	Stimulation of the lips results in deviation of the head toward the stimulus.
Tonic neck	With the neonate supine, turning the head to one side results in extension of the arm and leg on that side and flexion of the opposite arm and leg.
Startling	A loud noise or jarring of the bassinet results in abduction and extension of the neonate's arms and legs and the fingers assuming a "C" position. The neonate then brings in both arms and legs.
Placing	Touching the anterior surface of the neonate's leg to a table results in her or him making a few quick lifting motions as if to step onto the table.
Stepping	Holding a neonate in a vertical position with the feet touching a hard surface results in the neonate taking a few, quick, alternating steps.

Considerations for the Pediatric Patient

- While eliciting the history of a pediatric patient, obtain the following information:
  - Immunizations
  - Childhood illness or injury; health problems
  - Achieving developmental milestones
  - Performance of self-care activities, such as dressing or feeding
  - Progress in school
  - Favorite activities
- The evaluation of children should follow the same sequence of events as for adults with minor adjustments.
- Examine neuromuscular progress and skills displayed with spontaneous activity.
- Assess social/adaptive skills, such as interactions with other children, or independence of adults.
- Test various language skills, such as referring to self by name and using two- to three-word phrases.
- Inspect visual fields and hearing (drop a toy on the floor).
- Evaluate touch (sensory not normally evaluated before age 5) by having child close his or her eyes and point to area of sensation ("tickling").
- Test CN VII by asking the child to make "funny faces" similar to the practitioner (**Figure 16-19**).
- Assess fine and gross motor skills:
  - Gait while walking backward
  - Balance
  - Grasping of toys (**Figure 16-20**)
  - Heel-to-toe walking (**Figure 16-21**)
  - Standing or hopping on one foot (**Figure 16-22**)
  - Jumping
- Note in particular the muscles of the neck, abdomen, and extremities. Abnormal findings include muscle hypertrophy, atrophy, weakness, or incoordination. Note weaknesses indicating problems with the pelvis.
- Identification of a developmental delay, or soft sign, indicates failure to perform age-specific activities possibly related to central nervous system deficits, or maturation delays. Determining the differences between varying stages of development and the "soft signs" indicating functional neurological findings can be challenging. Initially, these findings may be considered normal, but as the child matures, these signs should disappear.

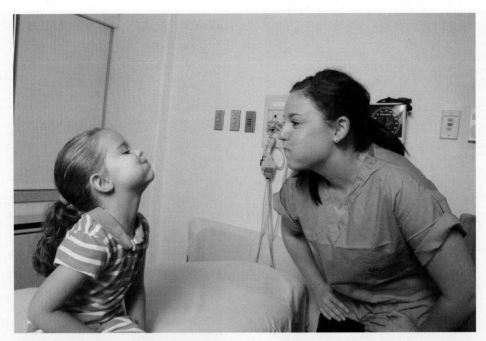

FIGURE 16-19 Testing CN VII: mimicking "funny faces."

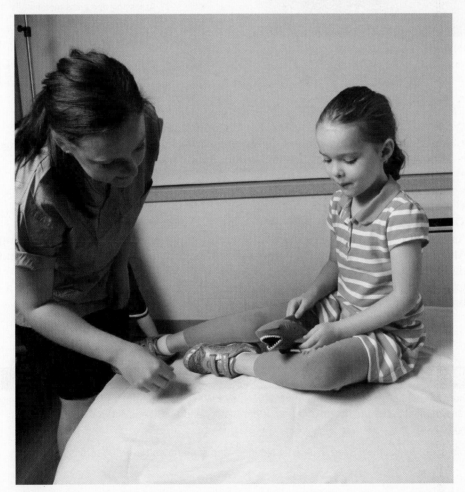

FIGURE 16-20 Assessing fine motor skills: grasping a small toy.

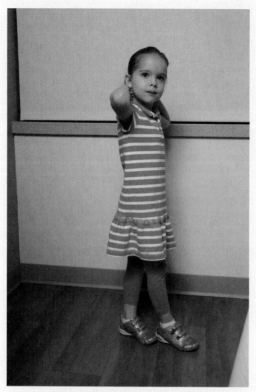

FIGURE 16-21 Assessing fine gross motor skills: heel-to-toe walking.

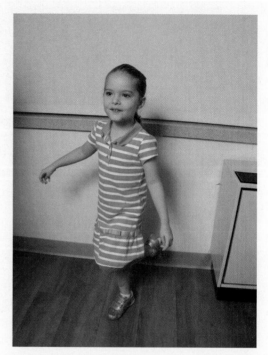

FIGURE 16-22 Assessing fine gross motor skills: standing on one foot.

Considerations for the Geriatric Patient

- While eliciting history, obtain the following information:
  - Ability to perform activities of daily living such as dressing, feeding, and bathing
  - Functional losses such as hearing, vision, or fine motor coordination
  - Incontinence
  - Intermittent neurological deficits
  - Pattern of falls, weakness, or imbalance
- The evaluation of the older adult is identical to the evaluation of the adult.
- Assessment of currently used medications could pinpoint certain causes of impairment.
- Alterations of the senses and changes in coordination and agility are not uncommon with the elderly.
- Changes in deep tendon reflexes also occur with aging. Reflexes are found to be less brisk, or even absent.

Case Study Review

Throughout this chapter, you have been introduced to KW. This section of the chapter pulls together her history and demonstrates the documentation of her history and physical examination.

Chief Complaint

"I have frequent headaches, keep losing my balance, and sometimes have difficulty speaking."

Information Gathered During the Interview

KW is a 48-year-old woman who presents to the clinic accompanied by her husband. Mrs. W reports that over the last 2 weeks she has experienced frequent headaches and periods of dizziness that resolved spontaneously. Mr. W states that early this morning he found his wife unresponsive. Shortly thereafter, she regained consciousness but had no recollection of the morning's events. She is currently having difficulty speaking and is unable to ambulate due to left-sided weakness and numbness. She denies a history of seizures and dysphagia.

Mrs. W denies a history of trauma. She states that she was diagnosed with hypertension 10 years ago but has been noncompliant with antihypertensive medications because of their adverse effects. Mrs. W also has a history of hyperlipidemia; she has been noncompliant with medication regimen because of the cost. Mrs. W had a right carotid endarterectomy 2 years ago.

Mrs. W denies any family history of coronary artery disease, diabetes, neurological disease, or cancer. She is an only child. Her father, age 78, has hypertension. Her mother, age 75, is alive and well. She does not have any children.

Mrs. W lives with her husband in a one-bedroom apartment and has worked as a receptionist for the past 20 years. Recently, she has had trouble completing tasks at work. She reports that she smokes one pack of cigarettes a day and has been smoking since she was 18 years old. Other than an occasional glass of wine with dinner, she does not drink. Mrs. W denies recreational drug use. She does not have a regular exercise regimen.

Clues	Important Points
Loss of balance upon ambulation	Associated with disease of the motor cortex and cerebellum and Parkinson's disease.
Difficulty speaking	Suggests dysfunction of the frontal or temporal lobes from tumor or stroke.
Left-sided weakness	Associated with cerebellar and motor cortex dysfunction.
Dizziness	Suggests decreased cerebral blood flow or problem with vestibular apparatus such as an inner ear infection or orthostatic hypotension.
Confusion	Associated with multiple pathological causes and requires further investigation.
Headaches	Associated with increased intracranial pressure resulting from hypertension, hemorrhage, tumor, or other causes.

Name KW	Date 1/17/15	Time 13:15
	DOB 6/10/67	Sex F

HISTORY

CC

"I have frequent headaches, keep losing my balance, and sometimes have difficulty speaking."

HPI

Over the last 2 weeks, a history of frequent headaches and periods of dizziness. Husband found her unresponsive this AM. Regained consciousness but does not remember the morning's events. Having trouble speaking and cannot ambulate, due to left-sided weakness and numbness. Denies seizures and dysphagia.

Medications

Novasc: 5 mg daily for HTN (Noncompliant due to adverse effects)

Lipitor: 20 mg daily for hyperlipidemia (Noncompliant due to cost)

Allergies

NKDA

PMI
Illnesses
Denies history of trauma; history of HTN and hyperlipidemia.
Hospitalizations/Surgeries
Right carotid endarterectomy 2 years ago.
FH
Negative for CAD, diabetes, neurological disease, and cancer; positive for HTN (father).
SH
Employed as a receptionist; has had difficulty completing work. 30 pack-year history of smoking. Occasionally uses alcohol. Denies history of recreational drug use. Denies exercise regimen.

ROS

General	Cardiovascular
Denies fever or chills.	Denies any problems.
Skin	**Respiratory**
Denies rash.	Denies any changes or problems.
Eyes	**Gastrointestinal**
Denies visual problems.	Denies any changes or problems.
Ears	**Genitourinary/Gynecological**
Denies hearing loss.	Denies any changes or problems.
Nose/Mouth/Throat	**Musculoskeletal**
Denies dysphagia.	Unable to ambulate.
Breast	**Neurological**
Denies lumps.	See HPI.

PHYSICAL EXAMINATION

Weight 178 lb	Temp 98.4	BP 210/108
Height 5'4"	Pulse 90	Resp 18

Skin
Warm, dry
HEENT
Scalp intact and symmetric. No lesions, lumps, or tenderness. Left ptosis. PERRL; EOM revealed left deviated gaze; visual acuity revealed left hemianopia. Auricles aligned with eyes without lesions, tenderness, or masses. Hearing grossly intact. Nose without discharge; nasal septum midline. No pain or tenderness upon palpation of the sinuses. Oropharynx is benign with no mucosal lesion; tongue midline without lesions or tremor. Gag reflex intact. Left-sided facial droop. Neck is supple and without adenopathy or thyromegaly.
Cardiovascular
Apical pulse palpated; regular rate and rhythm. S1 and S2 auscultated. No murmurs, rubs, or bruits.
Respiratory
Respirations even and unlabored. Chest excursion symmetrical. Vesicular breath sounds auscultated without adventitious breath sounds noted.
Gastrointestinal
Abdomen soft, nontender, and not distended. Normal BS × 4 quadrants.
Genitourinary
Not examined.
Musculoskeletal
Left-side hemiparesis; left shoulder lower than the right. Strength is 5/5 to upper and lower extremities on the right side. Strength is 0/5 to upper and lower extremities on the left side. No involuntary movements noted.

Neurological

A J O X 3; slurred speech; aphasic; follows commands; GCS, 13. CNII, left homonymous hemianopia; CNIII, IV, and VI, EOM, impairment in gaze to left; CNV, decreased sensation to superficial pain and light touch on left, intact on right; CNVII, left facial droop, lower face; CNVIII, no abnormalities detected; CNIX and X, no abnormalities; CNXI, left shoulder weak to shrug; CNXII, tongue midline. Proprioception, absent on left and intact on right. Vibration sense, noted deficit on left and intact on right. Stereoagnosis, graphesthesia, two-point discrimination; extinction: intact on right and impaired on left. Coordination (finger to nose, rapid alternating, heel to shin), impaired on left side. Gait, not tested due to hemiparesis. Meningeal irritation, negative. Cortical, intact on right and impaired on left.

Other

Lab Tests

Na: 140 mEq/mL	Hgb: 13.6 g/dL	Ca: 8.2 mEq/L
K: 4.1 mEq/mL	Hct: 38%	Mg: 1.4 mEq/L
Cl: 101 mEq/mL	WBC: $7.2 \times 10^3/mm^3$	Phos: 2.7 mg/dL
CO_2: 37 mEq/L	Neutros: 54%	PT/INR: 13.0/1.3
BUN: 8 mg/dL	Bands: 4%	PTT: 34
SCr: 0.8 mg/dL	Lymphs: 28%	Platelets: 268
Glu: 90 mg/dL	Monos: 5%	

Special Tests

Brain CT scan: suggested evidence of right frontal lobe infarct. Cerebral angiogram: revealed embolus and decreased perfusion to the right frontal lobe. Carotid ultrasound: 92% stenosis right carotid, 79% stenosis left carotid.

Final Assessment Findings

History of multiple TIAs

Presently CVA right frontal lobe, ischemic due to right carotid stenosis and embolization

Bibliography

Alpers, B. J., & Mancall, E. (1981). *Alpers and Mancall's essentials of the neurologic examination* (2nd ed.). Philadelphia, PA: F. A. Davis.

Detsky, M. E., McDonald, D. R., Baerlocher, M. O., Tomlinson, G. A., McCrory, D. C., & Booth, C. M. (2006). Does this patient with headache have a migraine or need neuroimaging? *Journal of the American Medical Association, 296*(10), 1274–1283.

Deyo, R. A., & Weinstein, J. N. (2001). Low back pain. *New England Journal of Medicine, 344*(5), 363–370.

Ferri, F. (2015). *Ferri's clinical advisor: Instant diagnosis and treatment.* St. Louis, MO: Mosby.

Goadsby, P., Lipton, R. B., & Ferrari, M. D. (2002). Migraine: Current understanding and treatment. *New England Journal of Medicine, 346*(4), 257–270.

Gorson, K. C. (2001). Case 9-2001: A 64 year old woman with peripheral neuropathy, paraproteinemia and lymphadenopathy. *New England Journal of Medicine, 344*, 917–923.

Haerer, A. F. (1992). *Dejong's: The neurologic examination* (5th ed.). New York, NY: J. B. Lippincott.

Hickey, J. V. (2014). *The clinical practice of neurological and neurosurgical nursing* (7th ed.). Philadelphia, PA: Lippincott Williams & Wilkins.

Katz, J. N., & Simmons, B. P. (2005). Carpal tunnel syndrome. *New England Journal of Medicine, 346*, 1807–1811.

Louis, E. D. (2001). Essential tremor. *New England Journal of Medicine, 345*, 887–991.

Rao, G., Fisch, L., Srinivasan, S., D'Amico, F., Okada, T., Eaton, C., & Robbins, C. (2003). Does this patient have Parkinson disease? *Journal of the American Medical Association, 289*(3), 347–353.

The Anatomical Chart Company. (2001). *Atlas of human anatomy.* Springhouse, PA: Springhouse.

Appendix A

CAGE Assessment

The **CAGE Assessment** tool/pneumonic is used to help determine if a patient's use of alcohol or other drugs is injuring him or her or his or her loved ones.
1. Have you ever felt you ought to **Cut** down on your drinking?
2. Have people **Annoyed** you by criticizing your drinking?
3. Have you ever felt bad or **Guilty** about your drinking?
4. Have you ever had a drink first thing in the morning or to get rid of a hangover **(Eye-opener)?**

Appendix B

Providing Care for Diverse Patient Populations

Patient populations are becoming increasingly diverse. All healthcare providers must provide competent care to patients from varied cultural and spiritual backgrounds. They must also provide care to patients with a variety of physical attributes.

Culture is a group of learned behaviors common to a given human society. "Cultural competence" is the phrase that refers to the knowledge base and interpersonal skills that allow healthcare providers to understand, appreciate, and work effectively with individuals from cultures that differ from their own. We live in a culturally complex world and in order to give competent care to our diverse patients, we must first recognize our own bias toward other cultures and respect the differences. It is important to be cognizant of others' beliefs and value systems when assessing them. Cultural awareness will improve patient satisfaction and could potentially correct the disparity in healthcare provision to diverse populations.

In addition, normal findings may vary among different groups. For example, normal findings related to hair texture vary according to racial background.

General Cultural Awareness Tips

Be sure to listen to the patient and learn about his or her culture. Be aware of and sensitive to the patient's body language. Remember never to assume anything and to avoid stereotyping the patient. In order to provide an effective assessment of patients, the healthcare provider should elicit the following:

- With what culture does the patient identify him- or herself?
- Does the patient strictly adhere to the cultural norms associated with that culture?
- What are the patient's social, ethnic, and religious affiliations/beliefs?
- What is the patient's perception of health, illness, and healthcare providers? Does the patient use alternative treatments?
- Are there any religious practices that may affect health care when the patient is ill?
- How does the patient describe his or her family and relationships? Does the patient have a support system nearby?
- Would the patient be more comfortable being interviewed by someone of the same gender?

Considerations During Health Assessment

Mental Health Assessment

Communication, space, social organization, time, environmental control, and biologic variations affect the interview and mental status assessment. Be aware that a certain stigma may be associated with mental illness in many cultures.

Skin Assessment

Findings range greatly depending on the patient's background:

- Lightly or nonpigmented skin may show more pigmentary reaction following trauma than darkly pigmented skin.
- Individuals whose skin tolerates the sun well often do not follow protective measures.
- Hairstyling methods used by some patients of African American and Caribbean descent may affect the hair follicle or hair growth cycle. Traction alopecia and hot comb folliculitis are common hair loss findings in these patients.
- Pseudofolliculitis barbae and keloid de nuchae, more commonly found in African American males, are disorders arising from follicular inflammation related to hair texture.
- African Americans are more likely to develop keloids.
- Native Americans have a higher incidence of scleroderma than Caucasians.

Eye Assessment

Keep the following in mind when assessing risk factors:

- African Americans, Hispanics, Native Americans, Asian Americans, and Pacific Islanders are at increased risk of developing glaucoma.
- Open-angle glaucoma is the leading cause of blindness in American Hispanics.
- African Americans are more likely to develop glaucoma that results in blindness than Caucasians are.
- Primary closed-angle glaucoma is more prevalent in East Asians.

Ear Assessment

Findings may range depending on the patient's background:

- Dry cerumen is found is 84% of Asians and Native Americans, including Eskimos. Wet cerumen is found in 97% of Caucasians and 99% of African Americans.
- African Americans are less susceptible to noise-induced hearing loss.
- African Americans have better hearing at high and low frequencies after age 40 years compared to Caucasians; Caucasians have better hearing at mid-range frequencies.

Nose and Mouth Assessment

The gums of patients who have darkly pigmented skin are darker and have blotches.

Respiratory Assessment

Respect the modesty of the patient. Some patients may prefer to have a same-sex healthcare provider assess breath sounds.

Cardiovascular Assessment

Findings and disorders are more prevalent in some patient populations than in others:

- Cardiovascular disease is the number one killer of African Americans. Cardiovascular disease includes heart disease, stroke, hypertension, congestive heart failure, and other atherosclerotic diseases.
- Among Mexican Americans, 27% of males and 29% of females have cardiovascular disease.
- Of non-Hispanic Caucasians, about 30% of males and 24% of females have cardiovascular disease.
- Asian Americans and Pacific Islanders have less incidence of cardiovascular disease than Caucasians.

Gastrointestinal Assessment

Keep the following in mind when assessing risk factors:

- People of lower socioeconomic status tend to buy foods that are high in fat and sodium and low in nutrition because they are less expensive. These eating habits can predispose the patient to obesity, diabetes, hypertension, and cardiovascular disease.
- Gastroesophageal reflux is more prevalent in Caucasians than African Americans.
- The incidence of *H. pylori* gastritis is higher in African Americans and Hispanics than Caucasians. *H. pylori* gastritis can be a precursor to gastric carcinoma.
- Native Americans, Hispanics, and African Americans have a higher incidence of colon cancer than the general population.

Male Genitourinary Assessment

This is a sensitive examination. Remember:

- Patients of Mediterranean, South American, Scandinavian, and non-Moslem Asian descent do not routinely practice circumcision.
- Many patients may be hesitant to answer questions truthfully about sexually transmitted disease risk factors, sexual dysfunction, and genitourinary dysfunction. Ask questions in a nonjudgmental manner.

Keep the following in mind when assessing risk factors:

- African American men have the highest incidence of prostate cancer and Asian Americans have the lowest.
- Incidence of bladder cancer is higher in whites than in African Americans but the mortality is the same due to the delay in seeking health care. Native Americans, Asians, and Hispanics have a lower incidence of bladder cancer than African Americans.
- African American men have a high incidence of chronic kidney failure.

Female Genitourinary and Breast Assessment

Offer a chaperone to the female patient when doing a genitourinary and/or breast assessment.
   When assessing risk, remember that Caucasians have the highest incidence of breast and cervical cancer and Native Americans have the lowest.

Endocrine Assessment

Keep the following in mind when assessing risk factors:

- African Americans have a higher incidence of diabetes and complications of diabetes (e.g., heart disease, lower extremity amputations, diabetic retinopathy, and kidney disease).
- Native Americans have a higher incidence of diabetes than non-Hispanic Caucasians and suffer from the same complications of diabetes as African Americans.
- Caucasians and Asians are more likely to develop hyperthyroidism.
- Native Americans have the highest incidence of hypothyroidism and Caucasians have the lowest. The Pima Indians in Arizona have up to a 70% incidence of hypothyroidism in the age group of 55 to 74.

Musculoskeletal Assessment

Keep the following in mind when assessing risk factors:

- The highest incidence of rheumatoid arthritis is in some groups of North American Indians (Yakima, Pima, Chippewa).
- Gout is most prevalent in Pacific Islanders and least prevalent in African Americans.

- Primary osteoarthritis is more prevalent in Native Americans than the general population.
- Sarcoidosis is most prevalent in African American females.

Neurological Assessment

Generally, the structure and function of the neurological system is consistent among the different ethnic groups. Slight variations have been observed in early motor development. For example, African American children typically develop motor skills more rapidly than children of other racial groups.

Appendix C

Considerations for Global and Unique Populations

Advanced Assessment of Special Populations

- Cultural values
- Gender/Gender identity
- Beliefs and practices
- Religion
- Philosophical or spiritual beliefs
- Economic factors
- Language

Culture and Lifestyle Assessments

There is a growing realization among healthcare professionals that the impact of culture and lifestyle on patient-centered care is significant. Not all groups assimilate into the mainstream culture; they instead retain unique features of their cultures, which has led to growing visibility and appreciation of different ethnocultural groups. Understandably, many healthcare professionals are increasingly concerned with providing culturally sensitive, patient-centered care and education, whether in their homeland or on medical assignments across the globe. Rather than taking on the virtually impossible task of learning about all possible cultures, it is more practical and helpful for advanced practice nurses to use a generic approach in performing a cultural and lifestyle assessment.

Providers must be willing to consider whether there are any issues that are critical to the success of the healthcare encounter that have not been addressed. Clinicians must remember that issues like the following may be present in their patients:

- A general lack of trust in healthcare providers or the healthcare system in general
- A fear of medical research or experimentation
- Fear of medications and potential side effects
- Discomfort with the Western biomedical belief system
- Fear of being judged or ostracized by clinicians who do not respect their lifestyle or beliefs

Cultural Values

"Andrews and Boyle (2008) formulated various health belief models/systems that different cultural groups use to explain health and illness. For example, familism and individualism determine whose needs are held as priority in the context of health care. In familistic cultures, the family unit is valued over the individual; healthcare decision making and problem solving are executed by the family. In contrast, individualism prioritizes independent problem solving and achievement as part of patient-centered care.

Time orientation dictates whether an individual will focus on the past, present, or future, with the latter two most applicable to health care. Time orientation influences how patients respond to situations; it can impact how well a patient adheres to an appointment time or medication instruction, and this nonadherence can be misinterpreted as a lack of comprehension. Present orientation may preclude preventive health practices, as it prioritizes survival and managing crises over avoiding future problems. In contrast, American health care focuses on the future, with an emphasis on preventive care, new technology, progress, and change; in this orientation, time is very specific and promptness is important to people. People from agriculture-based cultures tend to be less time oriented than those living in industrialized cultures.

In high-context cultures, members possess group orientation (i.e., consistent connections with peers over longer periods of time). There is less need for formal, direct, and written communication, as communication is more about process and relationship than problem solving. In high-context cultures, the group has a strong external boundary, so outsiders must work harder to earn trust. Alternately, in low-context cultures, such as that of American society, members have many superficial connections in which the goal of communication is specific and task driven to ensure clarity of rules and procedures and solve problems" (Singleton & Krause, 2009).

Data obtained from a cultural assessment will help the patient and clinician formulate a mutually acceptable, culturally responsive plan of treatment. The key focus of the cultural assessment is that patients have a right to their cultural beliefs, individual preferences, values, and practices, and that these factors should be understood, respected, and considered when providing treatment. The first step in cultural and lifestyle assessment is to learn about the expectation of health and the meaning of illness in terms of the patient's unique culture and lifestyle.

QUESTIONS THAT MAY BE HELPFUL IN ASSESSING CULTURAL AND LIFESTYLE VALUES

- How would you prefer to be addressed while here?
- Do you have other family members who live close to you? Do any of them live in the home with you? How would you like them to be involved in your care?
- Are there others that you would like to be involved in your care? Who are these persons? How would you like them to be involved?
- Will anyone other than yourself be participating in decisions affecting your care?
- When thinking about yourself, what does the word "healthy" mean to you?
- Tell me what you believe caused your illness.
- Why do you think that your illness started when it did?
- Since you have had this illness, do you feel any different during any particular part of the day or night or on different days of the week?
- What do you call the illness that you are here for? Have you had this illness before? When did it start? How has it made you feel?
- How will this illness affect your life and the life of your family?
- What made you come here now to seek treatment?
- It can be frightening to be in a hospital (clinic, etc.). How are you feeling about having to be here?
- What fears do you have about your illness?
- What disturbs you most about being here?
- Tell me about your feelings about this illness and how you feel it may affect you?
- Tell me what good care means to you. How would you like for nurses and other healthcare providers to care for you while you are ill? What can we do while you are here that will lead you to feel that you have received good care?
- Where do you most often receive care when you are feeling ill or for routine checkups?
- Have you encountered any positive or negative experiences while receiving professional care that we need to know about to better care for you?
- Tell me about any prescription drugs that you are taking (include dosage, frequency, and the reason you are taking them).

NUTRITION
- How many meals do you normally eat per day? At what times?
- Tell me about the foods that you generally eat at meals.
- Are there foods that you do not eat or do not eat at certain times? Why?
- With whom do you usually eat your meals?

ENVIRONMENT

- Are you exposed to anything in the air, water that you drink, etc. where you live or work that you believe may be harmful to you and your family?
- Are you allergic to anything in the environment that you are aware of (e.g., chemicals, mold, etc.)?
- Do you have the following in your home: electricity, running water/well water, indoor plumbing, stairs, etc.?

SLEEP

- What is your usual bedtime? Is there anything that helps you to sleep better? Is there anything that disturbs your sleep?

Modified from Andrews, J. (2014). *Cultural, ethnic, and religious reference manual for healthcare providers* (4th ed.). Winston-Salem, NC: JAMARDA Resources.

Gender/Gender Identity

Access to health care may be challenging for those who identify with a gender other than that on their birth certificate. Health history must address both the risks associated with the biological gender as well as that of the expressed or chosen gender, along with other cultural considerations. Hormone therapies may factor into the health of such patients, along with diet and exercise, cardiovascular health, cancer, HIV, and STIs. Alcohol and tobacco use must be addressed, as with all patients. Depression, anxiety, and suicide risk are critical assessment points in this population. Along with these, the nuances of plastic surgery and injectable silicone may factor into the treatment plan of these individuals.

Transgender patients may reveal themselves to the clinician only in the examination room, and then only because they are forced to do so because of their medical history. Clinicians will not always be able to recognize a transgender patient without his or her self-disclosure, but in some cases a clinician may discover during an examination that a patient's body does not conform to his or her self-declared gender or to the gender the clinician expected to find.

QUESTIONS THAT MAY BE HELPFUL WITH ASSESSING TRANSGENDER PATIENTS, GENDER-NONCONFORMING PATIENTS, AND PATIENTS WHOSE GENDER IDENTITY DOES NOT COINCIDE WITH THEIR BIRTH GENDER

- Do you consider yourself to be transgender/gender-nonconforming in any way?
- What was your assigned gender at birth (meaning on your original birth certificate)? What is your gender?
  - Transgender man
  - Transgender woman
  - Transgender
  - Man
  - Woman
  - Agender (no gender)
  - Genderqueer/genderfluid
  - Not listed above (specify)
- What is your sexual orientation?
  - Lesbian, gay, or same-gender attracted
  - Straight or heterosexual (not gay or lesbian)
  - Queer
  - Bisexual or pansexual
  - Not sure, questioning
  - Other
- Have you had any transition-related surgery?
  - Vaginoplasty
  - Orchiectomy
  - Scrotoplasty
  - Scrotectomy

- Phalloplasty
- Metoidioplasty
- Ring metoidioplasty
- Bilateral salpingo-oophorectomy
- Hysterectomy
- Bilateral mastectomy
- Breast reconstruction/breast augmentation

Modified from Andrews, J. (2014). *Cultural, ethnic, and religious reference manual for healthcare providers* (4th ed.). Winston-Salem, NC: JAMARDA Resources.

Beliefs and Practices, Religion, and Philosophy

"Individuals from non-Western cultural groups may not conceive of illness in terms to which providers are accustomed. Some may have highly developed philosophies as to the retention of health and the cause of disease that may be contrary to the concepts the form the foundations of Western medicine. Some non-Western paradigms include beliefs that illnesses have spiritual causes or that disease results from imbalance among essential physical components. Others may believe health (or lack thereof) results from a person's actions in past lives. The more the clinician knows about specific traditions or beliefs, the more likely it is that potential problems can be avoided" (Brangman & Periyakoil, 2014).

"The clinician must also remain alert to the possibility that a patient's beliefs may lead them to use alternative remedies (rituals, herbals, etc.) that they may not mention in the course of the assessment. Questions about these practices should be included among other questions about the patient's history. It is not realistic to expect that patients will automatically "adapt" to Western approaches to health care. It is necessary to negotiate a common understanding of the term "health," causation of illness, diagnosis, and treatment while maintaining respect for traditional beliefs and practices" (Brangman & Periyakoil, 2014).[1]

QUESTIONS THAT MAY HELP THE CLINICIAN LEARN ABOUT BELIEFS, PRACTICES, RELIGION, AND PHILOSOPHY

- We are committed to honoring your values and beliefs. Are there any that you would like for us to know about to help you to regain/maintain your health?
- Do you seek help from anyone (other than a licensed medical provider) who helps you to stay well or helps you when you are not feeling well?
- What helps you to stay well?
- Tell me about things you do to help yourself feel better when you are not feeling well.
- Tell me about any herbal or vitamin supplements that you are taking (include dosage, frequency, and the reason you are taking them). How do you get the supplements, herbals, etc.?
- Tell me about any activities that you are involved in for your health and well being.
- Have you taken or done anything before coming here to seek treatment for your present illness? Did it make you feel better, worse, or has there been no change in how you feel?
- Both males and females work here; all are involved in caring for patients and may be entering your treatment room. Are there any special considerations that we should know about related to persons of the opposite gender being involved in your care?
- Tell me about any considerations that we should know about related to your religious beliefs/practices—diet, prayer/meditation times, etc.?
- Do you have any restrictions related to receiving blood/blood products?
- Is there anyone that you contact to offer you spiritual/religious support?
- How can we best support you spiritually with regard to your health care?
- With regard to personal objects/valuables (crosses, cloth bracelets/strings, charms, amulets, medicine bags, etc.): What meaning does it have for you? Do you feel that your well being will be affected if it is removed? How?
- What normally helps you to feel better if you are feeling down/"blue"/stressed?

Modified from Andrews, J. (2014). *Cultural, ethnic, and religious reference manual for healthcare providers* (4th ed.). Winston-Salem, NC: JAMARDA Resources.

[1] To access the complete *Doorway Thoughts: Cross-Cultural Health Care for Older Adults*, 2nd ed. (2014), please visit www.GeriatricCareOnline.org.

Economic Factors

The cost of treatment may be a factor in the patient's adherence to healthcare regimens, especially in settings where uninsured patients are served. In other countries, medications may be furnished by government agencies but the patient may lack access to transportation or sufficient income to obtain them, or supplies of certain medications may be limited. Clinicians may find that assessment protocols and treatment standards of the country in which they are working differ from those in their home country; it is important to learn these differences prior to providing services to patients in such settings. Regardless, asking about resources available to the patient is an important part of the cultural and lifestyle assessment.

QUESTIONS THAT MAY HELP THE CLINICIAN UNDERSTAND ECONOMIC NEEDS

- How do you normally get medications or treatments that you need?
- Do you get financial assistance/support services for any of your daily needs? For medical services? For medications?
- Do you have transportation to get your medical care? Medications? Food and other daily needs?

Modified from Andrews, J. (2014). *Cultural, ethnic, and religious reference manual for healthcare providers* (4th ed.). Winston-Salem, NC: JAMARDA Resources.

Language

Language is foundational for effective clinician–patient relationships and is important for interpersonal and cross-cultural communication. Communication with a patient is critical to completing an accurate and comprehensive patient and family assessment, formulating and implementing an efficacious treatment plan, determining the effectiveness of interventions, and evaluating outcomes of care provided. As result of dramatic demographic changes in the United States, clinicians are increasingly faced with the challenge of communicating with patients who cannot speak English or who speak English with limited proficiency. Clinicians working in the global arena will find themselves encountering similar challenges in providing effective medical and nursing services.

Sometimes the clinician will find it necessary to work through a translator or interpreter. There are important differences between a translator and an interpreter. A translator is a person who can speak both English and the patient's native language. However, the translator often does not have equal fluency in both languages and may lose important cultural nuances and meanings. In contrast, an interpreter is professionally trained to interpret the meaning of words and phrases from the healthcare provider's language to the patient's language and provides the same services on behalf of the patient to the healthcare provider. The latter, when available, is the best choice for providing culturally competent services to patients.

QUESTIONS TO ESTABLISH LANGUAGE PROFICIENCY

- What is your primary language? Are you able to speak and understand other languages? If so, which ones?
- Are you able to read and write? In what language(s)?
- How do you believe that you learn best?
- Do you use any equipment/technology at home to help you to maintain or learn about your health (phone, computer, tablet, etc.)?

Modified from Andrews, J. (2014). *Cultural, ethnic, and religious reference manual for healthcare providers* (4th ed.). Winston-Salem, NC: JAMARDA Resources.

Case Example: Culture and Lifestyle

HEALTH HISTORY, CULTURAL ASSESSMENT, AND LIFESTYLE

A detailed history of the present complaint in the context of culture is necessary to provide appropriate care for patients of known diversity. Including cultural and lifestyle questions in the interview process helps ensure that correct data are obtained.

Chief Complaint and History of Present Illness (HPI)

"I have frequent headaches, my stomach hurts, and I haven't been able to sleep well for the last couple of months."

Mrs. Aida Avendanio, a 69-year-old female Filipino American, is brought to the ambulatory care clinic by her daughter with a present problem of recurring headaches, stomach pains, and insomnia. Mrs. Avendanio came to the United States about 3 years ago after her oldest daughter, an accountant, petitioned for her to come as an immigrant. The patient lives with this daughter and her husband, who is a lawyer, and their 4-year-old daughter and 2-year-old son.

The clinician is Deidra Anderson, an FNP who has 5 years of experience in a group practice in family medicine in a large metropolitan area. She is well known and liked among Asian and Hispanic patients in the community and many of her patient referrals are by word of mouth.

Deidra greets Mrs. Avendanio and her daughter and invites them to have a seat in the exam room. Deidra introduces herself, shakes Mrs. Avendanio's hand, and asks her how she would like to be addressed. The patient replies, "Mrs. Avendanio." Her daughter interrupts and explains that they have been to two other providers who "drew all kinds of labs" and did examinations but "didn't find anything wrong." Deidra reviews the labs, which are all within normal ranges. The daughter continues to talk more loudly and rapidly; Mrs. Avendanio looks increasingly distressed. Deidra asks the daughter to wait in the next room as she prepares to examine Mrs. Avendanio.

As she completes the review of systems, Deidra asks some additional questions, one at a time, allowing the patient to reflect on each and formulate an answer:

"Do you have other family members who live close to you?"

"How would you like for them to be involved in your care?"

"Tell me about any considerations that we should know about related to your religious beliefs or health practices?"

Mrs. Avendanio answers the questions, relating her current living situation. But, as she does so, begins to cry. She shares that her husband passed away 3 years ago. She and her husband shared very close relationships with relatives who lived nearby; these individuals often participated in their healthcare decisions. She often sought the advice of a folk healer who offered rituals, herbals, and healing objects. When her husband died, she felt it necessary to move to the United States to be with her daughter and to help with the grandchildren. She has become increasingly lonely for friends and relatives she left in the Philippines, but knows that she cannot go back; she feels helpless and isolated. Her daughter and son-in-law work full time, so she tries to take care of the children, but feels exhausted. She is worried that she is becoming a burden to the family and laments that she no longer has access to the folk healer who was instrumental in keeping her well.

Physical Assessment and Action Plan

Deidra completes the physical exam, which is unremarkable. She carefully explains to the patient and her daughter that she believes that Mrs. Avendanio is depressed.

Deidra suggests that Mrs. Avendanio needs to have activities that prevent her from feeling isolated. She tells Mrs. Avendanio's daughter that she will provide some medication for depression and sleep, but involvement with other Filipinos in the area on a regular basis will be important in her recovery. She suggests a half-day a week at the local senior center where Filipinos gather. The daughter also notes that they could subscribe to a Filipino television channel to allow her mother to keep up with events in her homeland and "reconnect" with her culture. She further agrees to provide day care for half a day a week for the children to give her mother a break from childcare duties.

Deidra sends prescriptions to the pharmacy and writes out a simple list of instructions for Mrs. Avendanio to follow.

1. Take your pill every day for energy and sleep.
2. Go to the senior center every Tuesday morning from 9 to 12.

FOLLOW UP

When Deidra sees Mrs. Avendanio again in a few weeks, she is much better. She is attending church with new friends she met at the senior center and has a new "charm" from a folk healer who has relocated from a community near hers in the Philippines. She feels life is "coming together" for her once again.

DISCUSSION

The skill of conducting a cultural assessment allowed the nurse practitioner to deliver culturally competent and patient-centered care that incorporated the patient's values, beliefs, and practices into the treatment plan. Also, a meaningful and deliberate cultural encounter allowed the nurse to "connect" with the patient as a unique, individual person, and not as a stereotype of the patient's cultural group.

Case Example: Gender Identity

A 58-year-old transgender female patient presents to the clinic to establish care. She does not immediately reveal that she is transgender, but waits to communicate her status to the clinician in the exam room.

Chief Complaint and History of Present Illness (HPI)

"I am here to establish care and get a physical for work. I haven't been to the doctor in a few years, and I am new in the community."

The clinician completes the health history as customary for a general physical. During the course of the history, the patient reveals that she is a transgender female. She tells the clinician that she is receiving hormone therapy that includes anti-androgen therapy as well as estrogen therapy and sees an endocrinologist for management of the hormones. She has also undergone a gonadectomy and a breast augmentation within the last 8 years.

The provider is surprised at this revelation, but remains calm and asks additional questions, noting them in the patient's chart.

1. What is your current gender identity? (Check and/or circle ALL that apply)
   - ☐ Male
   - ☒ Female
   - ☐ Transgender male/Transman/FTM (female to male)
   - ☒ Transgender female/Transwoman/MTF (male to female)
   - ☐ Genderqueer
   - ☐ Additional category (please specify): _____
   - ☐ Decline to answer
2. What sex were you assigned at birth? (Check one)
   - ☒ Male
   - ☐ Female
   - ☐ Decline to answer
3. What pronouns do you prefer? __She__

The patient was assessed for immediate health needs and medical problems. Allergies were verified; past medical history collected; specialists being seen were noted; and chronic and episodic medication usage was recorded, including any cross-sex hormone medication and its source (prescription, "street" dealers, sharing with others, etc.), duration of use, and any complications. Family history, with special attention to cardiovascular disease, diabetes, and cancer, especially of the breast, prostate, or reproductive organs, was discussed. Psychosocial issues were considered; screening for depression, anxiety, and suicide risk was conducted. Healthcare maintenance was reviewed, including immunizations, TB screening, safety, and safer sex counseling.

Even if surprised, the clinician must remain calm and respectful of the person's body and self-declared identity. Patients may not return for follow-up care if they do not feel respected or safe.

Identifying a transgender patient is easiest if intake forms have a place for transgender patients to safely and confidentially identify themselves to the physician and office staff, and the staff must be trained to handle the information respectfully. The ideal patient intake form has both a "gender question" and an "assigned-sex-at-birth question," such as those shown above, and an optional "preferred pronoun" question.

Asking both a gender and a sex question instead of just one (either sex or gender), and offering many choices, allows for specific disclosure of a person's history and validates his or her current gender identity. Many transgender patients may not identify as transgender or transsexual for a variety of reasons. Some believe it is part of their past and not a present identification, while others may not identify with "trans" terms due to cultural beliefs, social networks, or linguistic norms in various geographic areas.

Physical Exam

The clinician performs the physical exam and notes the breast augmentation. Examination of genitalia and rectum are deferred at this visit.

Assessment and Plan

The clinician completes the exam and talks about some recommendations for preventive healthcare services for the patient. A mammogram was recommended, as the patient noted a first-degree relative was diagnosed with breast cancer. Baseline labs had been recently drawn by endocrinology; these were requested for the patient's chart.

Discussion

It can be uncomfortable to be confused about someone's gender. It can also feel awkward to ask someone what their gender is. However, if you let the person know that you are only trying to be respectful, your question will usually be appreciated. For instance, you can ask, "How would you like to be addressed?" or "What name would you like to be called?" In order to facilitate a good provider–patient relationship, it is important not to make assumptions about the identity, beliefs, concerns, or sexual orientation of transgender and gender nonconforming patients.

The most important principle to apply in general prevention and screening is to provide care for the anatomy that is present, regardless of the patient's self-description or identification, presenting gender, or legal status, and always to provide that care in a sensitive, respectful, and affirming manner that recognizes and honors the patient's self-description or self-identification. Access to affordable, quality health care is central to avoiding negative health consequences, yet many insurance companies exclude medically necessary care and services for transgender people, including mental health therapy, hormone therapy, and surgeries. In addition, some transgender patients have had negative experiences in healthcare settings. Providers and office staff may lack the knowledge necessary to provide sensitive services to transgender individuals. Discrimination in the provision of services may cause transgender patients to delay or avoid necessary health services, including acute care interventions that are not related to their gender status, sometimes putting their overall health at risk.

ADDITIONAL SCREENINGS TO CONSIDER IN OLDER TRANSGENDER PATIENTS

Transwomen patients on feminizing hormone therapy: Mammograms are recommended for transwomen when patients have been using estrogen for at least 30 years AND are at least 50 years of age, unless there is a strong family history of early breast or ovarian cancer. (Grade C) Follow USPSTF guidelines for prostate screening. PSA is not useful if patient is on estrogen. (Grade B)

Transmen without hysterectomy: Pelvic exams every 1–3 years for patients over age 40 or with a family history of uterine or ovarian cancer; increase to every year if polycystic ovarian syndrome (PCOS) is present. Consider hysterectomy and oophorectomy if the patient's health will not be adversely affected by surgery, or if the patient is unable to tolerate pelvic exams. (Grade B, C)

Transmen: Consider bone density screening if older than age 60 and if taking testosterone for 5–10 years or less; if taking testosterone for more than 5-10 years, consider at age 50+, earlier if additional risk factors for osteoporosis are present; recommend supplemental calcium and vitamin D in accordance with current osteoporosis prevention guidelines to help maintain bone density. Note that this may be applied to transmen at ages younger than typical starting age for osteoporosis prevention treatment due to the unknown effect of testosterone on bone density. (Grade B, C)

Transmen stopping testosterone will experience loss of libido, hot flashes, loss of body hair and muscle tone, and weight redistribution in a female pattern. (Grade C)

Bibliography

Andrews, M. M., & Boyle, J. S. (2008). *Transcultural concepts in nursing*. New York, NY: Wolters Kluwer/ Lippincott, Williams & Wilkins.

Andrews, J. (2014). *Cultural, ethnic, and religious reference manual for healthcare providers* (4th ed.). Winston-Salem, NC: JAMARDA Resources.

Brangman, S., & Periyakoil, V. S. (Eds.). (2014). *Doorway thoughts: Cross-cultural health care for older adults* (2nd ed.). New York, NY: American Geriatrics Society.

Campinha-Bacote, J. (2002). The process of cultural competence in the delivery of healthcare services: A model of care. *Journal of Transcultural Nursing, 13*(3), 181–184.

Feldman, J. (2007). Preventative care of the transgendered patient: An evidence-based approach. In R. Ettner, S. Monstrey, & A. E. Eyler (Eds.), *Principles of transgender medicine and surgery* (pp. 33–72). Binghamton, NY: The Haworth Press.

Keatley, G., Deutsch, M., Sevelius, J., & Gutierrex-Mock L. (2014). Creating a foundation for improving trans health: Understanding trans identities and health care needs. In H. J. Makadon, K. M. Mayer, J. Potter, & H. Goldhammer (Eds.), *The Fenway guide to lesbian, gay, bisexual, and transgender health* (2nd ed., pp. 459–478). Philadelphia, PA: ACP.

Singleton, K., & Krause, E. (2009). Understanding cultural and linguistic barriers to health literacy. *The Online Journal of Issues in Nursing, 14*(3). doi: 10.3912/OJIN.Vol14No03Man04.

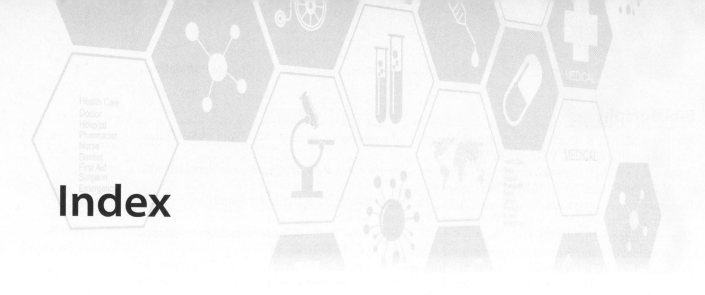

Index

Note: Page numbers followed by *b*, *f*, and *t* refer to boxes, figures, and tables respectively.

A

AAA. *See* abdominal aortic aneurysm
abbreviations, in documentation, 32
abdomen. *See also* gastrointestinal disorders and assessment
  anatomy and physiology, 241–242, 242*f*, 243*f*, 243*b*, 244*t*
  auscultation, 250–251, 259
  inspection, 250
  palpation, 254–257, 255*f*–257*f*, 297–298,
      307, 307*f*, 308, 308*f*
  percussion, 252–254
  physical examination, 27
  ultrasound, 234*b*
abdominal aortic aneurysm (AAA), 236, 241, 256, 257*f*
abdominal cavity, 241, 242*f*
abdominal girth, 250
abdominal pain, 244, 256–257
abdominal quadrants, 241, 243*b*, 243*f*, 254–255, 255*f*
abducens nerve (CN VI), 408*f*, 419
abduction
  hip, 386
  shoulder, 374, 375*f*
achilles reflex, 428, 429*f*
achilles tendinitis, 392*t*
achilles tendon
  palpation, 393
  rupture, 392*t*
AC joint. *See* acromioclavicular joint
ACL. *See* anterior cruciate ligament
acne, 81*t*, 86
acromioclavicular (AC) joint, 358–359, 373, 373*t*, 374*f*
ACTH. *See* adrenocorticotropic hormone
actinic keratosis, 82*t*
adaptive functioning, mental status examination, 54
adduction, shoulder, 374, 375*f*
adductors, 363
adipose tissue of breast, 315, 316
adrenal glands, 336
adrenocorticotropic hormone (ACTH), 333, 335*t*
adventitious breath sounds, 202–203, 202*t*–203*t*
aging, extrinsic and intrinsic, 87. *See also* geriatric patient
      assessments
alcohol use, social history, 15
Allen's test, 381
allergic contact dermatitis, 80*t*
allergic dermatitis, 83*t*
allergies, 11, 161–162
Allis' sign, 400
alopecia, 74

altered mobility, 412, 414–415
altered sensation, 368, 412
amblyopia, 101
amphoric breath sounds, 202
anatomy and physiology
  ankles, 364
  brain, 42, 42*f*, 407–411, 408*f*, 409*f*
  cardiovascular, 212–216
    arteries and veins, 213–214, 215*f*
    cardiac cycle, 214–216, 215*f*
    heart, 212–213, 213*f*, 214*f*
  ears, 117–121
  elbows, 360, 360*f*
  endocrine system
    adrenal glands, 336
    gonads, 336
    hypothalamus, 333, 409
    pancreas, 336
    parathyroid gland, 336
    pituitary gland, 334–336
    thyroid, 336
  external eye (extraocular structures), 92, 93*f*
  eyes, 92–94, 93*f*
  feet, 364, 365*f*
  forearms, 360–361, 360*f*
  gastrointestinal, 241–242, 242*f*, 243*f*, 244*t*
  hands, 361–363, 361*f*, 362*f*, 362*t*
  hips, pelvis and thighs, 363
  integument (skin and appendages), 62–64, 63*f*
  internal eye (intraocular structures), 92–94, 93*f*
  knees, 363–364, 364*f*
  musculoskeletal
    bones and connective tissues, 357–358
    elbows, 360, 360*f*
    forearms, 360–361, 360*f*
    hands, 361–363, 361*f*, 362*f*, 362*t*
    hips, pelvis and thighs, 363
    lower extremities, 363–365, 364*f*, 365*f*
    shoulder, 358–360, 359*f*
    spine, 365, 365*f*
    upper extremities, 358–363, 359*f*–362*f*, 362*t*
  neurological
    brain, 407–411, 408*f*, 409*f*
    central nervous system, 406, 407
    cranial nerves, 410
    neurons, 406–407, 407*f*
    peripheral nervous system, 406
    spinal cord, 411, 411*f*

myofascial pain, 373*t*
myometrium, 290, 290*f*

N
nail(s)
  beds, 224
  clubbing, 193, 224
  described, 64
  gastrointestinal examination, 250
  inspection, 75–76, 250
  palpation, 78
  structure and function, 64
nares/nostrils, 147
nasal cavity, 147, 156
nasal discharge, 149–151
nasal disorder. *See* nose/sinus disorders and assessment
nasal septum, 147
nasal turbinates (conchae), 147, 157
nausea, 245, 258
navicular fracture, 380*b*, 381
neck, physical examination, 26. *See also* mouth/throat disorders and assessment
Neer's sign, 377
neonatal patient assessments. *See also* pediatric patient assessments
  breasts, 328
  cardiovascular, 235
  ears, 140–141
  eyes, 113
  gastrointestinal, 258–259
  genitourinary, female, 310
  genitourinary, male, 282
  integumentary, 85
  mouth or throat, 178
  musculoskeletal, 399–400
  neurological, 435, 436*t*
  nose or sinus, 160–161
  physical examination strategies, 29
  respiratory, 205–207, 206*t*
  visual assessment of newborn, 29*b*
nephrons, 265–266, 292
nervous system
  anatomy and physiology, 406–411
  brain, 408*f*
  central nervous system, 406
  function of, 406
  peripheral nervous system, 406
  spinal cord, 411, 411*f*
neurofibroma, 82*t*
neurological assessment, 446
neurological disorders and assessment, 406–441. *See also specific disorders such as* headache
  anatomy and physiology, 406–411
    brain, 407–409, 407*f*, 408*f*
    central nervous system, 406
    cranial nerves, 410, 410*t*
    neurons, 406–407, 407*f*
    peripheral nervous system, 406
    spinal cord, 411, 411*f*
  case study review, 438–441
  diagnostic reasoning, 433–438
  differential diagnosis of headache, 434*t*
  function of nervous system, 406
  health history, 412–418
    chief complaint, 412–415
    family history, 416
    history of present illness, 412–415
    past medical history, 415–416

    review of systems, 417–418
    social history, 416–417
  level of consciousness alterations, 412
  physical examination, 28, 418–433
    actions and rationale, 419–432
    cortical sensation assessments, 427, 427*f*
    cranial nerve testing, 418
    equipment, 418
    inspection, 422–425
    motor function assessments, 422–425
    palpation, 422–425
    reflex testing, 428–430
    sensory function assessments, 425–428
  reflexes, 435, 436*t*
  special populations, 434–438
neurological systems, comprehensive ROS, 18
neurons, 406–407, 407*f*
neurotransmitters, 407
new/preexisting diagnoses, assessment finding categories, 38
nipple(s), 321*f*, 328
  anatomy and physiology, 315–316
  discharge from, 317, 318, 325
  inspection, 321–322, 321*f*
  palpation, 322–323, 323*f*
  supernumerary, 195
nocturia, 267
nodes of Ranvier, 407
nodule, 71*t*
normal blood pressure, 236*t*
normal heart rate, 236*t*
nose. *See also* nose/sinus disorders and assessment
  inspection, 205
  and mouth, assessment, 444
  in respiration, 183, 184*f*
nose/sinus disorders and assessment, 147–163
  anatomy and physiology, 147–149
  case study review, 161–163
  comprehensive ROS, 17
  diagnostic reasoning, 159–163, 160*t*
  differential diagnosis of congestion, 160*t*
  function of nose or sinus, 147
  health history, 149–155
    chief complaint, 149–153
    family history, 153–154
    history of present illness, 149–153
    past medical history, 153
    review of systems, 155, 155*t*
    social history, 154–155
  laboratory and diagnostic studies, 160*b*
  physical examination, 25, 155–159
    action and rationale, 156–159
    equipment, 155
    inspection, 156–157, 156*f*, 161
    palpation, 157–159, 157*f*, 158*f*
    percussion, 157–159, 159*f*
  special populations, 160–161
nuchal rigidity, 431
nummular dermatitis, 80*t*
nystagmus, 419

O
objective data, 3*b*, 37. *See also* physical examination
objective, SOAP format, 33
obturator test, 256, 257*f*
occipital lobe, brain, 42, 42*f*, 409
occupation, social history, 13
oculomotor nerve (CN III), 408, 419